ANATOMY and PHYSIOLOGY in HEALTHCARE

Other titles of interest

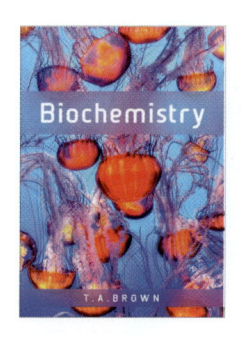

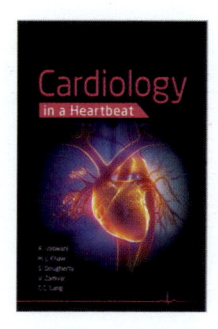

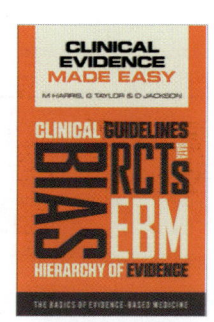

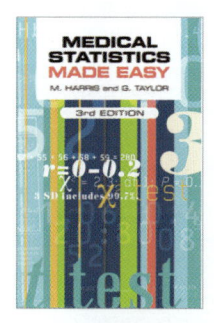

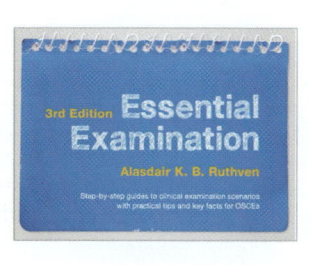

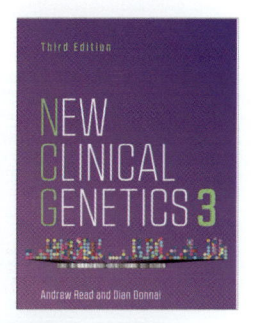

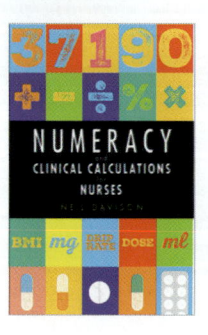

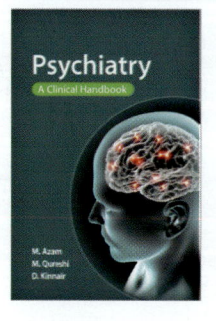

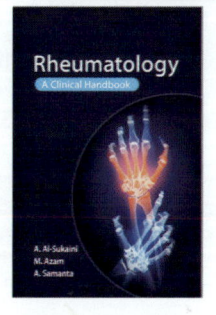

ANATOMY and PHYSIOLOGY in HEALTHCARE

P. MARSHALL
B. GALLACHER
J. JOLLY
S. RINOMHOTA

School of Healthcare
Faculty of Medicine and Health
University of Leeds, UK

Scion

© **Scion Publishing Ltd, 2017**

First published 2017

All rights reserved. No part of this book may be reproduced or transmitted, in any form or by any means, without permission.

A CIP catalogue record for this book is available from the British Library.

ISBN 978 1 904842 95 8

Scion Publishing Limited

The Old Hayloft, Vantage Business Park, Bloxham Road, Banbury OX16 9UX, UK

www.scionpublishing.com

Important Note from the Publisher

The information contained within this book was obtained by Scion Publishing Ltd from sources believed by us to be reliable. However, while every effort has been made to ensure its accuracy, no responsibility for loss or injury whatsoever occasioned to any person acting or refraining from action as a result of information contained herein can be accepted by the authors or publishers.

Readers are reminded that medicine is a constantly evolving science and while the authors and publishers have ensured that all dosages, applications and practices are based on current indications, there may be specific practices which differ between communities. You should always follow the guidelines laid down by the manufacturers of specific products and the relevant authorities in the country in which you are practising.

Although every effort has been made to ensure that all owners of copyright material have been acknowledged in this publication, we would be pleased to acknowledge in subsequent reprints or editions any omissions brought to our attention.

Registered names, trademarks, etc. used in this book, even when not marked as such, are not to be considered unprotected by law.

Last digit is the print number: 10 9 8 7 6 5 4 3 2

Illustrations by Matthew McClements at Blink Studio Ltd, www.blink.biz

Typeset by Evolution Design & Digital Ltd (Kent)

Printed in the UK

Contents

About the authors ... xv
Preface ... xvi
Abbreviations ... xvii

CHAPTER 01. Why is the human body the way it is? ... 1

1.1 Introduction and clinical relevance ... 1
Patient 1.1 – Amy 1
Patient 1.2 – Sylvia 2
Patient 1.3 – Francine 2

1.2 What you need to know – essential anatomy and physiology ... 3
   1.2.1 Why the human body is the way it is ... 3
   1.2.2 Single-celled and multicellular organisms ... 5
   1.2.3 Homeostasis and homeodynamics ... 6
   1.2.4 The internal environment and plasma ... 8
   1.2.5 The homeodynamic process ... 9
   1.2.6 The homeodynamic regulation of body temperature ... 12
      The homeodynamic response to cold ... 16
      The homeodynamic response to heat ... 18

1.3 Clinical application ... 19
Patient 1.1 – Amy 20
Patient 1.2 – Sylvia 20
Patient 1.3 – Francine 21

1.4 Anatomical language ... 21
   1.4.1 General anatomical terms ... 21
   1.4.2 Body cavities ... 24
   1.4.3 Body regions ... 24

1.5 Summary ... 26
1.6 Further reading ... 26
1.7 Self-assessment questions ... 27

CHAPTER 02. Cells and their environment ... 29

2.1 Introduction and clinical relevance ... 29
Patient 2.1 – Mary 29
Patient 2.2 – Sumina 30
Patient 2.3 – Sheila 30

2.2 What you need to know – essential anatomy and physiology ... 31
   2.2.1 Types of cell: the diversity of life ... 31
      Prokaryotes ... 32
      Eukaryotes ... 32
   2.2.2 Components of a eukaryotic cell ... 34
      Plasma membrane ... 34
      Membrane proteins ... 36
      Transport across plasma membranes ... 36
      Cell organelles ... 44

			Other cell structures	45
		2.2.3	Organization of cells in the body	46
			Tissues	48
	2.3	Clinical application		52
		Patient 2.1 – Mary 53		
		Patient 2.2 – Sumina 53		
		Patient 2.3 – Sheila 54		
	2.4	Summary		55
	2.5	Further reading		56
	2.6	Self-assessment questions		56

CHAPTER 03.   Genetics: how cells divide and introduce variation — 59

	3.1	Introduction and clinical relevance		59
		Patient 2.3 – Sheila 59		
		Patient 3.1 – Sarah 60		
		Patient 3.2 – Alexei 60		
		Patient 3.3 – Katherine 61		
		Patient 3.4 – Yasmeen 61		
	3.2	What you need to know – essential anatomy and physiology		61
		3.2.1	The genome	61
			Structure of the genome	63
			Function of the genome	64
			Gene expression: using the genetic code to make proteins	66
			Transcription: DNA makes RNA	66
			Translation: RNA makes protein	68
			What influences gene expression and what are the consequences?	71
		3.2.2	Chromosomes	74
			Sources of genetic variation: 'We are all different, aren't we?'	74
		3.2.3	Cell division	76
			Mitosis	76
			Meiosis	78
			Independent assortment	79
			Recombination	80
			Mutations	80
		3.2.4	Application of genetics to healthcare	81
			The importance of pedigree	81
			Patterns of inheritance	82
			Genes and cancer	87
			Diseases involving more than one gene	91
			Gene testing and issues for the individual and society	91
	3.3	Clinical application		92
		Patient 2.3 – Sheila 93		
		Patient 3.1 – Sarah 94		
		Patient 3.2 – Alexei 94		
		Patient 3.3 – Katherine 95		
		Patient 3.4 – Yasmeen 95		
	3.4	Summary		96

	3.5	Further reading	96
	3.6	Self-assessment questions	97

CHAPTER 04. Communication: short and fast — 99

4.1 Introduction and clinical relevance — 99
    Patient 4.1 – Bessie   99
    Patient 4.2 – Jade and Jordon   100
    Patient 4.3 – Graham   100

4.2 What you need to know – essential anatomy and physiology — 100
    4.2.1 Characteristics of a biological communication system — 100
    4.2.2 The nervous system: structural organization — 101
    4.2.3 Nervous tissue — 101
        Neuroglia — 101
        Neurones — 102
        The structure of a neurone — 103
    4.2.4 Functional organization of the nervous system — 104
        Sensory division of the nervous system — 104
        Motor division of the nervous system — 105
    4.2.5 The generation and propagation of an action potential — 105
        Neurotransmitters — 108
        Propagation of an impulse at the synapse — 108
    4.2.6 The central nervous system: the brain and spinal cord — 111
        Functions of the lobes — 112
        The diencephalon — 114
        The limbic system — 114
        The cerebellum — 115
        The brainstem — 115
        The midbrain — 116
        The pons — 116
        The medulla oblongata — 117
    4.2.7 Neuronal pathways and tracts of the brain and spinal cord — 118
        Direct (pyramidal) tracts or pathways — 118
        Indirect (extrapyramidal) tracts or pathways — 119
    4.2.8 Protection and nourishment of the brain and spinal cord — 119
        Meninges and CSF — 119
    4.2.9 The peripheral nervous system (cranial nerves and spinal nerves) — 122
        The reflex arc — 124
    4.2.10 The autonomic nervous system — 125
        Cholinergic receptors — 128
        Adrenergic receptors — 128
        Stress and adaptation — 129

4.3 Clinical application — 129
    Patient 4.1 – Bessie   130
    Patient 4.2 – Jade and Jordon   132
    Patient 4.3 – Graham   132

4.4 Summary — 133

	4.5	Further reading	133
	4.6	Self-assessment questions	134

CHAPTER 05. Communication: long and slow — 137

	5.1	Introduction and clinical relevance	137
		Patient 5.1 – David 138	
		Patient 4.2 – Jade and Jordon 138	
	5.2	What you need to know – essential anatomy and physiology	138
		5.2.1 The endocrine system	138
		5.2.2 Protein hormones	140
		Amino acid-derivative hormones	140
		Peptide-derivative and protein hormones	140
		5.2.3 Lipid-derivative hormones	140
		Steroid hormones	140
		5.2.4 How hormones exert an effect	141
		Protein hormone mechanism	141
		Steroid hormone mechanism	141
		5.2.5 Major endocrine glands and tissues	143
		Pineal gland	146
		Hypothalamus	146
		Pituitary gland	148
		Thyroid gland	150
		Parathyroid glands	151
		Thymus	151
		Adrenal glands	152
		Kidney	154
		Heart	155
		Pancreas	155
		Ovaries	157
		Placental hormones	158
		Testes	159
		Gastrointestinal tract	159
		Adipose tissue	160
	5.3	Clinical application	161
		Patient 5.1 – David 161	
		Patient 4.2 – Jade and Jordon 162	
	5.4	Summary	163
	5.5	Further reading	164
	5.6	Self-assessment questions	164

CHAPTER 06. How the external environment is interpreted — 167

	6.1	Introduction and clinical relevance	167
		Patient 6.1 – Sally 167	
		Patient 6.2 – Sadia 167	
		Patient 6.3 – Denzel 168	
	6.2	What you need to know – essential anatomy and physiology	168
		6.2.1 Sensation and perception	169

		6.2.2	Vision and the eye	169
			Physiology of vision	172
			Focusing of light onto the retina	174
			The retina and photoreceptors	175
			The visual pathway	176
			Control of eye movement	177
		6.2.3	Taste and smell	178
			The sense of taste	178
			The sense of smell: olfactory epithelium and neural pathways	179
		6.2.4	Hearing	179
			Structure of the ear	180
			Physiology of hearing	182
			The vestibular system and physiology of balance	184
		6.2.5	Touch	185
			Nociceptors and the perception of pain	186
	6.3	Clinical application		187
		Patient 6.1 – Sally 188		
		Patient 6.2 – Sadia 188		
		Patient 6.3 – Denzel 189		
	6.4	Summary		190
	6.5	Further reading		190
	6.6	Self-assessment questions		191

CHAPTER 07. Why food is needed: the chemical basis of health — 193

	7.1	Introduction and clinical relevance		193
		Patient 1.1 – Amy 194		
		Patient 1.3 – Francine 194		
		Patient 3.1 – Sarah 195		
		Patient 5.1 – David 195		
	7.2	What you need to know – essential anatomy and physiology		196
		7.2.1	The driving force behind cellular processes and activities	196
		7.2.2	Components of food	197
			Carbohydrates	197
			Proteins	199
			Fats	203
			Minerals	207
			Vitamins	210
			Non-starch polysaccharides (fibre)	214
			Water	214
		7.2.3	Making nutrients in food available	215
			Role of the gastrointestinal tract	216
			Processes of food digestion	217
			Digestion in the small intestine	220
			Role of the accessory organs	221
			Absorption of food	225
			Metabolism of food	231
	7.3	Clinical application		233

Patient 1.1 – Amy   235
Patient 1.3 – Francine   235
Patient 3.1 – Sarah   237
Patient 5.1 – David   237
7.4   Summary   238
7.5   Further reading   238
7.6   Self-assessment questions   239

CHAPTER 08.   The importance of water and electrolytes   241

8.1   Introduction and clinical relevance   241
Patient 8.1 – Marcus   241
8.2   What you need to know – essential anatomy and physiology   242
  8.2.1   Water and electrolytes   242
  8.2.2   Functions of the kidney   245
    Gross anatomy of the kidney   245
    Ureters and urinary bladder   246
    Urethra   248
    Formation of urine   248
    Homeodynamic regulation of water and sodium concentration   256
    The micturition reflex   260
8.3   Clinical application   262
Patient 8.1 – Marcus   262
8.4   Summary   263
8.5   Further reading   264
8.6   Self-assessment questions   264

CHAPTER 09.   Organs need to be perfused   267

9.1   Introduction and clinical relevance   267
Patient 2.3 – Sheila   267
Patient 3.3 – Katherine   268
Patient 3.4 – Yasmeen   268
Patient 9.1 – Robert   268
Patient 9.2 – Jane   268
9.2   What you need to know – essential anatomy and physiology   269
  9.2.1   Structure and function of blood vessels   269
  9.2.2   Blood flow and perfusion   272
  9.2.3   The heart: structure and function   274
    Anatomy of the heart   274
    Blood flow through the heart   277
    The heart as a pump   279
    The cardiac conducting system   280
    The cardiac cycle: integration of mechanical and electrical events   282
  9.2.4   Blood pressure   284
    Determinants of blood pressure   285
    Regulation of blood pressure   286
    Variation of blood pressure throughout the cardiovascular system   288
    Autonomic nervous system effects on the cardiovascular system   289

			Venous return	290
			Effects of postural changes on venous return	291
			Capillary fluid dynamics	291
		9.2.5	Blood composition and function	293
			Composition of blood	293
			Haemopoiesis	296
			Erythropoiesis	296
			Blood groups	297
			Haemostasis and blood clotting	300
	9.3	Clinical application		303
		Patient 2.3 – Sheila 304		
		Patient 3.3 – Katherine 305		
		Patient 9.1 – Robert 305		
		Patient 9.2 – Jane 306		
		Patient 3.4 – Yasmeen 306		
	9.4	Summary		307
	9.5	Further reading		308
	9.6	Self-assessment questions		308

CHAPTER 10. The body needs oxygen — 311

10.1	Introduction and clinical relevance		311
	Patient 2.1 – Mary 311		
	Patient 3.1 – Sarah 311		
10.2	What you need to know – essential anatomy and physiology		312
	10.2.1 Upper respiratory tract		313
	10.2.2 Lower respiratory tract		314
	10.2.3 Lung tissue and the bronchial tree		316
	10.2.4 Ventilation and the mechanics of breathing		318
	Factors that aid ventilation		320
	10.2.5 Respiratory volumes and capacities		321
	10.2.6 Exchange and transportation of gases		323
	10.2.7 Regulation of breathing by chemoreceptors		328
10.3	Clinical application		329
	Patient 2.1 – Mary 330		
	Patient 3.1 – Sarah 333		
10.4	Summary		334
10.5	Further reading		334
10.6	Self-assessment questions		334

CHAPTER 11. Protection from harm — 337

11.1	Introduction and clinical relevance	337
	Patient 1.3 – Francine 338	
	Patient 11.1 – Albert 338	
	Patient 11.2 – Jerry 338	
11.2	What you need to know – essential anatomy and physiology	339
	11.2.1 Lymphatic structures support immunity	341
	11.2.2 Innate immunity – physical defences	342

		11.2.3 Recognition of microorganisms by innate immunity	347
		11.2.4 Innate immunity – cellular defences	347
		Myeloid cells	349
		11.2.5 Innate immunity – humoral defences	351
		Cytotoxic factors in innate immunity	354
		Free radicals	356
		11.2.6 Acute inflammation	356
		11.2.7 Adaptive immunity	359
		Cells of adaptive immunity: small lymphocytes	360
		Antibody classes	363
		T-lymphocytes	364
		Concept of self and non-self: the major histocompatibility complex	366
		Acquiring immunity	366
		Immunity in neonates and infants	368
		Immunity in the older person	369
	11.3	Clinical application	370
		Patient 1.3 – Francine 371	
		Patient 11.1 – Albert 372	
		Patient 11.2 – Jerry 374	
	11.4	Summary	375
	11.5	Further reading	376
	11.6	Self-assessment questions	376

CHAPTER 12. Skin: our protective cover — 379

	12.1	Introduction and clinical relevance	379
		Patient 4.1 – Bessie 379	
		Patient 12.1 – Giuseppe 380	
		Patient 12.2 – Daphne and Joe 380	
		Patient 12.3 – Audrey 380	
	12.2	What you need to know – essential anatomy and physiology	381
		12.2.1 Structure of the skin	381
		Structure of the epidermis	382
		Structure of the dermis	383
		12.2.2 Factors affecting the skin	387
		Young skin	387
		Ageing	387
		Food	390
		Skin colour	390
		Sunlight and vitamin D	392
		Skin hygiene and vulnerability	394
		12.2.3 Wound healing	395
	12.3	Clinical application	397
		Patient 4.1 – Bessie 397	
		Patient 12.1 – Giuseppe 398	
		Patient 12.2 – Daphne and Joe 398	
		Patient 12.3 – Audrey 399	
	12.4	Summary	400

	12.5	Further reading	401
	12.6	Self-assessment questions	401

CHAPTER 13. Achieving movement — 403

	13.1	Introduction and clinical relevance	403
		Patient 4.1 – Bessie 403	
		Patient 4.3 – Graham 404	
		Patient 6.1 – Sally 404	
	13.2	What you need to know – essential anatomy and physiology	404
		13.2.1 Bones	404
		General structure of the skeleton	404
		Functions of the skeleton	405
		Classification of bones by shape	406
		Structure of bones	406
		Bone formation, growth and development	407
		Histology of bone	410
		The axial skeleton	412
		The appendicular skeleton	421
		13.2.2 The joints	427
		The synovial joint	428
		Types of synovial joints	429
		Forms of movement at synovial joints	431
		13.2.3 Muscles	431
		Characteristics of muscles	432
		Types, characteristics and functions of muscle	432
		Structure of skeletal muscle fibre, myofibrils and myofilaments	433
		The sliding filament theory of contraction	434
		Muscle biomechanics	436
		The neuromuscular junction	439
	13.3	Clinical application	440
		Patient 4.1 – Bessie 441	
		Patient 4.3 – Graham 442	
		Patient 6.1 – Sally 443	
	13.4	Summary	443
	13.5	Further reading	444
	13.6	Self-assessment questions	444

CHAPTER 14. From one generation to the next — 447

	14.1	Introduction and clinical relevance	447
		Patient 1.1 – Amy 447	
		Patient 2.3 – Sheila 448	
		Patient 4.2 – Jade and Jordon 448	
		Patient 5.1 – David 448	
		Patient 9.1 – Robert 448	
		Patient 14.1 – Jess 449	
	14.2	What you need to know – essential anatomy and physiology	449
		14.2.1 Structure and function of the male reproductive system	449

		Spermatogenesis	452
	14.2.2	Structure and function of the female reproductive system	455
		External genitalia	455
		Internal genitalia	456
		The ovarian cycle	462
		The menstrual (uterine) cycle	464
		Early hormonal changes associated with pregnancy	465
		The placenta	465
		Labour	468
		The menopause	469
		The breast and its development	469
14.3	Clinical application		472
	Patient 1.1 – Amy 473		
	Patient 2.3 – Sheila 473		
	Patient 4.2 – Jade and Jordon 473		
	Patient 5.1 – David 474		
	Patient 9.1 – Robert 474		
	Patient 14.1 – Jess 475		
14.4	Summary		475
14.5	Further reading		476
14.6	Self-assessment questions		476
	Glossary		479
	Index		499

About the authors

Dr Paul Marshall PhD, BSc (distinction), RGN, RMN, FHEA

Paul has many years as a nurse covering adult and mental health fields of practice. His PhD (1997) was in cardiovascular physiology with a focus on heart failure, and cardiovascular physiology and the impact of cardiac disorders remain the focus of his academic and research activity. Paul has for many years had a major commitment teaching biological sciences to nurses, midwives, radiographers and healthcare scientists and through the work of the special interest group 'Bioscience in Nurse Education' (BiNE) he contributes to enhancing bioscience education within nursing and more broadly, healthcare science education.

Mrs Beverley Gallacher BSc (Hons), RGN, MSc, PG Dip, FHEA

Beverley received a degree in Biology from the University of York in 1983, and trained as an RGN in Stoke-on-Trent, qualifying in 1986. She worked as a surgical nurse, on a variety of wards including gastroenterology, urology, gynaecology, general surgery, breast surgery and vascular surgery. She also worked as a research nurse in the gastroenterology unit at Leeds General Infirmary, specializing in the link between peptic ulcer disease and *Helicobacter pylori* infection. She entered teaching in 1995 and received a Postgraduate Diploma in Health Professional Education in 1998. She teaches on a variety of physiology modules in the School and has a special interest in infection prevention and control.

Dr Jim Jolly BSc (Hons), RGN, PGCE, PhD, FHEA

Jim served in the Royal Navy for 15 years as a medical assistant and then as a Registered Nurse. He then trained as a science teacher and has for the past 20 years been teaching biological sciences to nurses and allied health professionals at the University of Leeds. In the meantime, Jim completed a PhD in the Molecular Epidemiology Group at Leeds, investigating Barrett's oesophagus and oesophageal adenocarcinoma. Jim is a passionate advocate for the promotion of bioscience education within health professional education and is currently a steering group member for the special interest group 'Bioscience in Nurse Education' (BiNE).

Dr Shupikai Rinomhota PhD (Sheffield), MSc (Newcastle), BSc (Hons) (Leeds), RGN, RMN, PGCE, Registered Nutritionist, Associate Life Member - Royal Society of Medicine

Shupikai has many years' experience as a qualified Lecturer Practitioner in both Adult and Mental Health Nursing, with additional qualifications in Human Physiology, Biochemistry and Human Nutrition. He is a Registered Nutritionist with the Association of Nutrition (UK), a Member of the Nutrition Society (UK) and in 2016 was made an Associate Life Member of the Royal Society of Medicine (UK). His special interests are in neurophysiology and mental health issues, endocrinology, the gastrointestinal tract and nutrition. He has a strong belief in the adage 'Let food be your medicine' and believes many current health problems have a nutritional basis.

Preface

This book is a collaboration between four authors, each with a background in nursing and biological sciences, who have shared a similar professional journey. We are a diverse group with many years of teaching and clinical experience. We have been involved in teaching applied biomedical sciences within nursing, midwifery, audiology, radiography and cardiac clinical physiology programmes for many years, at all academic levels within the School of Healthcare at the University of Leeds. We firmly believe that knowledge of bioscience underpins decision-making in healthcare and is vital for the delivery of high quality care. First-hand experience with our students has taught us that many on healthcare courses find the bioscience sections challenging, particularly where there is an integrated curriculum, and this book was written with these students in mind.

It is our intention that the book supports readers in their learning by helping them to integrate their understanding of anatomy and physiology with clinically relevant examples, so that they can begin to apply their knowledge within their healthcare practice. Our primary audience are students on nursing, midwifery, radiography and healthcare science courses, but any student starting or revisiting a journey into the biosciences will find this book helpful. Our decision to integrate clinical cases throughout the book is intended to highlight the relationship between bioscience knowledge and real world practice. We are confident that the approach taken in this book will help stimulate a genuine interest in the biosciences and, ultimately, we hope that this will improve the competence of healthcare professionals to provide safe, high quality care to patients.

We are grateful to David Hames for his encouragement, guidance, and for being a critical reader during the early development of this book. We would like to thank the team at Scion Publishing Ltd for their support, diligence, patience and hard work guiding the development of this book; and without whom our idea would not have transformed into this book. Finally, we would like to thank the students who continue to challenge us, motivate us and whose experiences were the original catalyst for this book.

Paul Marshall, Beverley Gallacher, Jim Jolly and Shupikai Rinomhota

Leeds, 2017

Abbreviations

ABP	androgen-binding protein	GABA	gamma-aminobutyric acid
ACE	angiotensin-converting enzyme	GCS	Glasgow Coma Scale
ACh	acetylcholine	GFR	glomerular filtration rate
ADH	antidiuretic hormone	GH	growth hormone
ADP	adenosine diphosphate	GMP	guanosine monophosphate
AIDS	acquired immunodeficiency syndrome	GnRH	gonadotrophin-releasing hormone
AMP	adenosine monophosphate	GTP	guanosine triphosphate
ANP	atrial natriuretic peptide	HAART	highly active antiretroviral therapy
ANS	autonomic nervous system	HAI	healthcare-acquired infection
APC	adenomatous polyposis coli	HCAI	healthcare-associated infection
APC	antigen-presenting cell	hCG	human chorionic gonadotrophin
ATP	adenosine triphosphate	HCM	hypertrophic cardiomyopathy
AVN	atrioventricular node	HDL	high-density lipoprotein
BD	twice a day	HIV	human immunodeficiency virus
BMI	body mass index	HNPCC	hereditary non-polyposis colon cancer
BNP	B-type natriuretic peptide	hPL	human placental lactogen
BPH	benign prostatic hyperplasia	HPV	human papillomavirus
C	Celsius	Ig	immunoglobulin
CD	cluster of differentiation	IGF	insulin-like growth factor
CF	cystic fibrosis	INR	international normalized ratio
CNS	central nervous system	IRV	inspiratory reserve volume
COPD	chronic obstructive pulmonary disease	LDL	low-density lipoprotein
CRP	C-reactive protein	LH	luteinizing hormone
CSF	cerebrospinal fluid	MALT	mucosa-associated lymphoid tissue
CT	computed tomography	MAP	mean arterial blood pressure
CTL	cytotoxic lymphocyte	MDR	multi-drug resistant
DAG	diacylglycerol	MHC	major histocompatibility complex
DAMP	damage-associated molecular pattern	MI	myocardial infarction
DCIS	ductal carcinoma *in situ*	MRI	magnetic resonance imaging
DCT	distal convoluted tubule	mRNA	messenger RNA
DNA	deoxyribonucleic acid	MRSA	meticillin-resistant *Staphylococcus aureus*
DRE	digital rectal examination	MS	multiple sclerosis
DRG	dorsal respiratory group	MSH	melanocyte-stimulating hormone
DRV	dietary reference value	NADPH	nicotinamide adenine dinucleotide phosphate
DVT	deep venous thrombosis		
ECG	electrocardiogram	NICE	National Institute for Health and Care Excellence
ERV	expiratory reserve volume		
FAP	familial adenomatous polyposis	NK	natural killer
FAS	fetal alcohol syndrome	NSAID	non-steroidal anti-inflammatory drug
FGF	fibroblast growth factor	ORS	oral rehydration salts
FSH	follicle-stimulating hormone	PAL	protease, amylase, lipase

PAMP	pathogen-associated molecular pattern	RNS	reactive nitrogen species
PCT	proximal convoluted tubule	ROS	reactive oxygen species
PDGF	platelet-derived growth factor	rRNA	ribosomal RNA
PEFR	peak expiratory flow rate	SAA	serum amyloid A
PERT	pancreatin enzyme replacement therapy	SAD	seasonal affective disorder
PIH	prolactin-inhibiting hormone	SAN	sinoatrial node
PMC	pontine micturition centre	SER	smooth endoplasmic reticulum
PMNL	polymorphonuclear leukocyte	SNP	single-nucleotide polymorphism
PNS	peripheral nervous system	SPD	sensory processing disorder
PP	pancreatic polypeptide	SSRI	selective serotonin reuptake inhibitor
PRG	pontine respiratory group	TFA	*trans* fatty acid
PRN	as required	TGF	transforming growth factor
PRR	pathogen recognition receptor	TLR	toll-like receptor
PSA	prostate-specific antigen	TNF-α	tumour necrosis factor-alpha
PTH	parathyroid hormone	TPN	total parenteral nutrition
RAAS	renin–angiotensin–aldosterone system	TSH	thyroid-stimulating hormone
RER	rough endoplasmic reticulum	VLDL	very-low-density lipoprotein
RNA	ribonucleic acid	VRG	ventral respiratory group

CHAPTER 01 | Why is the human body the way it is?

Learning points for this chapter

After working through this chapter, you should be able to:

- Describe the general principles that underpin the theory of evolution
- Explain why organisms are required to adapt to their environment for survival in the short term and over longer evolutionary timescales
- Distinguish between the internal and external environment
- Discuss how the relative stability of the internal environment is a requirement for health
- Describe the homeostatic and homeodynamic processes that maintain the stability of the internal environment
- Outline, with specific examples, the homeostatic regulation of physiological processes
- Recognize the importance of using precise anatomical language in healthcare settings and identify key anatomical terms

1.1 Introduction and clinical relevance

Cases such as the ones below are presented throughout this book to demonstrate why it is essential that healthcare professionals understand the anatomy and physiology that underpin the practice of healthcare and the decisions made by healthcare practitioners.

Patient 1.1 | Amy | 1 | 20 | 194 | 235 | 447 | 473

- 18-year-old woman
- BMI 16.3
- Downy hair on face and arms
- Referred to eating disorder clinic

Amy is 18 years old and recently took her school exams. Just before her exams, Amy's parents, John and Megan, noticed that Amy was giving them excuses for not joining them to eat during family mealtimes. Initially, they thought that she just had too much homework to do, as part of her preparation for the exams. But as time went by, Amy's family noticed that she had lost weight, was going to school without eating breakfast and had started doing star jump exercises daily. Initially, Amy managed to disguise her weight loss by wearing baggy clothes or putting on many layers of clothing underneath a woolly jumper because she felt cold. During a conversation with her mother, Amy admitted that she had been dieting because she did not want to be fat. She divulged to her mother that her menstrual periods had become irregular and she had missed one completely the previous month. Amy and her mother agreed to go and see their family doctor. During the examination, the doctor measured Amy's weight and height. The doctor noticed that Amy's weight was 15% below the expected weight for her height and, with a body mass index (BMI) of 16.3 kg/m^2, she was beginning to look emaciated. Her skin was dry and beginning to develop fine brittle hair, visible on her arms and face. The doctor was so concerned that she arranged for Amy to be admitted to a local hospital for further assessment and for nutritional intervention. Amy now regularly attends an eating disorder unit as an outpatient.

Patient 1.2 — Sylvia — 2 — 20

- 81-year-old woman
- Hearing aid and cataract
- Dizzy and confused at audiology appointment
- Hyperthermia (37.9 °C) and heat exhaustion

Sylvia is an 81-year-old woman who lives in a small retirement community for elderly people who may require some support. She is fully mobile, has a hearing aid in her left ear and has a cataract in her right eye. She attended the outpatient audiology department for a routine hearing aid check, as she did on a regular basis. On the morning of the appointment, she took part in an exercise class provided within the community. She engaged fully in the exercises and, as usual, found that she was physically tired after the class. It was a very hot day and she was taken to the clinic by hospital transport. The journey took an hour longer than expected and there was no air conditioning in the vehicle. The side of the vehicle where Sylvia sat was bathed in sunlight throughout the journey and she could not open the window. Sylvia was wearing a woollen cardigan as she often felt cold. On arrival at the audiology department, it was clear that Sylvia was unwell. Sylvia felt dizzy when she stood up, and had to sit down again, before being helped into a wheelchair by the driver. Her skin was very moist and she felt warm. When the audiologist called her name repeatedly for her appointment, she did not answer, which initially he put down to difficulties with her hearing aid. However, when he introduced himself, Sylvia appeared confused and did not know where she was. As she was talking, the audiologist noticed that her mouth was very dry. On further assessment, her temperature, pulse and blood pressure were as follows:

- temperature: 37.9 °C
- pulse: 130 beats per minute
- blood pressure: 115/65 mmHg.

Patient 1.3 — Francine — 2 — 21 — 194 — 235 — 338 — 371

- 40-year-old woman
- Crohn's disease – on steroids
- Presents with inflamed bowel and anaemia

Francine is a 40-year-old woman who works as a financial management executive and has an inflammatory bowel condition called Crohn's disease. For many years, Francine had noticed that when she ate bread, oatmeal or creamed soups she experienced dyspepsia (indigestion) and abdominal pain with some distension, and this stimulated her to visit the toilet and to open her bowels more frequently. Her other symptoms included episodes of nausea and vomiting, diarrhoea and pale foamy stools, sometimes containing blood. She has experienced periods of relapse and remission over the years following the diagnosis of Crohn's disease. She has learned to live with the condition by avoiding certain foods and drinks that she knows will trigger her symptoms, such as spicy foods, milk and caffeine. She has been treated with steroid medications, including prednisolone and budesonide, antibiotics such as metronidazole and ciprofloxacin, and has also been provided with nutritional supplements during periods of relapse. Recently, her condition has become worse and she has been admitted to hospital with diarrhoea, blood in her stools, fatigue, pallor and weight loss. Following a clinical assessment, it has been suggested that Francine might require surgery because her bowel has been found to be very inflamed and her symptoms are no longer controlled adequately with medications. Her current BMI is 21 kg/m^2 and the results from a blood test revealed anaemia. As a new patient admission and candidate for potential surgery, Francine was screened to see if she is colonized with meticillin-resistant *Staphylococcus aureus* (MRSA).

You could easily meet patients similar to those described above in your role as a healthcare professional. In each of these cases, the patient's health and wellbeing are challenged. For example, both Amy (Patient 1.1) and Sylvia (Patient 1.2) may have difficulty in maintaining a stable and optimum body temperature, and Francine (Patient 1.3) may become dehydrated and also have an increased risk of infection. The next section will illustrate the importance of regulatory processes in the body, which operate in order to minimize the impact of challenges to health.

1.2 What you need to know – essential anatomy and physiology

1.2.1 Why the human body is the way it is

The form and function of our bodies are a result of hereditary information held in our cells (discussed in *Chapter 3*) and are also influenced by the environment we exist in. These two features underpin all life as we know it and provide a useful starting point from which the anatomy and physiology of the human body can be understood. Hereditary information is packaged into genes, which we inherit from our parents (see *Chapter 3*), and our genes determine our individual characteristics such as hair and eye colour. These characteristics are called traits (discussed in *Chapter 3*). Many of these inherited traits will offer no advantage to an individual, but some may be advantageous for survival in a particular environment, meaning that the individual is likely to live longer, have a greater time in which to reproduce and thus be more likely to pass their survival advantage on to their offspring. Over a long period of time, therefore, this trait will tend to spread throughout the population living in that particular environment. The term 'biological fitness' describes the ability of an organism to survive and reproduce. Differences in biological fitness mean that advantageous traits are selected naturally in particular environments. This 'natural selection' or 'survival of the fittest' is the basis of evolution.

Thus, the explanation for 'why the human body is the way it is' lies in evolution. Evolutionary theory describes how life evolved from common ancestors over successive generations. As we have seen above, central to the theory of evolution is the premise of natural selection, that is, differences between individuals develop and any difference that provides an advantage to survival will tend to persist, eventually becoming the norm over time.

The evolutionary outcome is determined by both the genes that are inherited by successive generations and the environment in which the organism exists, with the environment favouring the natural selection of particular genes. An example of this, in terms of human evolution, is the adaptation of people living at high altitudes (>2500 m above sea level).

Humans have lived at high altitudes for thousands of years according to the fossil record. Two frequently studied populations are those of the Andes mountains of South America and the Tibetan Plateau. When these populations are compared with lowland populations, a number of physiological differences are apparent. People from lowland populations, when placed in a high-altitude environment, frequently become ill with altitude sickness as a result of **hypoxia** (low oxygen levels in the tissues). The symptoms of hypoxia include fatigue, weakness, increased rate and depth of respiration, headache, tachycardia and light-headedness. High-altitude populations do not typically suffer from altitude sickness because they have adapted to the high-altitude environment.

The amount of oxygen in the atmosphere relates to the pressure exerted on it – 'atmospheric pressure'. There are more molecules of oxygen at sea level than at high altitude, because atmospheric pressure is greater at sea level due to the increased weight of the air. This weight reduces with increasing altitude, producing a lower atmospheric pressure. Although the percentage of oxygen molecules remains the same at approximately 21%, the number of oxygen molecules in a given volume is reduced due to the lower atmospheric pressure found at altitude. In other words, fewer oxygen molecules are breathed in with each breath at high altitude, as fewer molecules are available in the air. Thus, the amount of oxygen in this environment is potentially insufficient to meet the body's needs, which could result in hypoxia. However, high-altitude dwellers do not become hypoxic. They have met the physiological challenge of an environment where the availability of oxygen molecules is reduced by developing larger lung volumes, an increased number of red blood cells and a higher concentration of haemoglobin in their blood. They also use metabolic pathways at a cellular level that utilize oxygen more efficiently. These adaptations to hypoxia persist in the high-altitude population because individuals who possess the genes that improve survival at high altitude are more likely to thrive and become more prevalent by the evolutionary process of natural selection. Genes such as hypoxia inducible factor (*HIF*) genes have been naturally selected in this way in high-altitude dwellers, a process not seen in lowland dwellers.

Evolutionary timescales are observed to be greatly compressed in the rapid reproduction life cycle of microorganisms. Changes to genes or hereditary information can be observed to occur through successive generations, providing a direct observation of evolution in progress. For example, *Staphylococcus aureus*, a microorganism commonly found on the skin, causes no harm as long as it remains on the skin. At some stage, a random mutation (discussed in *Chapter 3*) occurred in a single *S. aureus* bacterium, which resulted in that bacterium becoming resistant to meticillin, an antibiotic that would normally kill it. In an environment where there is no meticillin, this mutation probably provides no positive benefit to the bacterium. However, if this bacterium is on the skin of a patient who is taking meticillin, the mutation will confer a survival advantage to it: it will survive while other *S. aureus* bacteria on the skin that lack this mutation will be killed by the meticillin. This elimination of the meticillin-sensitive *S. aureus* leaves more space available on the skin for the mutated 'resistant' bacteria to reproduce and spread. Therefore, these meticillin-resistant *S. aureus* (MRSA) bacteria are selected to survive.

MRSA is actually resistant not just to meticillin but also to many other β-lactam antibiotics, such as penicillin, ampicillin and a sub-group known as cephalosporins. Thus, although meticillin is no longer used in therapy, the term MRSA continues to be used to describe *S. aureus* strains resistant to this range of antibiotics.

Organisms such as MRSA that are resistant to multiple antibiotics are called multidrug-resistant (MDR) pathogens; their resistance to multiple antibiotics makes infections caused by them very difficult to treat (hence the precautions taken in hospitals to avoid the spread of MRSA – see Francine, Patient 1.3). Penicillin and other antibiotics are prescribed to millions of people each year, and a number of pathogens have developed resistance to these drugs. The emergence of MDR pathogens and the limited development by the pharmaceutical industry of new antibiotics that can treat MDR pathogens are becoming a major concern for health services globally.

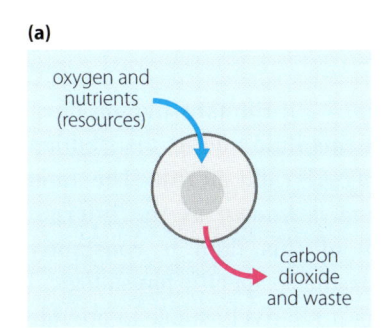

1.2.2 Single-celled and multicellular organisms

The evolution of all life from a single common ancestor is central to the theory of evolution, the common ancestor being a single-celled organism. It is from this very simple form of life that more complex forms such as humans have evolved. It is proposed that these early single-celled organisms originated in the seas around the Earth and that, over time, some single-celled organisms came together to form colonies (see *Figure 1.1*). Colony formation probably had survival advantages over existence as independent single cells. Eventually, colonies of single-celled organisms became interdependent, evolving into multicellular organisms.

Functionally, cells in a multicellular organism benefit the whole organism, rather than each cell working independently. An analogy here is of a car assembly plant. One way to produce a car would be for a single worker to accumulate all of the skills needed to build one completely from scratch. However, in a car assembly plant, different workers with different skills collaborate to build a car quickly and efficiently. For example, one worker adds the doors, another adds the windscreen and others add the bumpers (see *Figure 1.2*). This collaborative approach is replicated in multicellular organisms, where specific groups of cells perform specific functions. For example, the digestive system is responsible for processing nutrients, the respiratory system for accessing oxygen from the external environment and the renal system for the elimination of waste. Each system provides a survival advantage to the entire community of cells that functions as a coherent and interdependent multicellular organism.

Figure 1.1 – Evolving from (a) a single-celled organism to (b) a multicellular organism. Cells in the centre of the multicellular organism face potential problems as they are distant from the external environment and are surrounded by a small volume of fluid, the 'internal environment', which is naturally unstable.

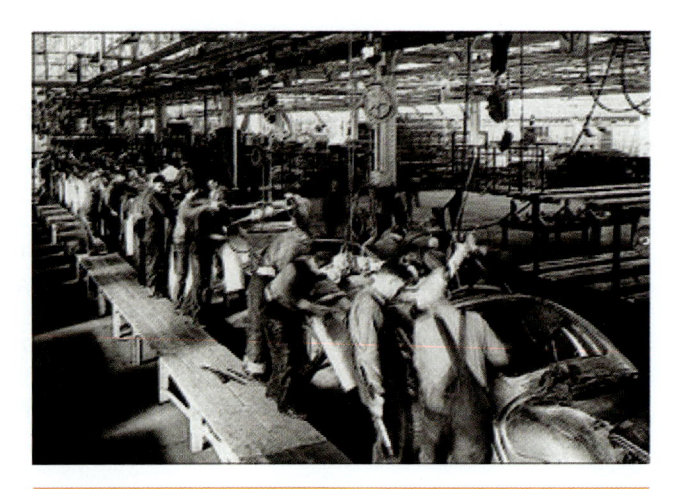

Figure 1.2 – **Assembly line in a car factory.**

All life as we know it depends on water (see *Chapter 2*). Humans live on land, but fluid exists within the body and the nature of this fluid and its distribution is essential for understanding physiological processes and health. The fluid surrounding cells within a multicellular organism is known as the **internal environment** of the organism. The composition of this fluid is constantly challenged by the activities of the surrounding cells and so specific physiological processes exist to regulate the composition, keeping it relatively stable to provide an ideal environment for the cells' survival. These processes are described by the concepts of homeostasis and homeodynamics.

1.2.3 Homeostasis and homeodynamics

Claude Bernard, a 19th century French physiologist, emphasized the importance of a stable internal environment for health and described how such stability could actually be achieved. In the early 20th century, Walter Cannon, an American physiologist, introduced the term 'homeostasis', meaning sameness (*homeo*) and to stand or stay (*stasis*). In his book written in 1932, *The Wisdom of the Body*, Cannon described various physiological processes that restore the normal state when it has been disturbed – the normal state being homeostasis.

However, biological systems are dynamic and nothing is ever completely stable; fluctuations in variables such as temperature and the concentration of dissolved substances are an inherent part of normal physiology and change over time. This has led to the emergence and development of an alternative concept of **homeodynamics**, which includes gradual adjustments and adaptations that organisms make to their internal environments, their physical organization and their physiological processes, in order to remain viable in the face of such constant change. Biological systems are homeodynamic because they have the ability to self-regulate and adapt, both structurally and functionally, over time when their chemical and physiological stability is challenged. These processes may occur rapidly between molecules, within a cell membrane or between cells, and within tissues and organs. As a dynamic process over evolutionary timescales, the process of homeodynamics can be used to explain how organisms adapt to their environment. The human organism has the property of 'robustness', that is, the ability to return to the normal functional state following a disturbance, such as increasing the heart rate in response to a sudden change in posture to help maintain a normal blood pressure. The processes involved in returning the internal environment to a stable state are at the heart of the concept of homeostasis. Biological systems, including human organisms, also exhibit the property of 'plasticity'; that is, the ability to change and develop their functional systems to maintain life processes when the physiological challenge is too great for a simple homeostatic response. This is certainly the case when thinking of how new neural connections develop in the brain following brain injury. In summary, recently the concept of homeostasis has been viewed as too restrictive and not fully encompassing the way organisms, including humans, function over time as they develop and age. A homeodynamic perspective of physiology encompasses more fully the processes involved in health and disease and will be employed within this book to illustrate what you need to know about anatomy and physiology and how it applies to healthcare.

The homeodynamic process ensures that the composition of the internal environment is kept within narrow limits, despite changes occurring inside and outside of the body. Some components (variables) of the internal environment that require regulation are listed in *Table 1.1*, together with their normal ranges. Within the normal range, there is an optimal value for each variable called the **set point**, around which the level of the variable will fluctuate, and to which adjustments are maintained via regulatory systems to maintain the variable close to the set point.

An awareness of all the normal ranges of physiological variables is extremely important in healthcare; *Table 1.1* shows just a selection. Values outside of the homeostatic range are typically associated with ill health and if allowed to remain so, or to deviate further, can lead to disease or death. In a clinical setting, it is relatively easy to extract a sample of venous blood (in essence a sample of the

Table 1.1 – The normal ranges of some variables within the internal environment

Internal environment variable	Normal range
Oxygen (O_2)	10.0–13.3 kPa
Glucose (fasting level)	4.0–5.9 mmol/L
Glucose (non-fasting level)	<7.8 mmol/L
Osmolality	285–295 mOsm/kgH_2O
Urea (a waste product of metabolism)	2.5–7.5 mmol/L
Sodium ions (Na^+)	135–145 mmol/L
Potassium ions (K^+)	3.5–5.0 mmol/L
Calcium ions (Ca^{2+})	2.2–2.6 mmol/L
Chloride ions (Cl^-)	98–108 mmol/L
Hydrogen ions (H^+) (pH)	7.35–7.45
Carbon dioxide (CO_2)	4.4–5.8 kPa
Core temperature	35.6–37.8 °C

internal environment), have the sample analysed in a clinical chemistry and haematology laboratory (e.g. sodium, potassium and blood glucose levels) and compare the results with the normal ranges; for example, a fasting blood glucose level over 7.0 mmol/L or a non-fasting level above 11.1 mmol/L are abnormal and are diagnostic of diabetes mellitus (discussed in *Chapter 5*).

1.2.4 The internal environment and plasma

Fluid inside a cell is called intracellular fluid, while the extracellular fluid surrounding the cell forms the internal environment. The extracellular fluid exists in several different 'compartments' in the body, two of which are interstitial fluid and plasma (the fluid part of the blood). **Interstitial fluid** surrounds tissue cells, while plasma is found in blood vessels. However, because blood vessels are themselves made of cells, plasma is outside of those cells and hence part of the internal environment (*see Figure 1.3*). In terms of quantity of fluid in an adult male of 70 kg, approximately:

- 3 L of the fluid is plasma (within the blood vessels)
- 10.5 L is located in the interstitial fluid (surrounding the cells)
- 28 L is located in intracellular fluid (within the cells).

Extracellular fluid is also found in a third compartment called **transcellular fluid**, which represents a collection of many different body fluids. These include cerebrospinal fluid, synovial fluid, fluid between the pleural membranes, the vitreous humour of the eye, urine, semen and gastrointestinal secretions

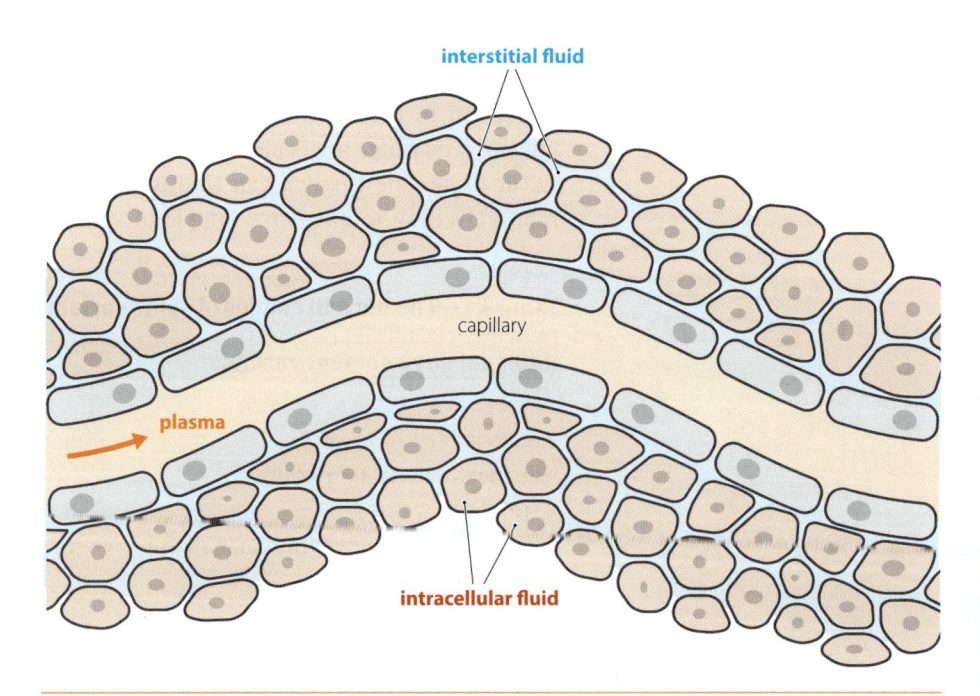

Figure 1.3 – **The internal environment comprising plasma and interstitial fluid (extracellular fluid).**

such as stomach acid, pancreatic juice and bile. The detailed composition of transcellular fluid obviously varies considerably. The volume of transcellular fluid is approximately 0.5 L. The total volume of water in an adult male is thus approximately 42 L, of which transcellular fluid makes up just 1%.

Understanding the role of body fluids in physiology and the part they play in health is essential to the practice of healthcare, because changes in the volume of these fluids (consider Francine, Patient 1.3, whose symptoms may lead to dehydration) or their composition can be associated with significant health problems. Identifying such changes and then correcting them is important for returning patients to biological health.

The external environment surrounding a human communicates with the internal environment through the body surface and orifices. For example, humans take food from the external environment and eat it. While it is in the gastrointestinal tract (see *Chapter 7*), this food remains in the external environment and it is not until the food is digested and the end products of digestion are absorbed into the plasma that they enter the internal environment.

Ultimately, the composition of the internal environment is influenced by conditions in the external environment. However, the external environment is not static, because the ambient temperature and the availability of water and nutrients constantly changes. Thus, the body has evolved mechanisms to constantly monitor and adjust the conditions of the internal environment, ensuring that any changes are brought back towards the optimal 'set point' in order to achieve an optimal environment for cell survival. This process is described as a **negative feedback**, whereby any deviation away from the set point is countered and brought back towards the set point.

For health, body temperature, blood pressure, extracellular and intracellular fluid concentration and blood glucose concentration are key variables regulated by a number of mechanisms. Taking blood glucose as an example, the concentration of glucose in the plasma is monitored constantly by glucose-sensitive cells in the pancreas. When the level of blood glucose falls, for example in response to missing a meal, the glucose-sensitive cells respond by initiating a chain of events leading to an increase in the level of blood glucose until the normal level is restored. This chain of events involves the release of the hormone glucagon from specialized cells in the pancreas and the breakdown of glycogen (the form in which glucose is stored) in the liver to glucose, which is released from the liver into the blood. As a consequence the initial fall in blood glucose is corrected and the secretion of the hormone glucagon is stopped. This is an example of negative feedback. However, negative feedback systems are not perfect, and an overshoot can occur whereby the correction causes a variable to fall too low or rise too high; homeodynamic mechanisms constantly work to correct this and maintain the optimal level.

1.2.5 The homeodynamic process

To maintain a stable internal environment, a basic system involves (*see Figure 1.4*):
- cells with a sensory function called receptors, which constantly monitor the internal environment for changes (a change is called a stimulus)

- organs known as effectors, which produce an effect to counteract the original stimulus.

In the earlier example of blood glucose regulation, the receptors are glucose-sensitive cells in the pancreas, the stimulus is the blood glucose concentration and the effectors are glycogen-containing liver cells. The receptors need to communicate with the effectors so that they respond to produce a sufficient effect at the appropriate time. The two main communication systems central to homeodynamics that facilitate this are the autonomic nervous system and the endocrine (hormonal) system. In the case of blood glucose regulation, it is the endocrine system working via the release of the hormone glucagon from the pancreas that signals the liver cells to break down glycogen into glucose and to release glucose from the liver into the plasma. The communication systems of the body and blood glucose regulation will be discussed further in *Chapters 4* and *5*.

An additional level of control between receptors and effectors is required so that physiological responses remain fully integrated for the optimal function of the

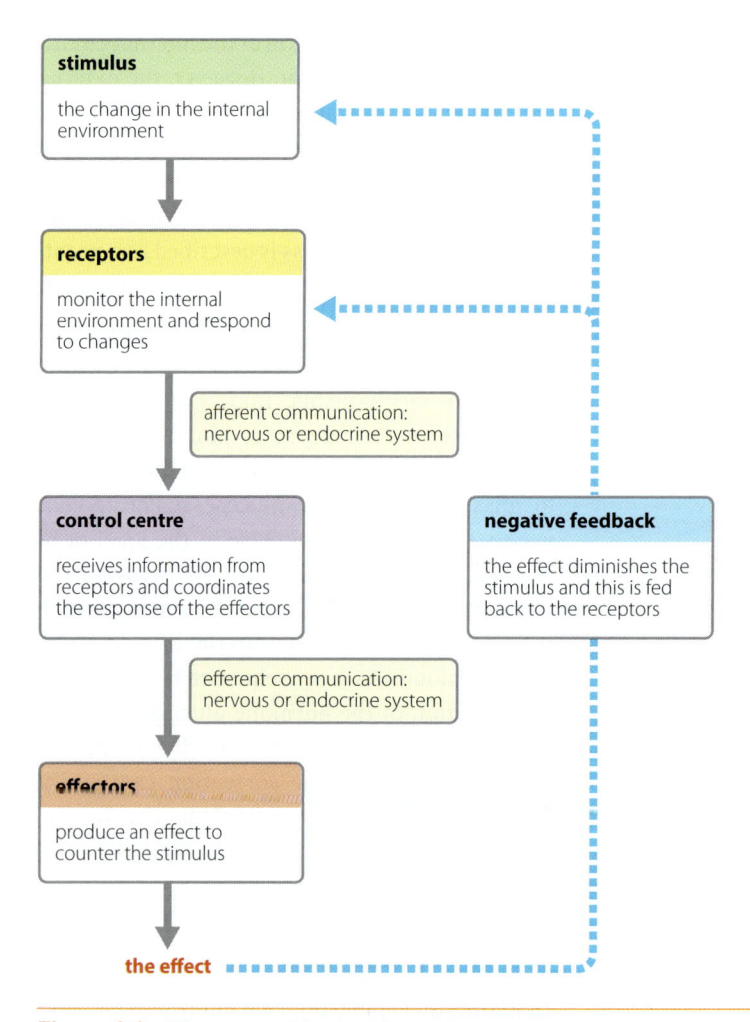

Figure 1.4 – The general homeodynamic process.
Illustrating how stimuli, receptors, a control centre, effectors and negative feedback maintain stability in the external environment.

whole body. This is achieved by a **control centre** between the two. Indeed, a control centre can coordinate the effects of a number of different effectors to a particular stimulus, and this is a more efficient way of achieving stability. In the case of blood glucose regulation, cells of the pancreas act as both control centres and effectors, but other examples exist where the control centre is part of the central nervous system, in particular the hypothalamus (discussed in *Chapter 4*).

Alterations in blood glucose concentration reflect the dynamic instability of the internal environment. Homeostatic control systems respond to changes in the blood glucose level by triggering various effectors to return the blood glucose level to normal. A summary of the regulation of blood glucose concentration is presented in *Figure 1.5*.

Scattered throughout the pancreas are specialized cells called **islets of Langerhans**, which are sensitive to changes in blood glucose concentration, and in response, secrete specific hormones. Two types of cells are located in the

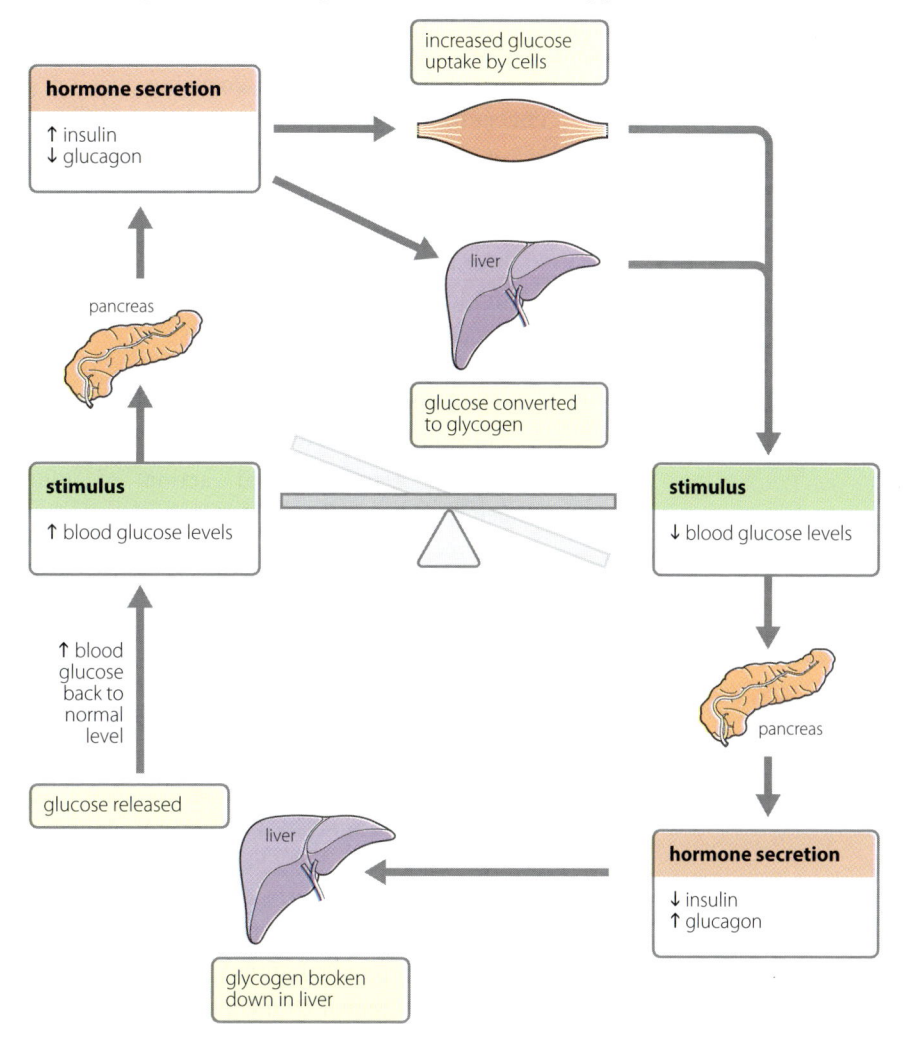

Figure 1.5 – **The homeodynamic control of blood glucose concentration by insulin and glucagon.**

islets of Langerhans: α-cells (pronounced alpha), which produce the hormone glucagon, and the more numerous β-cells (pronounced beta), which produce insulin. When the blood glucose concentration increases, for example following a meal, then:

- glucose-sensitive β-cells in the pancreas are stimulated and the hormone insulin is secreted from vesicles within these cells; at the same time, the secretion of the hormone glucagon is reduced
- insulin binds to insulin receptors located in the plasma membrane of liver cells and skeletal muscle cells and increases the rate of uptake of glucose into the cells (see *Chapter 2*); as a consequence, the blood glucose concentration falls towards the set point
- as the blood glucose level decreases, the initial stimulus (the rise in blood glucose) is corrected and insulin secretion is halted (an example of negative feedback).

When the blood glucose level decreases, for example if you have not eaten for a long time, this is corrected by a number of integrated mechanisms, including the autonomic nervous system (see *Chapter 4*) and the hormones adrenaline, thyroxine and glucagon. Focusing just on glucagon for simplicity, when the concentration of glucose in the blood falls too low:

- glucose-sensitive α-cells in the pancreas are stimulated and secretion of the hormone glucagon is increased; at the same time, the secretion of the hormone insulin is reduced
- glucagon acts on liver cells to stimulate the breakdown of glycogen to glucose, which is then released into the blood to increase the concentration of blood glucose
- as the blood glucose level increases, the initial stimulus (the decrease in blood glucose) is corrected and glucagon secretion is halted (an example of negative feedback).

Thus, the secretion and action of glucagon and insulin demonstrate homeodynamics whereby dynamic changes in the concentration of blood glucose are corrected.

1.2.6 The homeodynamic regulation of body temperature

Body temperature reflects the balance between heat production and heat loss. Fluctuations in core body temperature occur normally due to a number of factors such as diurnal variation, where the temperature is higher in the evening compared with the morning, extremes of age affecting the person's ability to respond to changes in the environmental temperature, eating, exercise and hormonal balance. For example, the metabolic rate (the rate at which chemical reactions occur, which generate heat) increases with the activity of specific hormones including adrenaline and thyroxine (see *Chapter 5*).

The homeodynamic regulation of body temperature relies on more than one effector coordinated by a control centre. Here, the effectors include:

- the skeletal muscles, which contract and relax repeatedly to produce heat (felt as a shiver)
- the smooth muscles of skin arterioles, which either constrict to conserve heat or dilate to lose heat
- the sweat glands, which produce sweat to cool the skin.

It is also important to recognize that subcutaneous fat acts as an insulator by reducing the temperature gradient between the body surface and the environment (consider Amy, Patient 1.1, whose eating disorder has resulted in a substantial reduction in her subcutaneous fat and therefore her ability to maintain her body temperature; as a result, she wears many layers of clothing underneath a woolly jumper).

The core temperature of the body must be maintained within a normal range around an optimal level (set point). The function of cells will be compromised if the temperature of the internal environment varies from the normal range. Cells rely on the function of **enzymes** – biological catalysts that help the chemical reactions of metabolism to occur, which generate heat. If body temperature becomes too high, the efficiency of enzyme function will be impaired. Likewise, as the core temperature decreases, enzyme-catalysed reactions slow down. In *Chapter 2*, the structure of the cell is discussed with particular reference to the proteins and lipids that make up the **plasma membrane**. Increases in body temperature can disrupt the normal structure of the plasma membrane, making the membrane less rigid, and the proteins are also **denatured** by higher temperatures. Such changes will impair normal cell function. The emphasis has been on the importance of maintaining a normal body temperature; however, an increase in body temperature due to an infection can be helpful. *Box 1.1* describes some important healthcare-related effects of increases in body temperature as a result of an infection.

Fever and infection

An increase in body temperature resulting in a fever may occur as a result of infection. Typically, the signs and symptoms of a fever include feeling cold and shivering (rigors) and elevated heart rate, respiratory rate and muscle tone, as well as the elevated body temperature. In this example, chemicals from infectious organisms and chemicals of the immune system (see *Chapter 11*) reach the hypothalamus from the body fluids and plasma and directly stimulate it. The hypothalamus functions as the control centre for thermoregulation and responds by resetting the set point to a higher value. In this context, the increase in temperature is a useful short-term response, because it improves the performance of the cells of the immune system and impairs the ability of the microorganisms to reproduce, and thus limits the infection within the body. Experiencing a prolonged fever, however, would have a detrimental effect on the body as it requires large amounts of energy to sustain, and it impairs normal physiological processes. An increase in body temperature and fever does not always occur in the presence of an infection. The temperature-regulating system of neonates, particularly premature babies, is not fully developed and so they might not develop a fever even if an infection is present. The lack of a raised temperature should not therefore be seen as indicating the absence of an infection in babies.

BOX 1.1

14 CHAPTER 01 | WHY IS THE HUMAN BODY THE WAY IT IS?

stimulus
DECREASE in body temperature

central receptors
hypothalamic (COLD) thermoreceptors excited

peripheral receptors
skin (COLD) thermoreceptors excited

↑ afferent impulses

control centre
hypothalamus activated

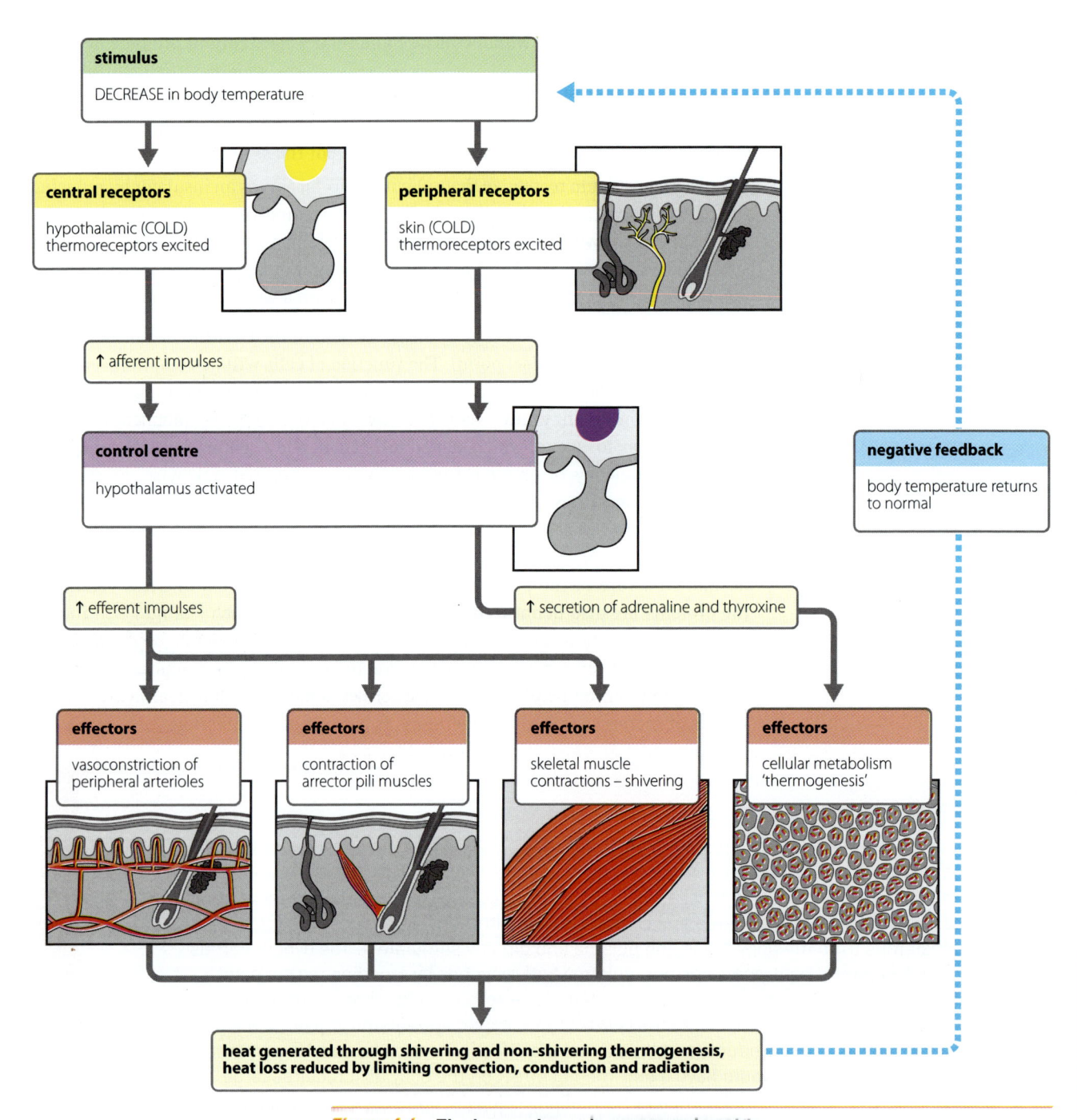

↑ efferent impulses

↑ secretion of adrenaline and thyroxine

effectors
vasoconstriction of peripheral arterioles

effectors
contraction of arrector pili muscles

effectors
skeletal muscle contractions – shivering

effectors
cellular metabolism 'thermogenesis'

heat generated through shivering and non-shivering thermogenesis, heat loss reduced by limiting convection, conduction and radiation

negative feedback
body temperature returns to normal

Figure 1.6 – **The homeodynamic response to cold.**
Note how the stimulus of a decrease in body temperature triggers heat generation and limits heat loss mechanisms by a variety of effectors.

The homeodynamic regulation of body temperature follows the schemes shown in *Figures* 1.6 and 1.7. Receptors for temperature (called thermoreceptors) are defined according to whether they respond to heat or to cold and also according to their location:

- *Central* thermoreceptors are located in the hypothalamus (a small area in the base of the brain) and constantly monitor the temperature of the plasma as it flows through the hypothalamus; this is known as the core temperature and reflects the temperature of the blood in the large blood vessels within abdominal and thoracic organs such as the heart, liver and brain.

stimulus
INCREASE in body temperature

central receptors
hypothalamic (HEAT) thermoreceptors excited

peripheral receptors
skin (HEAT) thermoreceptors excited

↑ afferent impulses

control centre
hypothalamus activated

negative feedback
body temperature returns to normal

↑ efferent impulses

effectors
sweat glands produce sweat

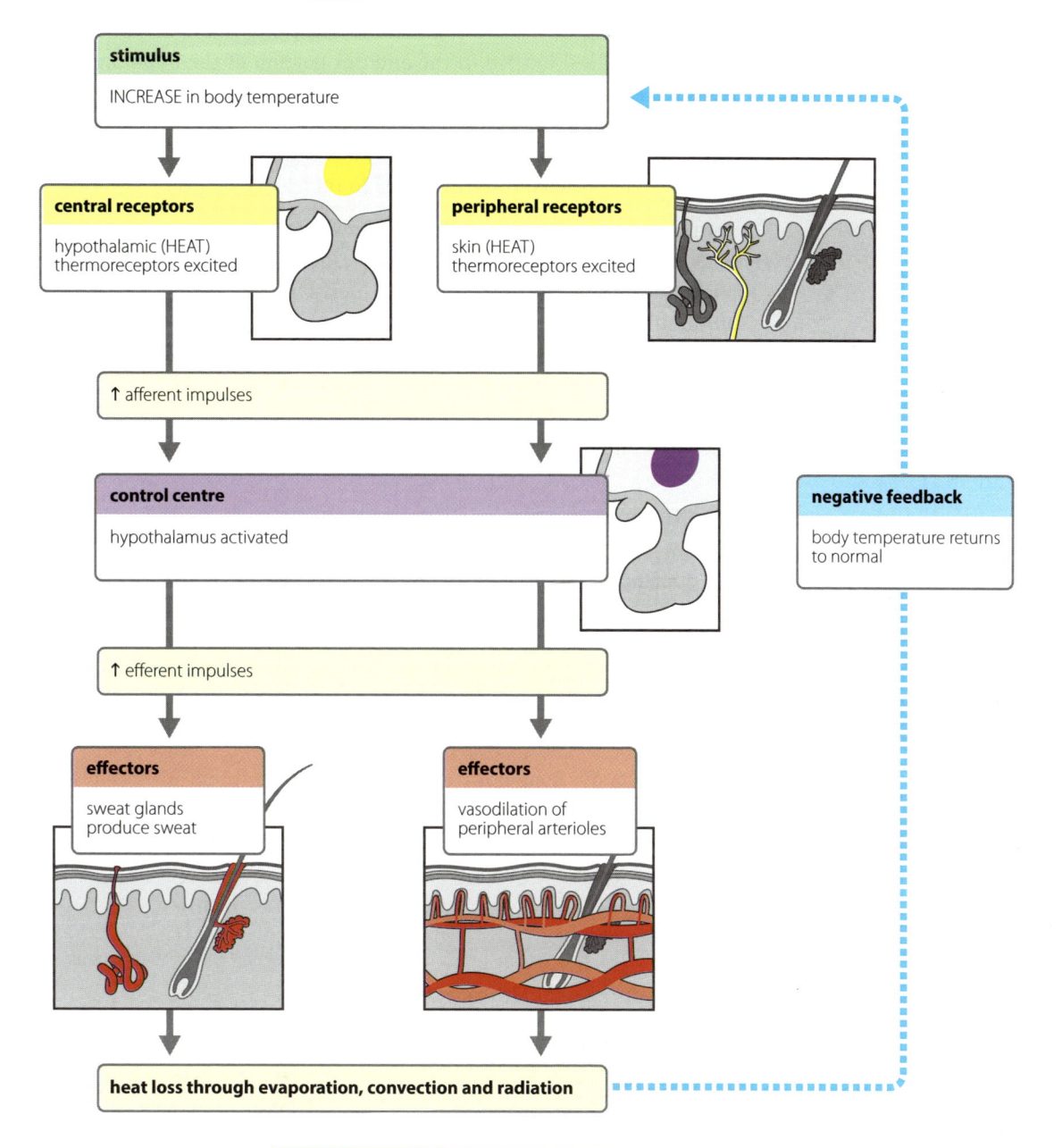

effectors
vasodilation of peripheral arterioles

heat loss through evaporation, convection and radiation

Figure 1.7 – **The homeodynamic response to heat.**
Note how the stimulus of an increase in body temperature triggers heat-loss mechanisms by a variety of effectors.

- *Peripheral* thermoreceptors are found in the dermal cells of the skin and monitor the temperature of the body at its surface; this is often called the shell temperature and is usually lower than the core temperature.

The hypothalamus has a number of roles including hormone production (discussed in *Chapter 5*) and, in the context of body temperature regulation, it acts as the control centre and communicates with a variety of different effectors to produce heat-generating or heat-losing actions. **Nuclei** (a name for a compact cluster of nerve cell bodies) located in the anterior portion of the hypothalamus (a specific region called the pre-optic area) receive signals from the thermoreceptors. The hypothalamus operates with a set point for temperature; this is generally regarded as being around 37°C and either initiates responses in effectors to produce more heat or sends signals to the effectors to increase heat loss.

The temperature of the blood flowing through the hypothalamus (core temperature) is maintained within narrow limits, despite large fluctuations in the peripheral temperature of the skin surface (shell temperature), which can vary widely from 20 to 40°C. Indeed, significant fluctuations in skin temperature occur as part of the homeodynamic response to maintain a stable core temperature. This is because the hypothalamus receives information from peripheral thermoreceptors, and this information is integrated into the homeodynamic response. The assessment of body temperature is considered in *Box 1.2*.

The homeodynamic response to cold

The homeodynamic response to cold is illustrated in *Figure 1.6*. Thermoreceptors detect changes in temperature and, as a result, the **neurones** they stimulate send messages to the brain where they are processed to provide the sensation of hot or cold; they are described as 'sensory' nerves. The direction of the impulse is *towards* the control centre and so these nerves can also be described as **afferent nerves**, in contrast to **efferent nerves**, which take messages *away* from the control centre.

A fall in body temperature to below the set point stimulates central and/or peripheral cold thermoreceptors, and these trigger sensory (afferent) nerve impulses to be sent to the pre-optic area of the hypothalamus. Nerve impulses are

---

BOX 1.2

Assessment of body temperature

The body temperature is frequently measured in healthcare environments because it is a good indicator of infection and altered health (discussed in *Chapter 11*) and it is easy to measure. Common sites for measuring body temperature are the mouth, rectum and ear, and electronic measuring devices are frequently used. Tympanic membrane thermometers are becoming more widespread because they are convenient and minimally invasive, and give an accurate approximation of core temperature. Tympanic membrane thermometers measure the temperature of the tympanic membrane, the warmest part of the ear canal. The temperature in this region reflects the core body temperature as the tympanic membrane lies close to the hypothalamus and shares the same core blood supply.

constantly sent from thermoreceptors to the control centre, but in the cold, more cold-sensitive receptors are stimulated.

Once the pre-optic area of the hypothalamus has been stimulated, the heat-promoting centres of the hypothalamus are activated and nerve impulses are sent to the effectors. The muscles and glands that constitute the effectors increase body temperature or reduce heat loss. The direction of the nerve impulses is *away* from the control centre, which means the nerves carrying the impulses are efferent nerves and, because the nerves stimulate or inhibit muscular and glandular function, they can also be described as **motor nerves**. Because the hypothalamus also regulates endocrine function, this process is also altered to increase heat production.

To understand how effectors are able to control heat loss and gain, we need to consider the four mechanisms of heat transfer, and these are presented in *Table 1.2*.

The process of heat production in an organism is called *thermogenesis*, and there are several mechanisms that can be used:

- *Shivering.* This occurs when muscles contract and relax rapidly as the core temperature falls. This rapid contraction and relaxation of muscles increases the amount of heat produced by muscle cells, which contributes to an increase in the core temperature. Shivering can be a very effective temperature-raising mechanism in the short term, with heat production increased fourfold in a matter of minutes.
- *Non-shivering thermogenesis.* Heat can also be created through an increase in metabolism. Adrenaline and thyroxine are two hormones that increase metabolism, in particular the metabolism of fat rather than glucose, and both hormones are released into the blood in greater quantities in response to exposure to cold.

Table 1.2 – Mechanisms of heat transfer

Radiation	The transfer of heat via electromagnetic waves, which are emitted from warm objects and travel through the air.
Conduction	The transfer of heat down a temperature gradient between molecules that are in contact. A hand on a warm radiator feels warm because thermal energy is conducted through the radiator into the cooler hand.
Convection	The transfer of heat by the bulk movement of free particles of air or fluid. As heat is transferred to the air molecules close to the skin, the air rises and is replaced by cooler air. This cycle is repeated and heat is lost to the air.
Evaporation	The conversion of liquid water on the surface of the skin to water vapour. This requires energy in the form of heat, and so heat is lost from the body as sweat evaporates from the surface.

- *Breakdown of brown fat.* This is a specific type of **adipose (fat) tissue** that is very efficient at producing metabolic heat. Brown adipose tissue is much more active in neonates and hibernating mammals than in adults, which is useful because neonates have not yet developed the ability to shiver effectively. Most adults appear to have very little active brown fat, as it is gradually lost throughout childhood.

In addition to thermogenesis, other responses to the cold to reduce heat loss are:

- *Goose-bumps.* The hairs on our skin rise from the surface and become erect when it is cold (see *Chapter 12*), and this is known as goose-bumps. This is because the arrector pili muscles to which they are attached in the skin contract in the cold, a process called **piloerection**, which causes the hairs to rise. The upright hair in fur-covered mammals effectively traps a layer of air next to the skin, and this acts as an insulator. Although humans have retained the piloerection function, it is not very effective because we have lost most of our body hair.
- *Vasoconstriction.* The narrowing of arterioles that supply blood to the skin also reduces the heat lost from the skin because blood is retained in the warmer core. This minimizes heat loss by radiation from the skin because the temperature gradient between the environment and the skin is reduced.

Finally, when people are exposed to the cold, in an attempt to preserve an optimum core body temperature, they typically respond with a range of behaviours, for example wearing additional layers of clothing or even curling up to reduce the surface area of the body.

Hypothermia is the term used when the core body temperature falls below 35 °C, causing the metabolic rate to decrease. Hypothermia is classified as mild (32–35 °C), moderate (28–32 °C) and severe (less than 28 °C).

The homeodynamic response to heat

The homeodynamic response to heat is illustrated in *Figure 1.7*. When the temperature of the internal or external environment rises, for example due to exercise or sitting out in the sun, more heat receptors are stimulated and sensory (afferent) impulses are sent to the hypothalamus. The hypothalamus responds by activating *heat-losing* mechanisms via motor (efferent) nerve impulses sent to effectors such as sweat glands and arterioles of the skin, which cool the body by increasing heat loss:

- *Vasodilation* Arterioles in the skin vasodilate (open up), which increases blood flow to the skin. As a result, the skin surface warms and may appear redder or flushed in fair-skinned people. Heat is lost via radiation, conduction and convection.
- *Sweating.* Sweat is produced by sudoriferous (sweat) glands in the skin (discussed in *Chapter 12*), and when it evaporates, heat is taken away

from the body, with the water molecules entering the air as vapour. As seen with Sylvia (Patient 1.2), when sweat evaporates, the skin cools down. When the air temperature is quite high and the ambient humidity of the air is low, then the evaporation of sweat provides a very effective additional mechanism for heat loss. However, there is a maximum level of water vapour that the air can hold, and as this is approached, it is more difficult for sweat to evaporate. The quantity of water vapour in the air is measured in terms of its humidity; on a hot day when the ambient humidity is high, sweating becomes a less efficient method of cooling the body because less vapour can move from the skin into the already moist air.

A range of terms are used when referring to elevated body temperature. **Pyrexia** refers to a raised body temperature due to resetting of the temperature-regulating set point in the hypothalamus and is associated with the signs and symptoms of fever (see *Box 1.1*), and occurs as a response to infection, injury to the hypothalamus and, rarely, as an adverse reaction to some drugs. **Hyperthermia** is elevation of the body temperature not associated with fever and resetting of the hypothalamic set point. Hyperthermia is due to impairment of thermoregulation, when the body absorbs or produces more heat than can be lost through normal homeodynamic mechanisms. However, due to activation of heat-losing mechanisms, one of the features of hyperthermia is the excess loss of water and sodium, which can lead to heat stroke.

1.3 Clinical application

Biological health can be understood in terms of the homeodynamic processes that maintain it. The homeodynamic process illustrates how adaptation and change over a long period of time contribute to the survival of living organisms. In this chapter, there has been a focus particularly on maintaining core body temperature. Understanding how a failure to maintain homeodynamics and the regulation of physiological function can lead to ill health is important in healthcare so that suitable explanations can be given to patients and appropriate management planned. The cases described in this chapter highlight how a failure to regulate body temperature can arise and how the development of resistance to antibiotics by microorganisms has significant health consequences:

- Amy (Patient 1.1) feels cold all the time and is unable to keep warm, a consequence of the significant loss of subcutaneous fat due to her eating disorder.
- Sylvia (Patient 1.2) developed a high temperature due to an inability to regulate her body temperature, a consequence of being exposed to direct sunlight and wearing inappropriate clothing.

- **Francine (Patient 1.3)** attended for planned surgery to correct problems associated with Crohn's disease. As part of routine screening pre-operatively, Francine was found to be colonized with MRSA. She needed appropriate treatment to decolonize the MRSA before her surgery.

Patient 1.1 | Amy | 1 | 20 | 194 | 235 | 447 | 473

- 18-year-old woman
- BMI 16.3
- Downy hair on face and arms
- Referred to eating disorder clinic

Amy wears many layers of clothing at home underneath a thick woolly jumper and tends to turn up the thermostat of the central heating system frequently. Amy's mother, Megan, is surprised at how cold Amy feels when she touches her. Megan has also noticed that the fine hair on Amy's face and arms appears more pronounced.

Amy's body is responding to starvation in a number of ways. She has lost weight because her energy stores (principally in fat but also in muscle) have been heavily depleted to compensate for her reduced food intake. Fat and protein, in particular, are broken down to provide her with the energy she needs for essential metabolism. This has resulted in her having a minimal layer of subcutaneous fat, which is inadequate to insulate her from the ambient air temperature. The homeodynamic response to starvation is to conserve as much energy as possible, and hence Amy's metabolic rate is lowered so that her energy stores may last longer. As discussed in *Section 1.2.6*, metabolism is the chief mechanism by which the body generates heat, and so her heat production is reduced. However, due to psychological factors contributing to the development of her eating disorder, Amy has adopted an intensive exercise regime with the deliberate intention of increasing her metabolism to cause the further breakdown of fat and protein. The increased fine layer of hair on her limbs is believed to develop in an attempt to keep her warm by reducing convection and conduction of heat.

Patient 1.2 | Sylvia | 2 | 20

- 81-year-old woman
- Hearing aid and cataract
- Dizzy and confused at audiology appointment
- Hyperthermia (37.9 °C) and heat exhaustion

Sylvia was displaying the clinical features associated with hyperthermia (see *Section 1.2.6*). Hyperthermia is an elevated core temperature above the normal set point of 37 °C and is associated with impairment of temperature-regulating mechanisms, when heat production and retention is greater than dissipation of heat. Sylvia's body temperature was measured using a tympanic thermometer, which provides a close approximation of the core temperature. In Sylvia's case, her tympanic temperature was recorded as 37.9 °C. Hyperthermia can be defined as a core body temperature between 37.5 and 38.3 °C. Sylvia exhibited mild confusion, dizziness and excess sweating; these signs and symptoms, alongside the elevated tympanic temperature, are consistent with the condition called heat exhaustion. Heat exhaustion with mild hyperthermia, as in Sylvia's case, is easily managed by ingesting cool drinks, removing clothing and moving to a cooler area. Extreme elevations in temperature, such as greater than 40 °C, require urgent medical treatment.

| Patient 1.3 | Francine | 2 | **21** | 194 | 235 | 338 | 371 |

- 40-year-old woman
- Crohn's disease – on steroids
- Presents with inflamed bowel and anaemia

The significance of MRSA was discussed in *Section 1.2.1*. To determine whether Francine was colonized with MRSA, a single swab was applied to both nostrils, another to both sides of the groin and a third to each axilla. These swabs were sent for analysis, and positive results were received, indicating that MRSA was present in her nostrils, axillae and groin, and is also likely to be present on the rest of her skin. Due to the potential risk of spreading MRSA to the surgical wound and causing an infection, Francine had to be decolonized prior to surgery. She was required to take daily showers for 5 days using the disinfectant chlorhexidine gluconate and to apply the antibiotic ointment mupirocin nasally three times a day prior to surgery. Decolonization was successful, and Francine commenced therapy with potent anti-inflammatory drugs in an attempt to improve her symptoms and avoid surgical removal of part of her bowel. Healthcare-associated infection imposes a significant burden on resources, and screening for MRSA is part of a broader strategy to reduce the incidence of healthcare-associated infection. In most hospital organizations, screening of elective surgery patients for MRSA is an established practice to reduce the incidence of wound and skin infections following surgery.

The concept of a homeodynamic process is useful as it provides a model that can explain how the body functions, i.e. its physiology. However, in biological sciences, function is often related to form, and it is important to bear in mind that the structure of the body (i.e. its anatomy) influences function. The following section introduces anatomical terms to help you understand body structures and their relationship to one another. This is particularly important in the healthcare setting, as precise and correct anatomical terminology is vital to ensure that appropriate care is given.

1.4 Anatomical language

1.4.1 General anatomical terms

As healthcare professionals, you need to be able to describe what you see when caring for patients, and be able to communicate this, via a common language, to other professional groups also caring for that patient. In a similar way, a universal language of communication is vital between anatomists and physiologists when describing the structure and function of the human body. Anatomists, in particular, need to describe what they see when they look at the human body, and also the relationship that exists between different parts of the body, in a consistent way. For example, would you say that the kidneys are above the bladder? This is certainly true when a person is standing or sitting upright, but not when they are lying down on their back; however, it *is* true if they are lying on their front. Can you see the difficulties already when trying to describe the relative positions of the kidneys and bladder? An obvious solution to this is for everyone to agree on a particular body position that can act as a consistent

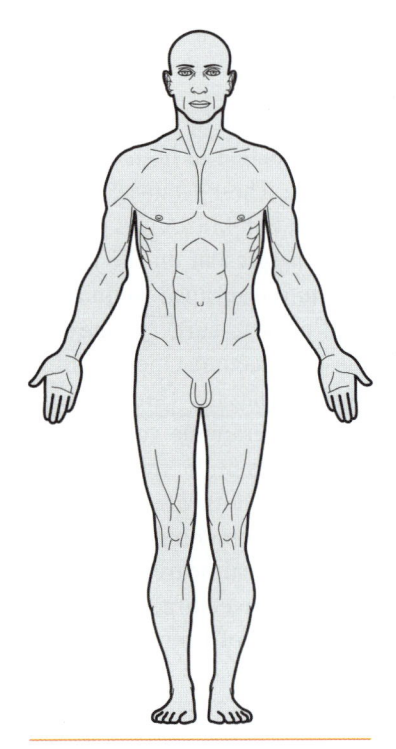

Figure 1.8 – **The anatomic position.**

starting point. This position is called the *anatomic position*, illustrated in *Figure 1.8*. In this position, the individual is represented by a figure standing erect with both feet flat on the floor and parallel to each other. The arms hang down by the sides of the body with the palms facing forwards and the head is level, with the eyes looking straight ahead. When the body is lying down rather than being in a standing position, it is described in two ways: *supine*, when the face is up, and *prone*, when the face is down.

As the human body is a three-dimensional object, it can also be viewed in three specific planes. A plane is an imaginary line that runs through the body in different directions (see *Figure 1.9*). The plane that divides the body into an upper and lower division is called the transverse or horizontal plane. The plane dividing the body into a front and back is called the *coronal* or vertical plane, and the plane dividing the body into equal right and left divisions is called the *midsagittal* or median plane. Any plane parallel to and on either side of the midsagittal plane is called a *sagittal plane*. Sagittal planes thus divide the body into unequal right and left sides.

A plane is an imaginary line; however, a section implies an actual cut through the body or an organ. Anatomists cut through the body and describe what they see, and again in order to standardize anatomical views and drawings, cuts are made that are parallel to the three body planes. Thus, we have transverse sections (also known as cross-sections), sagittal sections and coronal sections.

To be more specific and to indicate a perspective from a standardized viewpoint, we need to define the direction of the plane of view. A doctor may request a chest X-ray, to be taken as a coronal view, but does he want the X-ray taken from the front of the patient or from behind the patient? Both would be described as coronal views but produce very different images. The 'front' is thus termed *anterior* and the 'back' *posterior*. In practice, a doctor would request an AP (anterior–posterior) projection, which describes the direction the X-ray beam travels through the patient, entering anteriorly and exiting posteriorly. Anterior and posterior are both directional terms associated with a coronal view. The directional terms associated with a transverse section are *superior* or *inferior*, and those associated with a sagittal section are *medial* and *lateral*. In Chapter

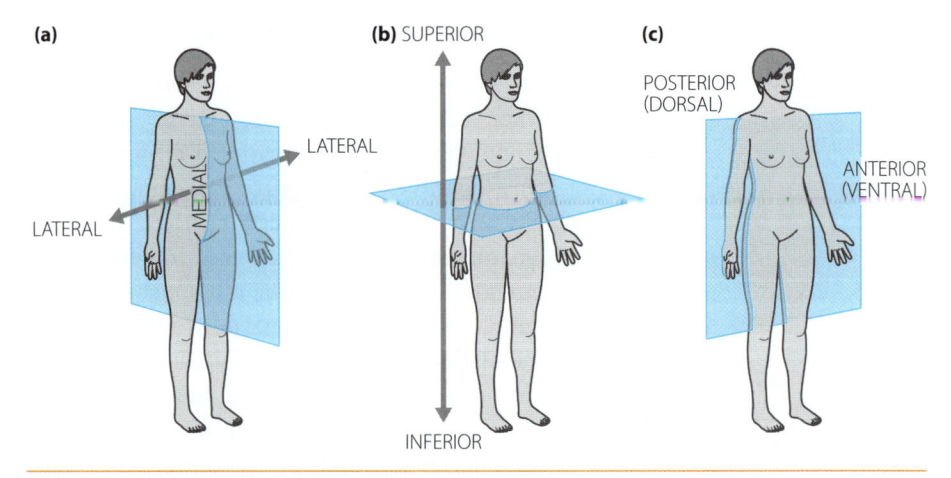

Figure 1.9 – **The planes of the body.**
(a) midsagittal; (b) transverse; (c) coronal.

10 of this book, *Figure 10.7* is an anterior coronal section of the thorax, *Figure 10.3* is a superior transverse section of the trachea and *Figure 10.6* is a sagittal section through the brain and respiratory centres. A list of common directional terms is shown in *Table 1.3*.

Traditional X-rays produce a two-dimensional image on a film or computer screen. In order to obtain an image of a patient's chest, for example, typically two images would be obtained: an anterior view and a lateral view. By looking at the two images together, an overall picture of the chest can be elucidated by the healthcare professional.

Table 1.3 – Common directional terms used in anatomy

Related plane	Term	Meaning	Example
Coronal plane	Anterior / ventral	The front of the body or body part	The trachea is anterior / ventral to the oesophagus
	Posterior / dorsal	The back of the body or body part	The spinal cord is posterior / dorsal to the heart
Transverse plane	Superior / cranial	Towards the head or upper part of a structure or the body	The kidneys are superior / cranial to the bladder
	Inferior / caudal	Towards the feet or lower part of a structure or body	The appendix is inferior / caudal to the stomach
Midsagittal plane	Medial	Towards or at the midline of the body; on the inner side	The heart is medial to the lungs
	Lateral	Away from the midline of the body; on the outer side	The arms are lateral to the liver
All planes	Proximal	Closer to the torso / trunk	The wrist is proximal to the fingers
	Distal	Further away from the torso / trunk	The hand is distal to the shoulder
	Superficial	Towards or at the surface of the body	The ribs are superficial to the lungs
	Deep	Away from the surface of the body	The uterus is deep to the skin
	Afferent	Carrying towards	Afferent nerves carry impulses towards the central nervous system
	Efferent	Carrying away	Efferent blood vessels carry blood away from the heart

Computed tomography (CT) scanners record transverse sections through the body, providing many images or slices through it, rather like the slices through a loaf of bread. The patient lies on their back, in the supine position, and slowly moves through the tunnel-like scanner. Low-density X-rays are passed through the body from one side of the scanner to the other and the image is processed by a computer. However, as multiple slices through the body can be obtained, the computer is able to reproduce three-dimensional images of the body. Thus, precise anatomical visualizations can be obtained that are not possible with conventional X-rays.

Magnetic resonance imaging (MRI) is able to picture the body in a similar way to CT scanning, by taking transverse sectional images that can collectively create a three-dimensional image. The tunnel-like scanner is similar to a CT scanner; however, the images are created using electromagnetic radiation and radio waves.

1.4.2 Body cavities

Body cavities are internal chambers within the body where specific organs, tissues and cells are found. There are four large cavities in the body: two are surrounded by bone (the cranial cavity and the vertebral canal) and two are surrounded by membranes (the thoracic and abdominopelvic cavities) (see *Figure 1.10*). Bone provides protection for the brain and spinal cord, which are found in the cranial cavity and vertebral canal. Similarly, the membranes surrounding the thoracic and abdominopelvic cavities also provide a degree of protection, but in addition enable organs to move within the cavity with minimal friction. Within the thoracic cavity, for example, the lungs increase and decrease in size with every breath. Similarly, within the abdominopelvic cavity, the stomach increases and decreases in size with every meal. This is made possible by the double membranes of these cavities. One membrane, the parietal membrane, lines the cavity itself, while the second, the visceral membrane, covers the organs within the cavity. Friction is minimized by the presence of serous fluid between the two membranes.

The diaphragm forms a physical division between the thoracic and abdominopelvic cavities. There is no physical division within the abdominopelvic cavity, although clinically healthcare workers do refer to the abdominal cavity and pelvic cavity. The imaginary separation between these cavities is a line drawn horizontally between the hip bones; superior to the line is the abdominal cavity and inferior to this line is the pelvic cavity.

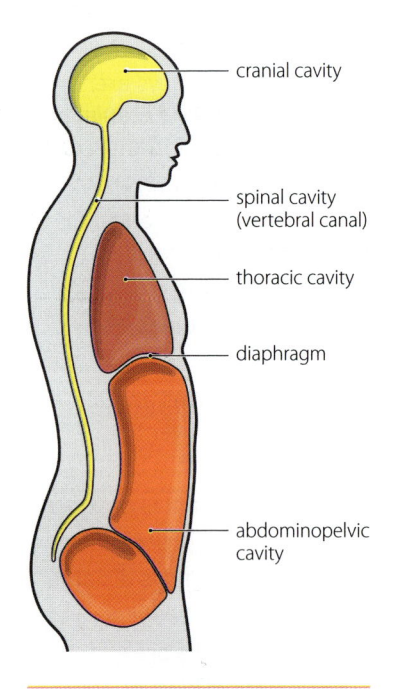

Figure 1.10 – The four large body cavities in the midsagittal plane.

Within the four large cavities already mentioned are smaller cavities such as the nasal cavity, oral cavity and pericardial cavity.

1.4.3 Body regions

The body can be divided into two broad regions: the axial region, which consists of the head, neck and trunk, and the appendicular region, which consists of the arms and legs or appendages.

Within the axial region is the abdominopelvic cavity. This is the largest of the cavities and also contains a large number of organs. In order to better describe the location of these organs, this cavity has been divided up into specific regions and quadrants (see *Figure 1.11*). As the name suggests, quadrants are achieved by dividing the abdominopelvic cavity into four areas around the umbilicus, using the midsagittal and transverse planes. These can thus be labelled the left upper, left lower, right upper and right lower quadrants; LUQ, LLQ, RUQ and RLQ, respectively, are how these are commonly written. In healthcare, these regions are extremely useful when describing the location of a patient's pain. For a more precise location, the abdominopelvic cavity can be divided into nine regions, using two transverse and two sagittal planes. Thus, for example, the gall bladder is found in the right hypochondriac region and the appendix is in the right iliac region. Some large organs are in more than one region; for example, the liver is found in the epigastric and right hypochondriac regions.

Humans are complex multicellular organisms who have evolved by the process of natural selection, a process that has facilitated their survival. Their ability to self-regulate their internal environment through the process of homeostasis has given them some capacity to withstand changes in their external environment. The concept of homeostasis helps to explain how the human organism regulates the function of cells and tissues within narrow limits. Recently, it has become increasingly recognized that this concept of 'stasis' might be limiting, because organisms and their physiological functioning develop over time, as is illustrated by human growth and development. Organisms are also governed by cyclic events, both in their cells (e.g. the cell cycle) and in their organ systems (e.g. the female reproductive cycle). The concept of homeodynamics is becoming more accepted, as it accommodates the recognition of adaptable, responsive systems that better characterize the processes of life.

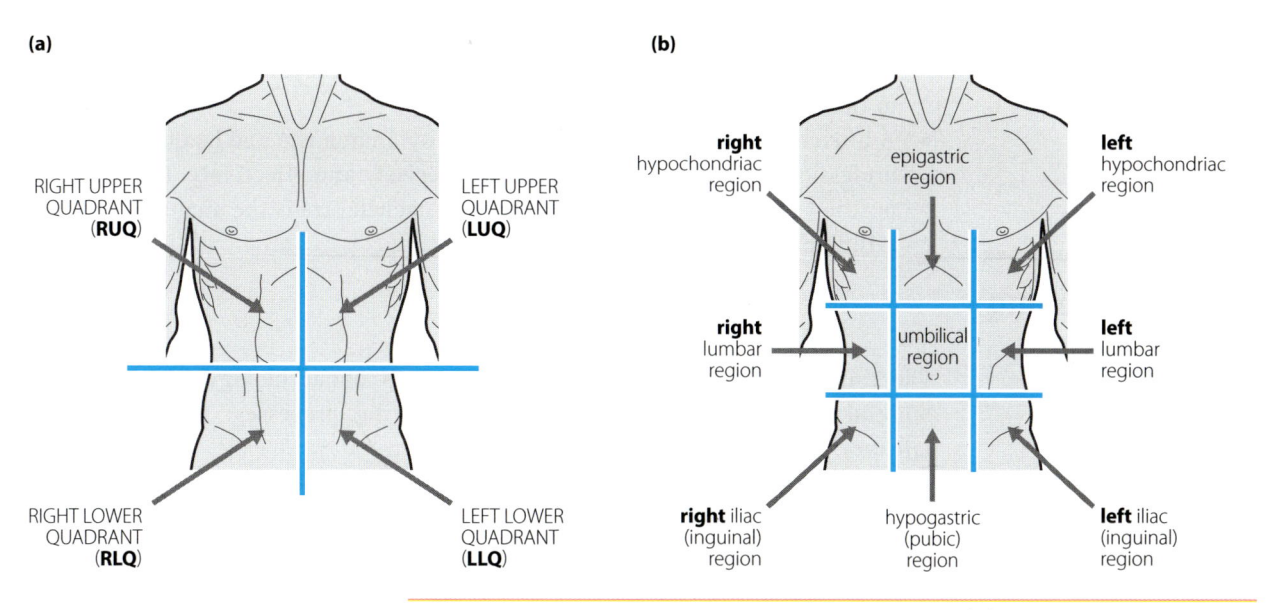

Figure 1.11 – The abdominopelvic cavity illustrating (a) the four quadrants and (b) the nine regions.

In this book, the primary focus is on biological health, which is vital to underpin and inform healthcare practice. As healthcare interventions may be required from conception until death, encompassing all states of health and human biological phenomena in between, it is important to recognize that human health is homeodynamic and, as such, healthcare must also be dynamic.

1.5 Summary

- Evolution by the process of natural selection provides a rationale for why the body is the way it is.
- Cell survival is reliant on a stable optimal composition of the internal environment. The process that maintains the stability of the internal environment is called homeodynamics and is achieved through the actions of receptors, a control centre and effectors (see *Figure 1.4*).
- The maintenance of normal blood glucose levels is an example of a homeodynamic process, achieved in part by regulating the secretion of the hormones insulin and glucagon from the pancreas (see *Figure 1.5*) and the storage and release of glucose by the liver.
- Peripheral and central thermoreceptors respond to temperature changes in the external and internal environments, respectively. Sensory impulses are conducted to the hypothalamus, which then initiates various responses via the autonomic nervous system and endocrine system (see *Figures 1.6* and *1.7*).
- Effectors for heat loss include skin arterioles, which vasodilate, resulting in warming of the skin and the loss of heat via radiation and convection, and sweat glands, which release sweat, causing heat loss as the sweat evaporates from the skin.
- Effectors that respond to cold involve the shivering response to generate heat, contraction of skin arteriolar muscles, causing vasoconstriction and thus reducing heat loss through the skin, and contraction of arrector pili muscles causing piloerection and the trapping of a layer of warm air next to the skin.
- A universal anatomical language is used by anatomists and healthcare professionals in order to communicate precisely and effectively. The position of reference for all anatomical nomenclature is the anatomic position.

1.6 Further reading

The following book challenges existing views about biology and discusses homeodynamics and the active nature of living processes: **Rose, S.** (2005) *Lifelines: Life Beyond the Gene*. Vintage, London.

The following article provides an interesting discussion about our ancestors and the genes we have inherited: **Stringer, C.** (2012) What makes a modern human? *Nature* **485**: 33–35.

1.7 Self-assessment questions

Answers can be found at www.scionpublishing.com/AandP

(1.1) Select the one correct answer. The composition of the internal environment comprises:
  (a) intracellular fluid
  (b) intracellular and interstitial fluid
  (c) interstitial fluid and plasma
  (d) intracellular fluid and plasma
  (e) transcellular fluid, interstitial fluid and plasma

(1.2) Select the one correct answer. Homeodynamic control mechanisms include a process where:
  (a) receptors are stimulated by effectors
  (b) the control centre sends afferent nerve impulses to effector organs
  (c) receptors, having been stimulated, send afferent nerve impulses to the control centre
  (d) the control centre switches off the receptor
  (e) effectors send efferent nerve impulses to the control centre

(1.3) Select the one correct answer. Francine is colonized with MRSA. This means that:
  (a) MRSA have passed into her blood
  (b) MRSA are destroying her skin
  (c) MRSA are living harmlessly on her skin
  (d) MRSA have stimulated an immune response
  (e) MRSA have been eradicated

(1.4) Select the one correct answer. If Francine remained colonized, she would have a higher risk of developing what sort of problem after surgery?
  (a) A colostomy
  (b) A wound infection
  (c) A deep vein thrombosis
  (d) A myocardial infarction
  (e) A chest infection

(1.5) Explain the terms homeostasis and homeodynamics.

(1.6) Outline the factors that have contributed to Sylvia developing hyperthermia.

(1.7) Match each numbered item with the most closely related lettered item:

1.	Midsaggital plane	a.	Lying face down
2.	Inferior	b.	Divides body into an upper and lower region
3.	Supine	c.	Contains the brain
4.	Epigastric region	d.	Towards or at the surface of the body
5.	Efferent	e.	Distal to the knee
6.	Coronal plane	f.	Divides the body into equal right and left halves

7. The hip
8. Cranial cavity
9. Left iliac region

10. Diaphragm
11. Transverse plane
12. Right lower quadrant

13. Prone
14. Superficial
15. The ankle

g. Towards the feet
h. Lying face up
i. Divides the thoracic and abdominopelvic cavities
j. Carrying away
k. Proximal to the knee
l. Divides the body into an anterior and posterior region
m. Superior to the umbilical region
n. Lateral to the hypogastric region
o. Inferior to the right upper quadrant

CHAPTER 02 | Cells and their environment

Learning points for this chapter

After working through this chapter, you should be able to:
- Outline the hierarchical organization of life
- Describe the composition and structure of a cell
- Describe the functions of organelles
- Explain how substances can be transported across the plasma membrane
- Describe the cellular and tissue organization of the human body

2.1 Introduction and clinical relevance

Each of the patients introduced in this chapter highlights how the function of cells can affect health. These cases also represent common situations likely to be encountered by healthcare professionals working in a clinical arena. They will be used to emphasize how knowledge of cells in terms of their structure, organization and function is useful to the practice of healthcare. We will return to these cases from time to time and introduce more cases as the book progresses in order to reinforce *what you need to know* about anatomy and physiology in healthcare.

Patient 2.1 | Mary | 29 | 53 | 311 | 330

- 57-year-old woman
- Chronic asthmatic on beclometasone dipropionate, salmeterol and salbutamol

Mary, aged 57 years, was diagnosed some years ago as having chronic asthma. She is currently treated with the following drugs:

- beclometasone dipropionate (200 micrograms (mcg) taken as two puffs twice a day (BD) via a volumetric spacer)
- salmeterol (50 mcg taken as one puff BD)
- salbutamol (100 mcg taken as two puffs as required (PRN)).

This combination of drugs improves her breathing by acting on the smooth muscle cells of the bronchioles within her lungs to relieve the narrowing of her airway (known as bronchospasm) which causes an expiratory wheeze, a common symptom of asthma.

| Patient 2.2 | Sumina | 30 | 53 |

- 2-year-old girl
- High temperature, D&V and tachycardia

Sumina is 2 years old and has developed a high temperature, diarrhoea and vomiting. She has become thirsty and irritable, looks very pale and has an increased heart rate (known as tachycardia) and her urine appears quite dark. Sumina is eager to drink, but is unable to retain any fluid she drinks. This is now the second day of symptoms and so Sumina's mother has obtained an urgent appointment with the family doctor.

| Patient 2.3 | Sheila | 30 | 54 | 59 | 93 | 267 | 304 | 448 | 473 |

- 47-year-old woman
- Recent diagnosis of breast cancer – biopsy shows cancer cells over-express HER2 protein

Sheila is 47 years old and has recently been diagnosed with breast cancer. A biopsy of her breast tissue revealed that her cancer cells over-express a protein on the plasma membrane called human epidermal growth factor receptor 2 (also known as HER2). She has been told by her doctor that she is a possible candidate for a form of cancer therapy with a compound that blocks the action of the HER2 receptor which will reduce the chances of the cancer reoccurring or spreading.

As outlined in *Chapter 1*, all living organisms are composed of cells and these cells are made of chemicals. The study of biochemistry focuses on the chemicals and chemical processes in living organisms. The chemicals involved in the many biochemical processes can be categorized into two main groups: an organic group, members of which always contain the element carbon, and an inorganic group, whose members do not contain carbon. All life synthesizes organic compounds because carbon is able to form very long interconnecting chain molecules, which form the basis of **macromolecules** – these include fats, carbohydrates, proteins and nucleic acids. Organic compounds can be small molecules, but inorganic compounds that do not contain carbon are typically small. It is important to recognize that both organic and inorganic chemistry is essential for life.

Simple organisms may be a single cell that reproduces by dividing into two cells, but more complex organisms comprise groups of cells that have specialized functions. These multicellular forms of life develop complex forms of communication, cooperation and reproduction in order for all the cells that make up the organism to survive. Humans are complex multicellular organisms, made up of trillions of cells. Because the cell is the fundamental unit or 'building block' of life, it is vital that you know about cells and how they function. If all the cells in an organism function in an optimal and stable manner, then the organism will be healthy.

The practice of healthcare involves looking after patients, but looking after biological health means looking after the cells too. The three cases explored within this chapter each need healthcare that addresses the activity of their cells in order to maintain a balanced, or homeodynamic, health status. For example, the symptoms of Mary's asthma (Patient 2.1) will be relieved by medication that relaxes the *smooth muscle cells* in her lungs. Sumina (Patient 2.2) will feel much better when her symptoms resolve as the distribution of *fluid between her body cells and tissues* is corrected. Finally, Sheila's breast cancer (Patient 2.3) is a disease of *uncontrolled cell growth*, and unless these abnormal cells can be removed, eradicated or brought under control, Sheila could become very unwell and possibly die. Each chapter of this book explores the essential anatomy and physiology and then highlights relevant clinical cases; an understanding of all of these cases requires you to know about cells.

2.2 What you need to know – essential anatomy and physiology

It is probable that the first cell was formed approximately 3.5–4 thousand million years ago, out of the spontaneous aggregation of chemicals on the primitive Earth into simple molecules. There is no fossil evidence for what happened in detail, but it is currently thought that some of these molecules were probably self-replicating and at some stage became surrounded by other molecules that formed an outer membrane. This membrane provided some protection for the chemical contents on the inside and maintained any differences between the inside and outside of the cell. The replicating molecules were probably nucleic acids (some ribonucleic acid (RNA) molecules today still have the ability to self-replicate with no other types of molecules such as proteins being required to help them) and eventually they gained the ability to direct the formation of proteins. Over time, these simple cellular structures evolved to gain the characteristics we recognize in the diverse forms of life on Earth today. This includes the ability to varying degrees to resist changing conditions in the environment and to use energy to perform activities such as movement, repair and reproduction.

2.2.1 Types of cell: the diversity of life

The current classification of life, often called the 'tree of life', is organized into three 'branches' or domains (see *Figure 2.1*):

- **Archaea** – these are prokaryotic, unicellular microorganisms often described as 'extremophiles' including, for example, those found living in high-temperature environments such as hot springs.
- **Bacteria** – simple prokaryotic bacteria.
- **Eukarya** – this domain includes a group of unicellular microorganisms as well as more complex organisms; all animals and plants are eukaryotes.

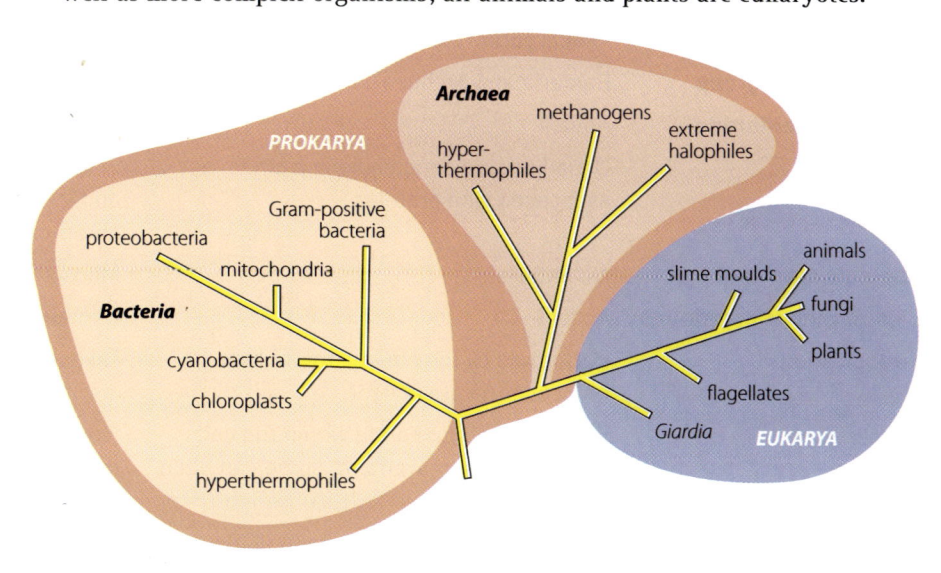

Figure 2.1 – The tree of life.
Note that the origin and evolutionary history of viruses is unclear; they are always found to be associated with life, but they do not reproduce or metabolize independently.

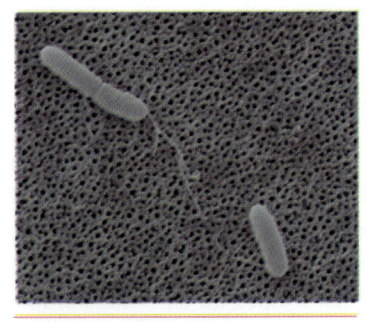

Figure 2.2 – Electron micrograph of *Salmonella enterica*, an example of prokaryotic cells.
This bacterium is responsible for causing gastroenteritis. Reproduced under a CC BY 4.0 International licence. Attribution: Mark Jepson, Wellcome Images.

Prokaryotes

Prokaryotic organisms (encompassing both the archaea and bacteria) are the simplest and most abundant forms of life (see *Figure 2.2*). They are small single-celled organisms lacking a membrane-bound nucleus; they range in size from 0.1 to 10 μm. They can be spherical (cocci), rod-like (bacilli) or spiral (spirilla) in shape. Different types of bacteria display different organizations of the individual bacterial cells. For example, staphylococci form clusters of cells, diplococci are arranged in pairs of cells and streptococci form chains of cells. Many prokaryotes have one or more tail-like appendages called flagella, enabling movement through an aqueous environment. Although prokaryotes are unicellular organisms, they are normally found living in aggregated colonies forming a 'biofilm'. Dental plaque, which causes tooth decay, represents a biofilm, and biofilms present on urinary or intravenous catheters can be responsible for urinary tract infections and sepsis.

Prokaryotic cells are surrounded by a cell membrane and a cell wall. The cell wall provides a strong coat around the cell, preventing rupture caused by osmotic pressure (osmosis is discussed in *Section 2.2.2*, below). Within the cell is a fluid (**cytosol**), which contains all the chemicals required for cellular metabolism. There are no organelles within the prokaryotic cell (see *Table 2.1* for a comparison of prokaryotes and eukaryotes), but within the cytosol the genetic material can be found. This is usually in the form of a circular molecule of DNA (deoxyribonucleic acid – see *Chapter 3*), condensed to form a body known as the **nucleoid**. Additional circular DNA molecules called **plasmids** that are not part of the nucleoid can also be present in the cytosol. Plasmids are not essential for growth and reproduction, but plasmid DNAs can provide additional selective advantages, because they often carry genes for resistance to specific antibiotics.

Table 2.1 – Comparison of prokaryotes and eukaryotes

	Prokaryote	**Eukaryote**
Phylogenetic group	Bacteria and Archaea	Animals, plants, algae, fungi and protozoa
Nuclear membrane	Absent	Present
DNA	Usually a single molecule in a circle, not associated with proteins	Linear molecule, together with proteins and in sufficient amounts to form several chromosomes
Cell division	No mitosis	Mitosis
Membranous organelles	Absent	Contain several
Respiration	Performed by the plasma membrane, mitochondria are absent	Takes place within mitochondria
Movement	Flagellin proteins rotate within the cell wall to provide movement; some can glide across a surface	Non-rotating flagella or cilia formed from microtubules
Approximate size	2–10 μm	2–100 μm

Adapted from Hayward, C.A. (2006) *Microorganisms*. eLS.

Prokaryotes reproduce 'asexually' by a process called **binary fission**. In this process, a copy of the genetic material is made and the **cytoplasm** is separated into equal halves by the formation of a new cell wall, with each new cell containing a copy of the genetic material.

Eukaryotes

The Eukarya domain includes all animals and plants. Eukaryotes (see *Figure 2.3*) can be unicellular but are usually multicellular organisms. These multicellular organisms are of course more than simply a collection of cells; the cells are *interdependent*, with specialized cells cooperating to maintain the whole organism.

Unlike prokaryotes, eukaryotic cells have a membrane-bound **nucleus,** which contains DNA packaged as chromosomes, along with a range of other membrane-bound organelles, each of which has a specific function. Eukaryotic cells are bound by a **plasma membrane**, but plant cells also have a relatively rigid cell wall surrounding their membrane.

Eukaryotic cells exhibit a greater variation in size than prokaryotic cells:

- the largest human cell is an **ovum** (see *Figure 2.4a*), which is approximately 100 μm in diameter
- the red blood cell (**erythrocyte**, see *Figure 2.4b*) is much smaller, approximately 7.5 μm in diameter
- the longest human cell is a nerve cell (a motor neurone, see *Figure 2.4c*) which can extend from the spinal cord to a toe, a distance that can reach over 100 cm. **Neurones** possess multiple branching extensions called dendrites, which participate in the generation of nerve impulses (discussed in *Chapter 4*). A hippocampal neurone (brain cell) is shown in *Figure 2.4c*.

The inside of the eukaryotic cell comprises the **cytoplasm**, a thick water-based fluid (cytosol) containing a variety of dissolved chemicals essential for life, together with a number of membrane-bound structures called **organelles**. These organelles include the nucleus, endoplasmic reticulum, mitochondria, Golgi apparatus, lysosomes, peroxisomes and, in plant cells, chloroplasts. The genetic material of eukaryotes (DNA) is contained within the **nucleus**. Reproduction requires coordinated division of the nucleus and the rest of the cell; in more complex eukaryotes, this can also involve sexual reproduction. A typical animal cell together with its internal structures is illustrated in *Figure 2.5*, although it is important to recognize that not all cells contain all of these structures. What marks out different types of cell found within a multicellular organism like a human is the number and type of organelles, together with the functional characteristics provided by the cell, such as the ability to contract (muscle cells; discussed in *Chapter 13*) and the ability to secrete hormones (cells of the endocrine glands; discussed in *Chapter 5*).

In the following section, each component of the cell is described to illustrate how cellular structure relates to its function in maintaining the viability and health of the organism, in our case the human.

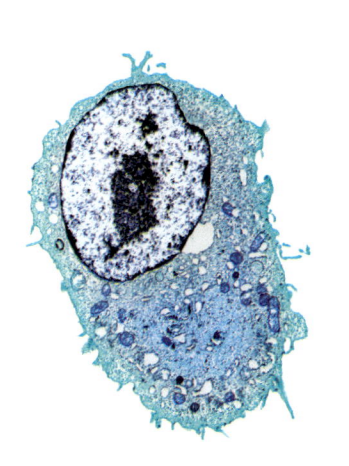

Figure 2.3 – **Coloured transmission electron micrograph (TEM) of a eukaryotic cell.**
Science Photo Library.

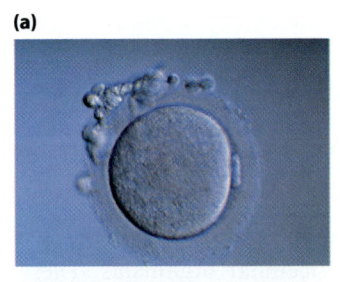

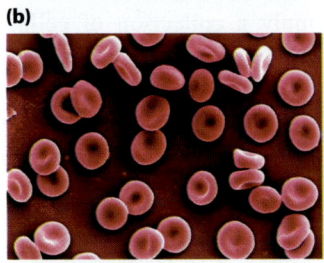

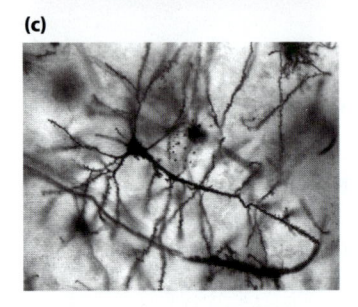

Figure 2.4 – Photographs of different cell types showing scale and form.
(a) An ovum with its first polar body (oval, centre right). Before ovulation the egg undergoes meiotic division to create two cells: a secondary oocyte and a polar body. The polar body will degenerate, while the larger egg develops in preparation for fertilization. Around the egg is the zona pellucida, a layer of glycoprotein which binds sperm; (b) erythrocytes, which are typically 7.5 μm in length; and (c) a hippocampal neurone from the brain showing multiple branching extensions called dendrites, which 'communicate' with other neurones. (a) Science Photo Library; (b) reproduced under a CC BY 4.0 International licence. Attribution: David Gregory & Debbie Marshall, Wellcome Images; (c) reproduced under a CC BY 4.0 International licence. Attribution: MethoxyRoxy.

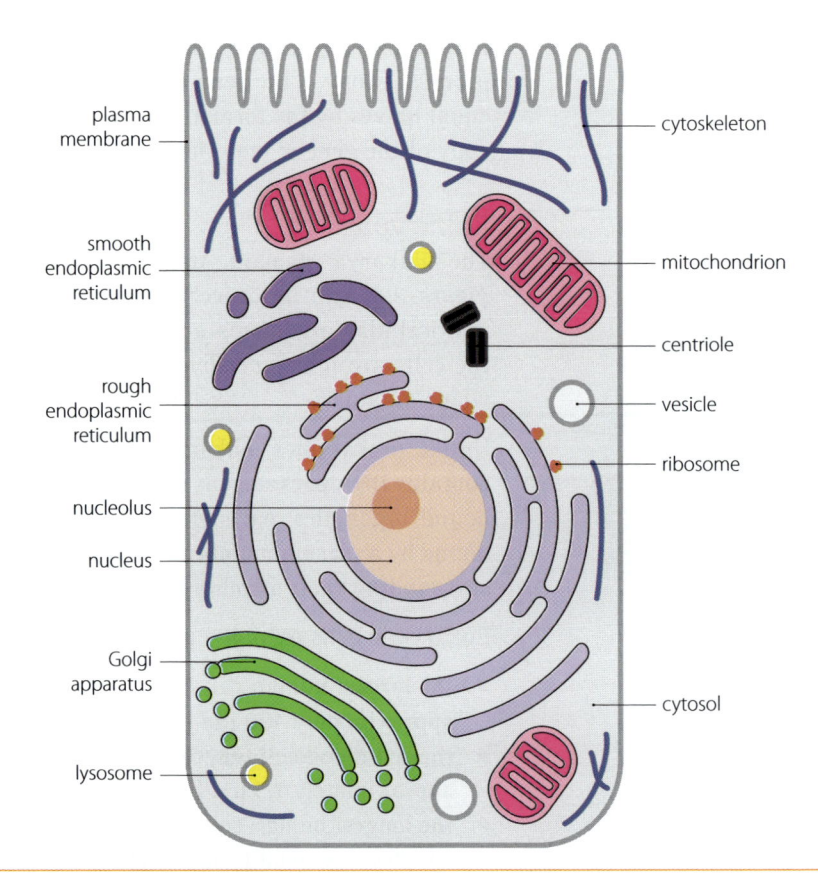

Figure 2.5 – A typical eukaryotic 'animal' cell.
The major organelles and cellular structures are labelled and include: nucleolus, nucleus, endoplasmic reticulum (rough and smooth), ribosome, lysosome, mitochondrion, Golgi apparatus, centriole, microfilaments (which form the cytoskeleton), cytosol and plasma membrane.

2.2.2 Components of a eukaryotic cell

Plasma membrane

A cell is delimited by its boundary, the plasma membrane, which obviously keeps the outside out and the inside in. Although this might sound very simple, being able to control the composition of the internal constituents of the cell, despite a constantly changing environment external to the cell, is vital for optimal cell function and survival. Other functions of the plasma membrane are that it:

- provides a mechanism for selective exchange of substances between the intracellular and extracellular environment
- contains receptor molecules to detect changes in the environment.

The structure of the plasma membrane is often described by the term '**fluid mosaic model**' (*Figure 2.6*). Visually, this can be likened to 'protein icebergs floating in a lipid sea'. In other words, the membrane is made up of a *mosaic* of large protein molecules embedded in and surrounded by a variety of phospholipid molecules. The phospholipids are themselves also able to move.

SECTION 2.2 | WHAT YOU NEED TO KNOW – ESSENTIAL ANATOMY AND PHYSIOLOGY   35

(a) PHOSPHOLIPID
- hydrophilic head
- hydrophobic tail

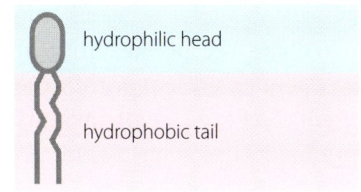

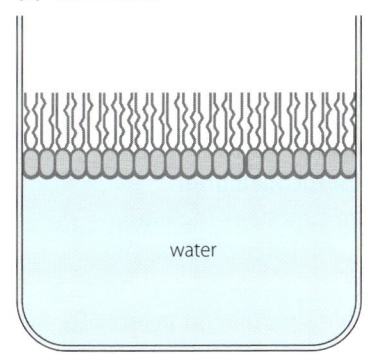

(b) MONOLAYER
water

(c) MICELLE

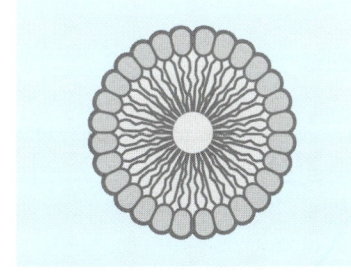

(d) BILAYER

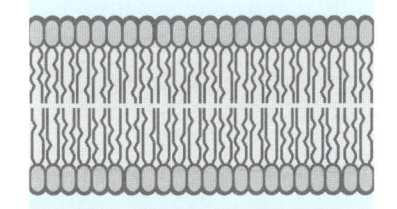

Figure 2.7 – The structure and arrangement of phospholipids.
(a) A single phospholipid molecule showing the hydrophilic head and hydrophobic tails; (b) a monolayer with the hydrophilic heads next to the water; (c) a micelle; and (d) a lipid bilayer.

[Diagram labels: carbohydrate, glycoprotein, peripheral protein, cholesterol, EXTRACELLULAR FLUID (watery environment), integral proteins, filaments of cytoskeleton, phospholipid non-polar tail, phospholipid polar head, CYTOPLASM (watery environment), phospholipid bilayer]

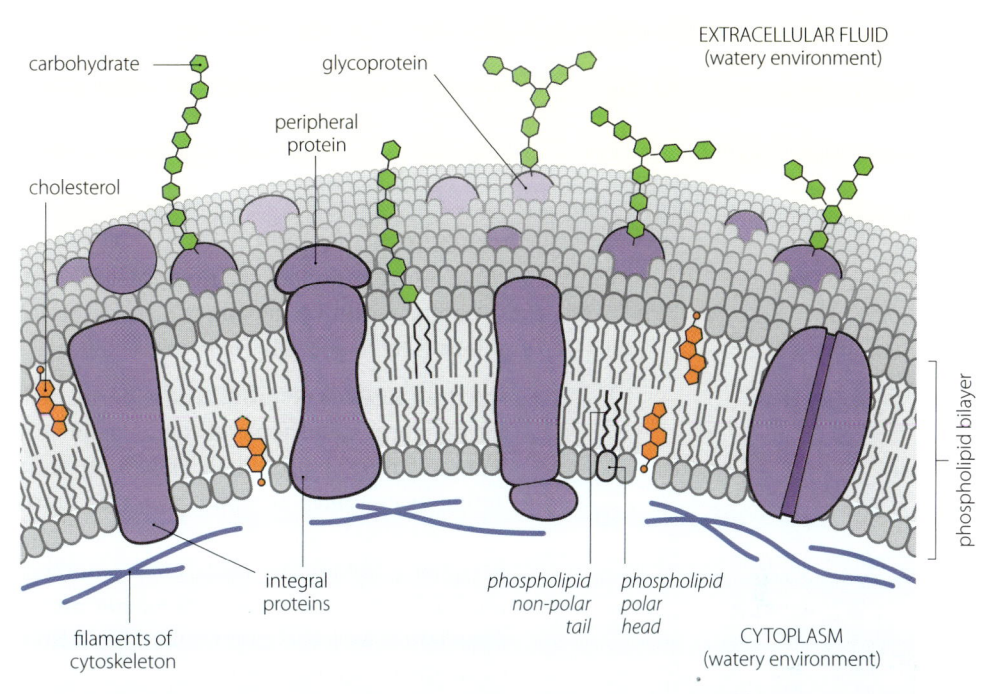

Figure 2.6 – The fluid mosaic model of membrane structure.
The plasma membrane separates and protects the inside of the cell from the extracellular environment. The phospholipid bilayer provides the cell's boundary: it is fluid at physiological temperatures. Proteins are embedded within the membrane.

The main part of the plasma membrane comprises phospholipid molecules arranged in two layers (a **lipid bilayer**). This arrangement occurs because the phospholipid molecules have two principal parts (see *Figure 2.7a*):

- hydrophobic ('water-hating') lipid tails
- a hydrophilic ('water-loving') head containing a phosphate molecule.

Two hydrophobic tails are connected to the hydrophilic head to create an **amphiphilic** membrane lipid, that is, a molecule that has both hydrophilic and hydrophobic properties. The phosphate head of the molecule readily interacts with water and the hydrophobic tails are repelled away from water (see *Figure 2.7b*). When placed in an aqueous environment, the membrane lipids spontaneously form a spherical shape known as a **micelle** (see *Figure 2.7c*) with the water-loving phosphate heads on the outside interacting with the water and the water-hating lipid tails clustering together on the inside, away from the water. The lipid tails are bulky compared with the phosphate head and so a micelle is not very stable, but the arrangement of lipid molecules becomes more stable when they are arranged in two layers, with the phosphate heads facing out towards the water and the lipid tails facing in towards each other. Thus, the plasma membrane is structured as a lipid bilayer (see *Figure 2.7d*).

The plasma membrane also contains other compounds, for example, cholesterol is usually present and interacts with the phospholipids to increase membrane packing and so reduce membrane fluidity; it also reduces the permeability of the membrane to water-soluble substances. Other compounds present within the plasma membrane may include glycolipids, glycoproteins and even small amounts of fat-soluble vitamins such as α-tocopherol (vitamin E, discussed in *Chapter 4*).

Membrane proteins

The lipid bilayer provides the fundamental structure of the plasma membrane, but the proteins within the membrane are essential because they provide a variety of functions (see *Table 2.2*). There are two broad groups of proteins:

- **Integral membrane proteins** are permanently embedded within the membrane and some of them completely span the membrane (**transmembrane proteins**). They have a range of functions including acting as enzymes, receptors and transporters for substances entering or leaving the cell, and adhesion to other cells.
- **Peripheral membrane proteins** are attached only to peripheral layers of the lipid bilayer or to integral membrane proteins and make a temporary association with the membrane. They also have a variety of roles, for example, in cell signalling.

Table 2.2 – General functions of membrane proteins

Function	Example
Adhesion	Binding cells together, e.g. β-catenin
Receptor	Hormone, e.g. thyroxine binds to the thyroxine receptor
Enzyme	ATPase catalyses the breakdown of ATP to ADP
Cell–cell recognition	Receptor for immune cells, e.g. T-cell receptor
Transport	Ion channels, e.g. the Na^+/K^+ pump regulates the transport of these ions across the plasma membrane
Cytoskeletal attachment	Actin filaments of the cytoskeleton attach to the plasma membrane

Receptors are protein molecules that bind a chemical and this induces a response by the cell. The chemicals are called signal molecules (**ligands**). Many types of receptors and many possible ligands exist. The range of ligands that can bind to a particular receptor is limited, providing control over the responses that cells can make to their chemical environment. **Agonists** are molecules (often synthetic drugs) that bind to receptors to mimic the effects that the natural ligand would produce when it is bound onto the receptor. Conversely, when an **antagonist** binds onto a receptor, it blocks the normal action of the receptor (see *Box 2.1*).

Transport across plasma membranes

The plasma membrane represents a *physical and chemical* barrier between the cytoplasm and the extracellular environment. It is a partial barrier (often described as 'selectively permeable' because it lets some molecules through but not others) that is able to control the passage of substances into or out of the cell. This control is based upon size, electrical charge, solubility, shape and chemical activity of the molecule to be transported. Transport can be a passive process, requiring no energy to be expended by the cell to allow transport of the molecule down a concentration gradient, or it can be an active process, which requires the cell to expend energy to *drive* a substance across the plasma membrane, often against a concentration gradient.

Passive transport

Passive transport occurs by diffusion, osmosis and facilitated (channel- or carrier-mediated) diffusion.

Diffusion. The movement of molecules by diffusion occurs in liquids and in gases. Imagine smoke in one part of a room. The particles of smoke will eventually, by

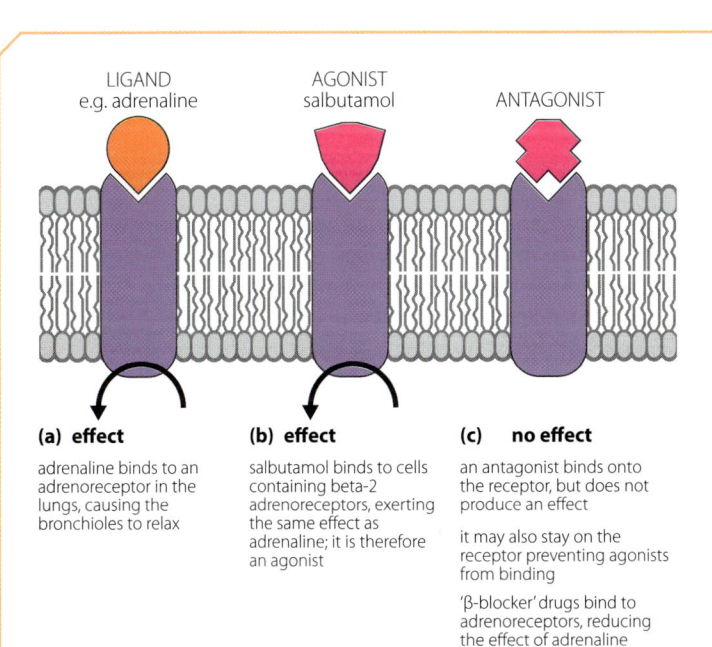

BOX 2.1

Agonists and antagonists

Agonists bind to receptors to mimic the effects of the natural signal molecule (ligand) and this ability is used by synthetic drugs such as the ones taken by Mary (Patient 2.1) and Graham (Patient 4.3). Antagonists are also able to bind on to a receptor where they block the normal action of the receptor; this ability can again be used in drug treatments.

(a) effect
adrenaline binds to an adrenoreceptor in the lungs, causing the bronchioles to relax

(b) effect
salbutamol binds to cells containing beta-2 adrenoreceptors, exerting the same effect as adrenaline; it is therefore an agonist

(c) no effect
an antagonist binds onto the receptor, but does not produce an effect

it may also stay on the receptor preventing agonists from binding

'β-blocker' drugs bind to adrenoreceptors, reducing the effect of adrenaline

Figure 2.8 – Action of agonists and antagonists.
The example shows adrenaline.

(a) Naturally occurring adrenaline binds onto a β_2-adrenoreceptor (pronounced beta-2) on the plasma membrane of a smooth muscle cell in the bronchiole and activates it – this causes the muscles to relax, allowing air to flow through the bronchiole more easily.

(b) Salbutamol (a synthetic drug) has a similar shape to adrenaline at the binding site and so is able to bind to the β_2-adrenoreceptor and activate it, causing the same relaxation in the smooth muscles of the bronchioles – it is therefore an agonist.

(c) Antagonists are also able to bind onto the receptor. They do not trigger the typical response (muscle relaxation in this case) but, by remaining bound onto the receptor, they can prevent the binding of a ligand such as adrenaline or an agonist such as salbutamol. For example, β-blockers are drugs that can bind to adrenoreceptors and inhibit the effects of adrenaline (discussed in *Chapter 5*).

the random movement of air particles, end up evenly distributed in all parts of the room. This occurs by diffusion, with the particles of smoke moving from a region where there is a high concentration to a region of lower concentration – this random movement of molecules continues even when equilibrium is reached. Diffusion occurs because molecules in gases and liquids are not bound to one another in a fixed manner and are in a constant state of random motion (known as **Brownian motion**) due to their inherent kinetic energy. This kinetic energy increases with increasing temperature and so diffusion will occur faster with increasing temperatures. Returning to the example of smoke, the random movement of smoke particles will not stop once equilibrium is reached, but overall the particles will remain equally distributed around the room. This can be described as a *dynamic* equilibrium.

Similarly, molecules of oxygen at a relatively high concentration, such as in the atmosphere, will diffuse down a concentration gradient to where there are fewer oxygen molecules, for example, in the lungs and blood, until a dynamic equilibrium is achieved (this is discussed further in *Chapter 10*). In this example,

---

BOX 2.2

Polar and non-polar molecules

In a non-polar molecule, the negatively charged electrons are equally shared between the atoms that make up the molecule, so that there is no local difference in charge between atoms. In a polar molecule, the negatively charged electrons are not shared equally by all the atoms and this produces small positive and small negative charges on different parts of the molecule. This has important consequences for the behaviour and interaction of the molecules because local charge differences can attract (positive attracts negative) nearby molecules and produce weak hydrogen bonds between the molecules.

For example, water (H_2O) is a polar molecule. The shared electrons are attracted more to the oxygen atom than the hydrogen atoms. Therefore, the slightly negatively charged oxygen atoms will be attracted to the slightly positively charged hydrogen atoms on other water molecules nearby (see *Figure 2.9*), or will tend to be attracted to and interact with other charged chemicals nearby. This interaction between molecules enables many substances to dissolve in water. Water has been termed 'the universal solvent' and is essential to all forms of life as we know it, which explains why scientists become very excited by the prospect of discovering water on other planets!

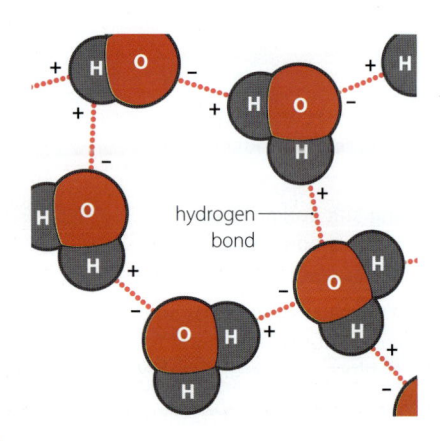

Figure 2.9 – Charge differences make water a polar molecule.
Weak hydrogen bonds are formed between the slightly negatively charged oxygen atoms and the slightly positively charged hydrogen atoms.

oxygen diffuses from the lungs (atmosphere), across the plasma membranes of cells within the lungs and blood vessels, and then across the plasma membrane of the **erythrocytes** (red blood cells) where it binds to the protein haemoglobin.

Substances able to diffuse across the plasma membrane generally include small non-polar molecules such as oxygen and carbon dioxide, and substances that can dissolve in lipids such as alcohol, lipid-soluble drugs, fatty acids and steroids. Specialized mechanisms exist to allow the selective transport of large polar substances such as amino acids across the plasma membrane, and these are described later on in this section. The use of the term polar and non-polar when describing molecules is outlined in *Box 2.2*.

Osmosis. Osmosis is the diffusion of water, a small polar molecule (see *Figure 2.9*), across a selectively permeable membrane such as the plasma membrane. The *relative concentration* of water inside and outside of the cell is vital for cell survival. The membrane also possesses special water channels called **aquaporins**, which regulate the rapid passage of water through the plasma membrane.

In order to understand osmosis, we have to remember that the diffusion of water is the movement of water from an area with a relatively high concentration of water towards a place where there is a relatively low concentration of water. When considering solutions and concentration, we refer to a substance (the solute) being dissolved in the water (the solvent). Within a fixed volume of solution, as the amount of a substance dissolved in the water increases, the relative concentration of water will decrease. All life needs water, but the water and the chemicals dissolved in the water need to be in the right amounts in a suitable volume and in the right place (inside and outside of the cell).

An imbalance in the distribution of water into or out of cells can have major implications for health. In cases of diarrhoeal disease (see Sumina, Patient 2.2), the excess loss of fluid from the body causes dehydration and this often causes a loss of electrolytes (such as sodium, potassium, chloride and bicarbonate ions) in plasma. If severe, electrolyte imbalance can disturb physiology in a variety of ways, including homeodynamic regulation of blood pressure and kidney function, or it can alter the function of the nervous system to cause confusion, and it can affect skeletal muscle tone. The correction of dehydration (see *Box 2.5*) requires not just the replenishment of the solvent (water), but also of solutes, especially sugar and sodium chloride (salt). Sugar and sodium chloride are readily absorbed across the cells of the gastrointestinal tract into plasma, creating an osmotic gradient that facilitates the absorption of water into the plasma; this leads to rehydration and is more effective than a drink of only water.

Imagine a container separated into two compartments by a selectively permeable membrane. In one compartment (A) is one volume of pure water. In the other compartment (B), there is the same volume of fluid, but dissolved in the water is a chemical, for example, glucose. Imagine also that the membrane contains tiny holes large enough to allow the small water molecules to pass through, but too small to allow the larger sugar molecules to cross the membrane (see *Figure 2.10*). Water molecules move randomly, allowing water to diffuse across the membrane from both compartments, but because compartment A has the highest concentration of water molecules, the net movement of water is greatest from compartment A into

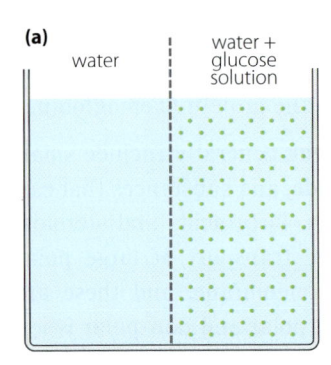

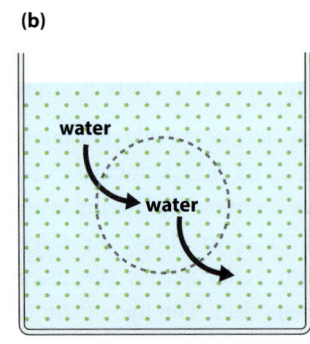

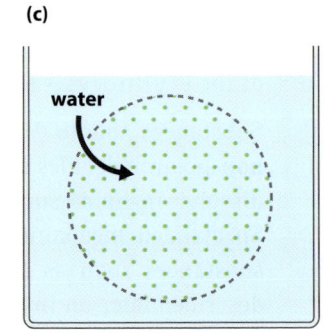

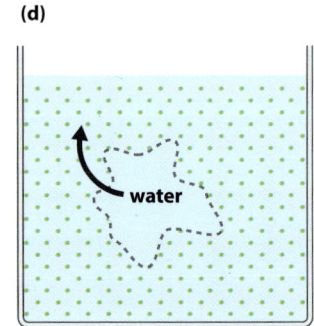

Figure 2.10 – Osmosis.
(a) Water is able to pass freely through a plasma membrane whereas larger solute molecules such as glucose cannot. (b) When the concentration of solute is the same on both sides of the plasma membrane, then water passes in and out of the plasma membrane at the same rate. (c) When the concentration of solute inside the cell is higher than the outside environment, then water flows into the cell in an attempt to equalize the water concentrations; the result is that the cell swells and may eventually rupture (cell lysis). (d) When the concentration of solute inside the cell is lower than the outside environment, then water flows out of the cell, causing the cell to shrink in volume.

compartment B; this movement continues, until a dynamic equilibrium of water in each compartment is reached. Remember, the movement of water molecules never stops, but equilibrium is maintained when the net movement in each direction is the same. Some of the consequences of an imbalance in water volume and concentration

---

BOX 2.3

The extreme effects of too much water on a patient

This true case study dramatically illustrates the effects of the movement of water molecules on cells. The case relates to an elderly diabetic patient admitted to hospital with pneumonia, congestive heart failure, respiratory failure and severe **hypernatraemia** (high concentration of sodium in the patient's plasma). As a consequence of the patient's existing conditions, the doctor treating him did not want to give him any more sodium or any other solutions that contained dextrose because the patient was diabetic, and so neither a standard saline intravenous infusion nor dextrose infusion could be used to keep the patient hydrated. Instead, sterile water was infused into the patient, partly to correct dehydration and also to reduce the hypernatraemia by diluting the sodium in the patient's plasma. Unfortunately, the patient developed acute renal failure and died.

The patient died because the medical intervention (in this case an infusion) had a harmful impact upon the patient's erythrocytes (red blood cells). The infusion of sterile water reduced the sodium concentration in the plasma by increasing the volume of water, but this meant that there was a lower concentration of water molecules and a higher concentration of sodium molecules inside the red blood cells compared with the plasma. So water moved, by osmosis, from the plasma into the erythrocytes down the concentration gradient (from a high concentration of water to a low concentration), eventually causing the erythrocytes to swell and then burst.

The destruction of erythrocytes (**haemolysis**) led to fragments of erythrocytes collecting in the small blood vessels of many organs, causing an obstruction to blood flow. This occurred in the small blood vessels of the kidney, causing kidney damage, and reduced the ability of the kidneys to make urine. In this case, homeodynamic processes were disturbed sufficiently to cause death.

This case study is taken from the United States Food and Drug Administration, Health and Human Services Patient Safety News.

of dissolved solutes are provided in *Box 2.3*, and *Chapter 8* will explore further the effects of gradual changes in water and solute concentration in body fluids and the homeodynamic adjustment to these changes.

Channel-mediated and carrier-mediated diffusion

Not all substances are able to diffuse through the plasma membrane without assistance:

- some are too large to pass through the pores
- others are polar molecules, which cannot cross the non-polar regions of the lipid bilayer.

In channel-mediated and carrier-mediated diffusion (see *Figure 2.11*), the movement of a larger or a polar substance still occurs by diffusion, that is, passively down the concentration gradient until dynamic equilibrium is reached, but the route it takes through the membrane involves specific proteins.

Channel-mediated diffusion involves **channel proteins** located within the plasma membrane. These proteins allow small polar molecules such as ions to cross the plasma membrane into or out of the cell. There may also be interaction between the channel proteins and the substance to be transported at specific binding sites on the channel protein. This interaction can open or close the channel and so control the transport of a particular substance from one side of the plasma membrane to the other.

Carrier-mediated diffusion involves the binding of the substance to be transported onto a **carrier protein**, such that the substance (typically larger polar molecules and small organic molecules such as glucose and amino acids) is essentially 'carried' in or out of the cell. The interaction of the carrier protein and substance to be transported is highly specific and a variety of different 'ports' of entry/exit can be found:

- a uniport transports one substance
- a symport transports two different substances in the same direction
- an antiport transports two different substances in opposite directions.

In each case, the movement of a substance across the plasma membrane is still a passive process down a concentration gradient (see *Figure 2.11*), but unlike simple diffusion, the rate of movement is regulated.

Active transport

There are times when a cell needs to acquire or excrete a substance, but cannot rely on diffusion because there is no favourable concentration gradient in the required direction. Moving a substance against a concentration gradient and accumulating a substance inside or outside of the cell requires the use of metabolic energy (discussed in *Chapter 7*). The substance to be transported is often a small polar molecule or an ion, but can also be a large polar molecule. Transport is via uniport, symport or antiport systems. Because these active transport systems often transport ions, they are sometimes called *solute pumps*.

Energy is provided in the form of adenosine triphosphate (ATP). The carrier protein has ATPase enzyme activity, which catalyses the conversion of ATP to ADP (adenosine diphosphate) and inorganic phosphate (P_i). The energy released from ATP hydrolysis alters the shape (known as the **conformation**) of the carrier protein, such that the substance bound to the carrier protein is moved across the plasma membrane.

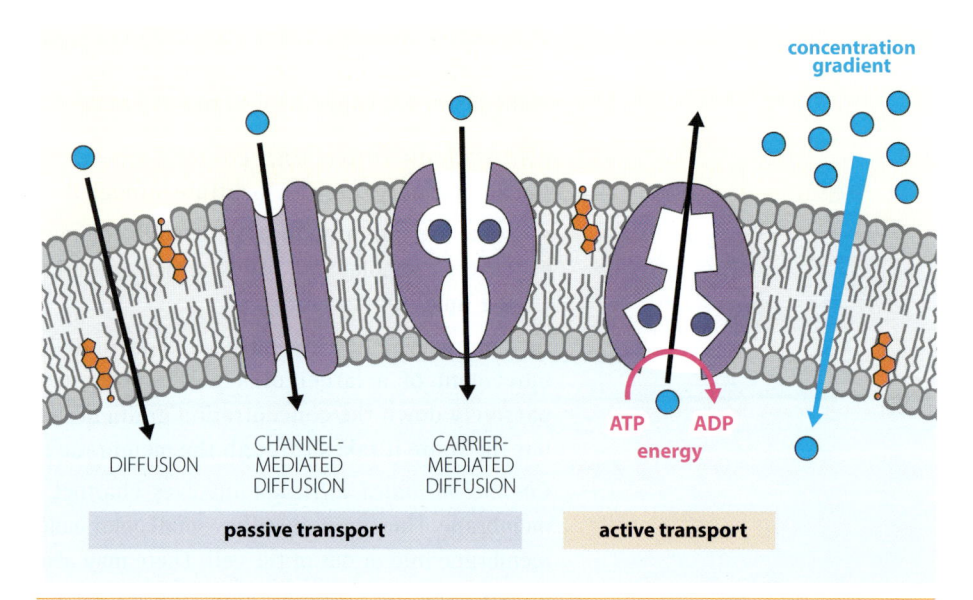

Figure 2.11 – Active and passive transport mechanisms across the plasma membrane.
Passive transport occurs across the plasma membrane down concentration gradients. Diffusion involves small non-polar and lipid-soluble molecules. Channel-mediated diffusion involves small polar molecules. Carrier-mediated diffusion involves larger, polar molecules and small organic molecules. Active transport occurs across the plasma membrane against concentration gradients. This process requires energy and is driven by energy-coupled transport proteins (the energy is derived from ATP hydrolysis).

An important example of an active transport system is the **sodium–potassium pump**. Most animal cells accumulate positively charged potassium ions (K^+) inside the cell, while maintaining low levels of sodium ions (Na^+). In order to achieve this, the cell must expel Na^+ from the cell and 'pump' K^+ into the cell, against the concentration gradient. The Na^+–K^+ pump is present on the plasma membrane of virtually all of our cells and requires the energy harnessed by the Na^+–K^+ ATPase.

The Na^+–K^+ pump involves the following steps:

- *three* intracellular Na^+ ions bind to the carrier protein (an ATPase)
- the binding of the Na^+ ions promotes an interaction between ATPase and ATP, and ATP is converted to ADP + P_i, which causes a conformational change in the ATPase
- this conformational change brings the *three* Na^+ ions to the outer surface of the plasma membrane, where they are released outside of the cell
- following the release of Na^+ ions, the carrier protein binds *two* extracellular K^+ ions and brings these across the plasma membrane into the cell as the carrier protein returns to its original conformation.

Remember, both sodium and potassium are positively charged ions, but *three* positive ions (from sodium) are lost from the intracellular fluid and *two* positive ions are gained (from potassium). Thus, the inside of the cell becomes increasingly electronegative. The maintenance of the correct amount of sodium and potassium and other electrolytes within body fluids, together with transport of these across plasma membranes, is vital for cellular and physiological processes (further examples will be discussed later: the active transport of sodium and potassium in the generation of nerve impulses will be discussed in *Chapter 4*, and the transport of water and electrolytes within the kidney to make urine is discussed in *Chapter 8*).

Vesicular transport

Large substances such as macromolecules are actively transported across the plasma membrane within a vesicle, which is a small membrane-bound structure that encloses the molecule to be transported. Vesicles are constantly forming from the plasma membrane and Golgi apparatus. Vesicular transport is called **ex**ocytosis for transport **ex**iting out of the cell and **en**docytosis for **en**try of substances into the cell (see *Figure 2.12*). A specific example of exocytosis and its clinical relevance is highlighted in *Chapter 4* and illustrated in *Figure 4.9*.

A type of endocytosis called phagocytosis transports large pieces of material such as bacterial cells into specialized immune cells called neutrophils and macrophages (this is discussed in *Chapter 11*); within these immune cells, the endocytic vesicle is known as a **phagosome** and it carries out the intracellular digestion of potential **pathogens**.

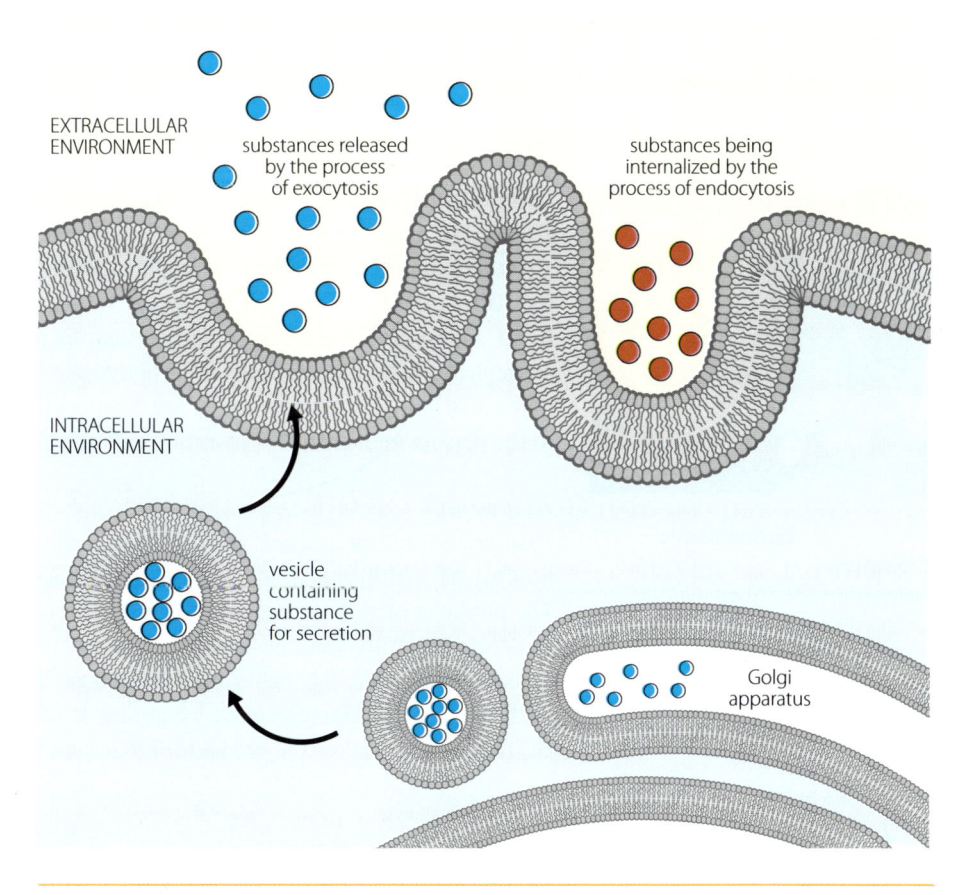

Figure 2.12 – Vesicular transport: endocytosis and exocytosis.
This is a complex transport process involving the plasma membrane, cytoskeletal filaments and the interaction of membrane proteins coupled to ATP hydrolysis; it requires metabolic energy.

Cell organelles

Nucleus

In somatic (body) cells of a human, the **nucleus** (see *Figure 2.13*) contains the complete genome, comprising the genomic DNA packaged into 46 chromosomes. In gametes (sperm and ovum), the nucleus contains only 23 chromosomes. The transcription of DNA to produce messenger RNA (mRNA) occurs in the nucleus – this is the first stage in the production of proteins (described in *Chapter 3*). The nuclear membrane (another lipid bilayer) selectively limits substances transported through it; its **nuclear pores** are sufficiently large to allow mRNA to pass through the nuclear membrane and out of the nucleus after synthesis.

Endoplasmic reticulum

The **rough endoplasmic reticulum (RER)** is a membranous mesh-like network of interconnected tubules studded with ribosomes on its outer surface (see *Figure 2.14*). Ribosomes are responsible for the synthesis of proteins in a process called translation (discussed further in *Chapter 3*) and may be found free in the cytoplasm or bound to the RER. Secreted proteins are synthesized by ribosomes on the RER and so the RER is particularly abundant in secretory cells.

The **smooth endoplasmic reticulum (SER)** has no ribosomes bound to it and so it does not make proteins. Instead, the SER synthesizes lipids, phospholipids and steroids, and also carries out drug detoxification. In muscle cells, the SER regulates calcium ion concentration.

Golgi apparatus

The **Golgi apparatus** is a series of flattened membrane-bound sacs (known as cisternae) and vesicles closely associated with the RER (see *Figure 2.15*). It acts as the sorting centre of the cell, accepting the contents of vesicles from the RER. The Golgi apparatus also makes modifications to proteins received from the RER; for example, to form a glycoprotein, carbohydrate is added to the protein (this is called **glycosylation**). The glycoproteins are then enclosed within vesicles and transported to the plasma membrane for insertion into the membrane or secretion by exocytosis.

Lysosomes

Lysosomes are specialized vesicular organelles containing a variety of enzymes (known as hydrolases) that catalyse the intracellular digestion of macromolecules. The products of this intracellular digestion can then be recycled for use by the cell. Enzymes generally work best within a narrow pH range, and the environment within a lysosome is acidic (i.e. below pH 7.0) because the lysosomal hydrolases work best in acidic conditions. The lysosomal membrane is adapted to retain the hydrolases within the lysosome but allow the products of digestion to leave the lysosome.

Mitochondria

Synthesis, repair, digestion, transport, cell division and other forms of 'cell work' require energy to be readily available. Energy is obtained by the metabolism of digested food. Glucose from food is a vital source of energy and this is catabolized (broken down) within the cytoplasm to pyruvate. Mitochondria continue the catabolism to produce carbon dioxide and water and release energy that is trapped

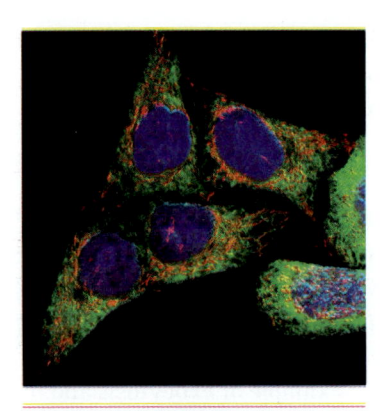

Figure 2.13 – **Nucleus.**
Composite confocal micrograph of human melanoma cells showing DNA of the nucleus (blue), mitochondria (red) and endoplasmic reticulum (green). Reproduced under a CC BY 4.0 International licence. Attribution: Paul J. Smith & Rachel Errington, Wellcome Images.

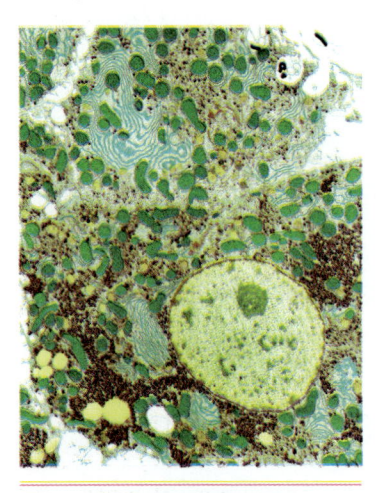

Figure 2.14 – **Endoplasmic reticulum.**
Coloured TEM of two liver cells. Organelles within the cells include: the nucleus (large yellow ovoid, lower right), rough endoplasmic reticulum (fuzzy blue lines at bottom centre), smooth endoplasmic reticulum (blue lines at left of nucleus), Golgi apparatus (blue lines at upper left), mitochondria (green), fat droplets (pale yellow), glycogen (brown) and lysosomes (yellow). The plasma membranes are pale green. Science Photo Library.

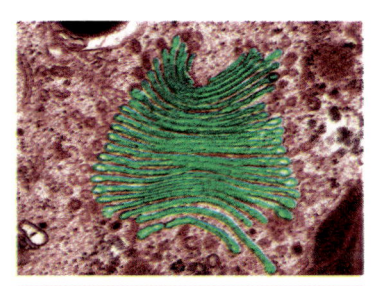

SECTION 2.2 | WHAT YOU NEED TO KNOW – ESSENTIAL ANATOMY AND PHYSIOLOGY 45

Figure 2.15 – Golgi apparatus.
Coloured TEM of a Golgi apparatus (green). Its primary function is post-translational processing of proteins to modify, store and transport proteins and lipids made elsewhere in the cell. The organelle's structure consists of a stack of flattened, membranous, disc-like structures called cisternae; these contain enzymes that help to modify proteins passing through the organelle. Science Photo Library.

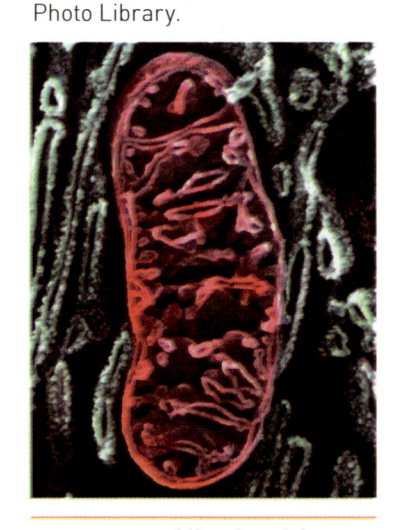

Figure 2.16 – Mitochondrion.
Coloured high resolution SEM of a single mitochondrion in the cytoplasm of an intestinal epithelial cell. The mitochondrion (pink, centre) has two membranes: an outer surrounding membrane and an inner membrane which forms folds called cristae. It is on the cristae that chemical reactions occur. Mitochondria are sites of cell respiration: sugars and fats are oxidized to produce energy which is then stored. Science Photo Library.

within ATP. However, the process is not 100% efficient and so some energy is released as heat, which explains why our bodies are at a temperature that is usually higher than ambient. The heat released contributes to the maintenance of the narrow temperature range required for the optimal working of the body.

The internal structure of a mitochondrion (see *Figure 2.16*) comprises highly folded internal membranes called **cristae**, which provide the mitochondria with a large surface area. The cristae are the site of energy-producing reactions, and the large surface area helps to maximize efficiency of this energy production. Details of mitochondrial function and their role in providing energy derived from food are discussed further in *Chapter 7*.

Other cell structures

Cytoskeleton

The cytoplasm contains an intricate network of microfilament proteins that form the cytoskeleton. There are three main types (see *Figure 2.17*):

- microfilaments
- microtubules
- intermediate filaments.

The filamentous proteins of the cytoskeleton provide strength and give shape to cells. This is particularly important, for example, in cells of the skin and heart muscle, which have to withstand mechanical stresses. Cytoskeletal proteins attach to the plasma membrane, providing an internal framework for the cell contents. For example, in red blood cells (erythrocytes), cytoskeletal proteins form a mesh-like network, which helps to maintain the large surface area required for gas exchange and also cell flexibility for travel through the narrow capillaries of the blood vessels. Microtubules are also key components of flagella and cilia.

Cilia

Cilia are protrusions of microtubules from the surface of the cell (see *Figure 2.18*). They are unique structures found only on certain types of body cells, for example, the cells lining the respiratory tract. Cilia have the ability to move, and it is the beating movement of the cilia that helps to trap foreign material, including bacteria, in mucus and cause it to be removed from the lungs. This combined action of the cilia and mucus is called the muco-ciliary escalator and it helps to protect the lungs from infection by keeping the respiratory membrane deep within the lungs unobstructed for gas exchange. Excess bronchial secretions that accumulate higher up the respiratory tract can then be removed by coughing.

Centrosome

The **centrosome** contains **centrioles,** which are a complex of proteins attached to cytoskeletal microtubules usually found close to the nucleus. The centrosome functions as an organizing centre for microtubular proteins and for organizing chromosomes in preparation for cell division (see *Figure 2.19*).

Ribosomes

Ribosomes comprise a complex of various ribosomal RNA (rRNA) molecules and proteins. Ribosomes are responsible for catalysing the production of proteins from

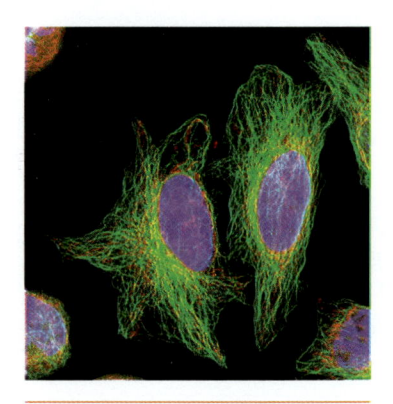

Figure 2.17 – Cytoskeleton.
Confocal light micrograph of two 'HeLa' cancer cells. The cell nuclei, which contain the cells' genetic information, are purple. Microtubules, protein filaments that make up the cytoskeleton, are green. The cytoskeleton maintains the cells' shape, allows some cellular mobility and is involved in intracellular transport. HeLa cells are immortal and so thrive in the laboratory. They are widely used in biological and medical research. Science Photo Library.

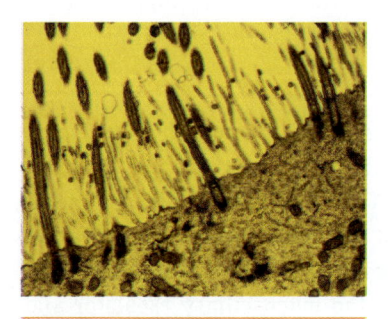

Figure 2.18 – Cilia.
Transmission electron micrograph, tinted yellow, of a section through a cell from the human trachea, showing influenza viruses (tiny black dots) filtering through the cilia which line the membrane surface. Science Photo Library.

amino acids using mRNA molecules as the template (discussed in *Chapter 3*); the mRNA molecules carry genetic information from the nucleus to the ribosome. In this way, information from the genomic DNA in the nucleus is used to direct protein synthesis. Many ribosomes are found free within the cytoplasm, but others are associated with the RER (ribosomes can be seen in *Figure 2.14* as dark blue dots).

2.2.3 Organization of cells in the body

The human body contains trillions of cells, which function in complementary ways, each contributing to homeodynamic processes within the following hierarchical system illustrated by *Figure 2.20*.

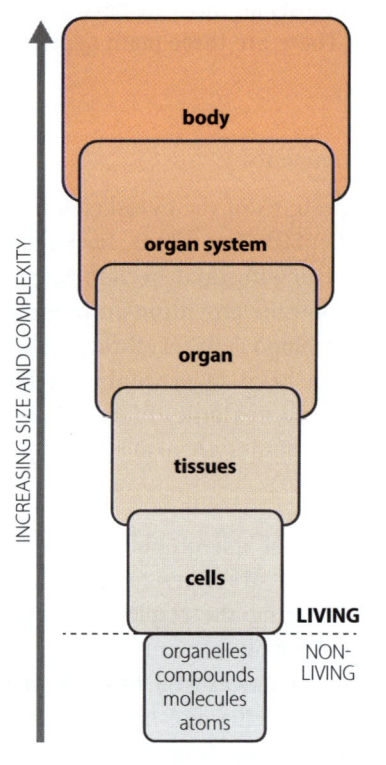

Figure 2.20 – Hierarchical organization of the body.
Cells are formed from chemical structures and these cells provide the fundamental living structure upon which all body structures are based.

There are approximately 200 types of cell in the human body. A group of similar cells that cooperate to perform a specific function can be described as a **tissue**. Physical groups of tissues, cooperating within the body to perform a specialized function that contributes to homeodynamic processes, are called organs. Groups of organs also cooperate to form the organ systems that together make up the human body (see *Table 2.3*).

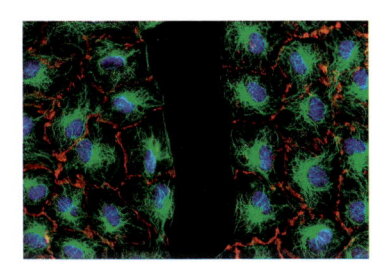

Figure 2.19 – Centrosome.
Immunofluorescence micrograph of a fibroblast monolayer that has been wounded. The cell nuclei, which contain the cells' genetic information, are blue. Microtubules, protein filaments that make up part of the cytoskeleton, are green. The cytoskeleton maintains the cells' shape, allows some cellular mobility and is involved in intracellular transport. The microtubule organizing centres (centrosomes) have orientated towards the wound. Cell–cell contacts are red. These allow communication between the cells and regulate cell growth. Science Photo Library.

Table 2.3 – Organ systems of the body

Organ system	General function
Skin/integumentary	Protection against mechanical stress, infection and dehydration
Skeletal	Support, resilience and locomotion
Muscular	Movement
Circulatory	Transport of nutrients and waste
Nervous	Communication and integration of homeodynamic processes via nerves
Endocrine	Communication and integration of homeodynamic processes via hormones
Excretory	Removal of waste
Digestive	Physical and chemical processing of food into nutrients
Reproductive	Specialized system for the generation of new organisms
Immune	Protection against infection and the repair of damaged tissue

Cell type is defined by morphology (what the cells look like) and also by function. All somatic cells contain the same genetic material and so cell type will be determined by which genes are expressed by that cell, leading to the specialized functions of different cell types. For example, liver cells usually contain many more mitochondria than skin cells, because more energy is required for the biosynthetic activity the liver is associated with, whereas skin cells accumulate much larger amounts of the insoluble protein keratin than liver cells. Specialized cells are also said to be differentiated.

Stem cells, for example those found in reproductive organs, in the bone marrow or within regenerative tissue such as the gastrointestinal tract or skin, remain undifferentiated. This means that they have not become specialized but can divide and produce new cells, which may later become differentiated.

Unlike somatic cells, which divide in a very controlled manner as and when required, cancer cells can divide repeatedly and without control, and so cancer has been described as a 'disease of the cell cycle'. Cancer cells often form an irregular accumulating mass and, because of abnormal gene expression, may also possess an altered function and morphology. A defining feature of cancer is the abnormal ability of the cells to invade other tissues, to spread to other parts of the body and to continue to divide (see Sheila, Patient 2.3). New 'biological therapies' are being used to treat cancer and chronic inflammatory disease (see *Box 2.4*).

BOX 2.4

'Biological therapies' to treat cancer

New 'biological therapies' are being used to treat chronic inflammatory diseases and cancer such as breast cancer.

Molecules that bind to specific receptors and stimulate cells to divide are termed **mitogens**. For example, the epidermal growth factor receptor (EGFR) is normally expressed on the surface of healthy epithelial tissue where it increases cell proliferation when activated by a variety of ligands. Over-expression of a key receptor may allow more of the mitogen to bind and stimulate cell division.

Over-expression of HER2 (a type of EGFR) and over-activity of this receptor occurs in the development of cancer at certain body sites, including the breast.

Antibodies have been developed to specifically block the binding of ligands to HER2 (*Figure 2.21*). Trastuzumab (trade name Herceptin) is a *monoclonal antibody* (an antibody synthesized by a single clone of antibody-producing cells) developed to bind to HER2 and is currently the most commonly used biological therapy for the treatment of breast cancer. Herceptin prevents the normal ligand, such as epidermal growth factor, binding to HER2 and acting as a mitogen. This reduces the rate of cell division in cells expressing the HER2 receptor. Where cells, such as the cancer cells in Sheila's breast (Patient 2.3), over-express the HER2 receptor, the growth of the cancer is slowed by Herceptin therapy and this should improve Sheila's prognosis.

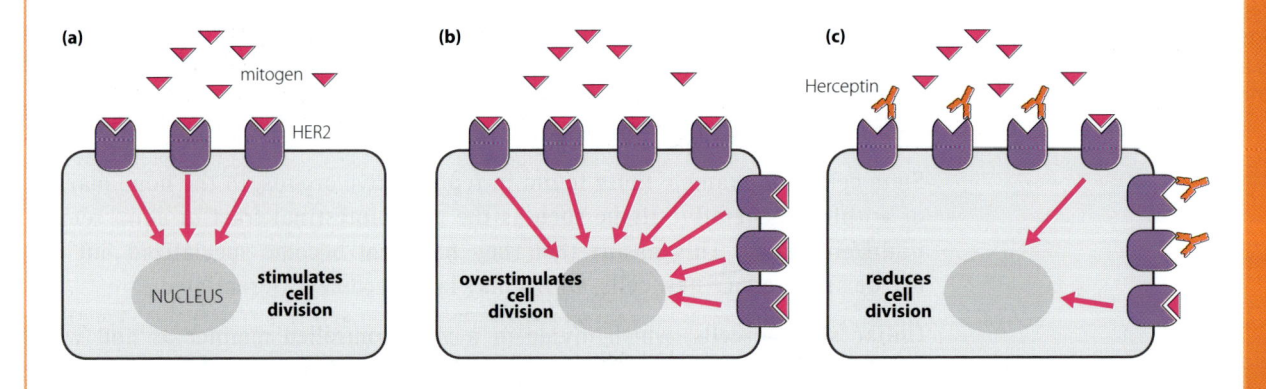

Figure 2.21 – The role of Herceptin in the treatment of breast cancer.
(a) Normal breast cell expressing HER2 receptors. (b) Too many HER2 receptors stimulate increased cell proliferation, leading to growth of a tumour. (c) A monoclonal antibody (Herceptin) binds to the HER2 receptor, blocking its action, and so reduces proliferation of cells.

Tissues

There are four main tissue types: epithelial, connective, muscle and nervous (*Figure 2.22*).

Epithelial tissue

Epithelial tissue provides a cover to the body surfaces and provides a lining to internal cavities, for example, the cells of the skin (discussed in *Chapter 12*)

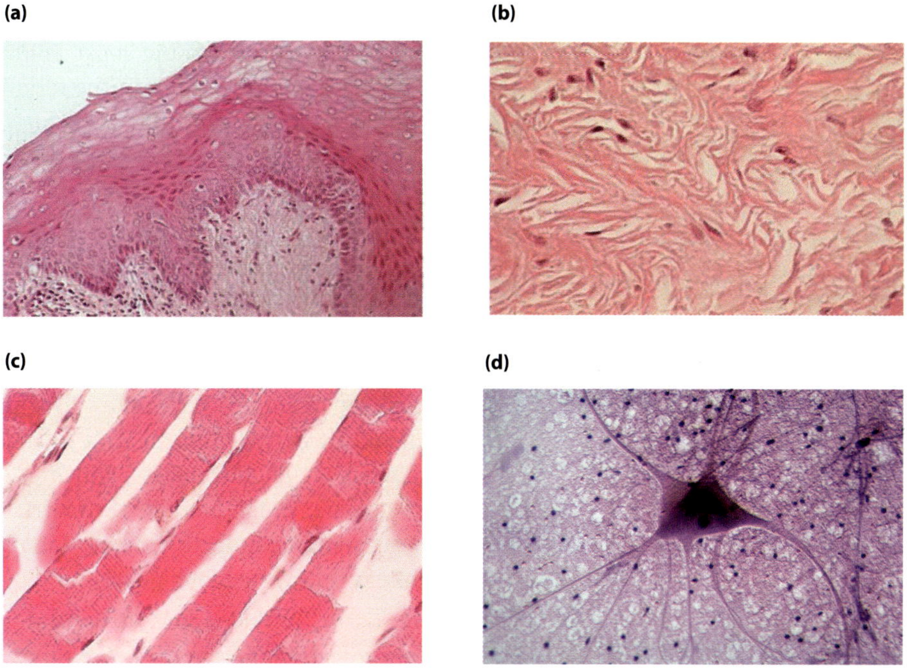

Figure 2.22 – Micrographs of the four main tissue types.
(a) Epithelial: note the multiple layers, which are important because this tissue provides a persistent covering to underlying organs. (b) Connective: note the irregular appearance of this dense tissue helping to provide resilience against mechanical stress. (c) Muscle: the organization of protein fibres within this striped skeletal muscle can shorten to provide muscular contraction. (d) Nervous: this light micrograph of a spinal cord motor neurone shows the cell body, dendrites and axon. (a) to (c) reproduced from www.pathguy.com/histo; (d) Science Photo Library.

or the cells lining the gastrointestinal tract (discussed in *Chapter 7*). There are different classes of epithelial cells:

- **Simple epithelia** – comprise a thin single layer of cells suitable for efficient absorption or secretion of substances.
- **Stratified epithelia** – contain multiple layers of epithelial cells, which form an abrasion-resistant covering in areas at risk of mechanical stress such as the skin.
- **Cuboidal epithelia** – found in areas where there is a need for secretion or absorption such as sweat glands, endocrine glands and the tubules in the kidneys.
- **Columnar epithelia** – usually possess additional adaptations, for example, intestinal cells may possess microvilli, which increase the surface area for absorption of nutrients, and some may be adapted for the production of mucus in the gastrointestinal or respiratory tract. In addition, columnar epithelial cells within the ventricles of the brain, uterus, Fallopian tubes and the respiratory tract possess cilia (ciliated columnar epithelial cells).

Connective tissue

Connective tissue represents the most abundant tissue found throughout the body. All connective tissues contain the following:

- A gel-like extracellular matrix called **ground substance**; this is a mixture of interstitial fluid, proteins for cell adhesion and glycoproteins (proteins with carbohydrate attached).
- Fibrous proteins – collagen fibres, elastic fibres (bundles of **elastin** protein) and/or reticular fibres (bundles of type III collagen); these provide a cross-linking mesh for additional structure and support.
- Connective tissue cells – these are widely distributed throughout the body where they secrete and maintain the extracellular matrix. **Fibroblasts** are found mainly in connective tissue where they secrete collagen and other elements of the extracellular matrix of connective tissue. Closely related to fibroblasts are **chondroblasts**, which produce the matrix of cartilage, and **osteoblasts**, which produce the matrix in bone. Other types of cell are also found within connective tissue, such as **adipocytes** (which store fat) and **leukocytes** (white blood cells).

Connective tissue provides the structural support for organs of the body, mechanical protection, an energy store in the form of fat within adipose tissue, and a fluid medium (blood) for the transport of substances. There are several types of connective tissue, which can be grouped into two main types.

True connective tissue

True connective tissue includes **areolar** tissue, which provides support and cushioning to surrounding organs. Within the areolar tissue, collagen, and elastic and reticular fibres are arranged loosely with a large amount of space-filling ground substance, which provides a medium for interstitial fluid, nutrients, waste and immune cells. Other true connective tissues include the following:

- **Adipose** – similar to areolar tissue, but the cells are specialized in accumulating fat and in providing a highly effective energy reserve. It is a very vascular tissue containing many small blood vessels, and provides thermal insulation and physical support for organs.
- **Reticular** – this contains loose reticular fibres only; these form an irregular mesh-like network of fibres and so it is more delicate than the other types. It contains many fibroblasts and provides a space for the cells within lymph nodes, spleen and bone marrow.
- **Dense** – contains large amounts of highly organized collagen fibres with rows of fibroblast cells. This provides a dense and very strong and elastic structure that is substantially less elastic than other connective tissues. It contains less extracellular matrix material and forms tendons and ligaments and, when the collagen fibres are organized into an irregular sheet such as in the skin and the fibrous covering of some organs and joints, it helps to provide significant resistance to tension. Dense connective tissue is often called fibrous connective tissue.

Specialized connective tissue

- **Cartilage** – this contains elastin and collagen fibres and chondroitin sulphate. The cells that make up cartilage tissue are called chondrocytes and are the mature cells of the cartilage found in small cavities called

cartilage lacunae. It is their function to produce and maintain the surrounding matrix. There are three types of cartilage:
  - Hyaline – this is extremely strong but also elastic and is found particularly at the end of long bones where it provides resilient cushioning for weight bearing.
  - Fibrocartilage – this is able to withstand large amounts of pressure and is found between vertebral discs.
  - Elastic – this is flexible and elastic; it is used to maintain the shape of flexible organs and is found in the epiglottis, larynx, Eustachian tube and pinna of the ear.
- **Bone** – this is exceptionally strong and has a complex structure with inorganic salts such as calcium deposited in the matrix. It has a good blood supply and contains osteocytes, which are responsible for regulating the composition of the matrix. The composition and structure of bone is described further in *Chapter 13*.
- **Blood** – the matrix of blood is plasma; the cells present within plasma are predominantly erythrocytes, leukocytes and thrombocytes (see *Figure 9.21*). This tissue does not provide any structural support, but has essential roles in transport, immunity and blood clotting (haemostasis).

Muscle tissue

Muscle is formed from cells that contain large amounts of the contractile proteins actin and myosin, and is responsible for movement of the skeleton and action of some of the internal organs, such as movement of the bowel for the digestion of food (see *Chapter 7*), contraction of muscles surrounding the bladder in the process of micturition (see *Chapter 8*) and the contraction of blood vessels to regulate blood pressure (see *Chapter 9*). Muscles require an extensive blood supply to provide a readily available source of energy and oxygen. There are three types of muscle:

- **Skeletal muscle** – under voluntary (somatic) control.
- **Cardiac muscle** – possesses an intrinsic ability to generate electrical impulses that lead to contraction of the heart muscle; this property is unique to the heart. It is a type of involuntary muscle stimulated by the autonomic nervous system that is unique to the heart. Within the cardiac muscle are cells that possess an intrinsic ability to generate electrical impulses that lead to contraction of the heart muscle.
- **Smooth muscle** – involuntary muscle also under the control of the autonomic nervous system.

Nervous tissue

Nervous tissue comprises two main types of cell:

- **Neurones** are conducting cells that transmit nerve impulses to and from the organs and nervous system. Neurones stimulate or inhibit organ function and are crucial in coordinating and integrating organ function, facilitating rapid responses to environmental stimuli and adjusting homeodynamic states.
- **Neuroglia** are specialized non-conducting cells within the nervous system that regulate and support neurones, the brain and the spinal cord (see *Chapter 4*).

The study of tissues is called **histology**, and commonly involves the microscopic examination of cells after suitable preparation, usually with a preservative and stains to highlight and reveal structural and chemical features of cells. **Histopathology** represents the study of diseased tissue. It is an important activity that contributes to accurate diagnosis and frequently guides clinical decisions. For example, a sample of tissue (a **biopsy**) can be examined by a pathologist to look for diagnostic information such as the presence or absence of cancer cells. Pathology results can also be used to direct treatment options; for example, a surgeon can decide how best to remove cancer cells and how much tissue surrounding the tumour should be removed.

2.3 Clinical application

Many factors influence the behaviour of cells, and much of healthcare practice is aimed at ensuring that homeodynamic processes (see discussion in *Chapter 1*) are optimized for achieving health, ultimately through the function of body cells. Correcting problems that lead to homeodynamic perturbation and the management or treatment of disease often involve altering the responses of cells and organs of the body.

The activity of cells and physiological activities of the body are affected by a diverse array of signal molecules such as hormones and neurotransmitters (discussed in *Chapter 5*). Understanding how these chemicals work at the cellular level to affect homeodynamic states is important to the practice of healthcare so that optimal health is achieved or maintained. The cases described in this chapter cover a range of different clinical problems, each reflecting a disturbance in cellular homeodynamic status.

- Mary (Patient 2.1) has asthma, a condition managed, but not cured, by the administration of drugs that bind to the cells of Mary's bronchioles. These drugs improve her breathing, ensuring that the transfer of the respiratory gases oxygen and carbon dioxide to and from her lungs is not compromised.
- Sumina (Patient 2.2) has an infection that has resulted in an overall loss of fluid from her body and an imbalance of fluid between her cells and the fluid circulating as plasma. Correction of this imbalance is vital to maintain the homeodynamic status of her organ systems. As a 2-year-old child, Sumina can only tolerate small fluctuations of fluid imbalance in her body, and fairly rapid intervention is likely to be required.
- Sheila (Patient 2.3) has breast cancer, with uncontrolled proliferation of cancer cells. In order to understand and manage cancer, we need to know how cells work, how they interact with each other and how they are influenced by genetics and the environment.

Patient 2.1 — Mary — 29 | 53 | 311 | 330

- 57-year-old woman
- Chronic asthmatic on beclometasone dipropionate, salmeterol and salbutamol

The salbutamol Mary uses to relieve the feeling of being short of breath is a β_2-adrenoreceptor agonist (see *Box 2.1*). The smooth muscle cells surrounding the bronchioles within the lungs possess receptors for adrenaline, and when adrenaline is released from the adrenal glands into the blood, it binds to integral proteins called adrenoreceptors (actually a subtype called β_2) present on the plasma membrane of cells that express the receptor. In the bronchioles, binding of adrenaline to the β_2-adrenoreceptor causes the bronchiolar smooth muscles to relax and so the bronchioles become less constricted and breathing becomes easier. Salbutamol is described as an adrenoreceptor agonist because it also binds to the β_2-adrenoreceptor and so exerts an effect similar to adrenaline (see *Figure 2.8*). Salbutamol is described as a reliever for symptoms of asthma. Mary always keeps it handy wherever she goes in case of unexpected bouts of breathlessness, sometimes triggered by allergies, exercise or even changes in the weather.

Patient 2.2 — Sumina — 30 | 53

- 2-year-old girl
- High temperature, D&V and tachycardia
- Given ORS to replace lost salts and sugar

The doctor explains to Sumina's mother that the rapid loss of body fluid from the gastrointestinal tract is known to disturb the concentration of important electrolytes such as sodium and potassium in the blood and that this can affect the function of nerve cells and the regulation of body systems. Caution must be exercised when encouraging Sumina to drink, because if Sumina takes large gulps of fluid in an attempt to ease her thirst, this can stimulate further diarrhoea and vomiting, increasing the loss of sodium and potassium.

After examination and investigation to ascertain the cause of the diarrhoea and vomiting, the doctor offered Sumina an oral hydration solution called Oral Rehydration Salts (ORS) (see *Box 2.5*). This contains sufficient salts and sugar to correct the electrolyte imbalance and rehydrate Sumina. This is offered to Sumina in the form of frequent small sips to avoid stimulating further vomiting and diarrhoea. The ORS is absorbed into the gut mostly by diffusion and osmosis. Electrolytes within the ORS can also be transported from the gut by active transport.

Diarrhoeal disease is responsible for nearly one in five deaths in children globally, and ORS can save lives and reduce this death rate. The United Nations Children's Fund (UNICEF) published a seven-point report in 2009 entitled *Diarrhoea: Why children are still dying and what can be done* (see *Box 2.5* and *Further reading*).

> **BOX 2.5**
>
> ### Ten things you should know about rehydrating a child
>
> 1. Wash your hands with soap and water before preparing solution.
> 2. Prepare a solution, in a clean pot, by mixing eight level teaspoons of sugar and one level teaspoon of salt in 1 L of clean water, **or** one packet of Oral Rehydration Salts (ORS) with 1 L of clean drinking or boiled water (after cooling). Stir the mixture until all the contents dissolve.
> 3. Wash your hands and the child's hands with soap and water before feeding the solution.
> 4. Give the sick child as much of the solution as it needs, in small amounts frequently.
> 5. Give the child other fluids alternately – such as breast milk and juices.
> 6. Continue to give solids if the child is 4 months or older.
> 7. If the child still needs ORS after 24 hours, make a fresh solution.
> 8. ORS does not stop diarrhoea. It prevents the body from dehydrating. The diarrhoea will stop by itself.
> 9. If the child vomits, wait 10 minutes and give it ORS again. Usually the vomiting will stop.
> 10. If diarrhoea increases and/or vomiting *persists*, take the child to a health clinic.
>
> **Figure 2.23** – **Oral rehydration salts packet.**
> Reproduced with kind permission of AGS Labs, Inc.

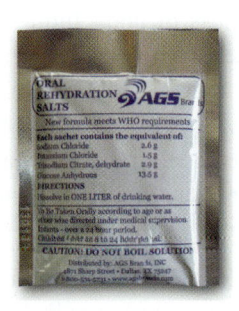

Patient 2.3 — Sheila — 30 **54** 59 93 267 304 448 473

- 47-year-old woman
- Recent diagnosis of breast cancer – biopsy shows cancer cells over-express HER2 protein
- Biological therapy with trastuzumab (Herceptin) to block HER2 action an option

Sheila is very worried about her diagnosis of breast cancer, but she is hopeful and is determined to understand more. She remembers learning about cells at school some 30 years ago, but knows nothing about receptors and organelles. She asks, 'Why can't they just take this HER2 thing out?' and 'Why do I have it anyway?'.

A number of options will be considered for the best management of Sheila, requiring coordination with a multidisciplinary team. Sheila's care will be considered further in *Chapters 3, 5, 8, 9* and *14*.

The suggested treatment is an example of a new type of 'biological therapy' that exploits elements of the immune system known as antibodies to block the action of (in this case) the HER2 growth factor receptor (see *Box 2.4*).

How would you go about helping Sheila understand how her body and cells operate so that she feels informed and not disempowered?

Informed decision making and consent can only occur when patients are provided with information and then actively involved with decisions about their healthcare.

The information must be offered at the right time, in the right amount and in a way that can be understood and managed by the patient. One-to-one discussion is the most common and powerful method of communication. However, it is often constrained by time and other work pressures. Family and significant others may not be present and so their information needs may be left unmet. Even after one-to-one discussion, information may not be retained, and so repetition or further input will be required. The use of diagrams and written information, including leaflets and internet-based resources, can help to support a patient's information needs, providing reinforcement and an opportunity to reframe understanding and seek clarification.

With reference to Sheila's specific needs, it is likely that she would benefit from one-to-one discussion. This would provide her with the opportunity to receive information, possibly supported by a trusted friend, and have the opportunity to reflect on it and then frame additional questions to help with her understanding and decision making. It is recognized that most people diagnosed with cancer want more information about their condition, and that positive outcomes for patients are linked to a good experience of care delivered safely and with clinical effectiveness. The ambition of the NHS is to achieve the best healthcare outcomes and one of the strategies employed is the process of '*shared decision making*'. More about this can be found online at www.england.nhs.uk/ourwork/pe/sdm/.

Health professionals must consider when and how to communicate relevant information to Sheila to ensure that she feels supported adequately and knows she can use the information given to her.

The fields of personalized medicine and of biological therapy continue to develop rapidly. Application of our knowledge of cells and tissues promises to be very useful for the management of healthcare in the future. This knowledge is sometimes contentious, raising social, ethical and legal issues for individuals and for society. Keeping up to date with the developments in cell biology as applied to healthcare is important for all health professionals and the *Further reading* section of this chapter has some suggestions to help you to do so.

2.4 Summary

- Humans are multicellular eukaryotes with their cells organized into larger structures as tissues, organs and organ systems. These provide a structural basis for physiological and homeodynamic processes.
- Our cells are metabolically active, contain subcellular structures called organelles (see *Figure 2.5*) and exist in a fluid chemical environment.
- The plasma membrane (see *Figure 2.6*) encloses the cell contents. It is a dynamic structure that interacts with the organelles and the intracellular and extracellular environment.
- The plasma membrane is a selectively permeable structure that can be described by reference to the 'fluid mosaic model' (see *Figure 2.6*).
- Transport of substances across the plasma membrane is dependent upon the physico-chemical characteristics of the substance being transported, such as size and charge, and its interaction with the plasma membrane, including membrane-bound proteins that act as selective carriers or create channels allowing transport to occur (see *Figure 2.11*).

- Proteins on and integrated within the plasma membrane provide a variety of functions important for cell survival and interaction with other cells, including cell–cell recognition, adhesion and signal transduction via receptors and their ligands.
- Tissues provide structure, mechanical resistance, form and function to the body. The nature of tissues is dependent upon the differentiated and collective activity of the cells that make them.

2.5 Further reading

The website of the Foundation for Genomics and Population Health is an excellent resource focusing on the application of biomedical science for health:
www.phgfoundation.org/

A useful resource about stem cells is the National Institutes of Health resource for stem cell research:
http://stemcells.nih.gov

The National Institute of General Medical Sciences (USA) provides a variety of interesting educational resources on science including cell biology.
https://publications.nigms.nih.gov

Diarrhoea: Why children are still dying and what can be done, provided by UNICEF and the World Health Organization, provides further reading and guidance on how managing fluid affects homeodynamic processes and saves lives.
www.7pointplan.org/

2.6 Self-assessment questions

Answers can be found at www.scionpublishing.com/AandP

(2.1) Mark each statement either true or false. The plasma membrane:
   (a) provides a completely impermeable barrier
   (b) is partially permeable
   (c) is fully permeable
   (d) is selectively permeable
   (e) is rigid

(2.2) Mark each statement either true or false. Phospholipids:
   (a) possess hydrophilic tails
   (b) possess hydrophobic heads
   (c) are amphiphilic molecules
   (d) possess hydrophobic tails
   (e) possess hydrophilic heads

(2.3) Mark each statement either true or false. Which processes involve the movement of water across a selectively permeable membrane, down a concentration gradient?
   (a) Diffusion
   (b) Osmosis
   (c) Facilitated diffusion
   (d) Active transport
   (e) Antiport

(2.4) Mark each statement either true or false. Ribosomes are:
    (a) membranous organelles that localize in the RER
    (b) involved with mitochondria for the release of energy from food
    (c) RNA–protein complexes involved in protein synthesis
    (d) proteins required for muscle contraction
    (e) ribbon-like sacs for storing glucose

(2.5) In humans, as red blood cells (erythrocytes) are formed, they 'lose' their nucleus. What is the consequence of this?

(2.6) Lactulose is a medicinal preparation containing an indigestible sugar, commonly used to treat constipation. It is broken down by colonic bacteria into metabolites that cannot pass through the gastrointestinal tissue. With this information, explain how lactulose might work and name the type of tissue that lines the gastrointestinal tract.

(2.7) Soap, like phospholipids, is amphiphilic. Describe the effect of soap on cells and explain why excessive washing of skin with soap could make it feel irritated and dry.

(2.8) In *Box 2.4*, the action of Herceptin to block the binding of EGF to its ligand (EGFR) was discussed. Use the following terms to outline, in a couple of sentences, the formation and location of EGFR:
integral, ribosomes, nucleus, protein, plasma membrane, rough endoplasmic reticulum, DNA, RNA.

CHAPTER 03 | Genetics: how cells divide and introduce variation

Learning points for this chapter

After working through this chapter, you should be able to:

- Understand the relevance and importance of genomics
- Detail the key steps in DNA replication and gene expression
- Describe the processes of cell division and provide examples of how genetic variation may occur
- Discuss, with specific examples, the implications of genetic knowledge for the practice of healthcare

3.1 Introduction and clinical relevance

The interaction of genetic and environmental factors is responsible for the development of the majority of disease, and in some cases the probability of developing a disease is known because the genetic factors can be traced through generations of families. In other cases, the exact contribution of genetic and environmental factors is less clear.

Each of the patients introduced in this chapter has a clinical condition strongly influenced by genetic factors. It is worth bearing in mind as you read this chapter that recent scientific and technological advances are rapidly altering our understanding of health and disease, and this is beginning to transform healthcare practice.

| Patient 2.3 | Sheila | 30 | 54 | **59** | 93 | 267 | 304 | 448 | 473 |

- 47-year-old woman
- Recent diagnosis of breast cancer – biopsy shows cancer cells over-express HER2 protein
- Biological therapy with trastuzumab (Herceptin) to block HER2 action an option
- Is still offered surgery, chemotherapy and radiotherapy
- Agrees to add trastuzumab to chemotherapy plan

As discussed in *Chapter 2*, Sheila has been told that she is a possible candidate for a form of cancer therapy with a compound that blocks the action of the HER2 receptor. She will continue to receive other recommended forms of treatment as necessary, including surgery, chemotherapy and radiotherapy. It is also expected that the addition of this form of 'targeted' therapy should significantly reduce the risk of the cancer reoccurring in the future.

| Patient 3.1 | Sarah | 60 | 94 | 195 | 237 | 311 | 333 |

- 17-year-old girl
- CF diagnosis at age of 1 year
- Frequent admissions for chest infections affecting breathing

Sarah, who is now 17 years old, was diagnosed at the age of 1 year with cystic fibrosis, a life-threatening inherited disease that clogs the lungs and digestive system with thick sticky mucus, making it hard for her to breathe and digest food. The fact that Sarah has cystic fibrosis was a surprise for her parents because no other family members were known to have the condition, although this is often the case with autosomal recessive conditions and especially when family histories are not well recorded.

Sarah leads as full a life as possible, enjoys dancing and skiing, and plans to go to university. Assisted by her mother, Sarah completes a daily series of physiotherapy exercises to clear her lungs of the viscous mucus secretions. Sarah has experienced very frequent admissions to hospital for exacerbation of her breathing problems due to the development of recurrent chest infections.

| Patient 3.2 | Alexei | 60 | 94 |

- 14-year-old boy
- Down syndrome – trisomy of chromosome 21
- Now withdrawn and disruptive; some breathlessness

Alexei is a 14-year-old boy with Down syndrome as a result of being born with an extra chromosome 21. He currently attends a mainstream school and has until recently enjoyed this. He has made firm friends and, with dedicated educational support, has made good progress. Recently, however, the teachers say his progress has plateaued and Alexei has been described as a bit withdrawn and occasionally disruptive. At home, Alexei's parents notice a change in Alexei's mood and that he is reluctant to engage in homework and attend school. Alexei really looks forward to a half round of golf with his friends and has surprised everyone with how good he is. However, for some weeks, he has not completed the round with his friends, preferring instead to catch his breath and rest for a few minutes with a drink and some chocolate.

Alexei's mother, Adelia, was 36 years old when she became pregnant with Alexei. The risk of Down syndrome increases with maternal age, and so her family doctor suggested she consider prenatal diagnosis. This would involve taking a sample of fetal cells from the fluid surrounding the developing fetus by a procedure known as amniocentesis. The procedure carries a small increase in the risk of miscarriage, but Adelia refused the procedure as she felt the information would not change her mind about her pregnancy. She preferred instead to provide a blood sample, which can estimate the extent of her increased risk, and underwent an ultrasound assessment of her developing baby (Alexei), which can also provide an estimate of the risk of Down syndrome.

> **Patient 3.3** — Katherine — 61 | 95 | 268 | 305

- 41-year-old woman
- Recent diagnosis of hypertrophic cardiomyopathy
- ECG shows arrhythmia and USS shows thickened left ventricle

Katherine is a 41-year-old woman recently diagnosed with hypertrophic cardiomyopathy (HCM), an inherited disease of the heart in which the muscle wall of the heart becomes thickened. Katherine has an older brother with HCM, diagnosed after he unexpectedly sustained a stroke. Her father has also been unwell for some years with a heart condition. She has started to experience a little shortness of breath, feeling 'light-headed' and frequent feelings of what she describes as 'fluttering' in her chest. She was referred to a cardiologist for investigations, and electrocardiography (ECG and ultrasound imagery of the heart) revealed an arrhythmia and thickening of Katherine's left ventricle consistent with HCM.

> **Patient 3.4** — Yasmeen — 61 | 95 | 268 | 306

- 17-year-old girl
- Has sickle cell disease but no long-term organ damage

Yasmeen is an active 17-year-old girl living with sickle cell disease, an inherited blood disorder in which red blood cells develop abnormally. After a period of denial and rebellious behaviour in her early teens, Yasmeen now regularly attends outpatient review appointments and employs a range of strategies and interventions to manage her condition. She has regular bouts of severe symptoms, but has not yet sustained any long-term organ damage.

The structure and function of our body, with its trillions of cells, complex physiological processes and varied form, rely on the inheritance and expression of the genetic material (nucleic acids) present within the nucleus of all our body cells. This hereditary material represents the physical link between generations and populations of people, helping to explain how people are similar and yet also different. When considered together with our adaptive physiological responses to the environment, this hereditary material, present within all of our cells, helps us to understand how we develop from a single cell into a fully formed human. Knowledge of genetics is therefore fundamental to understanding the basis of health and disease. Indeed, much of modern healthcare is being informed by a rapid explosion in genetic knowledge. This carries significant implications for the individual, families and society. In this chapter, we will explore the nature of this genetic material and how it functions to affect our lives and our health.

3.2 What you need to know – essential anatomy and physiology

3.2.1 The genome

The biological information required to make and maintain a living organism is present in all cells, encoded in the form of **deoxyribonucleic acid** (DNA). This, in its entirety within the nucleus of a cell, is termed the **genome**. During periods of cell division, the DNA can be seen under a microscope, organized within structures called **chromosomes**.

The genome represents the hereditary information in the form of **genes**, which provide the organism with a mechanism to function and to reproduce. A gene contains the information for the cell to make molecules called **ribonucleic acid** (RNA) and, through a type of RNA called messenger RNA (mRNA), to make the

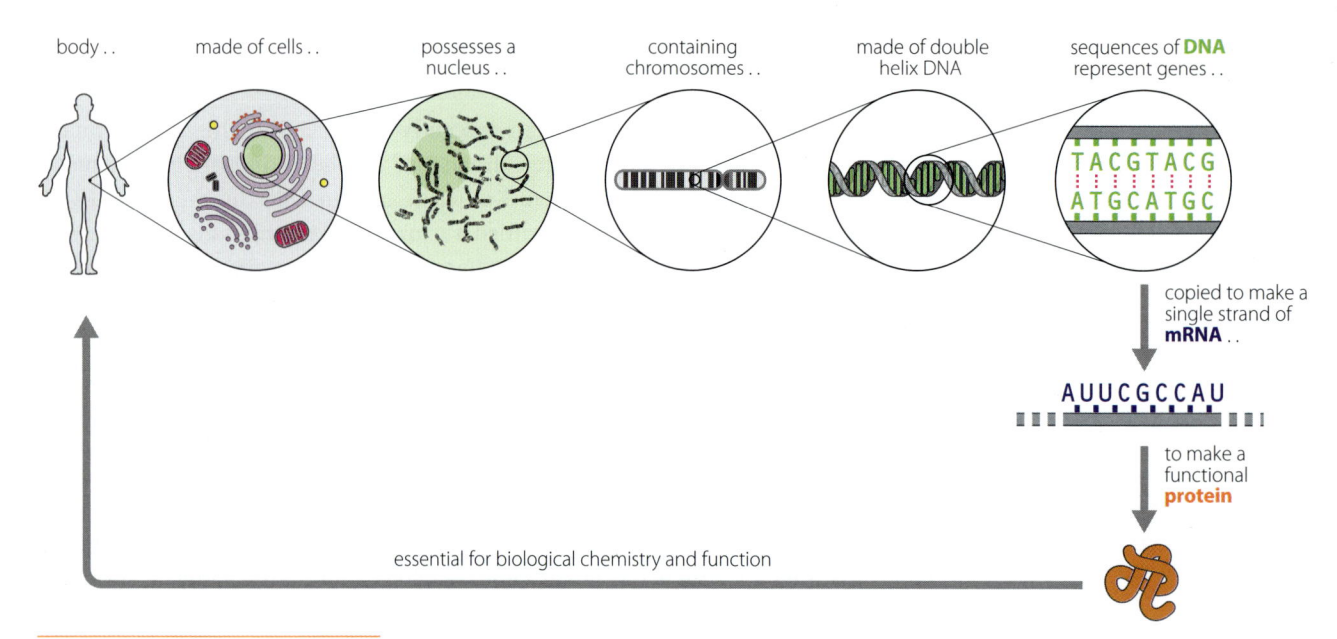

Figure 3.1 – The hierarchy of the genome.

The human genome contains all of the genetic information and is found in every cell, stored in the nucleus in the form of chromosomes. The chromosomes are tightly coiled DNA molecules, which contain genes that are transcribed to produce RNA, which is then translated to produce proteins.

proteins required by the body (see *Figure 3.1* and *Table 3.1*). It is estimated that in humans there are approximately 20 000–25 000 genes that code for proteins, although these genes represent only a small fraction of our genome. The remaining DNA does not directly code for proteins via the manufacture of mRNA. Instead, much of it is used to form a variety of *non-coding* RNA molecules that function as regulators, essential to the process of protein manufacture. Many thousands of proteins are required by the body and its cells. It is important that the amount of protein produced by individual and by different cells is carefully regulated by non-coding RNA. Protein turnover, affected by synthesis, protein stability and rates of degradation, is a crucial element for cell function.

Table 3.1 – Organization of the genome

Body	Made up of trillions of cells.
Cells	Every cell has a nucleus.
Nucleus	The nucleus contains chromosomes.
Chromosomes	There are 46 chromosomes in human somatic (body) cells and 23 in sex cells (sperm/ovum); they are made up of a complex of proteins and DNA.
DNA	Deoxyribonucleic acid (DNA) is the molecule that carries the 'genetic code'. The code is structured into individual genes.
Gene	A unit of inheritance (there are approximately 20 000 within each body cell), which is a specific segment of DNA that codes for the making of a polypeptide or a functional RNA molecule.
RNA	Ribonucleic acid (RNA) carries hereditary information transcribed from DNA. There are a variety of forms of RNA (including ribosomal RNA and transfer RNA), but it is messenger RNA (mRNA) that is used directly within the cytoplasm for making proteins.

Structure of the genome

The genome comprises all of the genetic information and is contained within 46 chromosomes in the nucleus of a somatic (body) cell; a small amount of (circular) DNA also exists within mitochondria, but this has a specialized role that is beyond the scope of this book. The chromosomes themselves are highly organized structures composed of DNA wrapped around histone proteins to form a coiled structure called **chromatin**. Chromosomes are normally only visible during cell division when the chromatin becomes tightly folded; throughout the rest of the cell cycle, chromatin remains in a more extended relaxed state.

DNA is synthesized from building blocks called nucleotides. There are three parts to a nucleotide used for making DNA (called a deoxynucleotide): a sugar molecule (2′-deoxyribose), a phosphate molecule and a molecule called a DNA base. There are four types of DNA base: **adenine (A)**, **thymine (T)**, **guanine (G)** and **cytosine (C)** (see *Figure 3.2a*).

To synthesize DNA from nucleotides, the sugar molecule of one nucleotide is joined to the phosphate molecule of another nucleotide by a **phosphodiester bond** to form a linear chain (see *Figure 3.2b*), which is several million nucleotides long. In all, there are approximately 6 billion DNA nucleotides within the genomic DNA of a human somatic cell. A DNA molecule in the nucleus of a human cell is double-stranded and forms a helical structure (see *Figure 3.2a*) – called the **DNA double helix** – with the DNA bases on one strand hydrogen bonded to the DNA bases on the other strand. This **base pairing** only occurs in two configurations:

- adenine (A) can bind to thymine (T)
- guanine (G) can bind to cytosine (C).

Thus, there are only two possible pairings (A–T and C–G) to bind the two strands of DNA; these are referred to as DNA base pairs. The weak **hydrogen bonds** holding together DNA base pairs are shown as dotted lines in *Figure 3.2b*; there

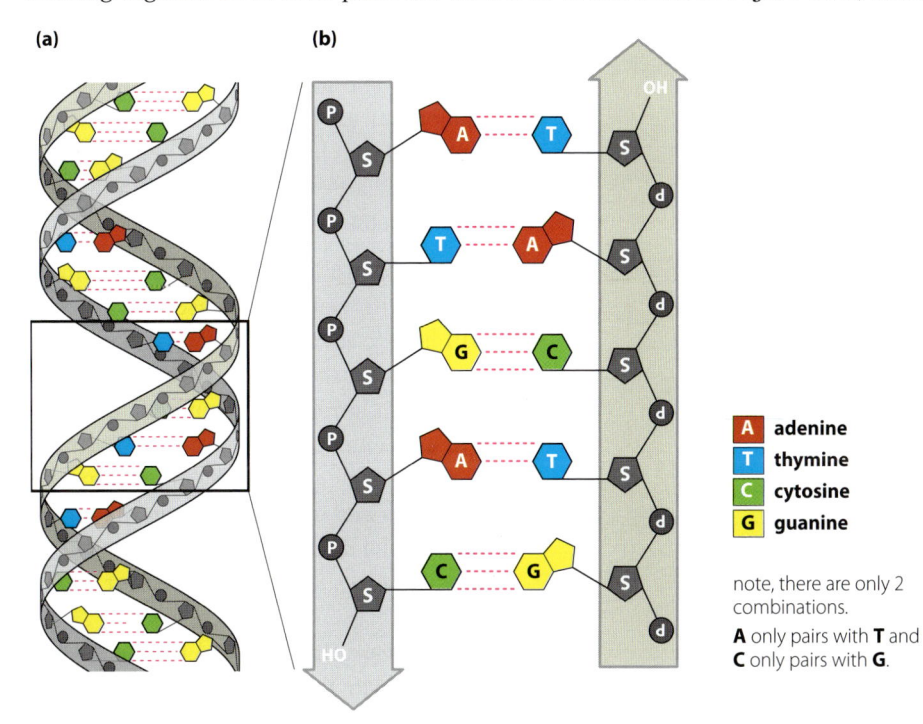

Figure 3.2 – The structure of a DNA molecule.
(a) Pairing of complementary base pairs. (b) The structure of the DNA double helix.

A adenine
T thymine
C cytosine
G guanine

note, there are only 2 combinations.
A only pairs with **T** and **C** only pairs with **G**.

are two hydrogen bonds between A and T and three hydrogen bonds between G and C. When a gene is expressed, specific enzymes separate the two DNA strands to allow mRNA to be made from the correct strand. The order of DNA bases along the entire length of the DNA molecule is crucially important, because it is the order of the bases that represents the 'genetic code' that is read during protein synthesis (see *Box 3.2*, later).

Function of the genome

The genetic material, in the form of DNA, must be able to:

- be repeatedly and accurately replicated, in order to create new and viable cells
- code for the development and function of cells as they grow and contribute to the maintenance of homeostasis
- change (a process called **mutation**), producing variations between individuals in a population so that the species can adapt for survival in its environment.

A specific sequence of DNA bases containing the information required to make a protein is called a **gene**. All the genes present in an individual's cells, responsible for coding for all the proteins to be made, are collectively referred to as the **genotype**. The **phenotype** of an individual is the observable characteristics, such as physical appearance, behaviour and biochemical activity, that arise as a consequence of protein synthesis following the reading of all the code in the genotype. The type and amounts of protein required by a living organism are dynamic and can change within minutes. Proteins govern and regulate cellular metabolism and so it is important that the amounts and types of protein available are tightly regulated. It is important to understand that the range and amounts of proteins synthesized (called the **proteome**) are highly dynamic, while the inherited genome remains static (except for the occasional mutation).

Modern technology is able to map and identify the genes held within a human cell and so is able to establish the genes that are expressed and translated into proteins. The aim of the **Human Genome Project** was to map and record the sequence of all of the 3 billion DNA base pairs within the haploid human genome (the term haploid will be explained later in this chapter). This was completed with an estimated accuracy of 99.9% in 2003 and is important for a number of reasons:

- It will enable an increased understanding of how genes interact and are involved with causing disease.
- It will help to identify who is susceptible to diseases and how they can be protected from them. This is especially pertinent to chronic diseases that exert a high burden and economic cost to patients and society.
- It will also enable a better understanding of how the expression of the genome is influenced by the environment. This will be important for populations and carries implications for public health programmes, including the development of strategies aimed at offering healthier lifestyle choices to people to limit or even prevent the development of disease.
- It will increase the potential for the development of gene therapies.
- It will stimulate the design of personalized therapies through the development

of drugs that act selectively on particular genetic variants (some of these are already available: see Sheila, Patient 2.3, with breast cancer).
- It will help improve the development of new diagnostic methods.

All organisms possess a genome, and efforts are under way to characterize the genome of a wide variety of species. Knowledge that emerges from these other genome projects can be extremely useful for humans; for example:

- Genes conserved among distantly related species can be indicative of important functions conserved through evolutionary time, suggesting how these particular genes may function in humans.
- Knowledge of plant genomics can be applied to the optimization of nutrition, food quality and supply.
- An improved understanding of microbial genomics can be applied to the clean-up of polluted environments, energy generation and the capturing of carbon released from human activity. Indeed, one application of

---

BOX 3.1

Genomic technology used to control outbreaks of infection in a hospital

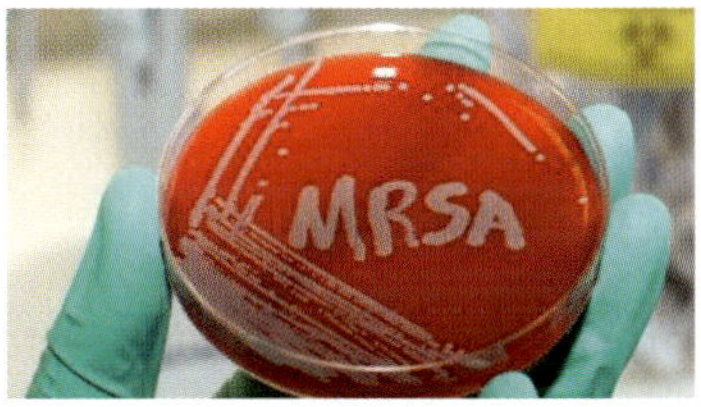

Figure 3.3 – MRSA colonies growing in a Petri dish.
Reproduced from www.med.cam.ac.uk.

Meticillin-resistant *Staphylococcus aureus* (MRSA) is a major cause of community- and hospital-acquired infection worldwide (MRSA was discussed in *Chapter 1*) (*Figure 3.3*). It is resistant to many antibiotics, is very difficult to eradicate and causes potentially lethal infection. The control of MRSA and healthcare-acquired infection is a patient safety issue and a public health priority.

Patients admitted to hospital are routinely screened for *colonization* with MRSA (see Francine, Patient 1.3) so that they can be treated before it causes infection in themselves or other people, especially vulnerable patients such as the young, the elderly and immunocompromised patients.

Researchers and clinicians from the Wellcome Trust Sanger Institute and the University of Cambridge and Cambridge University Hospitals in the UK used advanced DNA sequencing technology to identify specific strains of MRSA responsible for an outbreak of infection on a special care baby unit in real time. This allowed the researchers to identify whether an actual outbreak of MRSA infection was taking place. An unsuspected carrier of the bacterial strain linked to the outbreak was also identified and successfully treated. The study also revealed that the strain of MRSA responsible for the outbreak was being carried by, or was causing infection in, more people than previously recognized, having spread into the wider community; this conclusion could not be reached with traditional methods.

The DNA sequencing project was key in bringing the outbreak to an early end, possibly saving the hospital money and making patients safer.

Sir Mark Walport, then Director of the Wellcome Trust, was quoted as saying *'This is a dramatic demonstration that medical genomics is no longer a technology of the future – it is a technology of the here and now. By collaborating with NHS doctors, geneticists have shown that sequencing can have extremely important applications in healthcare today, halting an outbreak of a potentially deadly disease'* (http://www.sanger.ac.uk/news/view/2012-06-13-tracking-mrsa-in-real-time).

microbial genomics has recently been used to successfully control outbreaks of infection within hospitals (see *Box 3.1*).
- Knowledge of virus genomes and their infection strategies has also created the opportunity to vaccinate against specific forms of cancer caused by viruses, such as cervical cancer (see Jess, Patient 14.1).

It is clear that genomic technologies are likely to play an increasingly important part in our lives and not just in the healthcare environment.

Gene expression: using the genetic code to make proteins

The information stored in the form of a sequence of DNA bases in a gene has to be expressed in a physical form, which is that of the encoded protein. In humans, the DNA sequence representing the code for a particular protein is not stored in a continuous stretch of DNA bases in the gene. The gene actually comprises a number of protein-coding regions called **exons** (representing expressed sequences) interspersed with non-coding regions called **introns** (representing intervening sequences). A large amount of the human genome is composed of these non-coding introns, which have been shown to have a role in controlling gene expression.

There are several sequential steps involved in making a protein, and these are summarized quite simply by the so-called 'central dogma' of molecular biology (see *Box 3.2*).

Transcription: DNA makes RNA

Transcription involves copying one strand of double-stranded DNA into a single strand of RNA. Three main processes are required to make an RNA molecule: initiation, elongation and termination of an RNA chain (illustrated in *Figure 3.4*).

BOX 3.2

The central dogma of molecular biology

DNA ⟹ RNA ⟹ Protein
   transcription   translation

The central dogma of molecular biology represents a one-way sequential process whereby genetic information in the form of DNA is used to make RNA (in the form of mRNA for protein-coding genes), which is used to direct the synthesis of its corresponding protein.

However, we now know that in some limited biological circumstances the process can be reversed; that is, RNA can be used to synthesize DNA. For example, some viruses such as human immunodeficiency virus (HIV) contain RNA, rather than DNA, together with an enzyme called reverse transcriptase. When HIV infects a cell (as has happened to Jerry, Patient 11.2), its reverse transcriptase is used to make viral DNA from its RNA (the reverse of the central dogma of molecular biology). This viral DNA can then be integrated into the host genome.

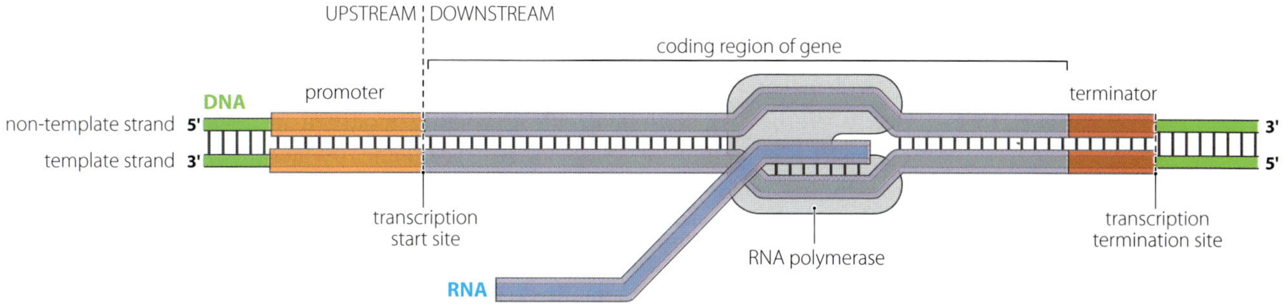

Figure 3.4 – Transcription of a gene.
The transfer of genetic information from DNA starts with the making of RNA, known as transcription of a gene.

Initiation

Regulatory proteins called transcription factors interact with chromatin (as described earlier, a complex of DNA and histone proteins) to unwind the DNA helix and reveal specific nucleotide sequences of DNA to which an enzyme called **RNA polymerase** can bind. These DNA sequences are located at a site called the promoter region, which is close to the gene to be transcribed. This region often contains a DNA sequence known as a TATA box, comprising the DNA nucleotide bases thymine (T) and adenine (A), marking the start of transcription. Once bound to the DNA, and assisted by a number of protein transcription factors, RNA polymerase begins to unwind and separate the two strands of DNA. The exposed DNA bases on a separated single strand of DNA (A, T, G and C) then become available for copying. The strand of DNA that is actually used to make an RNA copy is known as the **template** or **antisense strand**. The RNA produced has the same sequence as the non-template strand of DNA, called the **sense strand** or **coding strand** (except that the RNA contains U instead of T; discussed in the following paragraph).

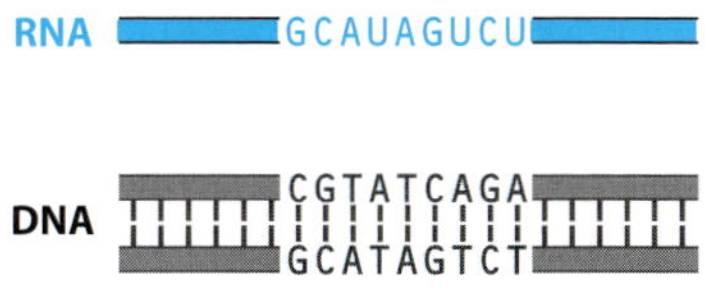

Figure 3.5 – Base pairing in DNA and RNA.
It is the order of the DNA nucleotide bases that represents the genetic information. Note that in the RNA, thymine has been replaced by uracil. G is guanine, C is cytosine, A is adenine, T is thymine and U is uracil (found only in RNA).

Elongation

RNA polymerase travels along the template strand of DNA, interacting with the exposed DNA bases. As it does so, RNA polymerase catalyses the formation of a long polynucleotide chain from RNA nucleotides. The order of the growing chain of RNA nucleotides is matched according to the order of A, T, G and C present on the DNA: if guanine is present on the DNA, then the complementary nucleotide in the RNA will be cytosine; if it is thymine, then adenine is added. However, the RNA molecule is slightly different chemically from DNA, in that RNA contains the base **uracil** (U) instead of thymine, and so when the RNA polymerase finds adenine on the DNA template, it adds uracil to the growing polynucleotide chain. The replacement of thymine by uracil does not change the *order* of nucleotide bases and so the encoded information remains the same (see *Figure 3.5*).

Termination

As the RNA polymerase travels along the DNA, copying it, the growing strand of RNA detaches from the DNA, which reforms as a double-stranded molecule. The newly synthesized RNA molecule is usually modified in a variety of ways; for example, each end of the RNA molecule is chemically modified. Most importantly, non-coding intron sequences from the gene are removed by post-transcriptional processing mechanisms called **RNA splicing**, which cut the RNA molecule at the exon–intron junctions and then join together the RNA coding for exon sequences. The RNA transcript then contains a continuous stretch of nucleotides coding for the corresponding protein with all intron sequences removed; at this stage, it is referred to as messenger RNA (mRNA). The mRNA molecules then leave the nucleus through pores in the nuclear membrane and enter the cytoplasmic compartment of the cell, where they attach to ribosomes and are *translated* into protein. Ribosomes can be found free within the cytoplasm, but are most frequently found within the extensive mesh-like network of the rough endoplasmic reticulum (see *Chapter 2*).

Other forms of RNA, for example ribosomal RNA (rRNA) and transfer RNA (tRNA), play important roles in the process of translation, although they do not code for proteins.

Translation: RNA makes protein

The process of reading an mRNA and using the coding information to synthesize a functional protein is called **translation**.

Proteins are macromolecules made of amino acids. In order to make a functional protein, the correct amino acids have to be covalently bound together in the correct order. The order of amino acids is crucial because this ultimately determines the protein's physical and chemical properties. Translation occurs in the cytoplasm using ribosomes (discussed in *Chapter 2*), tRNA molecules and amino acids; it also requires the presence of specific proteins called translation factors.

Three nucleotide bases in mRNA are required to specify a particular amino acid; this triplet of bases is known as a **codon**. Four different nucleotide bases are used to make up mRNA, and so 64 different codon combinations are possible ($4 \times 4 \times 4 = 64$). There are only 20 amino acids in total and so there are more than enough codons to represent all the amino acids. In fact, 61 codons represent the amino acids and the remaining three act as stop signals to terminate protein synthesis. The relationship between the codons and the amino acids they represent is called the **genetic code** (see *Box 3.3*).

Transfer RNA (tRNA) plays an important role in the process of translation, although it does not code for proteins. At one end of any given tRNA molecule is a site for the binding of just one of the 20 amino acids; after it forms a covalent bond with that amino acid, it is called aminoacyl-tRNA. The tRNA also contains a nucleotide sequence of three bases called an **anticodon**, which matches a complementary codon on mRNA and is able to hydrogen bond to it. This is the basis of how the genetic code is translated: a tRNA molecule recognizes a specific codon, has the correct amino acid already bound to it and so is ready to be incorporated into the protein to be synthesized. The process of protein synthesis also requires a ribosome that associates with the aminoacyl-tRNAs and the mRNA molecule.

Protein synthesis can be summarized as three main phases (see *Figure 3.6*).

BOX 3.3

The genetic code

The genetic code can be interpreted by reference to a codon table (see *Table 3.2*). Each triplet of RNA nucleotides is a codon and the order of codons on a strand of mRNA specifies which amino acids will be added to a polypeptide chain during protein synthesis.

Table 3.2 – A codon table

1st base in codon	2nd base in codon				3rd base in codon
	U	**C**	**A**	**G**	
U	Phe	Ser	Tyr	Cys	U
	Phe	Ser	Tyr	Cys	C
	Leu	Ser	STOP	STOP	A
	Leu	Ser	STOP	Trp	G
C	Leu	Pro	His	Arg	U
	Leu	Pro	His	Arg	C
	Leu	Pro	Gln	Arg	A
	Leu	Pro	Gln	Arg	G
A	Ile	Thr	Asn	Ser	U
	Ile	Thr	Asn	Ser	C
	Ile	Thr	Lys	Arg	A
	Met	Thr	Lys	Arg	G
G	Val	Ala	Asp	Gly	U
	Val	Ala	Asp	Gly	C
	Val	Ala	Glu	Gly	A
	Val	Ala	Glu	Gly	G

Some amino acids such as serine and arginine have multiple codons, whereas tryptophan and methionine have only one each. AUG doubles as the initiator codon and as the codon for internal methionines. Note the three stop codons.

Abbreviations

Ala	Alanine	Leu	Leucine
Arg	Arginine	Lys	Lysine
Asn	Asparginine	Met	Methionine
Asp	Aspartic acid	Phe	Phenylalanine
Cys	Cysteine	Pro	Proline
Glu	Glutamic acid	Ser	Serine
Gln	Glutamine	Thr	Threonine
Gly	Glycine	Trp	Tryptophan
His	Histidine	Try	Tyrosine
Ile	Isoleucine	Val	Valine

The codon AUG specifies the amino acid methionine. This codon also acts as the start codon, and so all polypeptides start with the amino acid methionine. Protein synthesis ends when one of the three stop codons (also called termination codons: UAA, UAG and UGA) is presented to the ribosome. The stop codons do not specify amino acids; instead, when the ribosome encounters a stop codon, a protein called a release factor binds and causes translation to end.

BOX 3.3 (continued)

The genetic code – continued

Note that the genetic code is *degenerate*, i.e. there are more codons than necessary for the 20 amino acids so there are often multiple codons coding for the same amino acid. Therefore, although a single nucleotide change in a DNA sequence (a mutation), and hence to the corresponding mRNA sequence, will change the codon to a different codon, this may still encode the same amino acid. In this case, therefore, the mutation will not alter the amino acid sequence of the final protein.

Each of the 20 amino acids has its own standard abbreviation, making it easier to compile a list of the amino acid sequence that makes a protein (see *Table 3.2*). This is useful for understanding how alterations in the genetic code or the amino acid sequence of a protein affect function and thereby influence health and disease (see Sarah, Patient 3.1, and Yasmeen, Patient 3.4). In the case of Sarah with cystic fibrosis, the genetic code is frequently altered by deletion of three DNA nucleotides in just one specific gene. This changes the amino acid sequence of a particular protein, which causes cystic fibrosis (discussed later in this chapter). In the case of Yasmeen with sickle cell disease, just one DNA nucleotide in the β-globin (pronounced beta-globin) gene changes from adenine to thymine (A to T), altering the polypeptide chain by just one amino acid, resulting in glutamic acid being substituted by valine (see *Chapter 7*) to cause sickle cell disease.

The amino acids highlighted in red in *Table 3.2* are essential amino acids that cannot be synthesized in the body and so they must be obtained from food (see *Chapter 7*).

Initiation

Initiation of protein synthesis requires a **start codon** (AUG) in the mRNA, which encodes the amino acid methionine (see *Table 3.2*). The corresponding aminoacyl-tRNA molecule (with methionine attached and an **anticodon** (UAC) complementary to the start codon) binds to the start codon and a ribosome also binds to form an initiation complex.

Elongation

Another aminoacyl-tRNA molecule, together with its complementary anticodon, binds to the next codon on the mRNA. With the help of the ribosome and a variety of enzymes, the two amino acids become joined together with a **peptide bond**. This process occurs repeatedly along the length of the mRNA molecule to form a growing polypeptide chain of amino acids that correspond to the codons in the mRNA. Many ribosomes can simultaneously interact with an mRNA molecule along its length forming a structure known as a **polysome**, to produce more than one copy of the protein at a time, ensuring that protein synthesis can occur rapidly and efficiently.

Termination

This occurs when a stop codon is reached. The polypeptide chain then leaves the mRNA and the ribosome. After translation, many proteins need to be chemically modified (in a wide variety of ways called 'post-translational modification') before they can become fully functional.

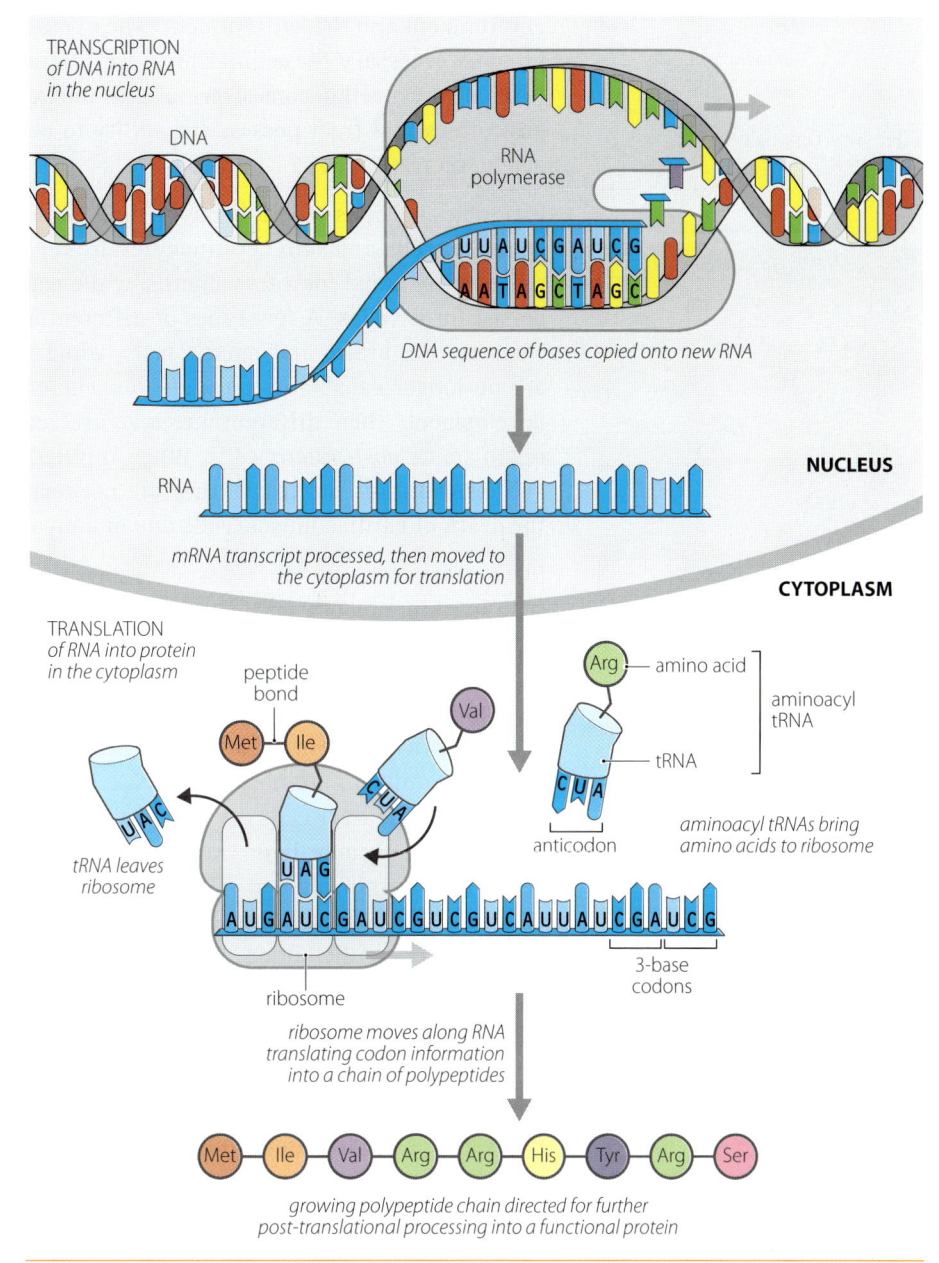

SECTION 3.2 | WHAT YOU NEED TO KNOW – ESSENTIAL ANATOMY AND PHYSIOLOGY 71

Figure 3.6 – **Summary of transcription (in the nucleus) and translation (in the cytoplasm).**
For further information see the text.

What influences gene expression and what are the consequences?

It is tempting to think that, because all cells contain the same genomic DNA, they are all the same type of cell. In fact, there are over 200 different types of body cells that give rise to our organs, grouped into the four main types of tissue (discussed in *Chapter 2*). The differentiation of cells into the different types is determined by which genes are expressed and when they are expressed. It is important to recognize that cells and tissues are responsive to their local environment and this will influence the expression of genes, which then make the proteins necessary for cellular processes. Gene expression, therefore, determines in what way a cell becomes specialized; for example, many of the cells lining the gastrointestinal tract possess the ability to absorb nutrients, whereas others are able to secrete mucus.

Differentiated cells generally have a limited lifespan; for example, gastrointestinal epithelial cells and skin keratinocytes are replaced every few days, erythrocytes remain functional for a few months, while neurones and memory T-lymphocytes persist for decades. A few types of differentiated cells, such as neurones, which comprise the brain, and muscle cells, which form skeletal and cardiac muscle, are no longer capable of cell division. These cells, produced during embryonic development, then differentiate, and are retained throughout the life of the organism as *post-mitotic* cells. When injured, they are capable of limited repair and regeneration, but if lost, they are not replaced. An example of this would be the death of cardiac muscle cells due to a myocardial infarction (heart attack).

In contrast, cells of other tissues, especially those with a rapid cell turnover such as skin, smooth muscle, fibroblasts, endothelial cells of blood vessels and the epithelial cells of most internal organs are able to proliferate as needed throughout life to maintain the homeodynamic state of tissues and organs. For example, keratinocytes and fibroblasts proliferate rapidly to repair tissues after injury, participating in the process of wound repair, while liver cells (hepatocytes), which in adults do not normally divide, can be induced to proliferate when large numbers of the liver cells are removed (for example, by surgical removal of part of the liver). Human liver transplants can be successful with only a part of a donated liver transplanted. This ability of hepatocytes to divide and regenerate to form a fully functioning liver makes liver transplants from living donors a realistic therapeutic option. However, it requires major surgery, with a high risk of morbidity and a small risk of death to the healthy donor, and so the procedure is restricted to specialist centres.

Stem cells – cells that are able to self-renew and remain undifferentiated while producing progeny that do differentiate (introduced in *Chapter 2*) – are of great interest in scientific and clinical research because they retain the potential for manipulation of gene expression, particularly in those genes involved in cell division and differentiation. The process of differentiation involves several stages as cells become increasingly specialized; this is influenced by external signals such as molecules in the local microenvironment, which influence which sets of genes are expressed, appropriate for the tissue they arise within. Stem cells hold great promise for the treatment of diseases that might best respond to the replacement and transplantation of cells or tissue; this represents the field of regenerative medicine.

Genetic factors mean that some people may be more or less susceptible or resistant to the development of specific diseases, such as cardiovascular disease or infection. However, the extent of their risk of developing the disease can be modified by environmental and lifestyle factors. For example, the risk of experiencing a heart attack – a blockage of a blood vessel in the heart causing heart muscle to die (discussed further in *Chapter 9*, see Robert, Patient 9.1) – is known to be influenced by inherited variations within genes on chromosome 9. However, recent findings from a large study of these genetic variations and lifestyle factors revealed that consuming a diet rich in raw fruit and vegetables reduced the risk of a heart attack. Cardiovascular diseases represent the leading cause of death in Western societies and have complex causes influenced by smoking, activity levels and diet. It is important to recognize that genetic inheritance may *predispose* a person to an increased risk of development of disease, but does not necessarily *determine* future health, as lifestyle and environmental factors play an important part in this. Globally, the most common chronic diseases are caused by four well-known and modifiable risk factors:

- tobacco use
- physical inactivity
- unhealthy diet
- being overweight.

Therefore, avoiding exposure to tobacco, participating in regular exercise and eating a healthy diet to maintain a healthy weight are simple but effective measures for improving population health, regardless of genetic inheritance. Promoting health through education and support is an important element of healthcare professional practice. To illustrate this, Robert (Patient 9.1), introduced in *Chapter 9*, will reduce his risk of further complications and possibly avoid an early death from heart disease if he is able to adjust his lifestyle.

In addition, people sometimes respond differently to therapeutic drugs depending on their genetics. The new discipline of 'pharmacogenetics' aims to understand individual responses to drugs based on an individual genotype. It is anticipated that personalized pharmacological therapy will increase as knowledge from the Human Genome Project is exploited.

The control of gene expression is influenced by many factors and by mechanisms that are still not fully understood, but it involves both transcription and translation. For example, the close interaction of histone proteins (a part of chromatin) with DNA affects the accessibility of DNA sequences available for transcription. Chromatin also controls the availability of regulatory proteins such as transcription factors to DNA, thereby regulating transcription. Given that a large number of protein-coding genes are estimated to be present in the genome, there is a requirement for the majority of these to be inactive until needed, and therefore tight control of gene expression is essential.

The availability of transcription factors to influence gene expression is often under the influence of external and internal environmental factors. The external environmental factors include stressors acting on the cell, such as heat, injury and light, while the internal environmental factors include changes in the local chemical environment such as the presence of reactive oxygen species and pro-inflammatory cytokines (see *Chapter 11*). The latter also includes the actions of hormones; for example, the hormone oestrogen produced in the ovaries binds onto oestrogen receptors present on cells within the uterus or breast. The receptor itself is a protein and, as such, is a product of gene expression. Activated oestrogen receptors bind to

DNA and influence the expression of many genes, some of which are required for the proliferation of uterine or breast cells, regulation of the menstrual cycle and the development of female secondary sexual characteristics (see *Chapter 5*).

Direct modification of DNA itself also influences gene expression, such as the addition of methyl groups (hypermethylation) to cytosine nucleotides within regulatory sequences of DNA, or the modification of histone proteins associated with DNA. The hypermethylation of DNA does not involve changing the order of DNA bases (A, T, C or G), but it does influence transcription, determining which proteins can be synthesized. This is an example of an **epigenetic** change (a change to the phenotype that is not caused by a change in the DNA sequence) that often results in suppression of gene expression. For example, if hypermethylation of DNA occurs within genes that regulate cell division, then rates of cell proliferation might change. Among many triggers, methylation of DNA is now recognized to occur in response to changes in the diet and exposure to environmental chemicals over the lifespan. Maternal nutrition is observed to influence the health of her offspring, not only at birth but also much later in life, affecting the risk of heart disease and obesity. The exact mechanism is not fully understood, but evidence is emerging indicating that epigenetic modification of DNA is involved. Epigenetic changes are now recognized to be a feature in a wide variety of clinical disorders, including cancer, type 2 diabetes mellitus, rheumatoid arthritis, Alzheimer's disease and neurodevelopmental disorders.

Understanding and mapping epigenetic changes is of great interest today because it represents chemical features of the genome that are important to gene expression and are therefore important in gaining a fuller understanding of the processes involved in health and disease. Where epigenetic changes occur in germ cells, these can be inherited and will be reflected in the phenotype of offspring. Studies of identical (monozygotic) twins show that although they share a common genotype, making them 'genetically identical', they are observed to develop clinical conditions such as rheumatoid arthritis or schizophrenia at different rates. Some of these differences can be accounted for by epigenetic changes that occur as identical (monozygotic) twins gradually age, live different lifestyles and begin to live apart as adults. Indeed, studies of twins over time provide very important information about the role of genetics and epigenetics in health and disease. A multinational project, similar to the Human Genome Project, is currently under way to map the human 'epigenome'. This project is likely to increase our understanding of how genes are regulated and involved in the development of disorders as diverse as cancer and neurodevelopmental disorders such as autism.

3.2.2 Chromosomes

Sources of genetic variation: 'We are all different, aren't we?'
Each somatic cell in humans is known as a **diploid** cell because it has two copies of each chromosome, that is, 46 chromosomes organized into two sets of 23 pairs. Twenty-two of these pairs of chromosomes are called **autosomes** and the remaining pair is referred to as the **sex chromosomes** (X and Y) because they carry genes that determine the sex of the individual. Germ cells that produce the gametes (sperm and ovum) undergo **meiosis**, a form of cell division that reduces

the number of chromosomes by half, so that each gamete contains only one copy of each chromosome and the gametes are described as **haploid** cells. Fertilization of an ovum with a sperm cell to produce a **zygote** restores the chromosome complement to a diploid state, that is, a full set of 46 chromosomes. **Mitosis** (a type of cell division that maintains the diploid state of reproduced cells) creates all future somatic cells that will develop into a full human being.

The 23 pairs of chromosomes found in every somatic cell are termed **homologous chromosomes**. The two chromosomes in a pair are similar in that they carry the same set of genes and can be recognized to form a pair with each other during the process of cell division. It is important to recognize that the genes are also inherited in pairs, but that these two genes are not identical. There are different forms of genes, called **alleles**, which usually provide a range of phenotypes; for example, there are three main alleles that determine the major blood groups (discussed in *Chapter 9*). The importance of alleles to heredity will be discussed later in this chapter.

During fertilization, when the haploid sperm and ovum join, one of each of the 23 pairs of chromosomes is inherited from the father and the other from the mother. We therefore inherit two copies of each gene. The sex chromosomes are an exception because they are not the same and are termed X and Y chromosomes. A human that inherits two X chromosomes will become a woman, whereas a man possesses one X chromosome and one Y chromosome (XY). Expression of genes located on the Y chromosome causes the formation and development of sexual and other organs that provide a male phenotype (see *Figure 3.7*).

Figure 3.7 – Distribution of the sex chromosomes during fertilization.
Diploid germ cells with 22 pairs of homologous autosomes and one pair of sex chromosomes divide to produce a haploid sperm or ovum, each containing one sex chromosome. When fertilization occurs, the zygote becomes diploid. There is an equal probability of a zygote containing two X chromosomes, or one X and one Y chromosome. In this way, the probable ratio of girls and boys is naturally maintained at approximately 50 : 50.

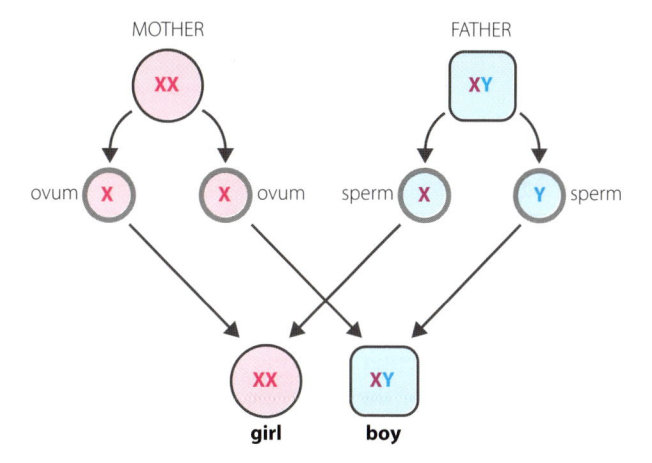

The transfer of genetic information from DNA starts with the making of RNA – transcription of a gene.

The chromosomes present within a cell can be observed under a microscope during a phase of cell division called **metaphase**. When stained with dyes and placed in order, the characteristic structure, number and staining pattern of chromosomes is revealed; this is called a **karyotype** (see *Figure 3.8a*). Any abnormality observed in a karyotype represents gross alterations to the genome and may indicate serious consequences for an individual's phenotype (an abnormal karyotype containing

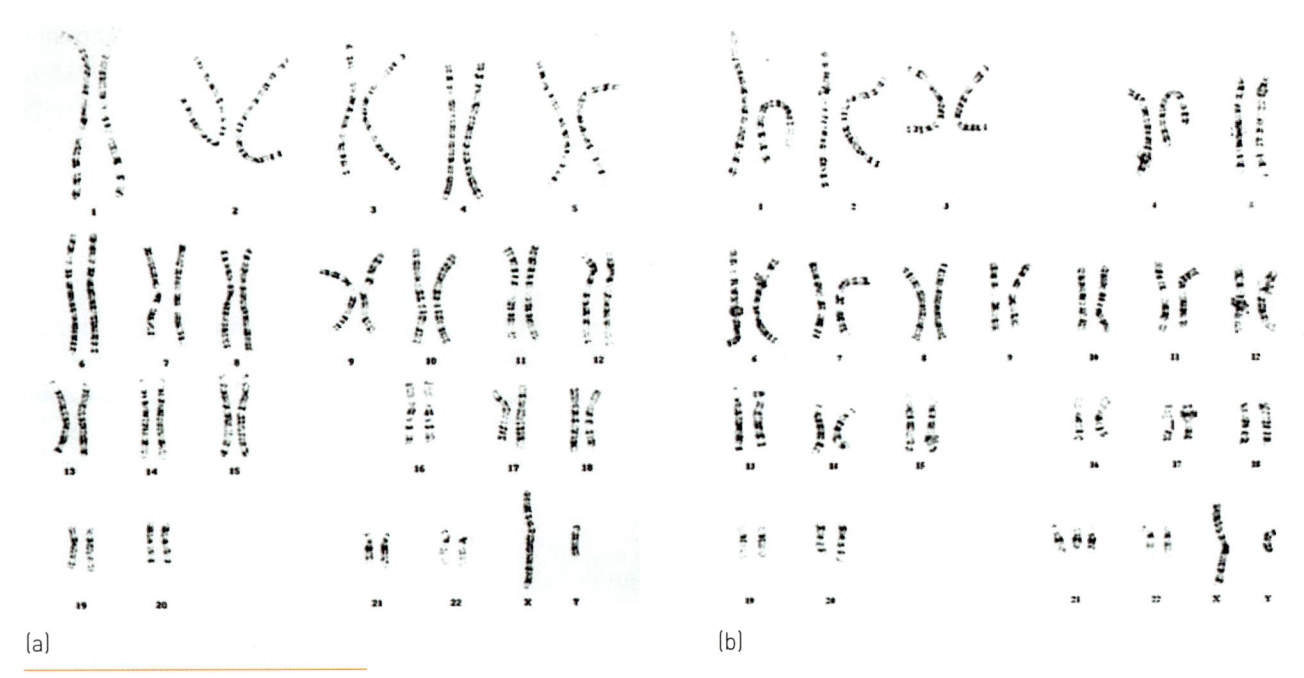

Figure 3.8 – (a) Normal female karyotype and (b) karyotype of an individual with Down syndrome.
(a) Note that the autosomes are grouped in similar pairs, with a single pair of sex chromosomes – in this case, the karyotype is described as 46,XX, meaning 23 pairs of chromosomes with two of them being X chromosomes. (b) This karyotype is described as 47,XX,+21 and is characteristic of an individual with Down syndrome – there is an extra copy (known as trisomy) of chromosome 21. Reproduced from Binns, V. and Hsu, N. (2001) Prenatal Diagnosis, eLS, © 2001 John Wiley & Sons, Ltd.

an extra chromosome representing Down syndrome is shown in *Figure 3.8b* and Alexei (Patient 3.2) has Down syndrome). Chromosomal abnormalities usually occur during the cell division process of meiosis, which occurs exclusively within germ cells, or during mitosis within somatic cells. The karyotype is a useful tool for the clinical geneticist in the diagnosis of genetic disorders and birth defects. Chromosomal abnormalities are sometimes, but not always, lethal to the individual.

3.2.3 Cell division

Mitosis
Dividing somatic cells form a population or 'clone' of genetically identical cells. This is because the process of somatic cell division (called **mitosis**) results in two genetically identical 'daughter' cells. Mitosis can be thought of as a cycle with a series of distinct phases (see *Figure 3.9*). When a cell is formed after mitosis, it may either enter a resting state or begin to enter another round of cell division. The stages of the cell cycle are as follows.

Resting
- G_0: this is the gap 0 or resting stage and represents the stage in which most of our body cells can be found as they metabolize, express genes and function normally. In this phase, the tightly coiled chromosomes relax and are not visible under a light microscope. In G_0, the cell may have temporarily or permanently left the cell cycle.

Interphase
A cell preparing to divide enters a period of growth and metabolism called **interphase**. Within interphase are three discrete phases called G_1, S and G_2:

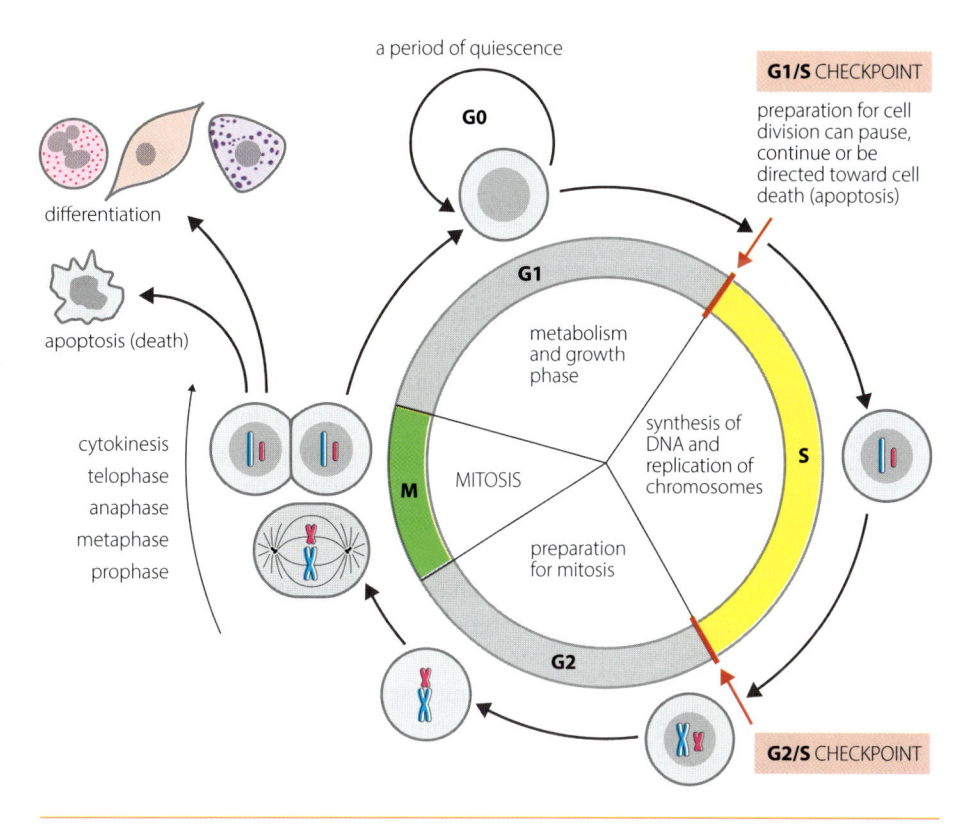

SECTION 3.2 | WHAT YOU NEED TO KNOW – ESSENTIAL ANATOMY AND PHYSIOLOGY

Figure 3.9 – The cell cycle.
Cell division represents a brief period in the cell cycle and is subdivided into five short phases. When cells escape the cell cycle, they enter G0 until division is required again. Alternatively, they may become terminally differentiated or may die through a process known as apoptosis.

- G_1: during this first **gap** phase, the cell grows and prepares to express proteins necessary for DNA synthesis; from here, the cell can continue round the cycle or can enter the resting phase, G_0
- S phase: during this *synthesis* phase, replication of DNA occurs to produce two identical copies of DNA (as 92 chromosomes)
- G_2: during the second **gap** phase, the cell organizes the structures required for the separation of the replicated DNA (in chromosomes) between the two daughter cells.

As the cell moves from one part of interphase to another, it passes through various **checkpoints**. The boundaries between the G_1 and S phase and between the G_2 and S phase are known as the G_1/S and G_2/S checkpoints, respectively. These checkpoints are sensitive to conditions of stress, allowing a cell to halt cell division and undergo repair; that is, they *check* that conditions are favourable for replication and allow DNA repair processes to occur if necessary. If the cellular stress is too great, the cell can undergo a self-destruct process called **apoptosis**. The molecular processes involved within these checkpoints are of great interest because they are informative about clinical conditions involving altered processes of cell division, such as occurs in cancer.

Mitosis

The actual act of division, the M or <u>m</u>itosis phase (*Figure 3.10*), represents only a relatively short period in the life of the cell, but it contains four main phases, culminating in the final act of cell division known as cytokinesis.

- **Prophase:** within the nucleus, replicated chromatin becomes highly organized and tightly coiled to form condensed chromosomes. Each of the original 46 chromosomes is paired with its duplicated copy and held close together at the **centromere** as **sister chromatids**. During prophase, two centrioles within the cell initiate the organization of cytoskeletal microtubular proteins into a complex called a spindle. The nuclear membrane then breaks down and the centrioles migrate to each end of the cell; the sister chromatids attach to the spindle at the centromere.
- **Metaphase:** chromatid pairs can be seen to be pulled by the spindle through the cytoplasm towards the middle of the cell where they become aligned.
- **Anaphase:** contraction in the spindle apparatus attached to the sister chromatids causes the centrosome holding the chromatid pairs to break down and the sister chromatids begin to separate (each forming a separate chromosome) and move towards opposite ends of the cell, pulling apart the replicated chromosomes so that one complete set (23 pairs of chromosomes) can be found at either end of the cell.
- **Telophase:** the spindle apparatus disintegrates, a new nuclear membrane forms around each set of chromosomes and these begin to uncoil.

Finally, the process of **cytokinesis** occurs. The plasma membrane invaginates, separating the two newly formed nuclei and forming two new **genetically identical** cells, which can then separate. During the process, organelles such as the Golgi apparatus and endoplasmic reticulum become fragmented, but others such as mitochondria are preserved and become distributed between the newly formed cells.

Meiosis

This form of cell division is reserved for the production of the gametes, the sperm and ovum (a process known as gametogenesis). Gametes are haploid, containing half the number of chromosomes (23) of our diploid body (somatic) cells. There are some important differences in the process of division between mitosis and meiosis (see *Figure 3.11*):

- meiosis generates haploid cells
- each haploid gamete produced by meiosis will contain just one chromosome obtained from each of the 23 pairs of chromosomes
- meiosis consists of two consecutive divisions of the nucleus to produce daughter cells
- each gamete cell produced through meiosis is genetically unique – this is the basis of genetic diversity.

PROPHASE
chromatin condenses into chromosomes

METAPHASE
nuclear envelope disappears
chromosomes align at the equatorial plate

ANAPHASE
sister chromatids separate
centromeres divide

TELOPHASE
chromatin expands
cytoplasm divides

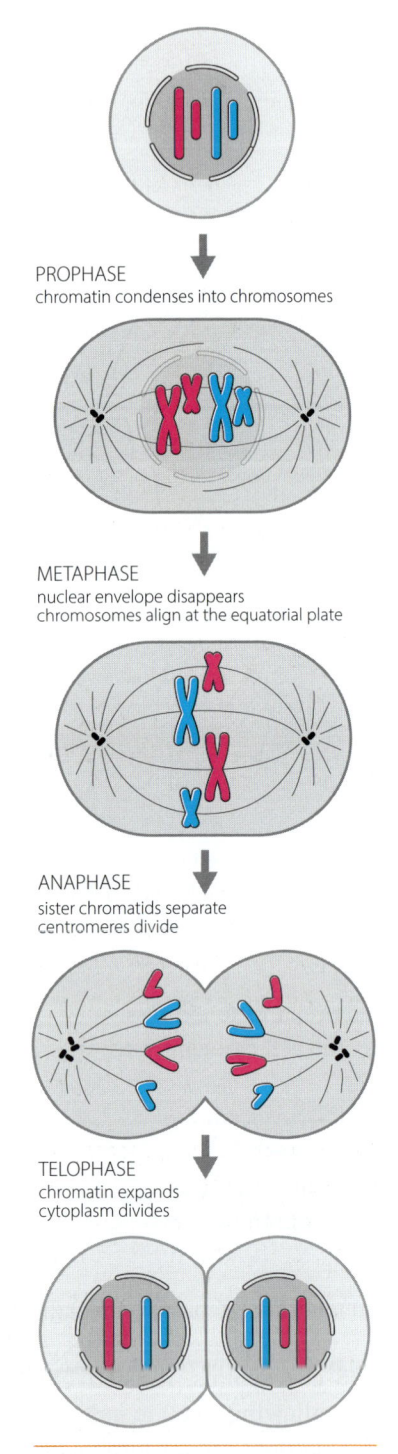

Figure 3.10 – **The stages of mitosis.**
Note that the number of chromosomes present in the figure has been reduced for clarity.

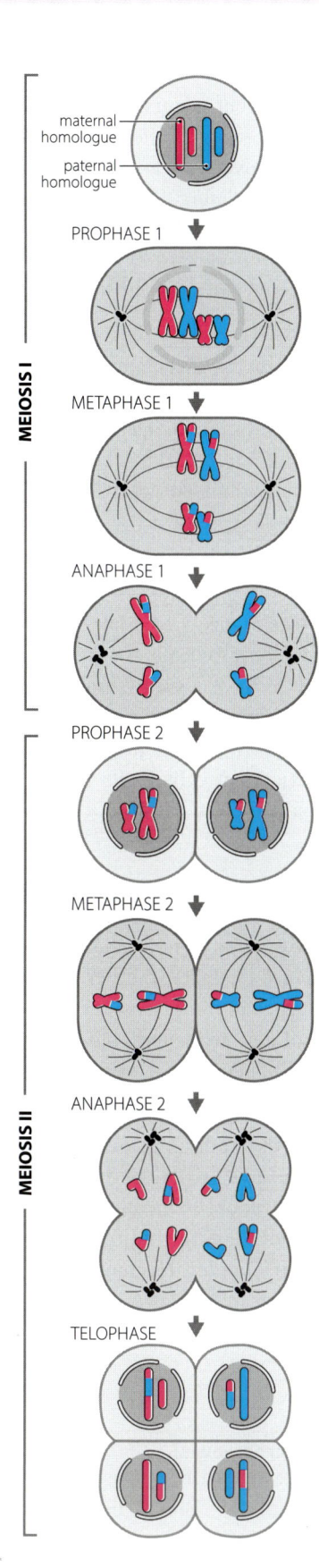

Meiosis I
During prophase of the first division (meiosis I), each pair of replicated chromosomes align together to form four chromatids known as a 'tetrad'. During this event, the chromosomes become very tightly bundled together, and this close association allows segments of DNA from homologous chromatids to be exchanged; this crossing-over of DNA between paternal and maternal arms of homologous chromosomes is known as recombination and it is this process that generates DNA sequence variation (described below). When chromatid pairs align across the middle of the cell during metaphase, they do so regardless of whether the chromosome was maternally or paternally inherited. When anaphase occurs, the centromeres remain intact so that the chromosomes do not separate, but remain as a pair of chromatids pulled towards each end of the cell. This gives rise to another source of genetic variation called **independent assortment** (sources of genetic variation are discussed below). As anaphase ends, the cytoplasm organizes into two parts and a nuclear membrane forms around the chromosomes.

Meiosis II
The second phase of meiosis is very much like mitosis, except that there is no S phase; that is, chromosomes are not replicated but the previously duplicated copies are instead separated further to make a total of four daughter cells. Each new cell is haploid and contains half of the total genetic material; importantly, these cells are no longer genetically identical and contain a mixture of maternal and paternal chromosomes.

Genetic variation
Meiosis is used to generate genetic diversity and it achieves this is in two ways: the random distribution of maternal and paternal chromosomes between daughter cells (independent assortment), and the exchange of DNA between maternal and paternal chromosomes (recombination).

Independent assortment
During the process of making the sperm and ovum by meiosis, the gametes will end up with only one chromosome from each chromosome pair (one chromosome no. 1, one chromosome no. 2, etc.). Depending on the alignment of the homologous chromosomes at the middle of the cell during anaphase, the chromosome could be either maternal or paternal (*Figure 3.12*). This process of separation is called **independent assortment** because the process is thought to be a random or independent event. The sperm and ovum will contain a combination of maternal or paternal chromosomes; the number of possible combinations is huge – because there are 23 chromosome pairs, there are 2^{23} ($2 \times 2 \times 2 \ldots 23$ times = >8 million) possible combinations of maternal/paternal chromosomes that could be distributed to each gamete. This helps to explain why closely related members of a family with the same parents, although genetically similar, are also different.

Figure 3.11 – The stages of meiosis.
Note that in meiosis II, chromosomes are not replicated, but are separated into newly formed haploid sex cells (sperm and ovum). Compare this with mitosis (*Figure 3.10*) where the end result is diploid somatic (body) cells.

Figure 3.12 – Independent assortment.
Twenty-three pairs of chromosomes undergo meiosis to produce two haploid gametes. Each gamete inherits one chromosome from each pair – each chromosome could be a maternal or a paternal one, so there are millions of potential combinations.

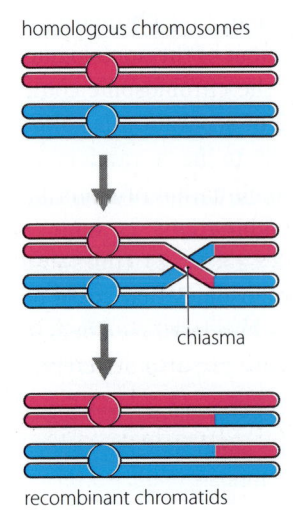

Recombination

During prophase in meiosis I, before independent assortment occurs, homologous chromosomes become closely aligned together in a process called **synapsis**. Sometimes, a segment of DNA on one chromosome crosses over onto another closely aligned chromosome and DNA is physically exchanged (see *Figure 3.13*). This event generates new sequences of DNA and the reorganization of maternal and paternal alleles. It is a complex process that occurs frequently on certain chromosomes and less frequently on others. It is an important source of variation in the human genome responsible for variety in the types of genes (alleles) that exist.

Recombination can also occur within somatic cells. It occurs frequently among chromosomes containing genes involved with immunity to infection. For example, the diversity of alleles present within the human population that code for the major histocompatibility complex (MHC) (discussed in *Chapter 11*) has been used to explain why people appear to have different individual susceptibilities to infectious diseases.

Mutations

Mutations represent a change in the DNA sequence (see *Figure 3.14*) and they are either inherited from a parent or acquired during a person's lifetime. If a mutation occurs in a differentiated somatic cell, it is unlikely to have a significant effect on the observable phenotype, because it is the overall population of cells present within an organ that exerts an overwhelming effect on an organ's physiological function. However, if mutations occur within somatic stem cells (cells that are capable of cell division), then the mutation can be passed on to daughter cells, as occurs in the development of some cancers.

Mutations that occur within germ cells are arguably the most important because (following fertilization) these can be passed on to the cells of future generations. The consequences depend on whether the mutation (altered genotype) actually has an effect on the phenotype and, if it does have an effect, whether this is beneficial or deleterious. There are many different types of mutations, including deletion of DNA bases or the addition and insertion of new sequences, but a more detailed examination of these is beyond the scope of this book.

Mutations can be induced by physical or chemical agents (known as mutagens), which increase the frequency of mutations above the spontaneous mutation rate. Common mutagens include the radiation from X-rays or radioactive decay, ultraviolet light, and chemicals such as those in tobacco smoke or alcohol, or those that occur as a result of human industrial activity. In addition, the highly reactive free radicals generated by mitochondria (discussed in *Chapter 11*) may also act as mutagens. Mutations can also occur through errors in the DNA replication process itself, although these are rare events.

Figure 3.13 – Genetic recombination (sometimes called cross-over).
The arms of homologous chromosomes cross over and exchange DNA nucleotides. This generates a new sequence of DNA code. Sometimes this alters the code for making proteins and has biological consequences.

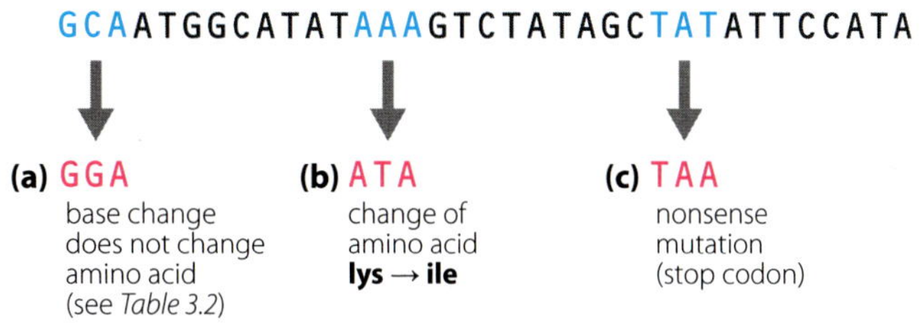

GCAATGGCATATAAAGTCTATAGCTATATTCCATA

(a) **GGA**
base change
does not change
amino acid
(see *Table 3.2*)

(b) **ATA**
change of
amino acid
lys → ile

(c) **TAA**
nonsense
mutation
(stop codon)

Figure 3.14 – Effect of single base mutations.
Sometimes a base change has no impact such as in (a) where a single change from GCA to GGA still codes for glycine (see *Table 3.2*), or it can change the amino acid coded, such as in (b) where a change from AAA to ATA changes the amino acid from lysine to isoleucine, or it can actually stop further production of the polypeptide, such as in (c) where a change from TAT to TAA produces a stop codon, which is likely to have a significant effect on protein synthesis.

It is important to recognize that the mutations that occur within germ cells represent a driving force behind evolution. Mutations sometimes cause disease, but they can also lead to advantageous changes. The generation of new genotypes containing beneficial mutations increases the probability of successful survival and reproduction, and such mutations are essential for the survival and evolution of all species, including humans.

Over evolutionary time, an accumulation of mutations within the genome can give rise to many genetic variants within genes. Gene variants occurring in gametes that represent single nucleotide changes detectable within at least 1% of the population are referred to as **single nucleotide polymorphisms (SNPs)**. These SNPs are useful in healthcare because they can act as markers for the location of genes associated with disease, indicating an individual's susceptibility to disease. Knowledge about SNPs is likely to inform future healthcare by influencing strategies for improving public health and personalized healthcare.

3.2.4 Application of genetics to healthcare

The importance of pedigree

An accurate record of a family history (drawn out as a pedigree diagram) is important in clinical genetics because it provides valuable clues for clinicians about a likely genetic diagnosis. It also provides background information to guide further exploration and counselling for family members affected by clinical disorders arising out of chromosomal abnormalities or genetic disease.

There are about 4000 known genetic disorders caused by mutations in single genes. These are classified as 'Mendelian' or single-gene disorders because a predictable pattern of inheritance of these disorders can be traced through generations within families. They are observed to follow the general principles of inheritance first elucidated by Gregor Mendel in the 19th century. Mendelian disorders arising from mutations in a single gene can be seen relatively easily in a pedigree chart, and the probability of them occurring in future generations can be quantified.

A pedigree diagram (see *Figure 3.15*) shows family relationships using symbols and connected lines (parents by a vertical line and siblings by a horizontal line). Those affected by a genetic condition are usually recorded as a 'filled-in' symbol. If possible, three generations are recorded, including all grandparents, parents and siblings of affected members. An internationally agreed set of symbols and instructions are used to create the pedigree. The information is interpreted according to Mendelian principles, to reveal whether the phenotypic trait was inherited and, if it was, the pattern of inheritance.

Patterns of inheritance

As described above, genes are inherited in pairs, but each gene can be inherited as one of a variety of forms called alleles. Different alleles may cause different phenotypes, sometimes called traits or characteristics. If both genes of a pair are identical, an individual is said to be **homozygous** for the gene. If the pair of alleles is not identical, then the individual is **heterozygous** for the gene. When an individual is heterozygous for a gene, it is the 'dominant' characteristic that is expressed – note that it is the characteristic or phenotype that is dominant and not the gene or allele. A 'recessive' characteristic will only be expressed when an individual is homozygous for the gene that produces that characteristic. Thus, an individual can exhibit dominant or recessive traits, depending on whether they are homozygous or heterozygous for the particular gene. Two important points to recognize are as follows:

- Individuals expressing dominant traits (perhaps a feature of a specific disease) will also have an affected parent (this will be evident from a pedigree chart), because the parent will have passed this allele on to their children (see *Figure 3.15a*).
- Individuals who possess recessive traits might have parents and grandparents who are not affected (see *Figure 3.15b*), but both of their parents would be carriers of the recessive allele. The offspring of two affected parents will all express the trait, because in order to express the condition, both parents will be homozygous for the recessive allele.

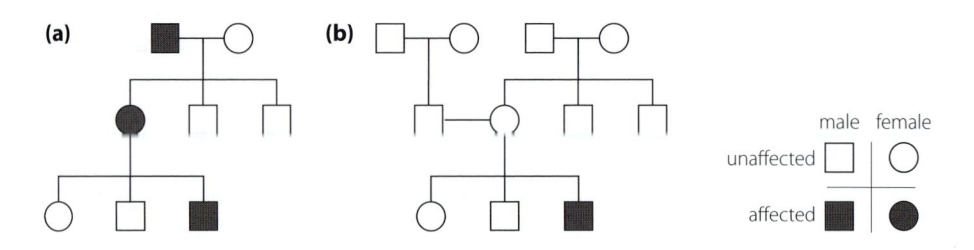

Figure 3.15 – Examples of pedigree charts.
(a) Typical autosomal dominant inheritance; note that the condition occurs in every generation. (b) Typical autosomal recessive inheritance; note that the condition can be observed to 'skip' generations – the allele for the recessive condition may be present, but it is the allele for the dominant condition that is expressed to provide an observable phenotype.

The pedigree is a useful tool, but interpretation of it is not always clear-cut. Some traits are not completely dominant, giving rise to a variable expression, and sometimes a number of genes may interact to modify the expression of alleles. The extent of an allele's effect on a specific trait, both within an individual and within the population, can in part be measured and explained by the concepts of penetrance and expressivity; although these concepts are beyond the scope of this book, suggestions for further reading are provided at the end of the chapter.

Not all disorders caused by alterations to DNA are inherited; for example, when genetic abnormalities occur only in somatic cells and not in germ cells, they will not be passed on to the next generation. Some disorders are caused by new mutations not previously present within a family, and so a pedigree chart will be uninformative. Chromosomal disorders can be inherited, but often they are not, because they are frequently caused by a problem in the process of cell division involving meiosis in germ cells, or mitosis in a developing embryo.

A chromosomal disorder: Down syndrome

An abnormal number of chromosomes in a cell is termed **aneuploidy**. This represents a gross abnormality and tends to have significant effects on phenotype. Down syndrome is caused by **trisomy** of all or part of chromosome 21 (see Alexei, Patient 3.2). The extra chromosome can be observed (see karyotype in *Figure 3.8b*) free or fused onto another chromosome. Chromosome 21 contains at least 300 genes; some of these code for several proteins that affect how cells function and influence development – the function of the remainder is not yet known. A wide range of phenotypic consequences of this chromosomal abnormality are observed, including altered neurological development, altered development of morphology and intelligence, earlier development of Alzheimer's disease, decreased muscle tone and increased risk of congenital heart disease.

There can be a great deal of phenotypic variation in people affected by Down syndrome and this can sometimes be explained by the concept of **mosaicism**. Mosaicism (illustrated in *Figure 3.16*) represents a mixture of genetically

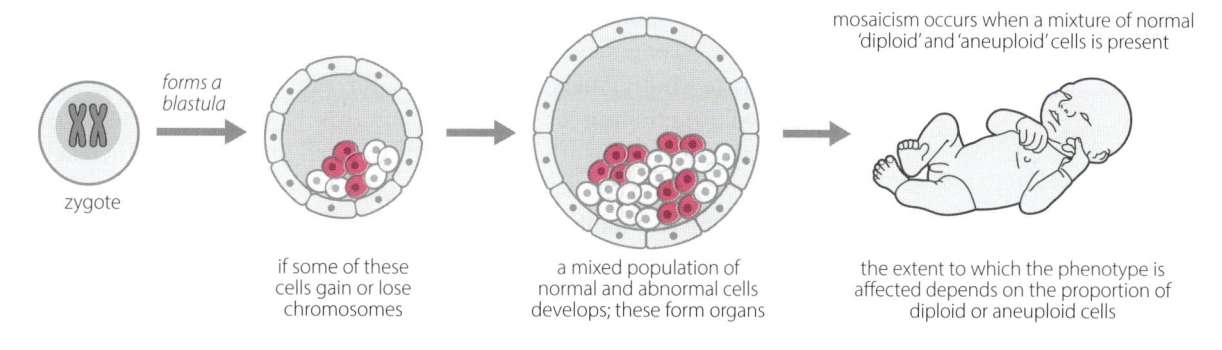

Figure 3.16 – Mosaicism.
Mosaicism can occur when the chromosomal number of some cells is altered during the early stages of embryonic development. The fetus then develops with a mixture of diploid and aneuploid cells. The phenotype of organs can be affected, depending on the proportion of diploid or aneuploid cells.

abnormal and normal cells present in an organism. If the event that causes an extra chromosome 21 occurs during an early stage of development of an embryo and *not* during meiosis, then a child will be born with some normal and some abnormal cells within the tissues, causing the expression of a range of phenotypes. This might involve more or less intellectual impairment or degrees of impairment in organ function. There is no known treatment for Down syndrome, but sequencing of chromosome 21 was an early and important goal of the Human Genome Project, in the hope that the molecular basis for Down syndrome could be better understood.

An autosomal recessive single-gene disorder: cystic fibrosis

In cystic fibrosis (see Sarah, Patient 3.1), the disease is the result of a mutation in a single gene on an autosome and not on a sex chromosome. As a single-gene disorder, the clinical condition is caused by only one faulty gene and is not reliant on the interaction of other genes. Cystic fibrosis is a recessive condition and so the disease is only expressed in individuals homozygous for the affected allele; in other words, two copies of the mutated gene must be present.

Cystic fibrosis is one of the most common inherited life-threatening conditions, affecting approximately 5% of the general population. It is caused by a mutation in the gene that codes for the 'cystic fibrosis transmembrane conductance transporter' (CFTR) protein. This protein is particularly expressed on intestinal and airway epithelial cells, but also in other tissues. It provides a channel for the transport of chloride ions across the plasma membrane. In patients with cystic fibrosis, the CFTR protein is not expressed and patients usually present with intestinal and breathing problems; for example, viscous mucus accumulates in the lungs and reduces lung function, causing breathing difficulties and respiratory tract infections. Digestive glands also become blocked, interfering with digestion and the absorption of nutrients (see Sarah, Patient 3.1). Cystic fibrosis is a lethal disorder, but improved clinical management of the condition has resulted in patient survival now commonly over 30 years of age.

For a lethal condition, the frequency of carriers with the affected *CFTR* allele within the population is relatively high. This suggests that the mutated gene might have some benefits in certain environments; this is called 'heterozygote advantage'. Individuals heterozygous for the mutated *CFTR* gene might have reduced functioning of the gene, but this is insufficient to cause clinically recognizable disease. It has been hypothesized that reduced efficiency of chloride transport across the epithelial wall of the gastrointestinal tract, as occurs in cystic fibrosis, might provide a survival advantage against diarrhoeal diseases such as cholera. Thus, mutations can be beneficial depending on environmental conditions. It is important to consider phenotype as a product of the genotype interacting within an environmental context.

A change to a single DNA base: sickle cell disease

Sickle cell disease is the most common genetic condition in the UK, estimated to affect 12 500 people. Approximately, 240 000 people are estimated to be carriers of the condition and about 300 babies per year are born with the condition in the UK. It occurs most frequently in people with a black African or Afro-Caribbean ancestry. Symptoms can be mild, highly variable and episodic, the most common symptom being pain, especially in the bones (see Yasmeen, Patient 3.4). However, complications can be life-threatening and include stroke (bleeding into the brain), damage to the spleen and acute lung syndrome. Sickle cell disease is caused by the formation of abnormal haemoglobin, which causes erythrocytes (red blood cells) to become sickle-shaped, fragile and unable to carry oxygen efficiently; their altered shape means that they can also become stuck within small blood vessels, further reducing the amount of oxygen that can reach tissues.

Sickle cell disease is another example of an autosomal recessive condition. However, although heterozygotes usually do not experience significant clinical symptoms, they can be affected. Heterozygotes produce a mixture of normal and abnormal haemoglobin because they possess one normal and one abnormal allele; as both alleles are expressed this is an example of *codominance*.

The haemoglobin protein used to carry oxygen and carbon dioxide within erythrocytes (discussed in *Chapter 10*) contains a polypeptide chain called ß-globin consisting of 146 amino acids. In normal haemoglobin, the sixth codon on mRNA coding for the ß-globin chain codes for the amino acid glutamic acid. A single change to a nucleotide within the codon for glutamic acid can alter the codon to represent instead the amino acid valine (see *Figure 3.17*) and it is this single amino acid change that is responsible for altering the function of the haemoglobin protein to the sickle condition.

An autosomal dominant disorder: hypertrophic cardiomyopathy

With dominant disorders, an affected gene will always be expressed, even if the individual is heterozygous and also carries a 'normal' gene. A general feature of autosomal dominant disorders is that if a parent possesses the mutated gene they will have the condition and any children will have a 50% chance of inheriting the mutated gene.

(a)

NORMAL □-HAEMOGLOBIN

ATG–GTG–CAC–CTG–ACT–CCT–GAG–GAG–AAG–TCT–GCC–GTT–ACT——— RNA code
start val his leu thr pro glu glu lys ser ala val thr ——— amino acid sequence

ABNORMAL □-HAEMOGLOBIN

ATG–GTG–CAC–CTG–ACT–CCT–GTG–GAG–AAG–TCT–GCC–GTT–ACT
start val his leu thr pro val glu lys ser ala val thr

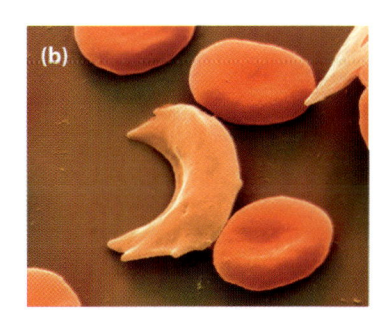

Figure 3.17 – Sickle cell disease.
(a) In this example of a mutation, a single nucleotide change has caused a change in the code for an amino acid (from glutamine to valine), altering the structure and function of the protein and resulting in sickle cell disease. (b) Sickle cell anaemia. Coloured SEM showing normal and sickle erythrocytes. Science Photo Library.

Hypertrophic cardiomyopathy (HCM; see Katherine, Patient 3.3) is the most common inherited cardiac condition, affecting approximately 1:500 of the general population. It is caused by a large variety of mutations in several genes encoding sarcomere proteins, which are normally expressed in cardiac muscle cells. The mutations cause the cardiac muscle to become enlarged and disorganized, and so patients with this disease may experience a variety of symptoms, including chest pain, sudden loss of consciousness and heart failure. HCM is recognized as the primary common cause of heart-related sudden death in young people, and secondary to the primary disease is an increased risk of abnormal heart rhythms and stroke.

Clinical presentation of HCM is very variable, with little consistent presentation of symptoms by patients, even within affected families. Some patients may not have any obvious disease, while other affected family members experience severe symptoms. Many factors probably act together to influence the disease, but much of this variability can be explained by the variability of mutations involved in several genes. In addition, polymorphisms in hormones that directly or indirectly influence the circulatory system (so-called 'modifier genes'), diet, exercise and blood pressure may also act together to influence development and progression of the disease.

Diagnosis often follows the sudden unexplained death of a relative, followed by examination of family histories and the construction of a pedigree. Management can involve medication, cardiac ablation, implantable cardiac devices and heart transplantation. Careful history taking, counselling, screening and surveillance of at-risk family members are important considerations that carry significant implications for those affected.

A sex-linked recessive disease disorder: haemophilia

Haemophilia is an X-linked inherited bleeding disorder, in which a protein required for blood clotting is reduced or missing, and so patients bleed for longer than normal. Small cuts or bruises do not cause significant problems, but larger cuts and traumatic injuries can be life-threatening.

The X chromosome is much longer than the Y chromosome and contains many more genes (most of which have nothing to do with sex determination). When alleles on the X chromosome are expressed to produce a trait or a disease, they are said to be **X-linked**. The majority of X-linked conditions are recessive, which means that a woman (who has two X chromosomes) will not usually develop the condition because she will also be carrying the dominant allele (from her other X chromosome), which will ensure normal function. However, if a male child inherits the recessive allele on the X chromosome, he will develop the condition because all genes on his single X chromosome will be expressed (he inherits a Y chromosome from his father). Two general patterns of X-linked inheritance can be observed:

- a non-affected father paired with a mother carrying the affected gene have a 50% probability of producing a son with the disease (see *Figure 3.18*)
- a non-affected father paired with a mother carrying the affected gene have a 50% chance of producing a daughter who carries the affected gene but does not have the disease (see *Figure 3.18*).

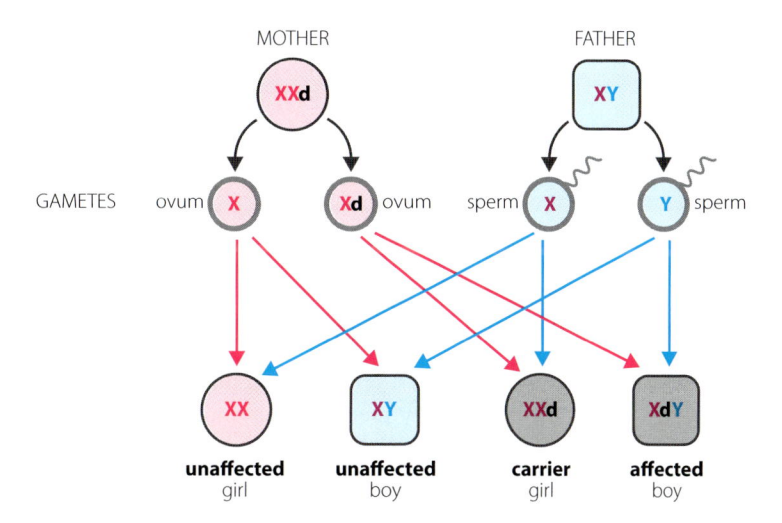

Figure 3.18 – Patterns of X-linked inheritance.
The affected allele (d) is present on the X chromosome, in this example carried by the mother. Note the expected frequencies of unaffected, carrier and affected children.

Blood clotting involves the interaction of blood cells and a variety of clotting proteins present in plasma in an extensive 'clotting cascade' to stop bleeding (haemostasis). Mutations in the genes coding for the clotting proteins reduce the efficiency of the blood clotting cascade. Haemophilia type A is the commonest type of haemophilia and is caused by a deficiency in a blood clotting protein known as factor VIII. The gene coding for factor VIII is found on the X chromosome and so the disease is usually found in the sons of female carriers of the mutated gene. The mutation responsible for haemophilia can occur spontaneously within germ cells in a family that does not have a previous history of haemophilia, but the mechanism by which this occurs is not known.

Four of the five clinical examples described earlier (the exception is HCM) refer to single-gene mutations that cause patterns of inheritance that are relatively easy to observe through successive generations. Clinical geneticists and genetic counsellors, by taking a family history and constructing a pedigree, are able to glean useful information for the management of affected and potentially affected relatives. This information is important for patients for decision making, such as whether or not to have children, and what lifestyle choices to make.

Genes and cancer

When mutations in somatic cells occur, they can sometimes provide cells with an abnormal ability to survive independently of normal regulatory mechanisms and to invade other tissues. When these abnormal cells accumulate, they form malignant **tumours**, commonly called cancers. A full discussion of the process of carcinogenesis is a complex subject beyond the scope of this text. However, it is worth understanding some of the key features that represent the 'hallmarks of cancer' (as proposed by Hanahan and Weinberg in 2000); they proposed the six hallmarks of cancer cells to be their ability to:

1. divide independently of positive regulatory controls
2. divide independently of negative regulatory controls
3. divide indefinitely, without growing old
4. avoid apoptosis (signals to self-destruct)
5. form a life-sustaining circulation (angiogenesis)
6. grow into other tissues and establish growth into distant tissues (invasion and metastasis).

More recently, in 2011, Hanahan and Weinberg proposed four additional hallmarks, as follows:

7. deregulated metabolism, for example, the use of abnormal cellular respiratory mechanisms to obtain energy
8. ability to evade normal regulatory controls of the immune system
9. ability to become genetically unstable
10. association with inflammation.

Mutations can assist with gaining these hallmarks in two main ways.

- Increased growth and survival advantage: if a mutation allows a cell to divide faster or more frequently and survive, then any abnormality will be retained by all mutated future cells. Cancer occurring in solid organs will form a larger mass of cells, recognizable as a lump or tumour.
- Increased genetic instability: if dividing cells accumulate mutations over successive generations, then the likelihood of generating abnormal cells that contribute to development of the hallmarks of cancer will be increased. When examined, cancer cells are observed to contain many more mutations and even gross chromosomal abnormalities in comparison with normal cells.

Colon cancer

Only 10% of colon cancers are inherited, with the majority of cases being due to the accumulation of genetic alterations over time in colonic epithelial cells (this occurs in approximately 1 in 20 people in the UK population).

Genetic abnormalities that accumulate within the epithelial cells of the colon occur in a multistage, stepwise manner, and so observation of the state of these cells can be used to gauge how far tissue in the colon has developed towards cancer (see *Figure 3.19*). One of the most commonly mutated genes found in colon cancer is the adenomatous polyposis coli (*APC*) gene. This normally functions as a tumour suppressor; that is, the protein encoded by the *APC* gene normally functions to suppress cell division by repressing the activity of a number of proteins that normally promote cell division (see 'hallmarks of cancer' discussed above). When the *APC* gene becomes mutated, it often codes for a protein that is shorter than the normal protein. Any somatic cell in the colon producing a shortened APC protein will no longer be able to suppress cell division and so growth of these cells continues unchecked; the overgrowths of the colonic mucosae that develop are called polyps. The polyps have gained a growth advantage and will have taken a first step towards the development of cancer. When mutation in the *APC* gene occurs in a stem cell, this will affect all future cells, which will all express abnormal APC protein. The affected cells are predominantly mucosal epithelial cells of the large intestine, and polyps develop along the whole of the large intestine (see *Figure 3.19*).

normal colonic mucosa → becomes hyperproliferative → multiple polyps develop → progress to carcinoma

mutations in key regulatory genes including cell cycle, DNA repair and others

increasing genetic instability

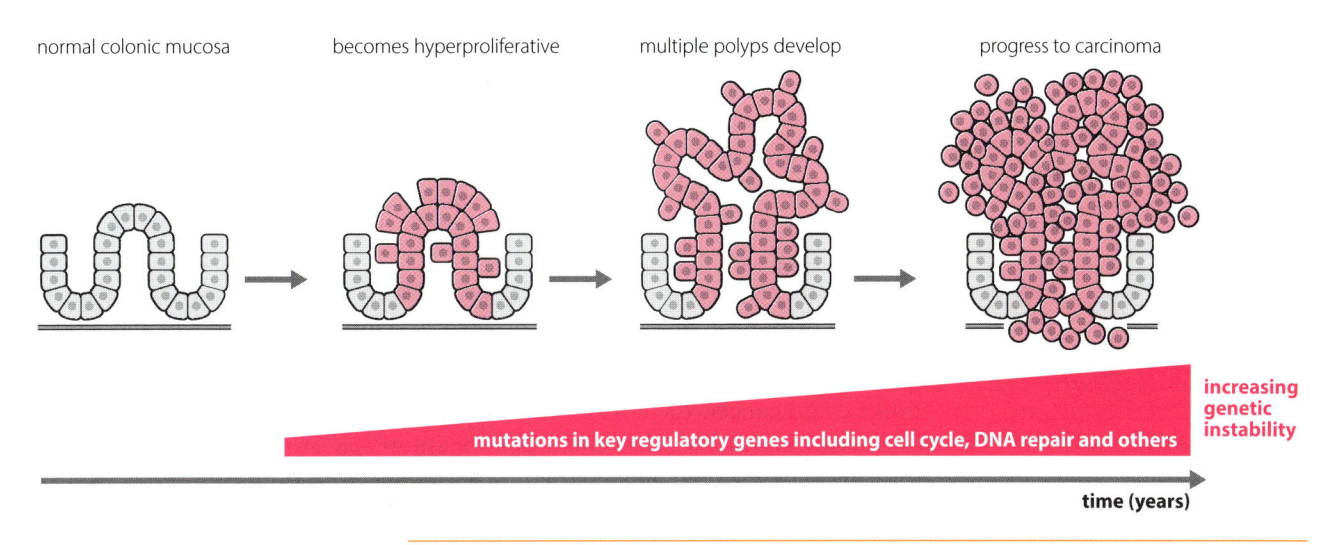

time (years)

Figure 3.19 – **Mutations in epithelial cells leading towards colon cancer.**
It is characterized as a stepwise process over many years, involving the gradual accumulation of mutations in key regulatory genes with increasing genetic instability.

A rare inherited disorder called familial adenomatous polyposis (FAP) causes colon cancer at a relatively young age in all individuals with a mutated *APC* (adenomatous polyposis coli) gene. A more common form of inherited colon cancer, affecting approximately 10% of all cases, is referred to as hereditary non-polyposis colon cancer (HNPCC). With HNPCC, the cancer tends to develop at a young age and polyps are also produced, not because of a mutated *APC* gene but because of the involvement of a number of other mutated genes. These are frequently genes that encode proteins involved in the repair of mistakes that occur during the replication of DNA – so-called DNA repair proteins. When mistakes are not repaired, genetic instability tends to increase in the affected cells and the risk of cancer consequently increases.

The treatment options for inherited colon cancer are limited, and most commonly prophylactic colectomy (removal of the colon) at a relatively young age is used to prevent the cancer becoming invasive and harder to eradicate; a colectomy significantly reduces the risk of cancer developing in affected individuals. A screening programme to identify people in the early stages of developing colon cancer is currently being implemented by the NHS and is being offered to anyone over the age of 60 years (see www.cancerscreening.nhs.uk/bowel/). The basis of this screening programme is examination of a small amount of faeces for the presence of 'occult blood' (blood present in tiny amounts not visible to the eye). If blood is detected, then patients are referred for endoscopic examination of their bowel (called a colonoscopy). If polyps are detected, these can usually be removed and examined for the presence of abnormal cells suggestive of cancer. This screening programme is expected to save thousands of lives in the UK annually.

Breast cancer

One in nine women in the UK is likely to develop breast cancer (making it the most common cancer affecting women), and it has become the leading cause of death in women between the ages of 34 and 54 years. It can also occur in men, but much less frequently. As with colon cancer, the majority of cases of breast cancer are sporadic (non-hereditary), but approximately 3% of cases are related to a known inherited breast cancer gene. Sheila (Patient 2.3) does not have a known family history of breast cancer. In the development of Sheila's cancer, her breast (somatic) cells have at some point in her life gained a mutation in the human epidermal growth factor receptor 2 (*HER2*) gene.

Unlike colon cancer, the development of breast cancer does not appear to follow a stepwise progression. The genetic abnormalities appear to accumulate in a more heterogeneous fashion, and a variety of histological types of cancer can develop within the breast. Multiple risk factors have been identified, including ethnicity, diet, exposure to alcohol and smoking. Reproductive factors are important, such as early onset of the menarche, late onset of menopause, giving birth to a first child after the age of 30 and possibly administration of oestrogenic contraceptives. The breast is sensitive to the effects of hormones, in particular oestrogen, progesterone and prolactin, and over-expression of oestrogen receptor genes is a common feature of breast cancer. Therefore, selective oestrogen receptor modulators, such as tamoxifen (a drug that blocks the oestrogen receptor), are used to treat breast cancer and also to prevent its development in women identified as being at high genetic risk for developing breast cancer.

Among others, two specific genes named <u>br</u>east <u>ca</u>ncer susceptibility gene <u>1</u> and <u>2</u> (*BRCA1* and *BRCA2*) have been identified as being important in the development of breast cancer – they are tumour suppressor genes involved in DNA repair, helping to maintain genomic stability and suppress uncontrolled growth of cells. Mutations in *BRCA1/2* inactivate their normal function of repairing damaged DNA and so increase the risk of developing breast cancer (they also may increase the risk of developing ovarian cancer) such that up to 80% of women with specific mutations in these genes will develop breast cancer in their lifetime. However, it is important to note that not all inherited mutations in these genes increase the risk of developing breast cancer. Also, even in families possessing a mutated *BRCA1/2* gene, these mutations will not necessarily be inherited by the daughters. Moreover, not every woman with harmful forms of the gene will go on to develop breast cancer. Although a family history of breast cancer doubles the risk of developing it, approximately 80% of women with a close family member with breast cancer will never develop it themselves.

Other altered genes are also known to influence the risk of developing breast cancer, and genetic tests to identify mutations in *BRCA1/2* and these other genes allow clinicians to estimate the cancer risk for an individual. These tests are generally only offered to individuals with a strong family history at specialist genetic clinics where genetic counselling can be offered to help patients make informed decisions and be supported with the consequences of the information provided to them.

As with many other forms of cancer treatment, treatment for breast cancer usually involves surgery and is often followed by radiotherapy and/or chemotherapy. Sometimes, hormones and biological treatments (as with Sheila, Patient 2.3) are also offered. Prophylactic mastectomy is sometimes considered for women at high risk, for example, those who have a strong family history and are positive for *BRCA1/2* mutations or other mutations.

Diseases involving more than one gene

So far, we have discussed the role of mutations occurring in a specific gene, or a few closely related genes, that have a major effect in causing clinically recognizable disease. These single-gene disorders are convenient to discuss because they provide relatively simple but stark examples of the role of genetics in health and disease. However, single-gene disorders are rare, affecting perhaps just 2% of the population. The majority of genetic disorders involve multiple genes and these are known as polygenic disorders.

Polygenic traits represent phenotypes produced by multiple genes, each exerting a small effect on the overall phenotype. Most human traits including eye colour, skin colour, height and weight are in fact polygenic traits. Some traits such as height and weight may also be affected by environmental factors and as such can be thought of as **multifactorial traits**. This interaction between multiple genes and environmental factors can make it very difficult to identify the alleles involved and the patterns of inheritance occurring within families. Each gene in combination with environmental factors confers a degree of risk or susceptibility towards a particular phenotype. Examples of polygenic and multifactorial diseases include coronary heart disease, diabetes, obesity, Alzheimer's disease and psychoses. Sometimes different combinations of genes produce related 'co-morbid' conditions; for example, a family history of rheumatoid arthritis is also associated with other autoimmune diseases such as systemic lupus erythematosus and multiple sclerosis. The variety of possible genetic alterations that might occur within genes, combined with the probability of inheriting specific combinations of genes, means that studying the effects of individual genes within polygenic disorders becomes complicated and problematic. Data from the Human Genome Project and population studies, integrated with advances in biotechnology and bioinformatics, should help to clarify the genetic contribution to disease.

Gene testing and issues for the individual and society

Currently, genetic testing is able to identify families at high risk of developing diseases such as specific types of cancer, for example colon or breast cancer. This allows affected family members to receive advice and recommended surveillance, and to make treatment and lifestyle choices, in order to minimize the risk of development of the disease.

Genetic alterations that occur in malignant tumours can also be investigated for the presence of specific gene mutations, and appropriate chemotherapeutic agents can then be targeted to the tumours. For example, some patients with advanced colon cancer can be treated effectively with a monoclonal antibody called cetuximab, but only if a gene in their tumour called *KRAS* is *not* mutated (the KRAS protein is a regulator of cell division); cetuximab therapy will not work in patients with a mutated *KRAS* gene in their tumours. Cetuximab therapy, often administered in combination with chemotherapy or radiotherapy, can prolong life and can even eradicate cancer from the body in patients with a specific cancer genotype.

For inherited conditions, identifying genes responsible for disease or those genes that indicate susceptibility can become useful markers of risk and can also be used for diagnosis. However, to date this knowledge has led to just a few limited examples of improved treatment.

Results from the Human Genome Project and the availability of genetic testing have stimulated a number of issues for society to consider including the following:

- Should a patient be screened to confirm the diagnosis of a disease that cannot be treated and does it matter how old the patient is?
- What will the impact of a diagnosis be on an affected person?
- Will a genetic diagnosis influence reproductive choices, or the ability to find work or obtain life insurance?
- Will a genetic diagnosis result in stigmatization and social exclusion?
- Does disability resulting from genetic variation represent disease, or simply difference between people?
- If an inherited condition is diagnosed in an individual, do the family members have a right to the information about it?
- If genetic susceptibility for a condition such as heart disease or obesity can be calculated and modified by a change in lifestyle, can this change be demanded, or even enforced?
- Can genetic information do harm?

Many more questions could be asked and, as our knowledge of the human genome increases, society will be required to respond to them. Clearly, genetic knowledge holds many ethical, legal and societal implications, and our legal system, social institutions and professional bodies are already struggling to keep pace with the rapid advances in genetics and biotechnology. The implications for healthcare practice are huge. The references at the end of this chapter will provide you with a starting point to consider these implications further.

3.3 Clinical application

As we have seen, genes can play an important part in the development of certain diseases. Understanding how genetics can result in particular diseases is important in healthcare in order that suitable explanations can be given to patients and appropriate treatment planned. The patients described in this chapter have covered a range of different genetic problems:

- Sheila (Patient 2.3) has developed breast cancer as a result of a somatic mutation that resulted in the over-expression of HER2 protein on the plasma membrane; it should therefore be possible to treat her cancer by selectively blocking the HER2 receptor and reducing cell division.

- **Sarah (Patient 3.1)** has cystic fibrosis, which has occurred as a result of her inheriting two faulty copies of the *CFTR* gene (remember, cystic fibrosis is an autosomal recessive disorder) and, as a result, Sarah requires daily physiotherapy to keep her lungs clear of viscous mucus, to aid her breathing and to reduce the risk of chest infection.
- **Alexei (Patient 3.2)** has Down syndrome as a result of a chromosomal abnormality (trisomy of chromosome 21). Alexei and his family will require ongoing support for a wide variety of social, psychological and physiological needs, with regular coordinated review of his care to enable Alexei to fully maximize his potential.
- **Katherine (Patient 3.3)** has hypertrophic cardiomyopathy, which is an autosomal dominant condition, and so it is important that Katherine and the rest of her family understand the implications of this for themselves and also for any future children.
- **Yasmeen (Patient 3.4)** has sickle cell anaemia, another autosomal recessive condition, and although she is managing her condition well, she is interested to discuss possible options for treatment.

Patient 2.3 | **Sheila** | 30 | 54 | 59 | **93** | 267 | 304 | 448 | 473

- 47-year-old woman
- Recent diagnosis of breast cancer – biopsy shows cancer cells over-express HER2 protein
- Biological therapy with trastuzumab (Herceptin) to block HER2 action an option
- Is still offered surgery, chemotherapy and radiotherapy
- Agrees to add trastuzumab to chemotherapy plan

Breast cancer cells that express too much HER2 receptor are often described as aggressive, because the cells grow very rapidly, become poorly differentiated and stimulate angiogenesis (see the earlier discussion of the 'hallmarks of cancer'). Over-expression of the HER2 protein is usually caused by multiple copies of the gene formed during the carcinogenic process (called gene amplification). A monoclonal antibody (antibodies are discussed fully in *Chapter 11*) called trastuzumab, when administered to patients, binds specifically to the over-expressed HER2 receptor, preventing it from exerting its effects on cells, reducing the rate of cell division and limiting the growth of new blood vessels (so the carcinogenic effects of HER2 will be reduced). Patients receiving trastuzumab therapy have been observed to demonstrate a significant decrease in the risk of breast cancer reoccurrence when compared with control patients in randomized clinical trials. The therapy is only effective on cancers caused by over-expression of the HER2 receptor, but, in combination with chemotherapy agents, trastuzumab has been shown to improve survival in patients with breast cancer. This is an example of personalized medicine that uses genetic information about the individual to tailor treatment. In consultation with her doctor and breast care nurse, Sheila chose to accept the addition of trastuzumab to the chemotherapy plan for her breast cancer (further discussion of Sheila's care is expanded in *Chapters 2, 9* and *14*). She experienced some minor side-effects, including flu-like symptoms, nausea and fatigue; these only lasted a couple of days and, with the support of her family and the multidisciplinary cancer support team, Sheila is looking forward to an improved prognosis, confirmed by the oncologist looking after her, and she has begun training for a 10K 'fun-run' in aid of cancer research.

Patient 3.1 — Sarah | 60 | **94** | 195 | 237 | 311 | 333

- 17-year-old girl
- CF diagnosis at age of 1 year via a sweat test
- Frequent admissions for chest infections affecting breathing

A sweat test that detects the elevation of salt in sweat was performed on Sarah when she was a baby in order to confirm a diagnosis of cystic fibrosis – remember that the lack of CFTR protein in cystic fibrosis disrupts chloride ion (Cl^-) transport across membranes and so excess salt (NaCl) is found in the sweat. This is a quick and painless procedure involving stimulation of a small patch of skin with the drug pilocarpine to promote sweating. Sweat is simply collected onto an absorbent card and the concentration of sodium chloride measured. Together with a clinical history, this is generally sufficient for a positive diagnosis to be made. In Sarah's case, genetic testing was also performed, and this provided useful information for advising Sarah's family members about their carrier status and will also be useful for Sarah when she starts to make future reproductive choices.

Today, screening for cystic fibrosis is routinely performed as part of the NHS newborn screening programme (https://www.gov.uk/topic/population-screening-programmes/newborn-blood-spot). Midwives generally take a small sample of blood from a newborn baby about 1 week after birth and place some spots of the blood onto a card, which is then sent for analysis. In addition to cystic fibrosis, a variety of other inherited conditions can be detected from this small blood sample, including congenital hypothyroidism, sickle cell disease and two enzyme deficiencies: phenylketonuria and medium-chain acyl-CoA dehydrogenase deficiency.

The carrier status of the relatives of a family member with cystic fibrosis can be discovered by taking a small blood sample or a swab of easily removed cheek cells from the inside of the mouth. This checking of the genetic status of family members is called **cascade screening** and helps to identify who might be at higher risk of being a carrier or of having a child with cystic fibrosis.

Patient 3.2 — Alexei | 60 | **94**

- 14-year-old boy
- Down syndrome – trisomy of chromosome 21
- Now withdrawn and disruptive; some breathlessness

Alexei lives a full and busy life, but recently, as he develops into a young adult, a variety of challenges have begun to present to him. Socially and educationally, Alexei probably will not develop at a comparable rate to his peers; as a result, he will be less able to keep up with his friends at school, and recently he has frequently been left out of activities. Alexei's real passion is for golf, but bouts of breathlessness have begun to interfere with this. Alexei is at risk of a wide variety of physiological challenges due to the altered expression of genes located on chromosome 21. He is due to receive a hospital appointment soon to assess his health status. This will include hearing and dietary assessments, X-rays to assess his skeletal development, a variety of blood tests including a measurement of haemoglobin concentration, and a cardiology assessment. His recent bouts of breathlessness while playing golf are worrying his mother, Adelia, who knows heart defects are common in children with Down syndrome.

Patient 3.3 — Katherine

- 41-year-old woman
- Recent diagnosis of hypertrophic cardiomyopathy
- ECG shows arrhythmia and USS shows thickened left ventricle
- Given warfarin to reduce stroke risk and anti-arrhythmic drugs
- Genetic tests on one daughter

Katherine has been prescribed the anticoagulant drug warfarin to reduce her risk of stroke, and anti-arrhythmic drugs to improve the altered heart rhythm and function of her heart. She has also been advised to have regular reviews with the specialist cardiology team.

Katherine was also referred to a clinical geneticist, and this consultation revealed a family history suggestive of heart disease inherited in an autosomal dominant manner. This led to the extended family getting together and discussing the history of health and early death in the family: one of Katherine's uncles on her father's side underwent a heart and lung transplant some years ago, and one of her cousins died suddenly at 17 years of age. DNA was collected from the family for a research project and Katherine was offered a gene test, but none of the commonly affected genes was identified. However, the clinical geneticist informed Katherine that this is not unusual because the condition is caused by the interaction of several genes, and not all genes implicated in causing the condition have so far been identified.

Katherine has two daughters aged 19 and 22 years; one has agreed to undergo annual electrocardiography and echocardiography to screen for HCM. Her other daughter has declined the offer of annual surveillance, saying, 'If I've got it and you can't cure it, I might as well forget it.' Her sister, on the other hand, is considering getting married and wants to know what the implications might be for her future children. The genetic nurse counsellor informs her that there is a 50% possibility that she has HCM, and if she does have it, there is a 50% chance that any of her future children will have it, but currently it is not possible to predict how unwell she or her future children might be, because the effects of the condition can be very variable, even within families. She provides her contact details to Katherine and her daughter so that they can arrange to discuss any issues that may arise in the future.

Patient 3.4 — Yasmeen

- 17-year-old girl
- Has sickle cell disease but no long-term organ damage
- Discussed bone marrow transplant as treatment option
- Referred to clinical geneticist to find out more

Yasmeen's family have heard that a bone marrow transplant can cure some people of certain genetic disorders, including sickle cell disease. They are also aware that most of the people around the world who have received a bone marrow transplant for sickle cell disease have survived disease-free. However, their family doctor said that it is a costly and potentially high-risk procedure that has been performed on only a few hundred people worldwide so far. He also cautioned that this would only be suitable if a close genetic match could be found from within the family. Yasmeen's mother told the doctor that she was planning to have another baby and so she wondered whether a new baby could be a suitable match for a bone marrow transplant to cure Yasmeen of sickle cell disease. The family doctor advised them that using unaffected family members to help cure an affected member raises a number of complex ethical and psychological issues for all those involved, including the unborn child. Yasmeen and her family agreed to accept a referral to a clinical geneticist so that they can explore and understand the implications further.

Knowledge of genetics is essential in order to understand biochemistry, cell biology and physiology, and the rapid expansion of the disciplines of genetics and genomics is already beginning to change the practice of medicine and healthcare. All health professionals need to be informed of these developments and be able to use their knowledge of genetics appropriately in their practice. Gene therapy might not yet be a realistic option, but personalized therapies, screening for genetic disorders and the use of reproductive technologies are a reality. Patients need informed professionals to help them make sense of this fast-moving discipline, and their explanations can help patients make decisions that are right for them and their families.

3.4 Summary

- All organisms possess a genome. This is the entire DNA content of a cell and represents the hereditary information. Knowledge about the human genome and also the genomes of other organisms is immensely valuable. Genomic and genetic knowledge, driven by the development of associated technologies, provides many ethical, legal and societal implications for individuals, families and populations.
- The human genome is located physically within the nucleus (although some DNA also exists within mitochondria). The human genomic DNA must be accurately copied and reproduced in every cell of the organism.
- DNA contains four types of DNA nucleotide with four types of base. It is the sequence of bases in DNA that carries the genetic information (see *Figure 3.2*). DNA is **transcribed** within the nucleus to produce mRNA, which is **translated** into proteins by ribosomes (see *Figures 3.4* and *3.6*).
- A gene codes for functional RNA or protein molecules. RNA molecules are important in the process of protein synthesis and in regulating gene expression. The activity of cells is mostly determined by the activity of proteins.
- Genetic variation is an important feature of life and occurs via independent assortment of chromosomes, recombination and mutation, which are crucial events in the processes of meiosis and sexual reproduction.
- Genetic traits can be observed within multiple generations of families. It is possible to construct a pedigree chart to record the transmission of relatively simple Mendelian traits.
- However, the majority of chronic diseases and long-term conditions can be described as polygenic (involving many genes) and multifactorial (involving interaction with environmental factors).

3.5 Further reading

Additional information to help you construct a pedigree can be found at: https://heartuk.org.uk/FHToolkit/ – click on Section 5 and download the pdf document 5C.

More information about the Human Genome Project and its ethical and societal implications can be found at:

www.ornl.gov/sci/techresources/Human_Genome/home.shtml

www.genome.gov/10001772

The following book gives further details of some of the topics covered in this chapter:

Read, A. and Donnai, D. (2015) *New Clinical Genetics*, 3rd edn. Scion Publishing, Oxford, UK.

3.6 Self-assessment questions

Answers can be found at www.scionpublishing.com/AandP

(3.1) Mechanisms of genetic variation include which one of the following?
　(a) Independent assortment and mutation
　(b) Somatic cross-over
　(c) Recombinant protein
　(d) Independent recombination
　(e) Short interfering RNA

(3.2) A mother has inherited an autosomal dominant genetic condition from her father, but her husband does not have the gene for the condition. Select the most appropriate statement that identifies how likely it is that one of their offspring will inherit the disease.
　(a) There is a 1 in 2 probability of one of the children having the disease
　(b) There is a 1 in 3 probability of one of the children having the disease
　(c) There is a 1 in 4 probability of one of the children having the disease
　(d) None of the children will inherit the disease
　(e) All children will inherit the disease

(3.3) During mitosis, metaphase represents which one of the following phases?
　(a) Condensation of chromosomes
　(b) Formation of two new cells
　(c) Separation of homologous chromosomes
　(d) Disappearance of the nuclear membrane
　(e) Alignment of homologous chromosomes around the middle of the cell

(3.4) Epigenetic changes include which of the following? More than one answer is possible.
　(a) Chemical modification of mRNA
　(b) Change in the sequence of DNA nucleotides
　(c) Non-heritable changes to DNA
　(d) Methylation of DNA
　(e) Acetylation of anticodons

(3.5) Mary smokes 20 cigarettes a day. She thinks that because her mother smoked and did not develop lung cancer, she is unlikely to develop it. Is this true or not true? Give reasons for your answer.

(3.6) Ian is only 24 years old and tells you he has seen blood in his stools after going to the toilet. He is worried he might have colon cancer. He thinks his father died of cancer when Ian was only 4 years old. What advice would you offer him?

(3.7) Complete the table to work out the sequence of amino acids coded by the DNA sequence below.

DNA	CAT	GGC	TTA	AAC	GCC	CGA	TAT	GTA	TAT
mRNA									
Amino acid									

(3.8) Name three types of RNA and state their role and location in the cell.

CHAPTER 04 | Communication: short and fast

Learning points for this chapter

After working through this chapter, you should be able to:

- Discuss the organization and components of the nervous system
- Describe the structure of a sensory and a motor neurone
- Discuss the generation of an action potential and the propagation of a nerve impulse
- Describe the structure of the synapse and synaptic transmission
- Describe the general and specific functions of neurotransmitters
- Discuss the coordinated function of the nervous system

4.1 Introduction and clinical relevance

The integration of a multitude of sensory stimuli is required for health. Bodily functions and activities are controlled and regulated by the nervous and the endocrine systems. These two systems work together in an integrated manner to ensure that we are aware of our environment and that the relevant mechanisms in the body are triggered to regulate homeodynamic processes. These processes are the gradual adjustments and adaptations that organisms make to their internal environment and those processes that make them remain coherent viable systems (see *Chapter 1*), influenced by environmental, developmental and genetic factors through time. The nervous system achieves this integration by the use of neurotransmitters, which are crucial signal molecules required to coordinate and direct cellular activity. Each of the patients introduced in this chapter demonstrates how the nervous system coordinates the activities of the body and highlights how injury to different parts of the nervous system can affect activities of daily living, thought processes, emotions, feelings and behaviour. The endocrine system is the focus of *Chapter 5*.

| Patient 4.1 | Bessie | **99** | 130 | 379 | 397 | 403 | 441 |

- 71-year-old woman
- Lifelong smoker – 20 cigarettes per day
- Found unconscious with stroke and hemiplegia

Bessie, a 71-year-old lady living independently on her own at home, was found unconscious on the floor of her kitchen by a neighbour. An ambulance was called, and Bessie was transferred as an emergency to the Emergency Department of a local hospital. On arrival in hospital, Bessie was diagnosed as having a left-sided stroke with right hemiplegia. For many years, Bessie had smoked 20 cigarettes a day, but she has been trying to cut down her smoking and now smokes five cigarettes a day.

| Patient 4.2 | Jade and Jordon | **100** | 132 | 138 | 162 | 448 | 473 |

- 6-year-old boy and 32-year-old mother
- Jade drank alcohol excessively while pregnant
- Jordon has dysmorphic facial features and behavioural issues

Jordon is a 6-year-old boy born to Jade, his 32-year-old mother. Soon after his birth, Jade noticed that her beautiful baby boy had a relatively small head with small and narrow eyes, and as he grew older, she observed that he had a thin upper lip and small teeth, and that the area between the nose and the upper lip (the philtrum) was smooth with no groove. When Jade was pregnant with Jordon, she used to drink one bottle of vodka and two bottles of white wine a week, and when she could not afford wine, she drank two bottles of cider instead. The alcohol affected Jordon's facial features. As he grew older, Jade noticed that Jordon was an anxious and nervous child, was a poor sleeper and could become very agitated. Now that Jordon is at school, his teachers have informed Jade that they have observed that Jordon has a short attention span as he gets bored very easily, his memory is poor and he has some difficulties with his peer group. Jordon's limited mental ability and behavioural problems at school are what alerted his teachers that something was wrong and to the possibility of a mental disorder. The behavioural support team were alerted to observe him at school. Jordon was also referred to the Child and Adolescent Mental Health Service (CAMHS).

| Patient 4.3 | Graham | **100** | 132 | 404 | 442 |

- 57-year-old man
- Gradual onset of trembling in left hand
- Family doctor referred him to neurologist
- Diagnosis of Parkinson disease led to depression

Graham is a 57-year-old man working as a carpenter. Over a period of 3.5 months, he noticed some trembling of his left hand at rest, which after 4 months progressed to the right hand as well. During this period, Graham had a couple of panic attacks while at work, and relationships at home became troubled because he was becoming withdrawn and was branded as becoming 'lazy' by his wife. With some encouragement from a friend, Graham was persuaded to visit his family doctor who referred him for assessment and evaluation by a neurologist. Graham was diagnosed with Parkinson's disease. Since his diagnosis with Parkinson's disease, Graham has become apathetic and withdrawn and has bouts of depression for which he takes prescribed medication in the form of selective serotonin reuptake inhibitors (SSRIs).

4.2 What you need to know – essential anatomy and physiology

4.2.1 Characteristics of a biological communication system

The characteristics of an effective communication system are illustrated in *Figure 4.1*. An effective communication system starts with a stimulus, which, in physiology, is a change in the internal environment or a deviation from the set point (see *Chapter 1*) that triggers a response. **Sensory receptors** that monitor changes occurring in the internal and external environments respond to the stimulus. When the stimulus exceeds a threshold, sensory receptors respond, resulting in information being conveyed by information carriers to a control centre where integration occurs. A response is then sent by the integration and control centre to effectors that trigger the homeodynamic mechanisms that will restore the stability

(a)

receptors — monitor the internal environment and respond to changes; changes act as a stimulus

↓

control centre — receives information from receptors and coordinates the response of the effectors

↓

effectors — produce an effect to counter the stimulus. This effect is constantly monitored and fed back to the receptors and control centre

negative feedback

(b)

receptors — PERIPHERAL AND CENTRAL RECEPTORS

↓

control centre — BRAIN AND SPINAL CORD

↓

effectors — MUSCLES, ORGANS AND GLANDS

negative feedback

communication (nervous and/or endocrine systems)

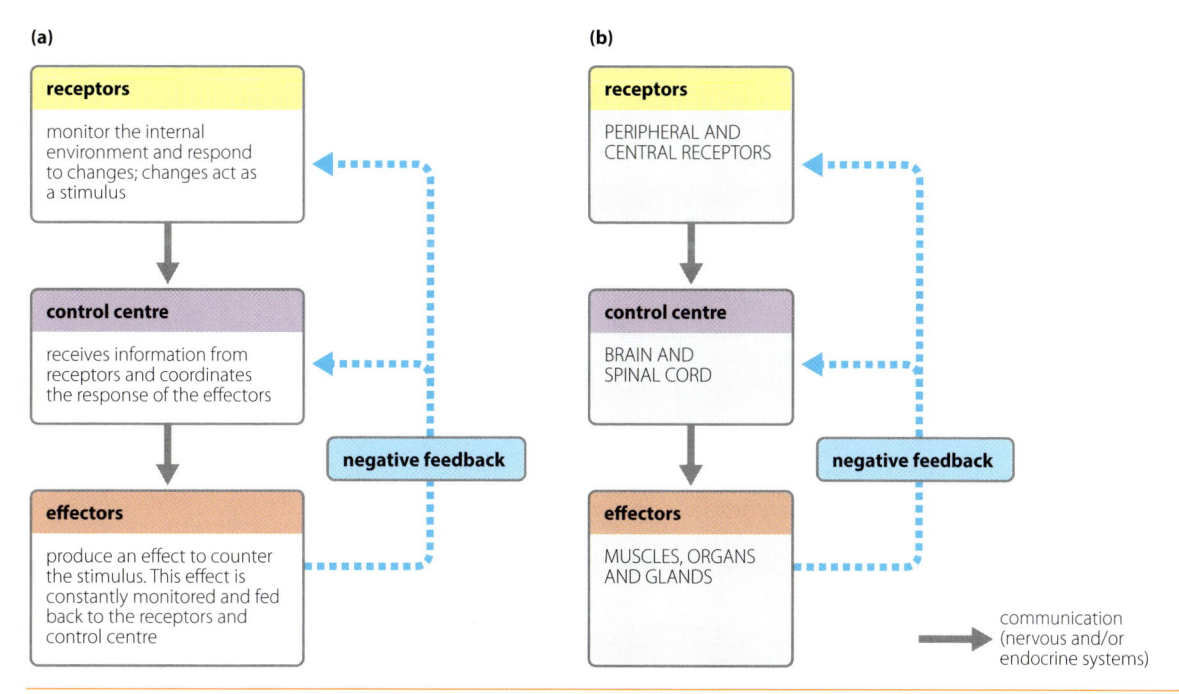

Figure 4.1 – **Communication systems in the nervous and/or endocrine system.**
(a) The main elements of a communication system and their role; and (b) the anatomical parts involved.

of the internal environment (see *Chapter 1*). In order to put this stimulus/response model into perspective, this chapter will focus on the nervous system.

4.2.2 The nervous system: structural organization

The nervous system can be divided into the central nervous system and the peripheral nervous system (see *Figure 4.2*). The **central nervous system** (CNS) consists of the brain and spinal cord, which integrate all the activities of the body. The **peripheral nervous system** (PNS) comprises nerves classified as sensory (afferent) nerves and motor (efferent) nerves. There are **31 pairs** of spinal nerves; all are mixed nerves that convey sensory impulses from different parts of the body to the CNS and motor impulses from the CNS to different parts of the body. Mixed nerves have both a sensory and a motor pathway.

4.2.3 Nervous tissue

Nervous tissue consists of two types of cell: **neurones**, cells that transmit electrical signals, and **neuroglia**, cells that support the neurones (see *Chapter 2*).

Neuroglia

Neuroglia are relatively small cells when compared with the neurones found in the CNS. They support, insulate and protect neurones from damage. There are four different types of neuroglia found in the CNS (see *Figure 4.3a*):

- **Astrocytes** form a selective barrier between neurones and capillaries, called the **blood–brain barrier**, thus protecting the brain from harmful substances such as toxins in the blood.

Figure 4.2 – The structural organization of the nervous system.

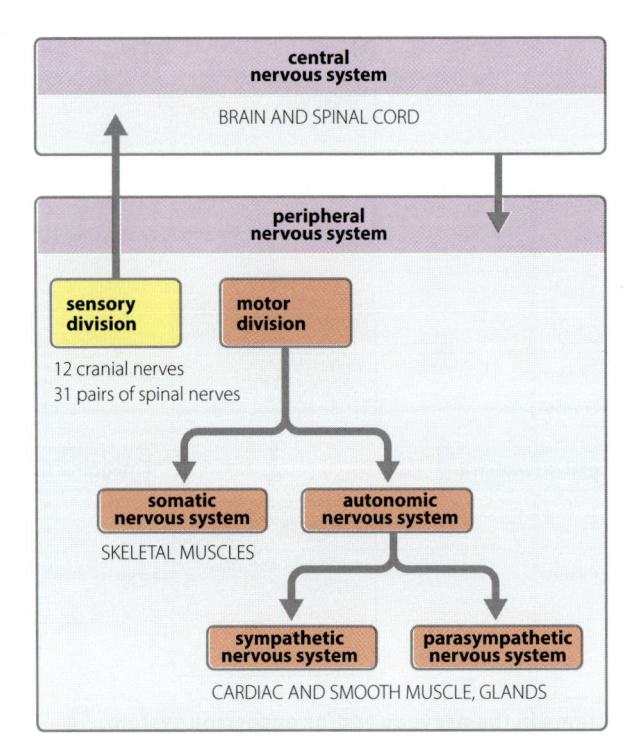

```
                    central
                nervous system
              BRAIN AND SPINAL CORD

                   peripheral
                nervous system

      sensory              motor
      division            division
   12 cranial nerves
   31 pairs of spinal nerves

                    somatic        autonomic
                nervous system   nervous system
                SKELETAL MUSCLES

                              sympathetic    parasympathetic
                            nervous system   nervous system
                      CARDIAC AND SMOOTH MUSCLE, GLANDS
```

- **Microglia** have a phagocytic role and remove dead brain cells and bacteria.
- **Ependymal cells** line cavities of the brain and spinal cord. Ependymal cells possess cilia, which facilitate the movement of **cerebrospinal fluid** in the cavities of the brain by the rhythmical movement of the cilia.
- **Oligodendrocytes** have extensions that wrap around many neurones and produce myelin sheaths that insulate the neurones.

There are two types of neuroglia found in the PNS: **Schwann cells** and **satellite cells** (see *Figure 4.3b*):

- Schwann cells are also known as **neurolemmocytes**. Their role is similar to that of oligodendrocytes in that they have extensions that wrap around an individual neurone and form a myelin sheath that surround the neurone in the PNS.
- Satellite cells are similar to astrocytes in the CNS. They anchor the neurones and surround the neurone cell bodies in **ganglia**. They regulate the environment of the neurone and allow the exchange of material between capillaries and neurones in the same way as astrocytes function in the CNS.

Neurones

Neurones, also called nerve cells, are the functional unit of the nervous system. They are highly specialized and conduct nerve impulses throughout the body. Due to differentiation (see *Chapter 2*), the majority of neurones lose the ability to divide and therefore are unable to be replaced when damaged in adults. However, in young people, **axons** have the ability to regenerate both in the PNS and CNS, while in adults, axons (discussed in *Section 4.2.4*) *can only regenerate in the PNS, not in the CNS*. Normally, we are born with sufficient nerve cells to maintain our activities and cognitive function and to accommodate the loss of neurones that occurs throughout life.

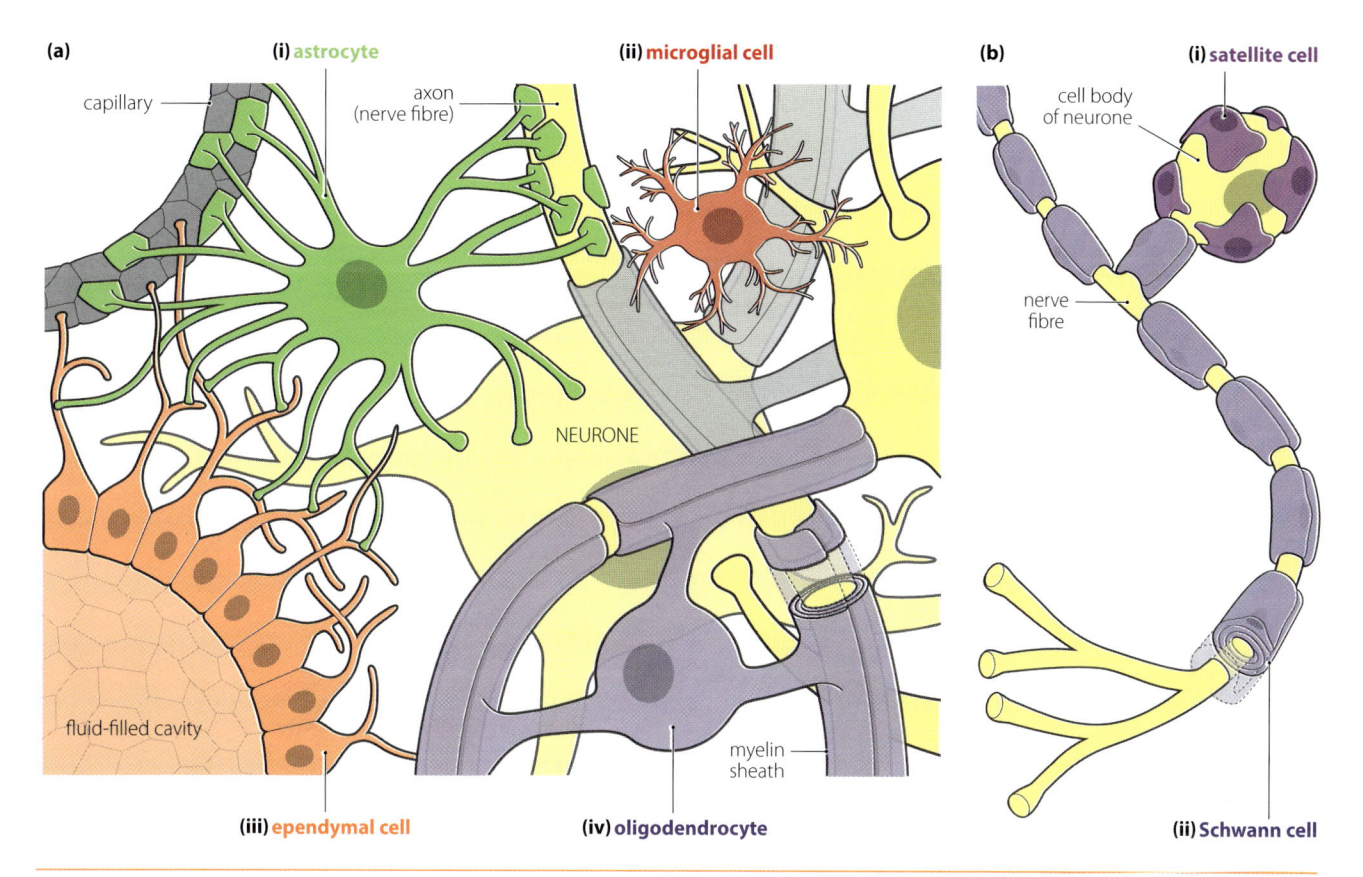

Figure 4.3 – Supporting cells.
(a) The central nervous system showing (i) astrocytes, (ii) microglial cells, (iii) ependymal cells and (iv) oligodendrocytes.
(b) The peripheral nervous system showing Schwann cells and satellite cells.

Neurones are classified as either sensory or motor neurones. Sensory (afferent) neurones conduct nerve impulses from the different parts of the body to the CNS while motor (efferent) neurones conduct nerve impulses from the CNS to effectors located around the body.

The structure of a neurone

The structure of sensory neurones and motor neurones differ, as illustrated in *Figures 4.4a* and *b*, respectively. The common features of all neurones are:

- **dendrites**, which are branching processes emanating from the cell
- the **cell body**, which is the control centre of the neurone
- the **axon** (also called a nerve fibre), which conveys information from the cell body to the axon terminals.

Dendrites are the main receptive region of the neurone and their role is to receive signals from other neurones and transmit these to the cell body. The cell body contains the organelles that are normally found in a somatic cell (see *Chapter 2*) with the exception of centrioles and hence neurones are unable to divide. Also present in the cell body are clusters of rough endoplasmic reticulum known as **Nissl bodies** (granules) that synthesize protein. Each neurone has a single long extension called an **axon** that arises from a specialized region of the cell body called the **axon**

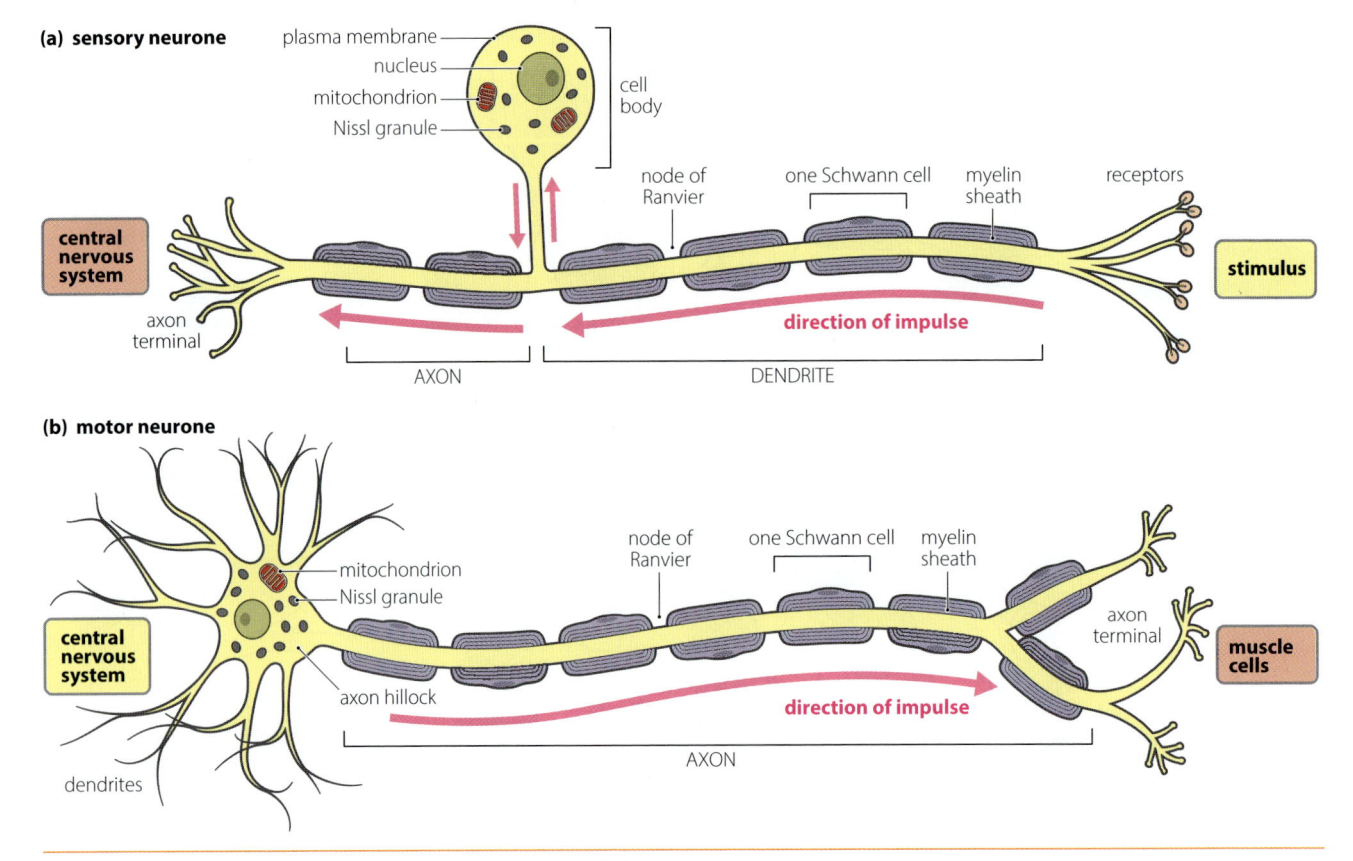

Figure 4.4 – Structure of (a) a sensory neurone, and (b) a motor neurone.

hillock. Axons vary in length but all terminate with many branches, each ending as an axon terminal, also called a synaptic knob. Some axons are covered by a sheath of myelin, a lipid substance that makes their appearance white. The myelin sheath is formed by oligodendrocytes in the CNS and by Schwann cells in the PNS. The myelin sheath has gaps at regular intervals along the length of the axon known as **nodes of Ranvier** (see *Figure 4.4a* and *b*). The function of the myelin sheath is to insulate the neurones and to speed up transmission of the nerve impulse (discussed later in this chapter). Other neurones have no myelin sheath and are called unmyelinated neurones. Most of these unmyelinated neurones are shorter than the myelinated ones found in the CNS, especially the brain, and they conduct impulses at a slower speed than myelinated neurones.

4.2.4 Functional organization of the nervous system

Sensory division of the nervous system

Sensory (afferent) neurones transmit nerve impulses from receptors in different parts of the body to the CNS. Somatic sensory neurones (somatic afferents) conduct impulses from the skin, skeletal muscles and joints, while visceral sensory neurones (visceral afferents) transmit nerve impulses from internal organs (the **viscera**). Thus, changes in both the external and internal environments are detected by sensory receptors, resulting in the conduction of sensory impulses to the spinal cord and the brain.

Motor division of the nervous system

Motor (efferent) neurones transmit nerve impulses from the brain and spinal cord to the muscles, organs and glands, which collectively are called effectors. The effectors produce actions that eventually produce the desired physiological effect, returning variables towards the set point.

The motor system is split into two divisions: the somatic (voluntary) nervous system and the autonomic nervous system. The somatic division enables conscious control of skeletal muscle activities, such as walking and running. The autonomic nervous system is divided into the sympathetic and parasympathetic nervous systems. The sympathetic division is stimulatory and prepares the body for acute stress, while the parasympathetic nervous system is inhibitory and is responsible for regulating physiological activity during periods of rest and for conserving energy. For example, the parasympathetic system activates visceral activity, such as digestion, which results in the release of energy from the breakdown of food. This energy can be stored in the body.

4.2.5 The generation and propagation of an action potential

Neurones generate and conduct an **action potential** (commonly called a nerve impulse) and are highly responsive to stimuli, a physiological state known as irritability. If a stimulus is strong enough, reaching a specific threshold, then an action potential is generated in the cell body and conducted along the axon to the axon terminals. The action potential is transmitted further to other neurones through synapses and to effectors (muscles, organs and glands) through **neuromuscular junctions** (see *Chapter 13*). If the stimulus is weak and insufficient to reach the threshold, an action potential is not produced. The strength or weakness of the stimulus is known as the '**all or nothing principle**'.

Action potentials are generated by the transport of ions across the plasma membrane of the neurone. This is possible because the plasma membrane contains specialized sodium and potassium pumps (see *Chapter 2*) that respond to changes in the electrical charge across the cell membrane. The potential difference in the electrical charge between the fluid outside the neurone and that inside the neurone generates a membrane potential (voltage) and is measured in millivolts (mV). The difference in electrical potential exists because a difference in ion concentration is created on either side of the plasma membrane. For example, in the extracellular fluid, there is a high concentration of sodium compared with inside the neurone. However, inside the neurone, there is a high concentration of potassium compared with the extracellular fluid. The effect of the differences in ion concentration is that extracellular fluid has a more positive charge compared with intracellular fluid, which is less positive. This difference in ion concentration creates a voltage, otherwise known as an electrical potential difference, across the membrane. When a neurone is in a polarized state (at rest), there are more sodium ions outside the plasma membrane of the nerve cell than inside it and more potassium ions inside the plasma membrane than outside it, creating an ionic gradient and therefore a voltage difference between the outer and inner parts of the membrane. This voltage difference is called the **resting membrane potential** and is typically −70 mV (see *Figure 4.5a,i*).

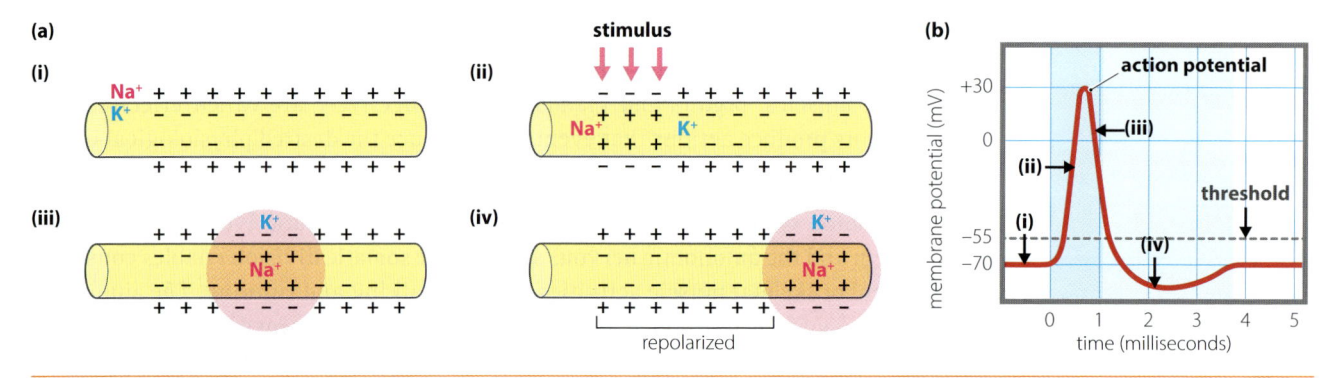

Figure 4.5 – **(a) Action potential and nerve impulse conduction along an unmyelinated neurone; and (b) the phases of action potential.**
(a) (i) Resting membrane (polarized state). (ii) Depolarized state (stimulus strong enough to initiate generation of an action potential). (iii) Propagation of the action potential. (iv) Migration of action potential along a neurone. The conduction velocity is slow. (b) (i) Resting state: both sodium (Na⁺) and potassium (K⁺) channels are closed. (ii) Depolarization phase: Na⁺ channels are open, K⁺ channels are closed. (iii) Repolarization phase: Na⁺ gates and channels close, K⁺ channels open with K⁺ flowing out of the cell. (iv) Hyperpolarization phase: Na⁺ channels and gates closed, but K⁺ channels remain open and K⁺ continues to leave the cell.

In response to a stimulus, Na⁺ channels in the plasma membrane of the axon and **axon hillock** (the cone-shaped elevation of the cell body where the axon joins the cell body) open, allowing Na⁺ to move into the neurone. This causes the inside of the neurone to become more positive, a reversal of polarity, which is called **depolarization**. If the movement of Na⁺ ions is sufficient to reduce the membrane potential so that the voltage reaches a critical value called the threshold, for example –55 mV, an action potential will be produced based on the 'all or nothing principle' (see *Figure 4.5a,ii* and *b*). Increasing numbers of open voltage-sensitive Na⁺ channels cause depolarization of the local axon membrane and the cell interior becomes progressively more positive. Depolarization lasts for only about 1 millisecond and is self-limiting. As the inside of the neurone becomes more positive, passing 0 mV, the Na⁺ channels close while the K⁺ channels, which are slower to respond, open to allow K⁺ to diffuse out of the neurone. As a consequence, the inside of the neurone becomes less positive, a process called **repolarization** (see *Figure 4.5b*). The movement of K⁺ out of the cell is typically prolonged as the K⁺ channels are also slower to close, causing the inside of the neurone to become even more negative, producing a dip in the voltage below the normal resting membrane potential. This dip is called **hyperpolarization** (see *Figure 4.5b*). The resting membrane potential is restored as primary Na⁺ and K⁺ channels are closed and the difference in ionic concentration across the membrane is established by the Na⁺/K⁺ pump transporting Na⁺ out of the axon and moving K⁺ into the axon.

The changes in permeability (depolarization) in adjacent parts of the axon membrane are conducted rapidly along the entire axon to the axon terminal. The propagation of the action potential along the neurone and the velocity at which this occurs vary between unmyelinated and myelinated neurones. In unmyelinated neurones, the action potential is propagated by continuous conduction (see *Figure 4.5a, iii* and *iv*). Sufficient depolarization of an axon to reach the threshold causes voltage-gated Na⁺ channels to open, resulting in the initiation of an action potential. A local current develops at an initial segment of the plasma membrane as Na⁺ moves from extracellular fluid into the cytoplasm inside the membrane. Once an action potential has been initiated, it can only be propagated in one direction. Changes in the membrane potential must occur at each local segment of the plasma membrane due to entry of the positive charge from the Na^+, resulting in propagation of the action potential at a relatively slow conduction velocity until the action potential reaches the axon terminal. Some neurones such as **pyramidal cells**, known as **projection neurones**, possess long axons that extend from one part of the brain to another, while others, such as **stellate cells** found in the cerebral cortex, have very short axons. In myelinated neurones, the conduction velocity is much faster as the action potential skips from one node of Ranvier to another, a process known as **saltatory conduction** (see *Figure 4.6*). This type of conduction occurs because there is an increased concentration of voltage-gated Na^+ channels in the membrane at the nodes of Ranvier. Thus, depolarization in the membrane in one node of Ranvier is sufficient to cause depolarization in the next node, resulting in propagation of the impulse. In addition to the presence of the myelin sheath, other factors that increase the speed of transmission of a nerve impulse are the size of the diameter of the axon, axon length and temperature. An axon with a large diameter has a faster conduction velocity than one with a small diameter, while long axons have slower conduction velocity to such an extent that an inverse relationship exists between axon length and conduction velocity in both sensory and motor nerves. An increase in temperature increases conduction velocity, while alcohol and other drugs such as anaesthetics slow down the conduction velocity of nerve impulses by preventing an increase in membrane permeability to Na^+.

The conduction of impulses between neurones is achieved by the release of chemical messengers called neurotransmitters from the axon terminals, and the point of connection between one neurone and other neurones or effectors is called the synapse (see *Figure 4.7*). Synapses may inhibit or enable the conduction of the nerve impulse.

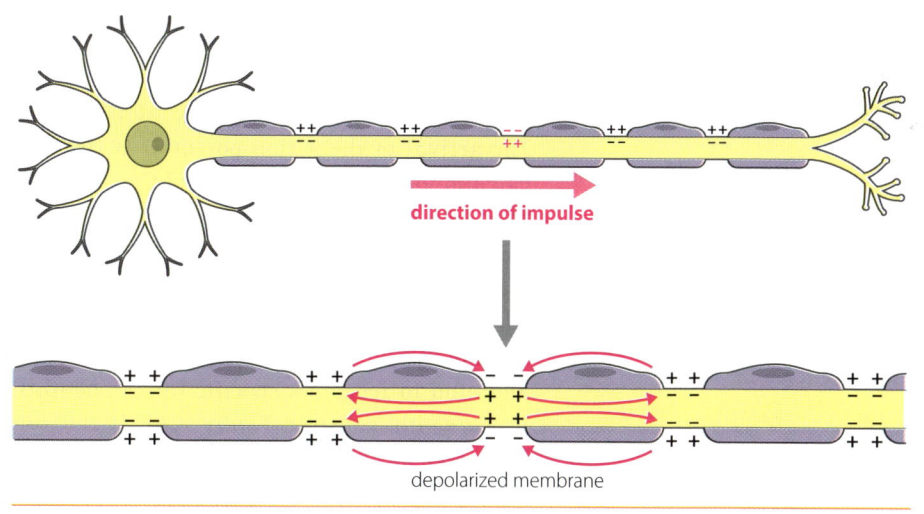

Figure 4.6 – Saltatory conduction showing nerve impulse conduction along a myelinated neurone.
Conduction velocity is fast because the impulse jumps from one node of Ranvier to another. The depolarized region, showing the creation of local currents that enable the spreading of the depolarization wave, is indicated.

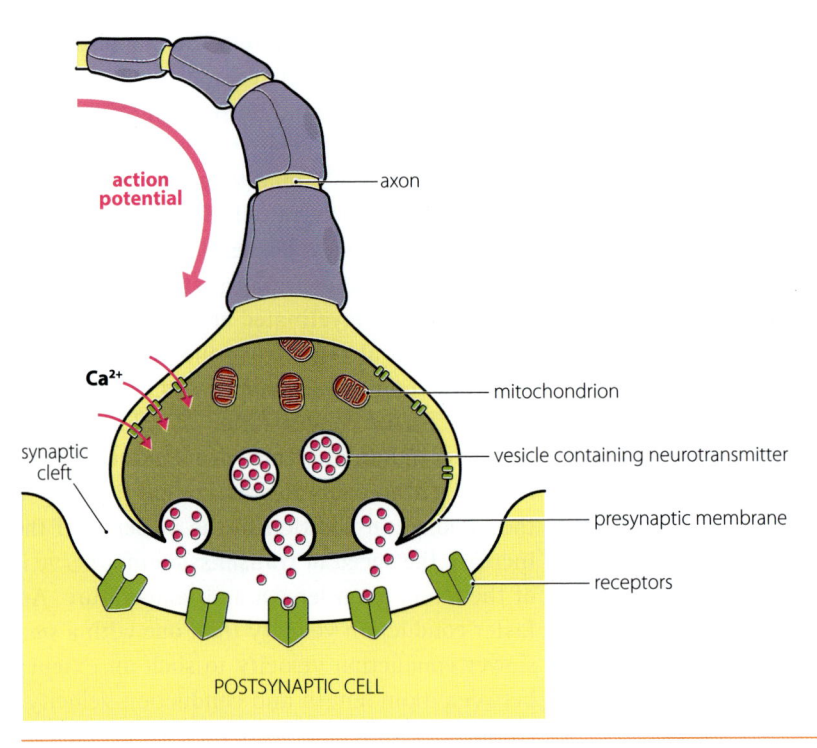

Figure 4.7 – **The synapse.**

Neurotransmitters

Neurotransmitters (see *Table 4.1*) are a structurally diverse group of compounds synthesized from amino acids. Some neurotransmitters such as acetylcholine and noradrenaline (also known as norepinephrine) are widely distributed in the body, and others such as dopamine are found in large quantities, predominantly in the brain. Many drugs – both therapeutic and illicit drugs – enhance or inhibit the function of neurotransmitters.

Propagation of an impulse at the synapse

The arrival of the action potential at the synaptic knob opens voltage-sensitive calcium ion (Ca^{2+}) channels, and Ca^{2+} moves from the surrounding extracellular fluid into the synaptic knob (see *Figure 4.7*). The entry of calcium ions activates vesicles containing a specific neurotransmitter to move towards the presynaptic membrane. The vesicles fuse with the presynaptic membrane and release the neurotransmitter into the synaptic cleft (a microscopic gap between the neurones) by exocytosis. The neurotransmitter molecules diffuse across the synaptic cleft and bind to receptors specific for the neurotransmitter on the membrane of the postsynaptic cell (see *Figure 4.8*). If the synapse is excitatory, binding of the neurotransmitter to the complementary receptor on the postsynaptic membrane will open the Na^+ channels to generate an action potential.

Soon after the binding of the neurotransmitter and receptor, the neurotransmitter is broken down by enzymes specific for that neurotransmitter. For example, **acetylcholine** is broken down by **acetylcholinesterase**, while the catecholamines (adrenaline (epinephrine), noradrenaline (norepinephrine) and serotonin

Table 4.1 – Neurotransmitters, their functions and related pathology

Neurotransmitter	Location in the brain	Function and examples of related pathology
Acetylcholine	Cerebral cortex pyramidal pathways, reticular activating system, thalamus	Cognition, consciousness, memory, skeletal muscle movement, e.g. dementia
Adrenaline (epinephrine)	Medulla oblongata, hypothalamus, thalamus	Appetite, arousal, body temperature, mood, sleep, e.g. depression
Dopamine	Basal ganglia (extrapyramidal pathway), hypothalamus, limbic system, medulla oblongata, midbrain	Skeletal muscle movement, behaviour, regulation of prolactin secretion, e.g. Parkinsonism, schizophrenia
Gamma-aminobutyric acid (GABA)	All regions	Inhibitory motor control, consciousness, memory, e.g. anxiety
Glutamate	Cortex, basal ganglia, other brain regions	Learning and memory, e.g. schizophrenia, bipolar states
Noradrenaline (norepinephrine)	Amygdala, hypothalamus, reticular activating system	Appetite, arousal, body temperature, mood, sleep, e.g. depression, eating disorders, insomnia
Serotonin	Hypothalamus, reticular activating system	Appetite, arousal, body temperature, mood, sleep, behaviour, pain transmission, e.g. depression, schizophrenia

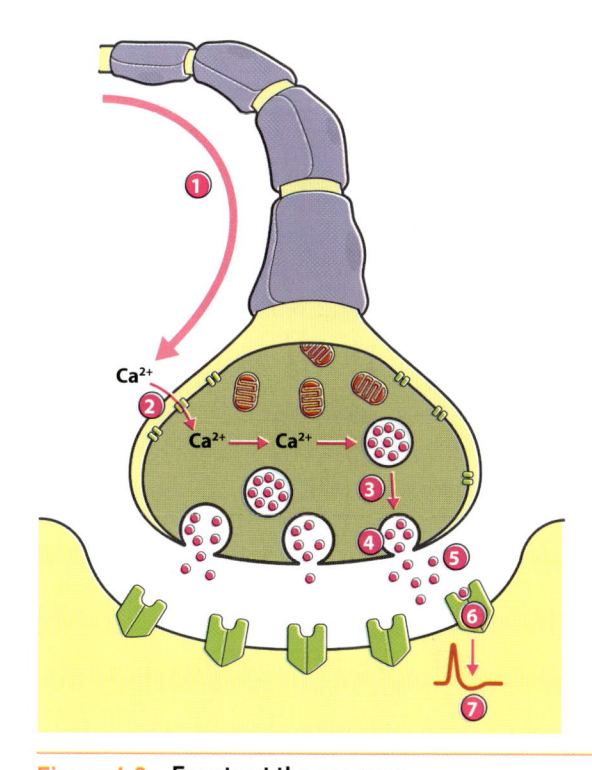

Figure 4.8 – Events at the synapse.
(1) Arrival of an impulse or action potential. (2) Ca^{2+} enters plasma membrane. (3) The vesicle is activated by Ca^{2+} to move towards the presynaptic membrane. (4) The vesicle fuses with the presynaptic membrane and releases the neurotransmitter by exocytosis. (5) The neurotransmitter diffuses across the synaptic cleft. (6) The neurotransmitter binds to receptors. (7) An action potential is regenerated.

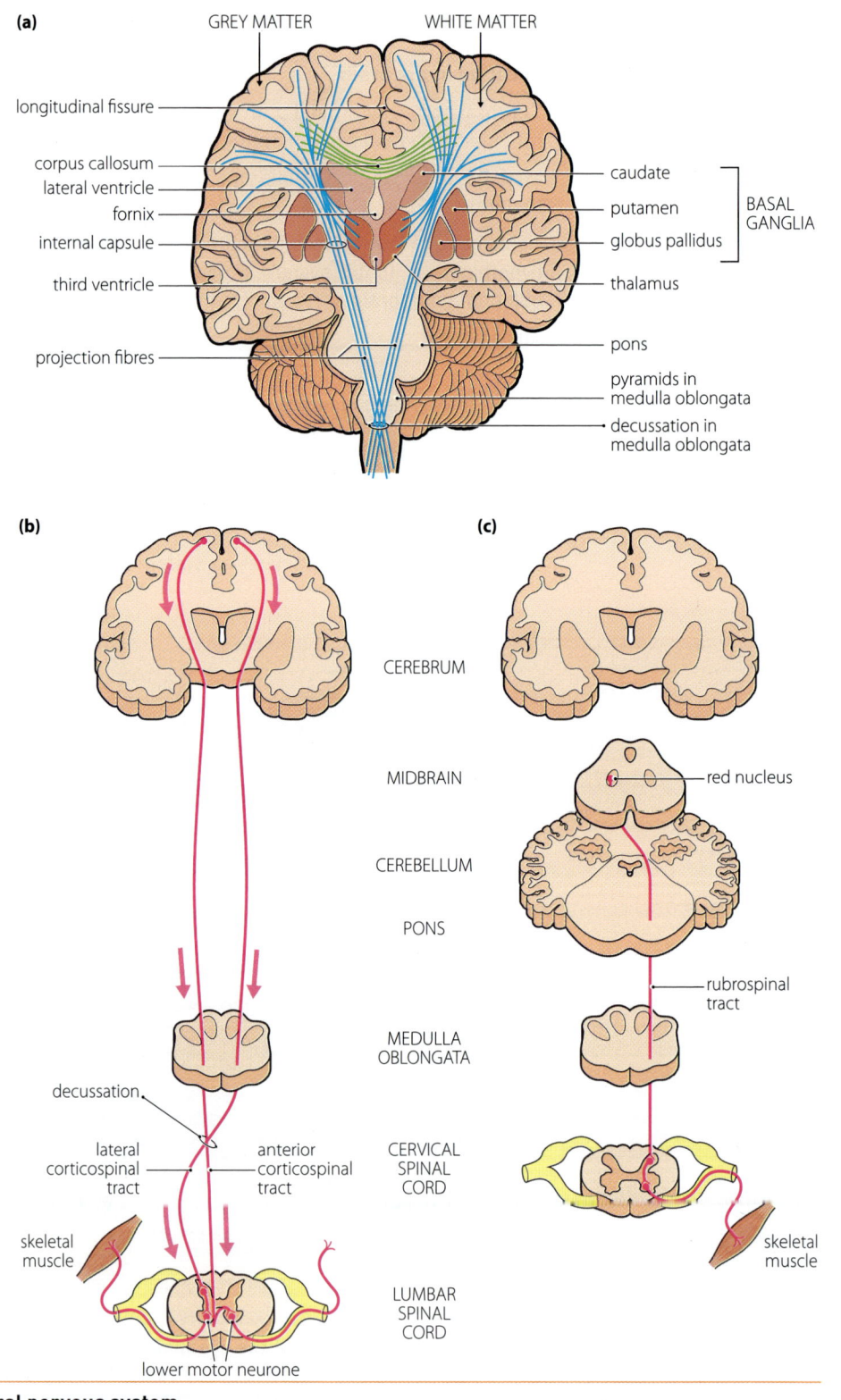

Figure 4.9 – Structure of the central nervous system.
(a) Cross-section of the brain showing the corpus callosum, internal capsule, basal ganglia and projection fibres, with decussation in the pyramids of the medulla oblongata. (b) Direct (pyramidal) pathways that carry motor nerve impulses to skeletal muscle. (c) The indirect (extrapyramidal) tract, which regulates muscle tone on the opposite side of the body.

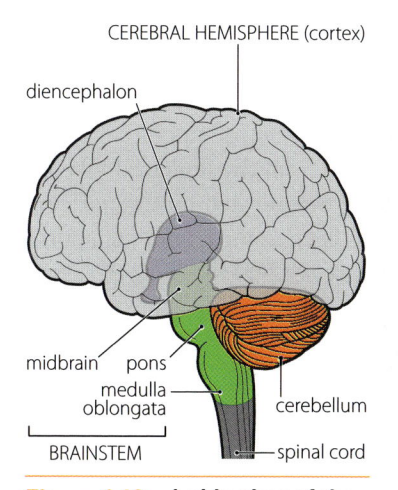

Figure 4.10 – A side view of the brain.

(5-hydroxytryptamine)) are broken down by **monoamine oxidase**. **Gamma-aminobutyric acid (GABA)** is inactivated by GABA transaminase. The components of the neurotransmitter are reabsorbed back in the presynaptic membranes where the neurotransmitter is resynthesized.

4.2.6 The central nervous system: the brain and spinal cord

The brain and spinal cord make up the central nervous system (CNS). The adult brain weighs approximately 1.5 kg (3 lbs) wet weight. The ratio between the brain and body weight in humans exceeds that of most other animals. The human brain is made up of left and right cerebral hemispheres, which are separated by a deep fissure, called the longitudinal fissure. A band of white fibres (myelinated axons) known as the **corpus callosum** connects the two hemispheres (see *Figure 4.9a*).

The four main regions of the brain are (i) the **cerebrum** (comprising the cerebral hemispheres); (ii) the **diencephalon**, which is sometimes referred to as the **between brain**, and comprises the thalamus and hypothalamus; (iii) the **cerebellum**; and (iv) the **brainstem**, which is made up of the midbrain, the pons and the medulla oblongata (see *Figure 4.10*). Most of the brainstem is covered by the cerebrum, which constitutes about 83% of the total brain mass. **Grey matter**, which is composed of cell bodies and dendrites (see *Figure 4.4*), without myelin sheaths, is found covering the surface of the cerebral hemispheres as a thin layer called the cortex and is also found deep within the brain, forming structures called nuclei (see *Figure 4.11a*). The rest of the brain tissue is formed of **white matter**, composed of connecting fibres (axons), which are myelinated, giving it its characteristic white colour (see *Figure 4.11a*). The cortex, which is approximately 2–4 mm thick, is highly folded in order to increase its surface area, with elevated ridges called **gyri** and shallow grooves called **sulci**. The outer layer of the cerebral cortex is called the **neocortex** and is responsible for higher functions such as sensory

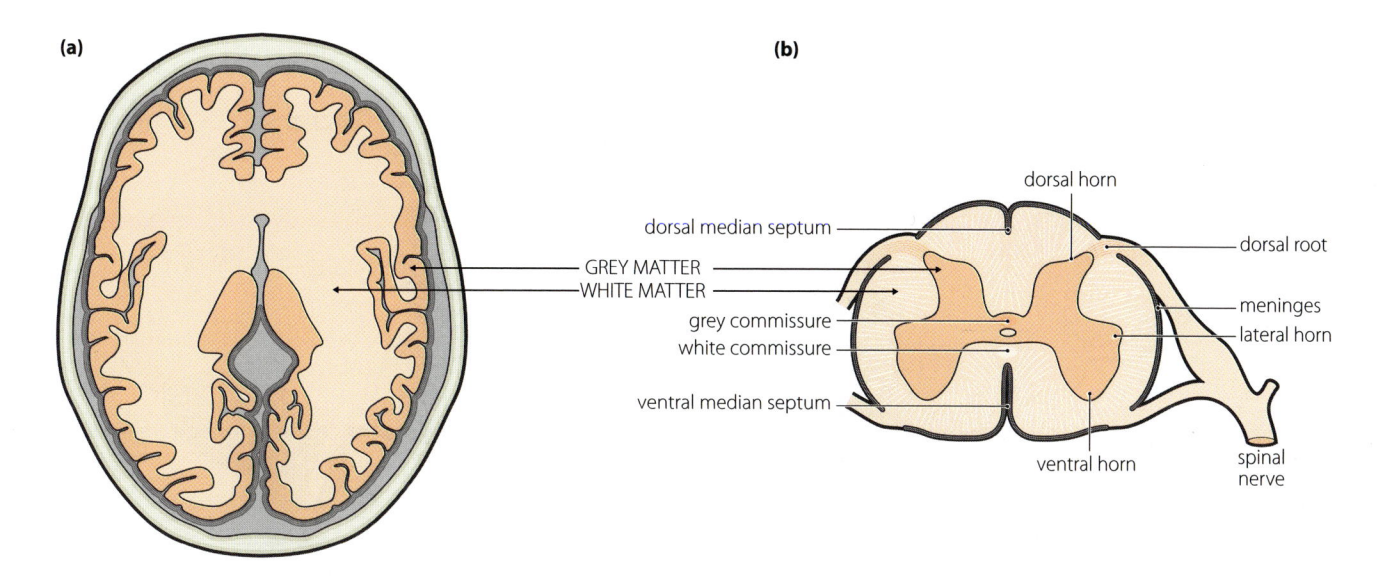

Figure 4.11 – The arrangement of grey and white matter in (a) the brain and (b) the spinal cord.

perception, conscious thought and reasoning. The cerebral cortex is divided into four main lobes (see *Figure 4.12a*): the frontal, parietal, occipital and temporal lobes, all of which have their names derived from the bones of the skull that cover them; they are separated from each other by sulci. The central sulcus separates the frontal and parietal lobes, and these are separated from the temporal lobe by the lateral sulcus. The occipital and parietal lobes are separated by the parieto-occipital sulcus. A fifth area known as the **insula** lies deep in the frontal, temporal and parietal lobes within the lateral sulcus (see *Figure 4.12b*).

Functions of the lobes

Motor (efferent) impulses originate from the primary motor area (**precentral gyrus**) lying in the frontal lobe, just in front of the central sulcus (see *Figures 4.12a* and *4.13*). Spatially, the whole body is represented within the brain in such a manner that neurones dedicated to the lower part of the body (toes and foot) are at the upper and middle part of the brain (*supermedial end*), while the head is at the lower region and side (*inferolateral area*) of the precentral gyrus (see *Figure 4.13*). The amount of the cortex that controls a particular body region such as the torso or face is proportional to and based on the sensitivity of that body region. For example, a smaller part of the cortex controls the lower limb and torso of the body when compared with the part of the cortex that controls the face, lips, jaw, tongue and neck (see *Figure 4.13*).

Sensory (afferent) impulses to the cerebral cortex are directed to an area in the parietal lobe that lies just behind the central sulcus called the primary somatosensory area or the **postcentral gyrus** (see *Figures 4.12a* and *4.13*). Sensory nerve impulses arising from different parts of the body due to stimulation by changes in temperature, posture and pain sensation (nociception) are brought to the somatosensory area of the cortex (postcentral gyrus) where the afferent impulses are interpreted. Certain parts of the body such as the face, lips and

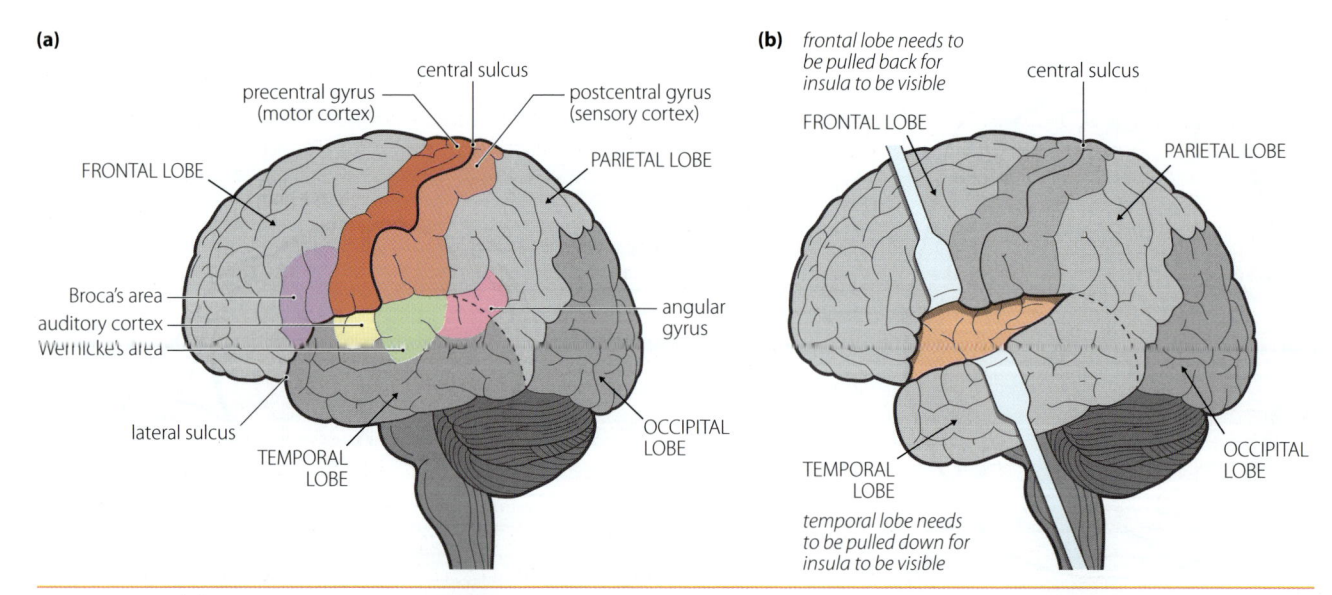

Figure 4.12 – (a) A lateral view of the cerebral hemisphere showing the lobes and the language centres, and (b) lobes of the cerebral hemisphere showing the position of the insula.

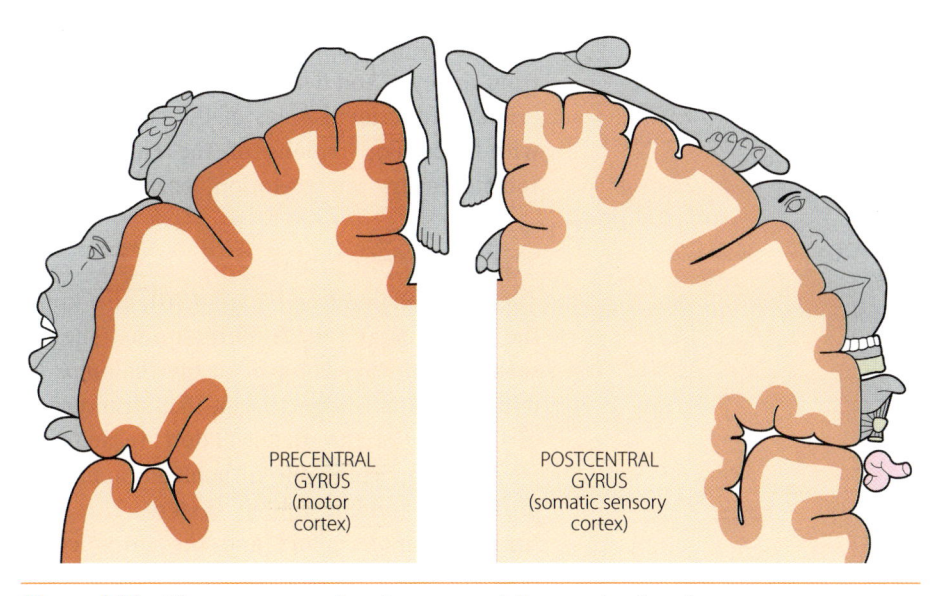

Figure 4.13 – The sensory and motor areas of the cerebral cortex.
The relationship between the cortical area and various body tissues can be seen. The precentral and postcentral gyri are also shown in *Figure 4.12a*.

fingertips are innervated with more receptors than other parts of the body, detecting information and transmitting it to the somatosensory area via the sensory neurones (see *Figure 4.13*). In some children, there is an inappropriate response to stimuli whereby the children are either hypersensitive or hyposensitive to environmental stimuli when they reach the CNS, resulting in a condition known as **sensory processing disorder** (**SPD**) causing an inability to organize sensory information into appropriate motor responses. In children with SPD, information received in the CNS is perceived and interpreted differently compared with in people without the disorder.

There are two language centres in the left hemisphere. Associated with the somatosensory area and located on the superior part of the temporal lobe in the left hemisphere is the auditory interpretation area known as **Wernicke's area** (see *Figure 4.12a*). Wernicke's area helps with the comprehension of verbal and non-verbal auditory information. Information received by Wernicke's area is transferred to **Broca's area**, another language centre also known as the **motor speech area** or **speech centre** (see *Figure 4.12a*), which is found in the frontal lobe of the brain and in the same hemisphere as Wernicke's area. Broca's area processes the received information for vocalization, and with the coordinated involvement of the motor cortex, speech is produced by movement of the lips, tongue and vocal cords.

The frontal lobe is responsible for intellectual processes, voluntary control of muscles, verbal communication and personality. People undergo changes to their personality when their frontal lobe becomes damaged. The temporal lobe processes auditory and visual experiences and stores memories of such experiences, as well as other information, and contains the centre for the interpretation of speech. The parietal lobe receives and processes information and interprets **somatosensory** inputs, which include all information received by the brain in relation to cold, heat, body position, pain and pressure. The occipital lobe receives impulses from the eyes and deals with perception of vision (see *Chapter 6*). Linked to the primary functional areas of the cortex are association areas that communicate with numerous regions of the cortex, having complex functions including somatosensory interpretation, learning and memory formation.

The diencephalon

The diencephalon (see *Figure 4.10*), also known as the between brain, comprises the **thalamus** and the **hypothalamus**. The thalamus acts as a relay station, and sensory pathways connect in the thalamus before passing to the cerebrum. The hypothalamus is a small pea-like structure at the base of the brain that is part of the floor of the diencephalon. In spite of its small size, the hypothalamus plays an important role in homeodynamics because of its connections with the **brainstem** and the **limbic system**. The hypothalamus controls water balance through osmoreceptors and the thirst centre (see *Chapter 8*), monitors and regulates body temperature via thermoreceptors (see *Chapter 1*), and plays an important role in metabolism through its involvement with the hunger and satiety centres. The hypothalamus regulates complex emotional and motivational states including anger, appetite, pain, pleasure, rage and sex drive, and it provides a link between these states and physiological responses. Its connections with the limbic system make it an important participant in emotionally driven behaviour. The hypothalamus has connections with the pituitary gland via a hypothalamo-pituitary stalk known as the **infundibulum**. Neuronal tracts that originate in the hypothalamus and pass down the infundibulum transport hormones that are synthesized in the hypothalamus to the posterior pituitary gland (see *Chapter 5*).

The limbic system

The limbic system exists as a group of nuclei and connections scattered around the brain that form a network (see *Figure 4.14*). These nuclei and connections of the limbic system form a border between the cerebrum and the diencephalon. The structures of the brain that form the limbic system include the amygdala

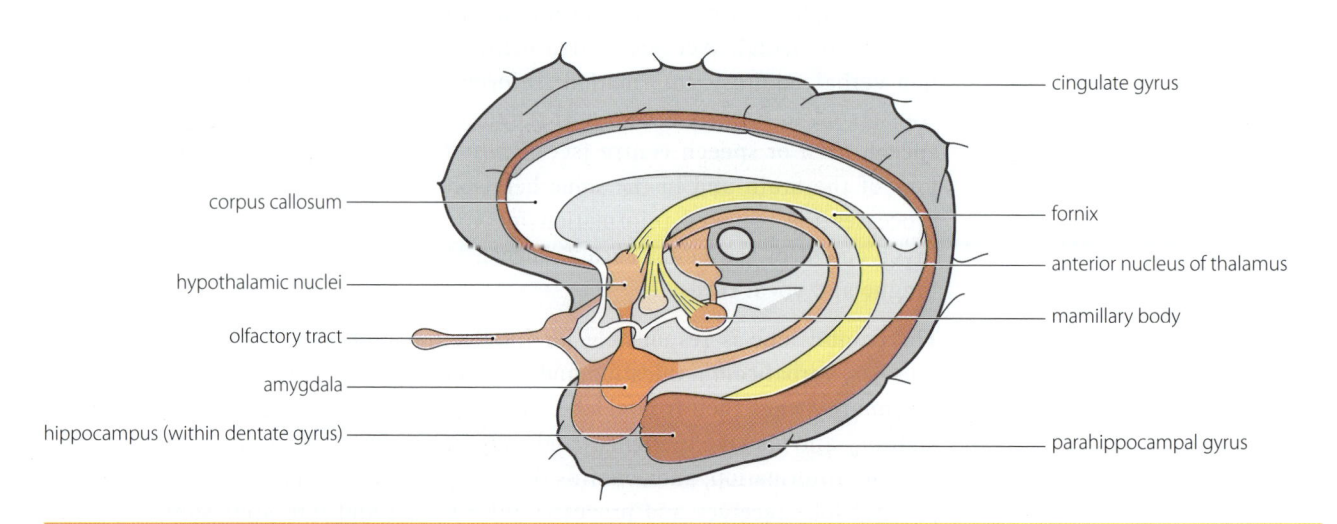

Figure 4.14 – **The limbic system.**

(links the cerebrum with the limbic system), corpus callosum, fornix (a band of white matter linking the hippocampus to the hypothalamus), hippocampus (involved in memory), neocortex and thalamus. There are three gyri (folds) that are part of the limbic system or lobe, namely the cingulate gyrus, which lies superior to the corpus callosum, the parahippocampal gyrus, which forms the inferior and posterior parts of the limbic lobe, and the dentate gyrus, which lies between the other two gyri. Gyri are important anatomical landmarks in addition to having a role in physiological function. For example, the cingulate gyrus links behaviour to motivation and is involved in the fear response predicting negative consequences. This suggests a role in depression and schizophrenia. The parahippocampal gyrus has a role in the coding and retrieval of memory, while the dentate gyrus contributes to episodic memory.

The limbic system links the autonomic functions of the brainstem, such as changes in blood pressure and respiration, with the conscious intellectual processes of the cerebral cortex; it deals with all emotional states and is concerned with storage and retrieval of memory. In addition, the limbic system deals with motivational aspects of behaviour. The limbic system communicates with the brainstem and the hypothalamus in order to maintain homeodynamics, and ensures that autonomic effects are part of a more complex phenomenon that encompasses emotional and behavioural aspects. For example, there are emotional and behavioural components associated with changes in blood pressure and respiration to support this perspective.

The cerebellum

The cerebellum is found at the back of the brain (dorsally) beneath the occipital lobe of the cerebral cortex (see *Figure 4.10*). It has both grey matter and white matter. It receives afferent inputs from **proprioceptors**. Proprioceptors are sensory receptors found in muscles, joints and tendons whose role is to detect the position and movement of the body. The function of the cerebellum is to coordinate muscle movement, thereby controlling both posture and balance. It monitors the position of the body, continually sending feedback to the cerebral cortex, which then sends motor responses to skeletal muscles for the necessary adjustments to be made to maintain balance and control movement.

The brainstem

The brainstem comprises the midbrain, pons and medulla oblongata. It is a pathway for ascending and descending tracts and within it is found the **reticular formation**, a band of grey matter that provides motor control to visceral organs. Part of the reticular formation (see *Figure 4.15*) controls the sleep–wake cycle,

---

BOX 4.1

Coma

Damage to the cerebral cortex (trauma), subarachnoid haemorrhage, tumours, subdural haematomas, meningitis, hypoglycaemia, opiate use and other drug poisoning, excessive alcohol intake and sepsis can lead to coma. Coma is a state of unresponsiveness in which it is difficult to arouse a person, and can be assessed by the Glasgow Coma Scale (see *Box 4.2*). The sleep–wake cycle is absent and the eyes remain closed.

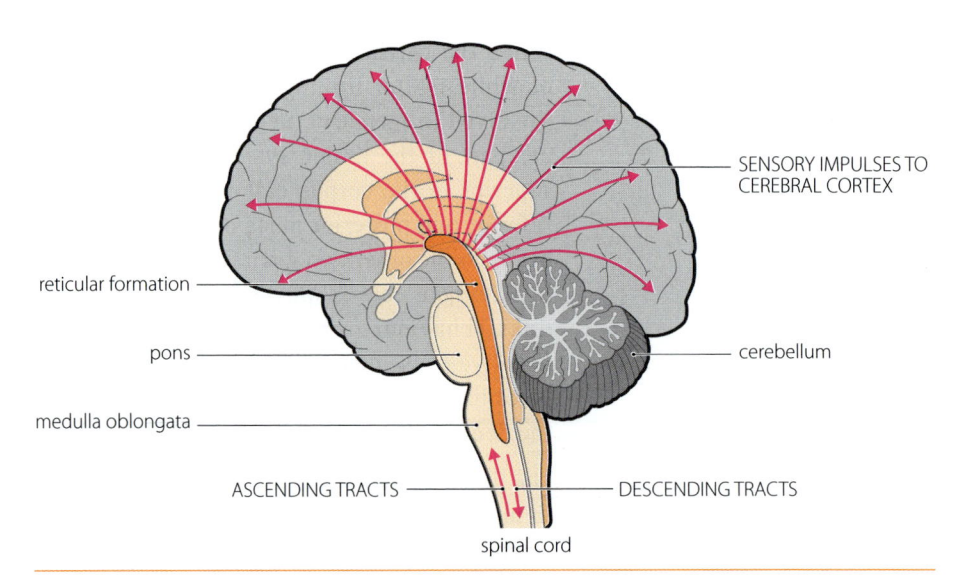

Figure 4.15 – **The ascending and descending tracts passing through the reticular formation of the brainstem.**

alertness and consciousness, and is known as the **reticular activating system**. The reticular activating system and its connections to the cerebral cortex control the state of arousal, and damage to this area of the brain can cause coma (see *Box 4.1*). Twelve cranial nerves (discussed later in this chapter) originate in the brainstem. The control of many vital functions such as heart rate, respiratory rate and rhythm, blood pressure, the maintenance of carbon dioxide and oxygen concentrations, deglutition (swallowing) and vomiting occurs in the brainstem, especially the medulla oblongata.

The midbrain

Lying superior to the midbrain are the thalamus and hypothalamus, and inferior are the pons and cerebellum. The nuclei (grey matter region containing the cell bodies) of cranial nerves III and IV, which carry sensory and motor information, are found in the midbrain. Damage to the midbrain can result in pupil dilation, diplopia (double vision) and sensory loss of the face and limbs. The midbrain contains ascending and descending tracts that connect the diencephalon to the pons and the cerebellum. Pupil responses to light are an indication of an intact midbrain if the optic nerves are also intact (see *Box 4.2*).

The pons

The pons lies below the midbrain and above the medulla oblongata. It has connections with the cerebellum, and contains tracts of nerve fibres as well as nuclei that control respiration. The nuclei are clusters or groups of nerve cells in the grey matter of the CNS and these nuclei constitute the origins of the cranial nerves. The nuclei of cranial nerves V, VI, VII and VIII and nerve fibres of the sympathetic nervous system that form the sympathetic chain (discussed later in this chapter) are found in the pons. **Lesions** in the pons can cause loss of facial sensation, facial weakness, pinpoint pupils and deafness. Damage to cranial nerve V, the trigeminal nerve, can result in trigeminal neuralgia (see *Box 4.3*).

> **BOX 4.2**
>
> ### The Glasgow Coma Scale
>
> The Glasgow Coma Scale (GCS) is a neurological scale that is used to assess a patient using set criteria by a first aider, in Emergency Departments, in high-dependency units and in intensive care units. The depth of coma is assessed by awarding points or scores on eye opening and verbal and motor responses. Coma is defined as an eye opening score of 2 or less, a verbal response score of 2 or less, and a motor response score of 4 or less. An overall score of 3 on the GCS indicates deep unconsciousness, while a score of 15 indicates full consciousness.
>
> | Characteristic | Score |
> | --- | --- |
> | **Eye opening** | |
> | Spontaneous | 4 |
> | To verbal command | 3 |
> | To painful stimuli | 2 |
> | No response | 1 |
> | **Verbal response** | |
> | Orientated | 5 |
> | Confused speech | 4 |
> | Inappropriate words | 3 |
> | Incomprehensible sounds | 2 |
> | No response | 1 |
> | **Motor response** | |
> | Obeys commands | 6 |
> | Localizes pain | 5 |
> | Withdraws to pain | 4 |
> | Abnormal flexion to pain | 3 |
> | Extends to pain | 2 |
> | No response | 1 |
>
> Examination of the pupils may suggest possible causes of coma. For example, pinpoint pupils suggest opiate overdose, damage or lesion in the pons, while dilated pupils may suggest raised intracranial pressure or damage to the midbrain. It is important to remember that there are many other causes of coma including hypoglycaemia, hyperglycaemia, kidney failure, stroke and liver failure.
>
> For further details, see:
>
> www.glasgowcomascale.org/
> www.sciencedirect.com/science/article/pii/S0140673674916390#

The medulla oblongata

The medulla oblongata is the lowest part of the brainstem and links with the pons superiorly and the spinal cord inferiorly. It also has fibres linking it to the cerebellum. It contains the nuclei for cranial nerves IX, X, XI and XII, and also contains connections to the sympathetic nerve fibres. Important nerve fibre tracts pass through the medulla oblongata, and within the medulla oblongata are found nuclei that control respiration, heart rate, blood pressure and deglutition

> **BOX 4.3**
>
> **Cranial nerve V and trigeminal neuralgia**
>
> The trigeminal nerve (cranial nerve V) is the largest of the cranial nerves, with fibres extending from the pons to the face. It has sensory and motor divisions with three branches: the ophthalmic, maxillary and mandible nerves. Sensory information relating to temperature, touch and pain is transmitted from the face to the pons.
>
> Trigeminal neuralgia is very severe pain, which lasts less than 2 minutes and may last only a few seconds, caused by inflammation and compression of the trigeminal nerve by blood vessels. The pain is felt in the cheeks, side of the face, ear, eyes, forehead, lips, nose, scalp and teeth. It is sometimes triggered by chewing, talking or shaving.

(swallowing). Damage to the brainstem can result in dysphagia (difficulty in swallowing), dysarthria (a speech disorder characterized by difficulty in articulation), nystagmus (uncontrolled or involuntary movement of the eyes from side to side) and vertigo.

4.2.7 Neuronal pathways and tracts of the brain and spinal cord

White matter is found inside the cerebrum. It is made up of nerve fibres linking the different parts of the brain, which also carry information to and from the brain. Communication between the two cerebral hemispheres is via the corpus callosum. Some fibres known as **projection fibres** link the cerebral cortex to the diencephalon, the cerebellum, the brainstem and the spinal cord. A collection of these ascending and descending neurones passes through an area known as the **internal capsule** (see *Figure 4.9a* and *b*). As the fibres continue to descend, 90% of them cross over to the other side in the medulla oblongata with the result that the left hemisphere of the brain will control the right side of the body, while the right hemisphere will control the left side of the body. The crossing over of nerve projection fibres in the medulla oblongata is known as **decussation** (see *Figure 4.9a*).

Direct (pyramidal) tracts or pathways

The neurones that enable the execution of skilled and precise voluntary movement of skeletal muscles are known as **pyramidal cells**. These are located in the motor cortex or the precentral gyrus of the frontal lobe. The long nerve pathways of the lateral corticospinal tracts start in the motor cortex and pass through the brainstem, extending into the spinal cord without forming synapses. They are known as **direct pathways** because of the lack of synapses and are organized into bundles as they pass through the medulla oblongata. As they do so, they appear to form a pyramid-like shape (see *Figure 4.9a* and *b*). Due to these 'pyramids' that form in the medulla, these voluntary corticospinal tracts were once known as the pyramidal system, although the term direct tracts or pathways is more accurate. Eventually, the motor neurones arrive in areas of the spinal cord (called the **ventral horn**) where they synapse with the motor neurones of the PNS that innervate the specific parts of the body whose movement they control. This direct pathway from the pyramidal cells of the cerebral cortex down to the ventral horn within the spinal cord constitutes the **upper motor neurone**.

Indirect (extrapyramidal) tracts or pathways

The **indirect** or **extrapyramidal pathways** are more complex and have many synapses. Different tracts including the rubrospinal tract (see *Figure 4.9c*) form these indirect pathways that control muscles involved in maintenance of posture and balance, and control limb, head and neck movements, as well as eye movements when following an object. The specific roles of the different indirect pathways are:

- Corticobulbar tract – innervates cranial nerves.
- Reticulospinal tract – maintains posture.
- Rubrospinal tract – controls flexor muscles.
- Spinothalamic tract – transmits information from the spinal cord to the thalamus.
- Vestibulospinal tract – controls muscle tone and balance during standing and moving.

Some psychotropic drugs used in the management of psychoses such as schizophrenia affect indirect pathways. The motor neurones arising from the ventral horn of the spinal cord to the skeletal muscles are known as the **lower motor neurone**.

4.2.8 Protection and nourishment of the brain and spinal cord

There are three main lines of protection of the brain and spinal cord. The first line of protection is provided by the **skull and the vertebral column**. The second is provided by the membranes surrounding the brain called the **meninges**, while the third is provided by the **blood–brain barrier** and **cerebrospinal fluid (CSF)**. CSF mixes with the interstitial fluid that bathes the neurones and neuroglia of the brain. There is no free access of substances to the brain because of the presence of the blood–brain barrier and the **blood–CSF barrier** that isolate the CNS from the general circulation. Arterial blood flow to the brain is via the internal carotid arteries, which supply the cerebrum with more than 80% of its blood needs, and the vertebral arteries. Selective directional movement of nutrients such as glucose, fatty acids, amino acids, vitamins and minerals occurs from brain capillaries through the blood–brain and blood–CSF barriers into cells within the brain and spinal cord. Waste products from the CNS move back into the CSF and eventually back into the general circulation. Astrocytes, described earlier in this chapter, secrete chemicals that maintain the specific permeability properties of the blood–brain barrier.

Meninges and CSF

The meninges consist of three membranes: the **dura mater**, the **arachnoid mater** and the **pia mater** (see *Figure 4.16*). The outer membrane is the dura mater and the middle membrane is the **arachnoid mater**, which has specialized protrusions that form the **arachnoid villi**. It is through the arachnoid villi that CSF is absorbed back into venous blood. The pia mater is the innermost membrane and lies next to the brain and spinal cord. Two spaces are found between the meninges, the **subdural space** and the **subarachnoid space**.

CSF is a clear fluid with a pH of 7.35 and a composition similar to plasma, made in the choroid plexuses of the lateral ventricles (see *Figure 4.16*). It circulates around the brain and spinal cord, carrying oxygen and nutrients and removing metabolic wastes such as carbon dioxide, which eventually are taken back into the general circulation via the arachnoid villi. CSF acts as a shock absorber, cushioning the brain and spinal cord. In clinical practice, a sample of CSF obtained via a procedure known as a 'lumbar puncture' can be analysed to help in the diagnosis of some conditions such as meningitis and brain injury. Strokes can result from burst blood vessels due to a weakness in the wall of a blood vessel in the brain, and such a weakness is known as a brain aneurysm. Following a stroke, blood may collect in the subdural space to form a subdural **haematoma** and in the subarachnoid space to form a subarachnoid haematoma.

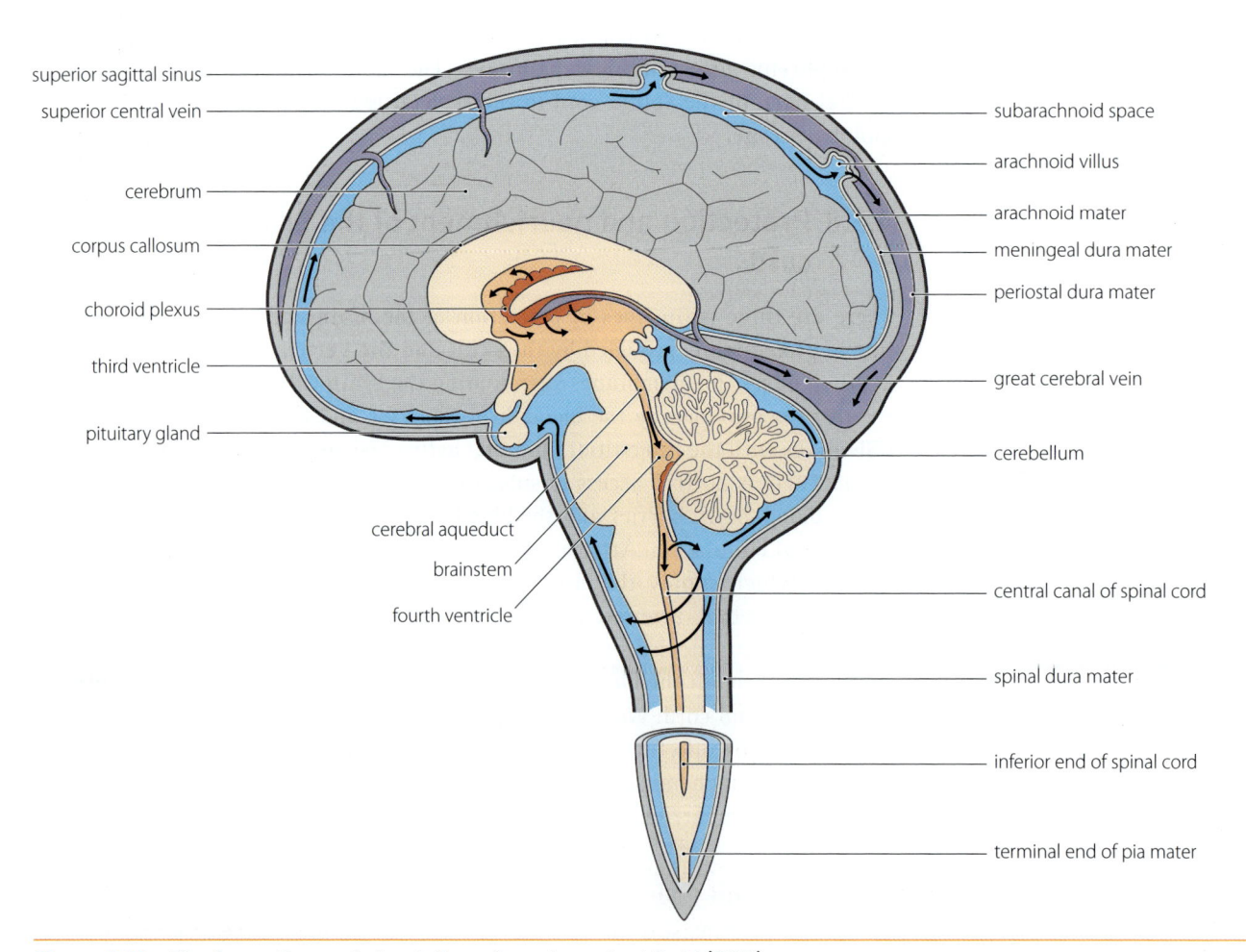

Figure 4.16 – **The formation and circulation of cerebrospinal fluid (CSF).**

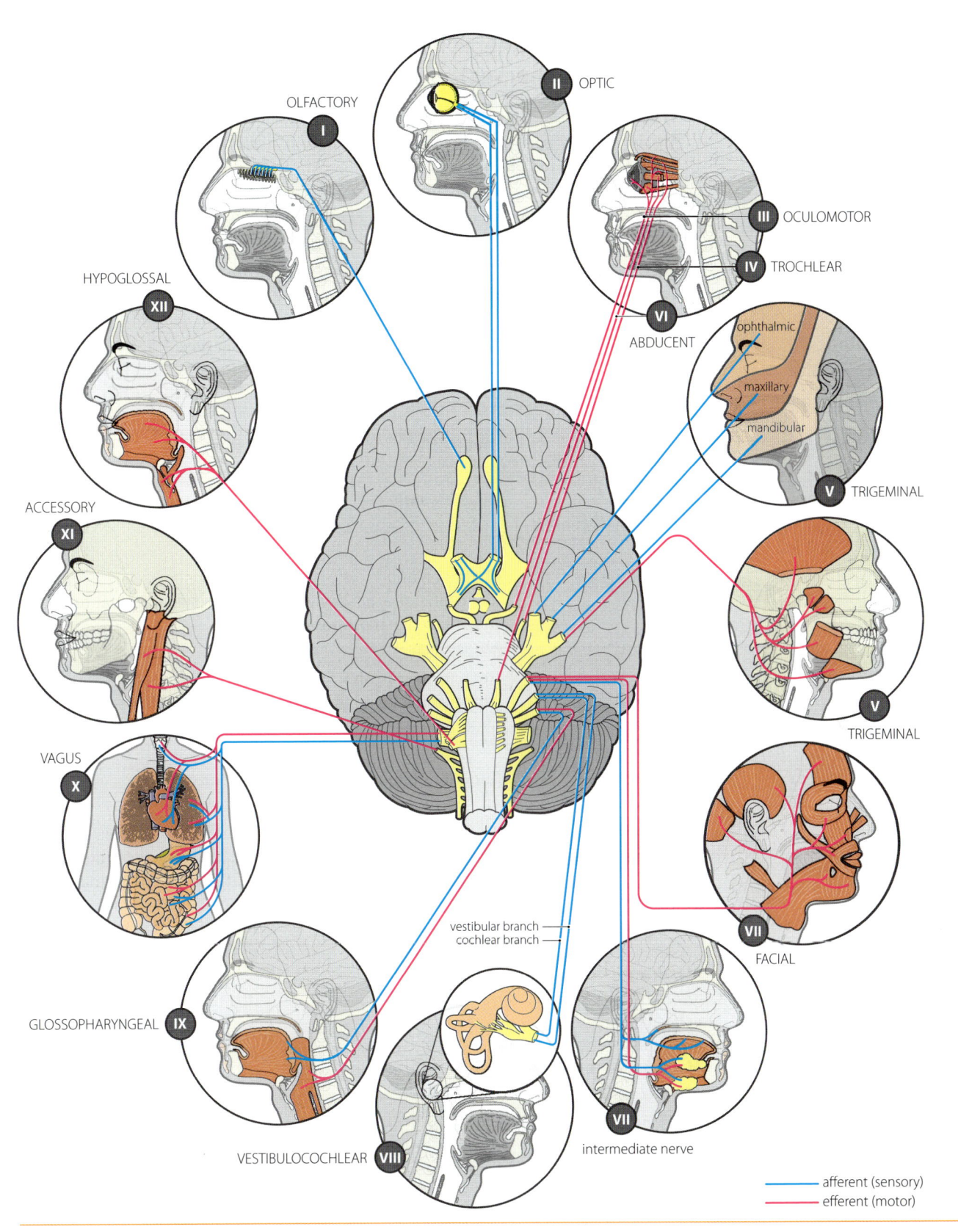

SECTION **4.2** | WHAT YOU NEED TO KNOW – ESSENTIAL ANATOMY AND PHYSIOLOGY 121

Figure 4.17 – **The cranial nerves.**

4.2.9 The peripheral nervous system (cranial nerves and spinal nerves)

When discussing the brainstem, reference was made to the cranial nerves. There are 12 cranial nerves (see *Figure 4.17*), some of which are sensory, some motor and others mixed (both sensory and motor). The cranial nerves are identified with Roman numerals by convention. Eleven of these cranial nerves remain in the head or neck; the exception is the cranial nerve X, known as the **vagus nerve**, which innervates many organs in the thorax and abdomen such as the heart, lungs and gastrointestinal tract. The cranial nerves are summarized in *Table 4.2*. Cranial nerves I, II and VIII are purely or mostly sensory. Cranial nerves III, IV, VI and XI are mostly or primarily motor in function but do also have sensory fibres. Cranial nerves V, VII, IX, X and XII are mixed nerves.

Table 4.2 – The cranial nerves

Cranial nerve	Name of cranial nerve	Origin	Destination	Function
I	Olfactory	Receptors are in olfactory epithelium	Olfactory bulbs	Purely sensory Carries information for the sense of smell
II	Optic	Retina of the eye	Thalamus and diencephalon – passes via the optic chiasma where fibres cross	Purely sensory Carries visual information
III	Oculomotor	Motor – mesencephalon (midbrain) Sensory – eye muscle	Rectus, oblique and levator muscles of the eye Midbrain	Mostly motor Somatic and visceral motor eye coordination movements
IV	Trochlear	Mesencephalon (midbrain)	Superior oblique muscle of the eye	Mostly motor Allows eye to move downwards and sideways
V	Trigeminal	Has **three** main branches: **Ophthalmic** – (sensory) forehead, upper eyelid, nose **Maxillary** – (sensory) lower eyelid, cheek, upper lip, palate, gums, teeth, nose **Mandibular** (mixed) Sensory – gums, lips, tongue, teeth, palate Motor – pons	Sensory – nuclei in pons Motor – muscles of mastication by mandibular branch	Mixed (sensory and motor) Somatic sensory information from the head and face Motor information to muscles of mastication
VI	Abducens	Pons	Lateral rectus muscle	Mostly motor Sideways (abduction) eye movements

Cranial nerve	Name of cranial nerve	Origin	Destination	Function
VII	Facial	Sensory – taste receptors in anterior two-thirds of tongue Motor – pons	Sensory – nuclei in pons Motor: Somatic – facial expression Visceral – tear (lacrimal) gland, nasal mucosal glands, sublingual and submandibular salivary glands	Mixed (sensory and motor) Monitors pressure sensation in the face and taste information from the tongue. Motor fibres send information to the scalp and muscles of the face. Damage to this nerve can lead to facial muscle paralysis and loss of taste sensations
VIII	Vestibulocochlear	Receptors in inner ear (vestibule and cochlea) Motor – pons	Nuclei of pons and medulla oblongata Cochlea hairs	Mostly sensory Vestibular branch – balance and equilibrium Cochlea branch – hearing
IX	Glossopharyngeal	Sensory – posterior one-third region of tongue Motor – nuclei in medulla oblongata	Sensory – nuclei in medulla oblongata Somatic motor – pharyngeal swallowing muscles Visceral motor – parotid salivary glands	Mixed (sensory and motor) Sensory nerves provide taste sensations from the tongue and monitor baroreceptor and chemoreceptor activity in the carotid sinus and carotid body (see *Chapters 9* and *10*) Motor nerves
X	Vagus	Sensory – pharynx, auricle and external auditory canal of the ear, visceral organs of the thorax (heart, lungs), diaphragm, visceral organs of the abdomen (stomach, liver, pancreas, spleen, kidneys, small intestines and colon) Motor – nuclei in medulla oblongata	Sensory – medulla oblongata Visceral motor – palate muscles, pharynx, gastrointestinal tract, cardiovascular system, respiratory system	Mixed (sensory and motor) Sensory – relays somatic information from the external ear and diaphragm. Visceral information is relayed from the gastrointestinal tract and respiratory system Motor – information carried to the heart and smooth muscles of the whole gastrointestinal tract and accessory organs. Coordination of the swallowing reflex is affected by damage to the vagus nerve
XI	Accessory	Spinal cord and medulla oblongata	Voluntary muscles of the palate, pharynx, larynx, neck muscles (sternocleidomastoid) and back muscles (trapezius)	Mostly motor
XII	Hypoglossal	Sensory – proprioceptors in tongue muscles Motor – medulla oblongata	Medulla oblongata Tongue muscles	Sensory – conducts nerve impulses for proprioception (the non-visual perception of position and movements) Motor – voluntary motor movements of the tongue

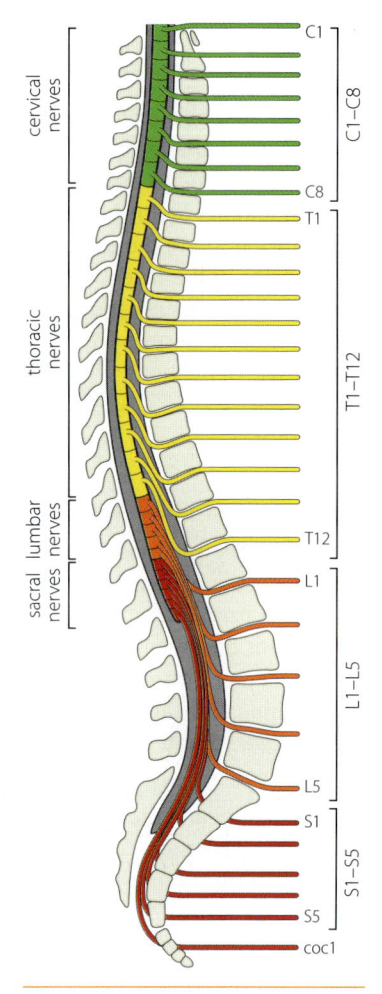

Figure 4.18 – **The arrangement of spinal nerves in the vertebral column.**

The names of the spinal nerves relate to the region of the vertebral column from which they originate (see *Figure 4.18*). Of the 31 pairs of spinal nerves, eight pairs are cervical, 12 pairs are thoracic, five pairs are lumbar, five pairs are sacral and one pair is coccygeal. Each spinal nerve is connected to the spinal cord by a **dorsal root** that contains sensory (afferent) fibres and a **ventral root** that contains motor (efferent) fibres. The spinal nerves divide into **dorsal and ventral rami** (branches), which form the cervical **plexus** (network), which serves the neck muscles and diaphragm; the brachial plexus, which supplies the upper limbs; the lumbar plexus, which supplies the abdomen, buttocks and lower limbs; and the sacral plexus, which serves the thigh and the foot. A plexus is a network of nerves that serves an area of the body. The sciatic nerve, which is the largest nerve in the body, is part of the lower lumbar (L4–L5) sacral plexus. Thus, the peripheral nerves that serve the upper limbs and lower limbs arise in the cervical and lumbar regions of the spine, respectively.

The reflex arc

The spinal reflex arc (see *Figure 4.19*) illustrates the ability of the nervous system to respond very quickly to unforeseen situations that demand an immediate response by producing a reflex action. Most of these situations suggest danger and, if there was no immediate response, could result in severe injury and sometimes death. Involuntary reflexes, also known as autonomic or visceral reflexes, affect smooth muscles, cardiac muscle and glands, while somatic reflexes are associated with skeletal muscles. A pinprick is an example of a somatic reflex called the withdrawal or flexor reflex and is initiated by a painful stimulus. Inflicting pain on a part of the body causes automatic withdrawal to that part of the body. Withdrawal reflexes are very important for survival and are protective against suspected or real injury.

Another example of a protective reflex is the stretch reflex, which prevents muscle from overstretching. The stretch reflex affects large muscles such as those of the arms, thighs and abdomen. The knee-jerk or patellar reflex is a good example of a stretch reflex that enables an upright posture to be maintained without the knees giving way. When the knees begin to buckle, the stretch reflex causes the thigh muscles known as the quadriceps to lengthen and the muscle tone is adjusted. As discussed under homeostatic mechanisms, a reflex arc has elements similar to a homeostatic loop (see *Chapter 1*) and includes a receptor, an input message carrier (the sensory or afferent neurone), an integration centre (the spinal cord), an output message carrier (the motor or efferent neurone) and an effector (muscle, organ or gland). Within the integration centre is usually found an interneurone or association neurone.

Spinal reflexes are initiated and completed at the spinal cord level, and many of these do not involve higher centres in the brain, although the brain is made aware of these spinal reflexes. For example, during clinical examination, a positive result for any stretch reflex test indicates that there are intact connections between the relevant muscles and the spinal cord. Where peripheral nerve damage exists, stretch reflexes tend to be hypoactive or absent.

4.2.10 The autonomic nervous system

The relationship of the autonomic nervous system (ANS) to other parts of the nervous system is illustrated by *Figure 4.2*. The ANS is part of the motor division of the PNS. The ANS controls activities not under voluntary control, such as smooth muscle contraction, cardiac function and the activity of glands. The ANS consists of the sympathetic and parasympathetic nervous system. These two divisions differ both structurally, in terms of location of ganglia, and functionally, in terms of the type of neurones that go to the effectors and the neurotransmitters they produce. Unlike the somatic nervous system, which has single neurones from the CNS to effectors, in both the sympathetic and parasympathetic nervous system there are two neurones between the CNS and the effector with a ganglion between the two neurones. The neurone from the CNS to the ganglion between the two neurones is called a **preganglionic neurone**. This preganglionic neurone is thin and its myelin sheath is light. The neurone between the ganglion and the effector is called a **postganglionic neurone**. It is thinner than the preganglionic neurone and is unmyelinated. Preganglionic neurones in both sympathetic and parasympathetic nervous systems produce acetylcholine. The postganglionic neurones in both systems are unmyelinated but they produce different neurotransmitters (see *Table 4.3* and *Figure 4.20*). Postganglionic neurones in the sympathetic nervous system

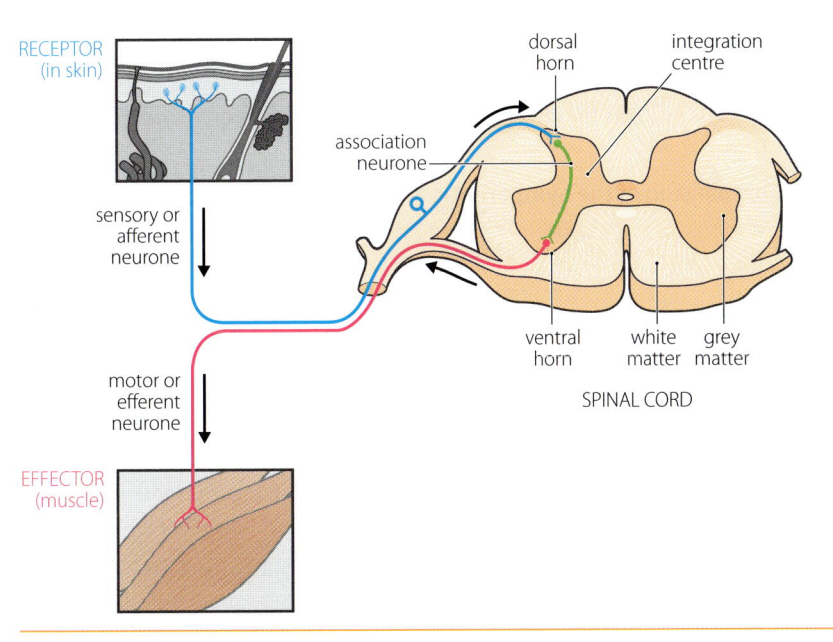

Figure 4.19 – **The reflex arc.**

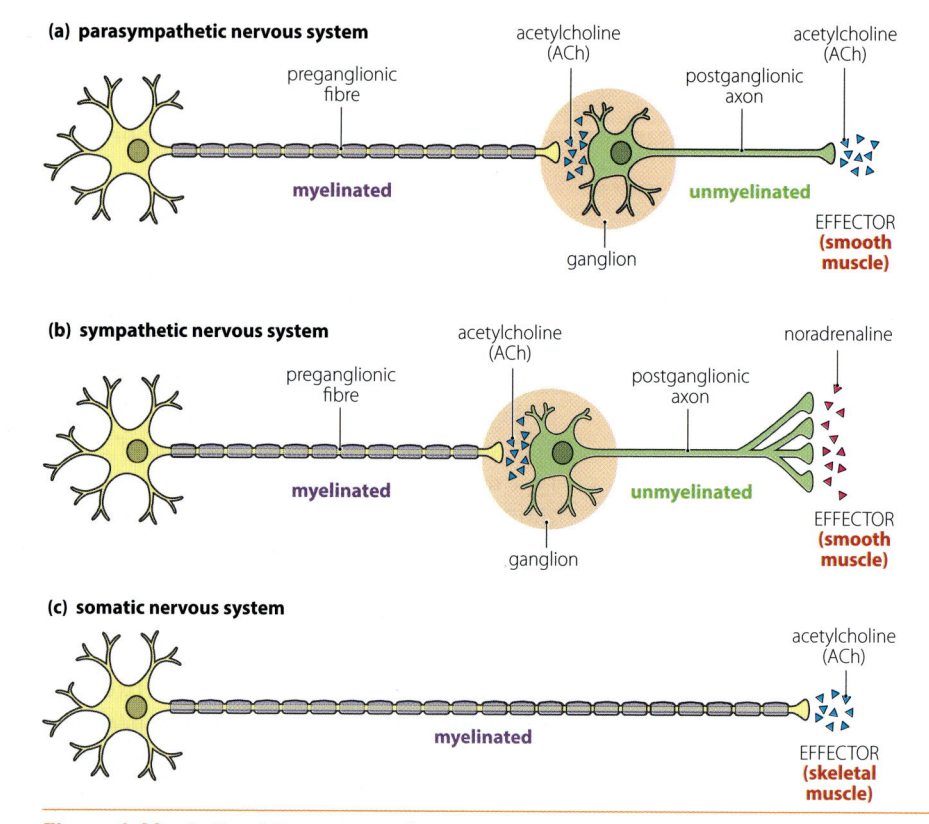

Figure 4.20 – Cells of the autonomic nervous system.
Cells of the autonomic nervous system showing myelinated preganglionic and unmyelinated postganglionic fibres and the neurotransmitters released in (a) the parasympathetic and (b) the sympathetic system; (c) the somatic nervous system releases acetylcholine only.

Table 4.3 – Comparison of the sympathetic and parasympathetic nervous systems and their activation

Characteristic	Sympathetic	Parasympathetic
Ganglia location	Located near spinal cord	Located on or near receptors
Appearance of ganglia	Chain of ganglia	No chain of ganglia
Neuronal fibres	Adrenergic	Cholinergic
Neurotransmitter	Preganglionic – *acetylcholine* Postganglionic – *adrenaline, noradrenaline*	Preganglionic – *acetylcholine* Postganglionic – *acetylcholine*
Effect	Speeds up activity and produces emergency response – fight-or-flight reaction (accelerator)	Produces the relaxation response (brake)
Blood	Withdrawn from gastrointestinal tract and skin and moved to vital organs and muscles	Moved to gastrointestinal tract
Pupils	Dilated	Constricted

produce noradrenaline (norepinephrine), while the postganglionic neurones in the parasympathetic nervous system produce acetylcholine. The effects of noradrenaline and acetylcholine on various organs and tissues are summarized in *Figure 4.21*. The preganglionic nerve fibres of the sympathetic nervous system leave the spinal cord from the thoracolumbar vertebral region (T1–L2). An interconnected chain of **ganglia** (the sympathetic trunk or sympathetic chain) in the sympathetic nervous system is located near the spinal cord on either side to produce a *whole-body response* (by virtue of the interconnections between the nuclei within the ganglia) when the system is activated. It is this sympathetic

PARASYMPATHETIC DIVISION

- **eye muscles** — contraction
- **salivary glands** — profuse watery secretion
- **heart** — decrease in heart rate, decrease in contractility
- **LUNGS** — bronchial muscles contraction; bronchial glands stimulation; arterioles dilation
- **stomach** — increase in motility, relaxation of sphincters, stimulation of secretions
- **pancreas** — increased insulin and glucagon secretion
- **liver and gall bladder** — contraction
- **small and large intestine** — peristalsis
- **urinary bladder** — contraction
- **genitals**

SYMPATHETIC DIVISION

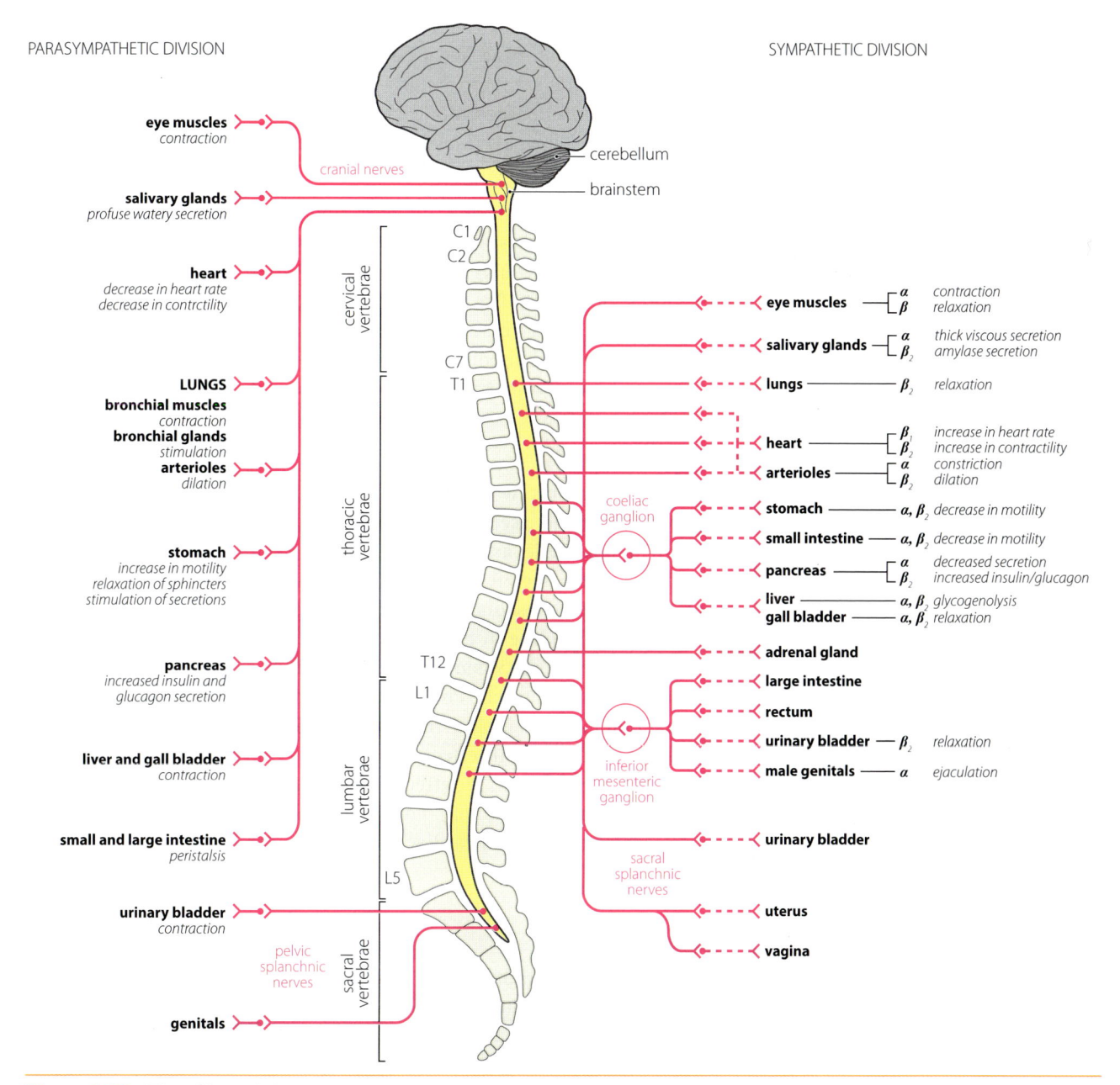

- **eye muscles** — α contraction, β relaxation
- **salivary glands** — α thick viscous secretion, β_2 amylase secretion
- **lungs** — β_2 relaxation
- **heart** — β_1 increase in heart rate, β_2 increase in contractility
- **arterioles** — α constriction, β_2 dilation
- **stomach** — α, β_2 decrease in motility
- **small intestine** — α, β_2 decrease in motility
- **pancreas** — α decreased secretion, β_2 increased insulin/glucagon
- **liver** — α, β_2 glycogenolysis
- **gall bladder** — α, β_2 relaxation
- **adrenal gland**
- **large intestine**
- **rectum**
- **urinary bladder** — β_2 relaxation
- **male genitals** — α ejaculation
- **urinary bladder**
- **uterus**
- **vagina**

Figure 4.21 – The effect of the autonomic nervous system on various parts of the body.

activation and production of adrenaline (epinephrine) that produce a whole-body response. The ganglia in the parasympathetic nervous system, however, are located on or near the effectors. The parasympathetic nervous outflow is referred to as craniosacral because the preganglionic fibres originate in the brainstem and arise from neurones in the grey matter of the sacral region (S2–S4) of the spinal cord.

Some of the preganglionic fibres that leave the spinal cord and go to the sympathetic trunk form plexuses or other ganglia from where branches are sent to different organs. For example, the cardiac and pulmonary plexuses have postganglionic fibres that innervate the heart and the lungs. The coeliac ganglion has postganglionic fibres that innervate the liver and gall bladder, stomach, spleen, kidneys, small intestine and part of the large intestine. Postganglionic fibres from the superior mesenteric ganglion innervate most of the large intestine, while those from the inferior mesenteric ganglion innervate the descending colon, sigmoid colon, rectum, urinary bladder and sexual organs, thus facilitating a whole-body response.

All ANS preganglionic fibres and *all* parasympathetic postganglionic fibres release acetylcholine at their synapses and are known as cholinergic, while *most* sympathetic postganglionic fibres release noradrenaline and are referred to as adrenergic fibres. However, a few sympathetic postganglionic fibres such as those that innervate some blood vessels and sweat glands release acetylcholine. The nature of the response that is produced in effectors depends on the neurotransmitter and on the type of receptor on the effector (see *Figures 4.20* and *4.21*).

Cholinergic receptors

The cholinergic system has two types of receptor called **nicotinic** and **muscarinic receptors**, which bind to acetylcholine. **Nicotinic acetylcholine receptors** are located in all sympathetic and parasympathetic ganglionic neurones, in the adrenal medulla, which secretes hormones (discussed in *Chapter 5*) and on cell membranes at the neuromuscular junctions of skeletal muscles (see *Chapter 13*). The binding of acetylcholine to nicotinic receptors stimulates all effectors with such receptors. For example, when acetylcholine binds to nicotinic receptors on the membrane of skeletal muscle, ion channels open allowing depolarization and muscle contraction to occur. **Muscarinic acetylcholine receptors** are found on all parasympathetic postganglionic effectors and some sympathetic effectors such as blood vessels and sweat glands; the effect depends on the subclass of the receptors and can be stimulatory or inhibitory. For example, the effect of acetylcholine on muscarinic receptors located on cardiac muscle is to inhibit or slow down heart rate.

Adrenergic receptors

Adrenergic receptors are slightly more complex in that the two major classes of alpha (α) and beta (β) receptors have further subclasses of α_1 and α_2 and β_1, β_2 and β_3, respectively. The effect of either adrenaline or noradrenaline on effectors can be excitatory or inhibitory and very much depends on the subclass of receptor the effector possesses. For example, *adrenergic stimulation* of β_1 receptors in the sinoatrial node (see *Chapter 9*) increases heart rate, while *adrenergic stimulation* of $β_2$ receptors in the ventricles of the heart increases contractility and conduction velocity of heart muscle. Similarly, stimulation of $β_2$ receptors on arterioles and urinary bladder detrusor muscle causes relaxation, while such stimulation in the stomach and small intestine decreases motility and tone (see *Figure 4.21*).

Stress and adaptation

The presence of a highly developed nervous system in humans has enabled us to adapt to changes and challenges in our environment and is consistent with homeodynamics. Stressors come in different forms and include injury, infection, exposure to harmful agents and chemicals, physiological disturbances, noise, pollution, relationships and work. When challenged by stressors, the nervous system is able to integrate the received information and initiate appropriate responses via motor (efferent) pathways in order to minimize the effects of the stressor.

In acute stress, which can be physiological, psychological or both, the autonomic nervous system activates the fight-or-flight response, which involves the mobilization of different body systems and mechanisms to deal with the challenge or threat. The body's responses and mechanisms will involve different tissues, organs and systems such as the endocrine glands (see *Chapter 5*), the liver (see *Chapter 7*), the kidneys (see *Chapter 8*), heart and blood vessels (see *Chapter 9*), the lungs and associated structures (see *Chapter 10*), the immune system (see *Chapter 11*), the skin (see *Chapter 12*) and the musculoskeletal system (see *Chapter 13*). During acute stress, increased activation of the sympathetic nervous system diverts blood from areas such as the skin and gastrointestinal tract to the heart, lungs and muscles, and this is coupled with increases in heart rate, blood pressure, and respiration rate and depth. There is breakdown of glycogen to increase blood glucose and increased breakdown of fats to form fatty acids and glycerol; all these substances are sources of energy. The kidneys retain sodium and water in order to increase blood volume. There is heightened cognition with increased alertness and vigilance due to increased arousal by sympathetic activation.

Continued exposure to the stressor or challenge triggers adaptive responses through stimulation of the endocrine system, which produces hormones such as adrenocorticotropic hormone and cortisol (discussed in *Chapter 5*) that enable us to manage the stress. Long-term stress and activation of cortisol can lead to health problems such as heart disease due to the increased release of fatty acids. The involvement of the endocrine system following acute responses by the nervous system demonstrates how the nervous and endocrine systems work in an integrated manner in order to maintain homeostatic and homeodynamic processes.

4.3 Clinical application

The nervous system has an important role in the effective coordination of physiological processes that are necessary for homeodynamic regulation and therefore for health. Impairment of this coordinated activity can arise from injury or disease processes, leading to impaired health. The patients described in this chapter highlight health problems that can arise from a range of factors that compromise and impair the functioning of the nervous system.

- **Bessie (Patient 4.1)** had a sudden stroke affecting the left side of her brain, leaving her with right-sided weakness and impairment of her speech. This is causing her problems with communication and in responding to her environment, and also in regulating physiological processes. Her inability to move and her incontinence will result in skin damage (see *Chapter 12*).
- **Jordon (Patient 4.2)** was diagnosed with fetal alcohol syndrome that he acquired while he was still in his mother's womb because Jade, his mother, used to drink excessively when she was pregnant with him.
- **Graham (Patient 4.3)** has Parkinson's disease, which started in his left hand and progressed to his other hand, giving him a tremor both at rest and during movement. He started having panic attacks, which affected his work and relationships, resulting in him becoming withdrawn.

Patient 4.1 — Bessie | 99 | **130** | 379 | 397 | 403 | 441

- 71-year-old woman
- Lifelong smoker –20 cigarettes per day
- Found unconscious with stroke and hemiplegia

The ambulance personnel applied the **FAST rule** (see *Box 4.4*) and noticed that Bessie's right arm was weak, her speech was slurred and she had saliva drooling from her mouth. Bessie's right-sided weakness, or **hemiplegia**, is due to her having a stroke on the left side of her brain. Stroke is a sudden focal or global neurological deficit that persists for more than 24 hours. The majority of the neuronal pathways from the right side of the brain cortex and other neuronal pathways from the left side of the brain cortex cross over in the medulla oblongata (decussation). This means that the right side of the brain controls movement on the left side of the body and the left side of the brain controls movement on the right side of the body. On admission, rapid assessment and investigations were carried out to ascertain the precise nature of the stroke and whether Bessie's stroke was due to bleeding or a clot (see *Chapter 9*) so that the appropriate interventions would be done to resuscitate and support her. Bessie's speech is affected because the speech centre is located on the left side of the brain in most people. Stroke can result in **receptive aphasia** characterized by poor comprehension when the damage is in **Wernicke's area**, and to **expressive aphasia** when the damage is in **Broca's area**. In expressive aphasia, the person knows what she or he wants to say but is unable to do so due to poor speech initiation and poor word forming and articulation, which is very frustrating to the individual. In receptive aphasia, the person is able to speak normally but is unable to understand spoken or written words. The causes and symptoms of stroke are summarized in *Boxes 4.5* and *4.6*, respectively. Bessie has cut down her smoking and is trying to quit smoking altogether. However, Bessie has smoked 20 cigarettes daily for many years. Smoking is one of the main causes of stroke (see *Box 4.5*) because it damages blood vessels such as arteries, interfering with blood flow and affecting blood pressure (discussed in *Chapter 9*).

BOX 4.4

Using FAST in suspected stroke

The Face, Arm, Speech Test (FAST) can help you recognize the symptoms of a stroke.

If you suspect a stroke, act FAST and call the emergency services.

Ambulance crews use FAST.

Face
Can the person smile? Has their mouth or eye drooped?

Arms
Can the person raise both arms?

Speech
Can the person speak clearly?
Can the person understand what you say?

Test all three
Test all three symptoms.
Time is of the essence

BOX 4.5

Stroke

Stroke leads to major disability and is the third most common cause of death in the Western world. It affects males more than it does females. The types of stroke include ischaemic (thromboembolitic) and haemorrhagic.

Causes of stroke include:

- Smoking
- Excessive alcohol intake
- An aneurysm
- Hypertension
- Diabetes mellitus
- High blood cholesterol
- Ischaemic heart disease
- Peripheral vascular disease

A stroke is a medical emergency and prompt action is required in order to prevent further damage to the brain.

Management of stroke:

Once a stroke is suspected, the individual needs to be taken to hospital quickly by the emergency services to receive appropriate treatment.

BOX 4.6

Symptoms of a stroke

- Sudden weakness or numbness of the face, arm or leg on one side of the body
- Sudden loss or blurring of vision
- Sudden difficulty in speaking or understanding spoken language
- Sudden confusion
- Sudden severe headache with no apparent cause
- Dizziness
- Dysphagia

Patient 4.2 — Jade and Jordon | 100 | **132** | 138 | 162 | 448 | 473

- 6-year-old boy and 32-year-old mother
- Jade drank alcohol excessively while pregnant
- Jordon has dysmorphic facial features and behavioural issues
- Jordon has fetal alcohol syndrome

Jordon suffers from fetal alcohol syndrome, which he acquired when he was in Jade's womb. Jade drank while pregnant with Jordon, compromising his health because alcohol is toxic to the brain and modifies CNS development. The development of the nervous system begins soon after the second week of life in the womb. Alcohol is a drug and has **teratogenic** effects in human tissues during embryological development.

The presence of a **teratogen** such as alcohol in Jade's blood suggests that development of the white matter (myelin-covered axons) of Jordon's nervous system was greatly affected. Furthermore, as a baby's facial features are formed between weeks 6 and 9 of pregnancy, some facial deformities affecting Jordon's nose and lips occurred and are noticeable as a result of damage by alcohol. Jordon's liver (see *Chapter 7*) was not developed enough to metabolize alcohol adequately. In addition to the facial birth defects, the effect of alcohol on Jordon's brain while he was still in his mother's womb caused functional impairment, and this is evident in him being an anxious and nervous child, his poor sleep pattern, his agitation, his poor attention span, his poor memory and his poor social skills in his interactions with his peers. It is important to recognize that some of the behavioural problems that are exhibited by individuals during childhood and later on in life are a result of developmental issues *in utero*, as is the case with Jordon, where exposure to alcohol during the gestation period (see *Chapter 14*) resulted in birth defects and functional impairment.

Patient 4.3 — Graham | 100 | **132** | 404 | 442

- 57-year-old man
- Gradual onset of trembling in left hand
- Family doctor referred him to neurologist
- Diagnosis of Parkinson disease led to depression
- MRI has excluded other causes
- Prescribed bromocriptine to help with Parkinson symptoms

The symptoms of Parkinson's disease in Graham did not develop suddenly but were insidious, beginning with trembling in his left hand, which progressed to the other hand. In addition, he began to experience panic attacks and become withdrawn. In order to exclude other causes, the neurologist referred Graham for magnetic resonance imaging (MRI) of the head (see *Chapter 1, Section 1.4*), and following clinical examination and further investigations, the neurologist concluded that Graham has *idiopathic* Parkinson's disease (Parkinson's disease whose cause is unknown), in which there is loss of neurones in the substantia nigra, a part of the basal ganglia. Dopaminergic cells in the substantia nigra produce the neurotransmitter dopamine. Parkinson's disease demonstrates how damage to neurones can result in disorders of other systems of the body such as movement (see *Chapter 13*). Graham was prescribed bromocriptine, a dopamine receptor agonist (see *Chapter 2, Box 2.1*), by his family doctor. He now takes bromocriptine 10 mg three times a day in order to increase the amount of dopamine in his brain. Parkinson's disease is a neurodegenerative disorder that usually affects people between the ages of 50 and 70 years. A diagnosis of Parkinson's disease can be accompanied by apathy and feelings of depression due to the change in an individual's life and circumstances. Depression, anxiety and dementia are common in Parkinson's disease and depression is often overlooked, and yet it interferes with quality of life. Graham's mood was very low most of the time such that, in addition to the dopamine agonist, his family doctor prescribed citalopram 10 mg daily initially, which was increased to 30 mg daily, and he now takes the latter dosage every morning. Selective serotonin inhibitors minimize the reuptake of serotonin from the synapse by the presynaptic membrane, thus allowing the concentration of serotonin in the synapse to increase within the CNS. Taking medication has helped Graham in that his mood has improved. This has helped in his relationship with his wife who has begun to understand Graham's forgetfulness and has realized he was not just lazy as she initially thought.

4.4 Summary

- Homeodynamic regulation of organ systems requires coordination and integration of activity, which is achieved by the nervous systems.
- The nervous system communicates through neurones and neurotransmitters, producing quick, immediate responses.
- The brain and spinal cord make up the central nervous system, while the cranial nerves and spinal nerves make up the peripheral nervous system.
- There are 12 cranial nerves and 31 spinal nerves (see *Figures 4.17* and *4.18*).
- The cholinergic system has two types of receptor called nicotinic and muscarinic receptors, which bind to acetylcholine.
- The two major classes of adrenergic receptors are α and β receptors, both of which have further subclasses.
- The function of neurotransmitters can be enhanced or inhibited by many therapeutic and illicit drugs.

4.5 Further reading

The National Aphasia Association (NAA) is an organization that promotes education, research, rehabilitation and support services for people with aphasia and their families. It is an excellent resource for raising awareness of aphasia for both professionals and non-professionals:
www.aphasia.org/

This resource is provided by the Stroke Association and covers many facets of stroke, including guidance on how to act when a stroke is suspected:
www.stroke.org.uk/

The National Institute for Health and Care Excellence (NICE) website provides the quality standard for the care of people who have had a stroke and is worth visiting as an authoritative resource:
http://guidance.nice.org.uk/QS2

Information on how to use the Glasgow Coma Scale in clinical practice and how to interpret and record the observations made can be found at the website below. There is a video with a narrative by Sir Graham Teasdale, who described the scale for the first time and published it with his co-author, Bryan Jennet:
www.glasgowcomascale.org

The original article, published by the authors who first described the scale in 1974 and how they had used it, can be found at the following website:
www.sciencedirect.com/science/article/pii/S0140673674916390#

The National Organisation for Foetal Alcohol Syndrome – UK (NOFAS-UK) supports people with fetal alcohol syndrome spectrum disorders and their families. Women who are pregnant or thinking about becoming pregnant are encouraged to contact the organization for information. NOFAS-UK also runs an accredited course on fetal alcohol syndrome for healthcare professionals in the UK. There is also a film for midwives on the website entitled No Alcohol, No Risk: www.nofas-uk.org/

4.6 Self-assessment questions

Answers can be found at www.scionpublishing.com/AandP

(4.1) Select the one correct answer. A reflex action:
   (a) originates in the cerebral cortex
   (b) terminates in the spinal cord
   (c) is a rapid automatic response to a stimulus
   (d) results from activity in two central nervous system synapses
   (e) is very slow and lasts forever

(4.2) Select the one correct answer. In which part of the brain does decussation of the descending motor neurones occur?
   (a) The pons
   (b) The internal capsule
   (c) The thalamus
   (d) The medulla oblongata
   (e) The spinal cord

(4.3) Select the one correct answer. Which parts of the nervous system comprise the brainstem?
   (a) The midbrain, medulla oblongata and internal capsule
   (b) The pons, medulla oblongata and basal ganglia
   (c) The medulla oblongata, basal ganglia and cerebellum
   (d) The hypothalamus, thalamus and cerebellum
   (e) The midbrain, pons and medulla oblongata

(4.4) Select the one correct answer. In trigeminal neuralgia, which cranial nerve is damaged?
   (a) Cranial nerve I
   (b) Cranial nerve V
   (c) Cranial nerve VI
   (d) Cranial nerve IX
   (e) Cranial nerve XII

(4.5) Mark each statement either true or false:
   (a) Damage to the midbrain can result in pupil dilation and diplopia
   (b) The responses of pupils to light are an indication of an intact midbrain, indicating that the optic nerve is intact
   (c) The effect of either adrenaline (epinephrine) or noradrenaline (norepinephrine) on effectors is only excitatory
   (d) The thinner the diameter of an axon, the faster the transmission of the action potential
   (e) The parasympathetic nervous system outflow can be referred to as craniosacral

(4.6) Select the one correct answer. Identify the structure that is not part of the limbic system.
(a) The amygdala
(b) The thalamus
(c) The hypothalamus
(d) The corpus callosum
(e) The pons

(4.7) Select the one correct answer. Receptive aphasia is due to damage to:
(a) Broca's area
(b) the basal ganglia
(c) Wernicke's area
(d) the precentral gyrus
(e) the corpus callosum

(4.8) Select the one correct answer. Which neurotransmitter is produced by the basal ganglia and is associated with the extrapyramidal pathway?
(a) Dopamine
(b) Gamma-aminobutyric acid
(c) Acetylcholine
(d) Serotonin
(e) Glutamate

(4.9) Describe the process of saltatory conduction.

(4.10) Describe the mechanism involved following a pinprick to the forefinger resulting in withdrawal of the forearm.

(4.11) Compare the activities of the sympathetic and parasympathetic nervous systems and explain how a whole-body response is produced by sympathetic activation.

CHAPTER 05 | Communication: long and slow

Learning points for this chapter

After working through this chapter, you should be able to:
- Describe the organization and components of the endocrine system
- Describe how hormones exert an effect
- Describe the general functions of hormones
- Discuss the functions of specific hormones
- Discuss the integrated function of the endocrine and nervous systems

5.1 Introduction and clinical relevance

Biological communication occurs by the release and transport of chemical messengers. Some of these have a local effect, while others are released directly into blood and have an effect at a distance. The endocrine system ensures that cellular and physiological mechanisms in the body are regulated to achieve homeodynamics through the release of **hormones**. As with neurotransmitters, hormones are crucial signal molecules required to coordinate and direct cellular activity. Some hormones promote growth and some enable metabolic processes to occur at the cellular level, while others ensure that the individual is able to respond and adapt to changes within the environment. Hormonal communication has a long duration of action and is slow to make cellular changes, which enables the body to respond to situations of long duration when the response of the nervous system alone would be inadequate. Thus, the endocrine system cooperates with the nervous system in the integration of a multitude of sensory stimuli to produce responses that enable the regulation of bodily function and activities in order to achieve homeodynamics. As discussed in *Chapter 4*, nervous system communication is via neurotransmitters and is fast and short lived, while endocrine communication is long and slow. Each of the patient studies in this chapter illustrates how the endocrine system regulates the activities of different organs and tissue in response to different stimuli in order to restore deviation from the norm.

| Patient 5.1 | David | **138** | 161 | 195 | 237 | 448 | 474 |

- 44-year-old man
- Increased urine output; thirsty and hungry
- Blood test: low thyroxine and raised blood glucose

David is a 44-year-old manager of a successful restaurant. David is a very sociable person and when diners come to his restaurant, he is very welcoming and excellent at making them feel at ease. Recently, David noticed that he was passing a lot of urine and was becoming more thirsty and feeling more hungry, which meant that he ate more. David noticed that he was feeling lethargic and he could not understand this. When David visited his family doctor, blood samples were taken to assess his blood composition, liver function, thyroid function and blood glucose levels. The results showed that David had an underactive thyroid gland and that the levels of both his random and fasting blood glucose were higher than normal.

| Patient 4.2 | Jade and Jordon | 100 | 132 | **138** | 162 | 448 | 473 |

- 6-year-old boy and 32-year-old mother
- Jade drank alcohol excessively while pregnant
- Jordon has dysmorphic facial features and behavioural issues
- Jordon has fetal alcohol syndrome

Jordon was born with fetal alcohol syndrome, and when his health visitor reviewed his developmental milestones such as crawling and walking, she observed that there was a developmental delay. From the age of 2 years, he had a small stature and his weight for age was lower than what it should be. Jordon was sent to see a paediatrician for an assessment and, following investigations, the results showed that he was producing low levels of growth hormone (GH). Jordon started receiving injections of GH and his stature has since improved, such that he is around the 60th percentile of stature for age.

The two patients explored in this chapter demonstrate how hormones influence body structure and physiological function. The symptoms of hunger, thirst and passing a lot of urine that David (Patient 5.1) is experiencing are due to his body not producing enough of the hormone insulin that enables glucose to enter cells where it can be utilized by cells to produce energy. David will need to change his lifestyle by changing his diet. Jordon (Patient 4.2) has a small stature because he is not growing as he should, as a result of not producing enough growth hormone (GH). Jordon will need GH injections to enable him to grow properly. Both David and Jordon illustrate how hormones work at the cellular level for good health and to allow normal growth and development to be achieved.

5.2 What you need to know – essential anatomy and physiology

5.2.1 The endocrine system

Coordination is achieved not only by the function of the nervous system but also by endocrine mechanisms. While the nervous system regulates bodily functions via neurones and neurotransmitters, the endocrine system signalling brings about changes in physiology by autocrines, paracrines and hormones. An autocrine signalling molecule has an effect on the cell that secreted it (self-signalling). An example of an **autocrine** signalling molecule is insulin (discussed later in this chapter), which can inhibit its own release from β-cells in the islets of Langerhans, while a **paracrine** signalling molecule stimulates a neighbouring cell. A **hormone** is a substance secreted by endocrine glands, organs or tissues (see *Figure 5.1*) directly into the blood and is distributed until it reaches a target organ, gland or tissue possessing specific receptors to that hormone. **Endocrine glands** have no ducts, unlike **exocrine glands** such as the salivary glands (see *Chapter 7*) and breasts (*see Chapter 14*), which secrete substances onto the surface of membranes into ducts, which carry the secretions to areas where they exert their function. A paracrine signalling molecule acts locally on cells other than the one that produced it (cell-to-cell signalling). An example of a paracrine signalling molecule is GH (see *Figure 5.2*). Chemically, hormones are either **protein hormones** made from simple amino acids, peptides or proteins, or lipid-based hormones, such as **steroid hormones** made from cholesterol.

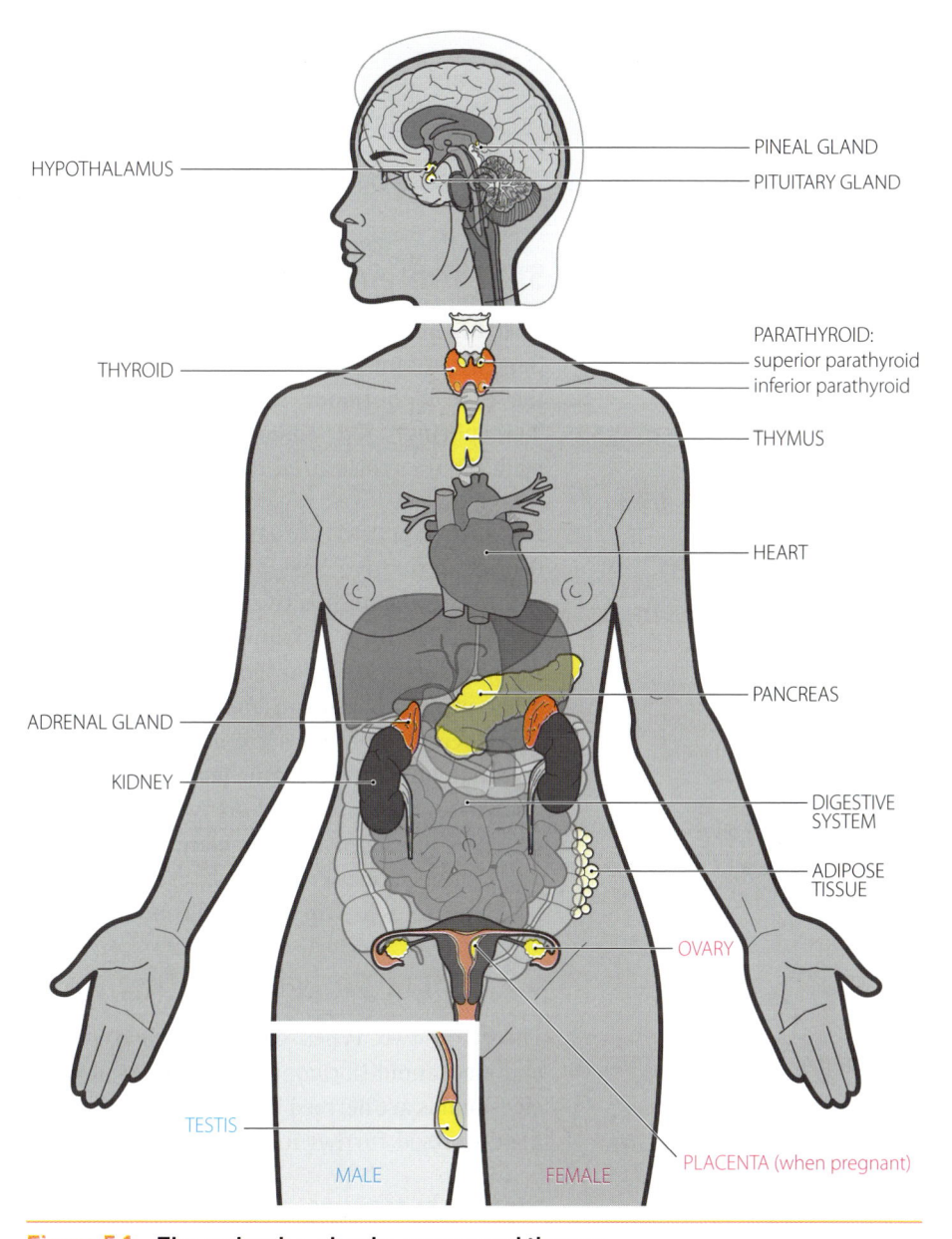

Figure 5.1 – **The endocrine glands, organs and tissues.**

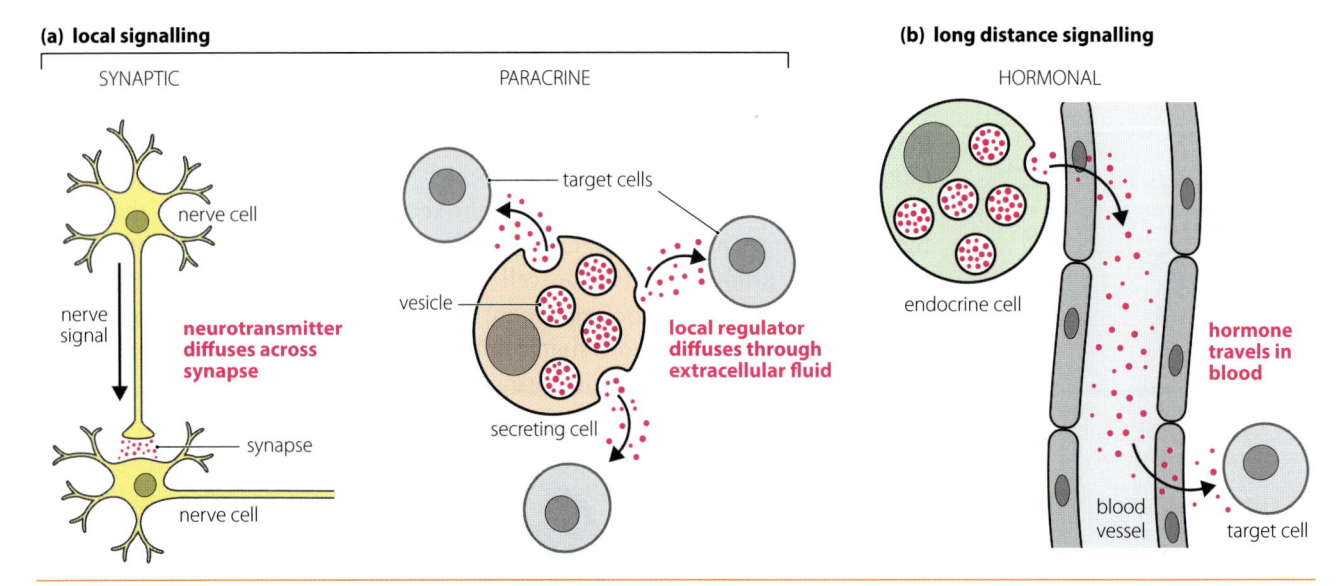

Figure 5.2 – Chemical signalling showing (a) local signalling by the synaptic and paracrine systems and (b) long-distance signalling by hormones.

5.2.2 Protein hormones

Amino acid-derivative hormones

Biogenic amines are small hormones derived from amino acids. For example, the thyroid hormone thyroxine and the catecholamine hormones adrenaline (epinephrine) and noradrenaline (norepinephrine) produced by the adrenal medulla are synthesized from the amino acid tyrosine.

Peptide-derivative and protein hormones

Peptide-derivative hormones are composed of chains of amino acids that are synthesized in an inactive form and later activated just before or after secretion. The inactive form is known as a **prohormone**. Some peptide-derived hormones such as antidiuretic hormone, oxytocin and insulin are small molecules, while other protein-based hormones such as GH and prolactin are large molecules. Some peptide hormones are made up of more than 200 amino acids and possess a carbohydrate side-chain, making this group more complex. These hormones, known as **glycoproteins**, are very large and include chorionic gonadotrophin, which is produced after implantation of the zygote in the uterus (see *Chapter 14*), and hormones from the anterior pituitary gland such as thyroid-stimulating hormone, follicle-stimulating hormone and luteinizing hormone.

5.2.3 Lipid-derivative hormones

There are two types of lipid-derivative hormones, namely steroid hormones and eicosanoid hormones. Steroid hormones are derived from cholesterol, while eicosanoids are derived from arachidonic acid, a long-chain fatty acid. Eicosanoids are discussed further in *Chapter 11*.

Steroid hormones

Steroid hormones include the male hormones (androgens), female hormones (oestrogens and progesterones) and those from the adrenal cortex of the kidney (glucocorticoids and mineralocorticoids). All are derived from cholesterol and differ only in the side-chain attached to the main ring structure. Once secreted, steroid hormones bind to specific plasma proteins and are transported in the blood to various parts of the body where they have their effect. The mechanism by which steroid hormones enter the cell and have their effect is discussed later in this chapter. They have a longer half-life than peptide hormones, which means that they tend to exert a more sustained action. Eventually, they are metabolized in the liver and excreted in urine or as part of bile.

5.2.4 How hormones exert an effect

Hormones bind to specific receptors, which are complex molecular structures. They travel long distances in blood, either bound to carriers or as free hormones, and work via two mechanisms depending on whether they are protein or steroid hormones.

Protein hormone mechanism

Peptide and protein hormones cannot cross plasma membranes as they are not lipid soluble, and for this reason, they bind to receptors located on plasma membranes of the target cells (see *Chapter 2*). The hormone is the first messenger. Once the hormone binds to its receptor, the receptor changes its shape and binds to G protein. G protein activates adenylate cyclase, which catalyses the conversion of adenosine triphosphate (ATP) to **cyclic adenosine monophosphate** (cyclic AMP), a **second messenger**. Cyclic AMP activates protein kinase enzymes to phosphorylate proteins and trigger cellular activity such as enzyme production and cellular secretion. Phosphorylation activates some proteins and inhibits others. The second messengers are located on the inner part of the plasma membrane and trigger a series of reactions catalysed by enzymes. The mechanism by which protein hormones exert their effect is summarized in *Figure 5.3*. As ATP is found in all cells where it drives many reactions and processes, the second messenger that is most commonly distributed in the body is cyclic AMP, which is the end product formed in the breakdown of ATP (see *Figure 5.3a*). The formation of cyclic AMP is catalysed by the enzyme adenylate cyclase, which is found on the inside of the plasma membrane. Other second messengers are **cyclic guanosine monophosphate** (cyclic GMP), the end product in the breakdown of **guanosine triphosphate** (GTP), and **calcium**. When some protein hormones bind to their receptors on the surface of plasma membranes, calcium channels open, allowing an influx of calcium ions into the cytoplasm of the cell, which act as an intracellular signal. The increase in intracellular calcium concentration activates a type of **G protein** (guanine nucleotide-binding protein) triggering the action of **phospholipase C**. Phospholipase C splits a plasma phospholipid known as **phosphatidyl inositol bisphosphate** (PIP_2) into **diacylglycerol** (DAG) and **inositol triphosphate** (IP_3), both of which act as second messengers (see *Figure 5.3b*). Further reactions that involve IP_3 occur enabling a protein called **calmodulin** to combine with calcium to form a calcium–calmodulin complex that mediates in intracellular metabolism.

Steroid hormone mechanism

Steroid hormones are lipid soluble and readily cross the plasma membrane. They bind to receptors in the cell cytoplasm or nucleus to form a hormone–receptor complex. When the hormone–receptor complex is formed in the cytoplasm, the complex enters

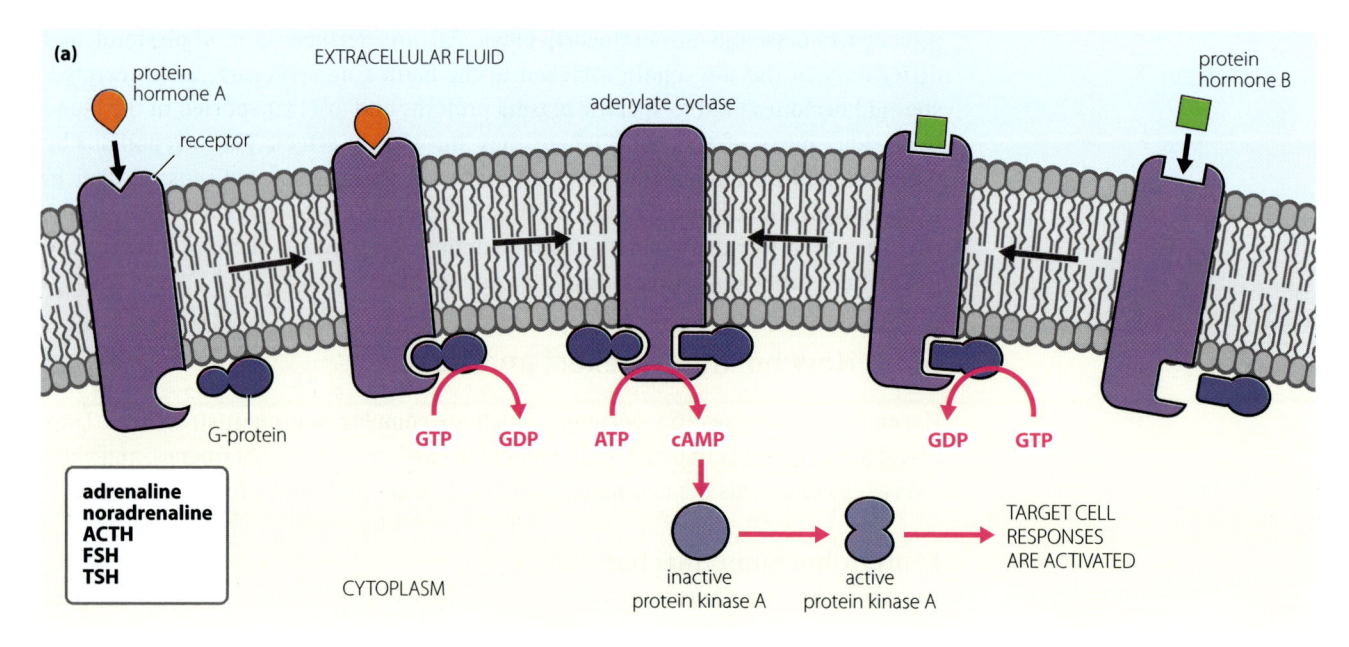

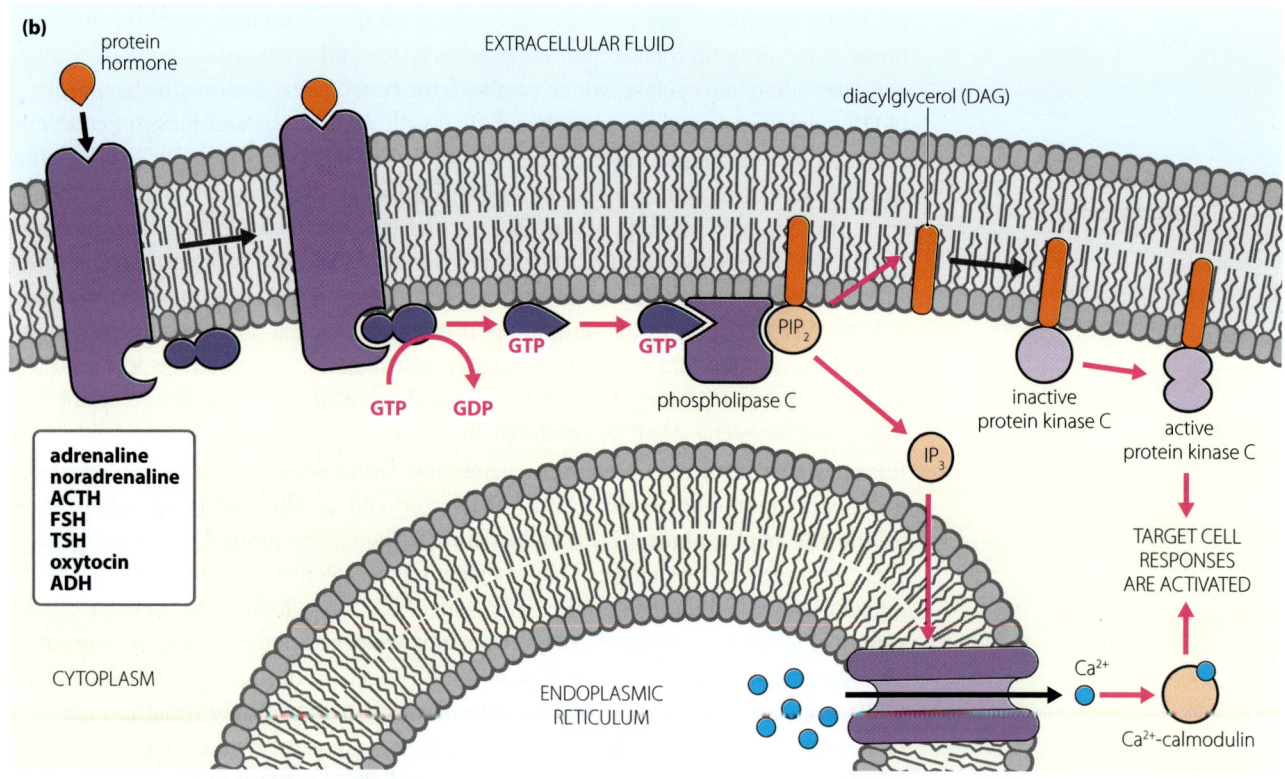

Figure 5.3 – Protein hormone mechanisms.
(a) Cyclic AMP second messenger mechanism. (b) Phosphatidyl inositol bisphosphate (PIP_2) second messenger mechanism.

the nucleus. Alternatively, the hormone can enter the nucleus via a nuclear pore to form the hormone–receptor complex within the nucleus. The hormone–receptor complex binds with DNA and activates or inhibits transcription factors. Mechanisms such as transcription and the production of messenger RNA and transfer RNA through to translation are activated, leading to protein synthesis (see *Chapter 3*). The mechanism of action of steroid hormones is summarized in *Figure 5.4*.

5.2.5 Major endocrine glands and tissues

Most hormones are secreted by endocrine glands but others are produced by endocrine organs and tissue. The main endocrine glands, organs and tissue are presented in *Figure 5.1* and the hormones they produce are summarized in *Table 5.1*. Some hormones are produced in response to neural mechanisms, discussed later in this chapter.

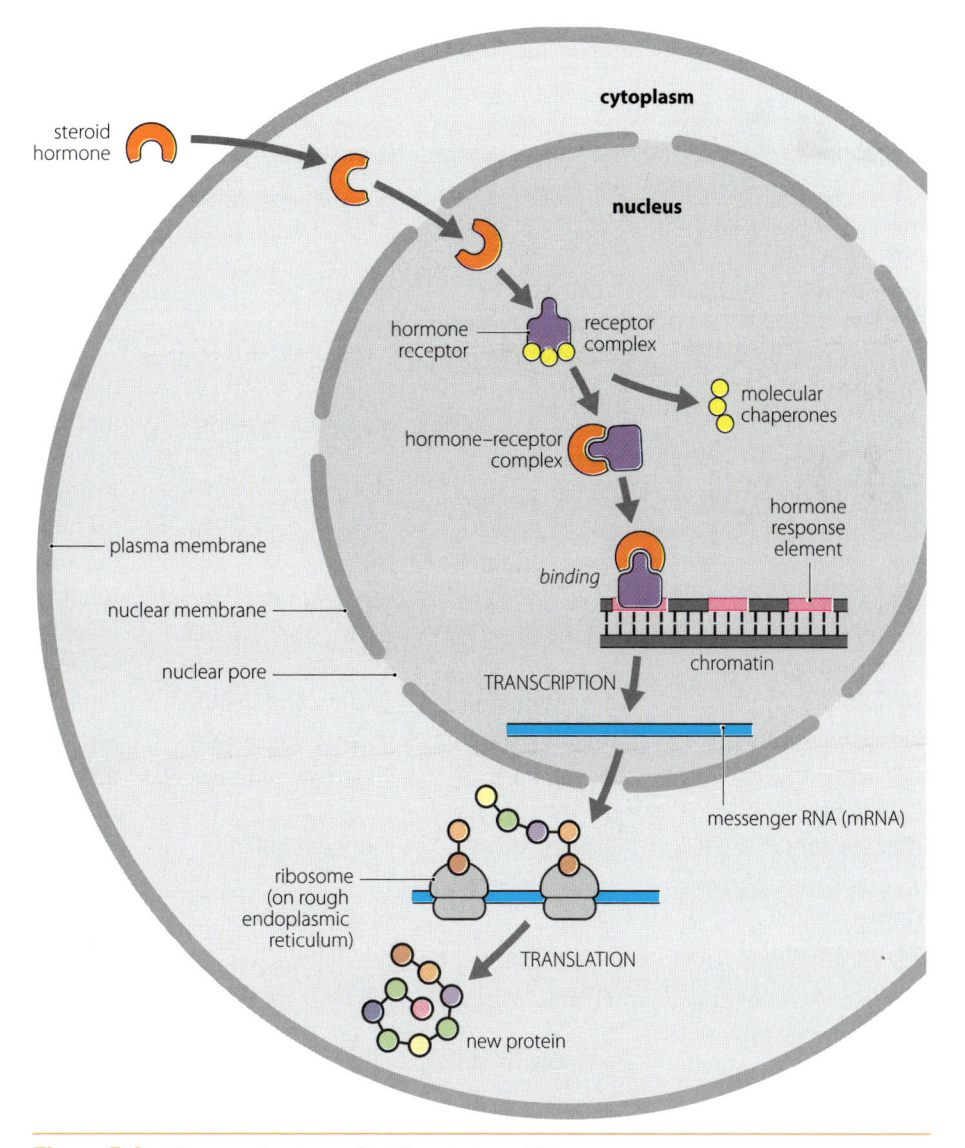

Figure 5.4 – **The mechanism of action of steroid hormones.**

Table 5.1 – Summary of hormones

Hormone	Producing gland or tissue	Target	Major action(s)
Thyroid-stimulating hormone (TSH)	Anterior pituitary gland	Thyroid gland	Production of thyroxine by thyroid gland
Adrenocorticotropic hormone (ACTH)	Anterior pituitary gland	Adrenal cortex	Production of glucocorticoid and mineralocorticoid hormones
Growth hormone (GH)	Anterior pituitary gland	Various tissues and organs (bone, cartilage, liver, muscle)	Growth of various tissues and organs Metabolism
Follicle-stimulating hormone (FSH)	Anterior pituitary gland	Gonads (ovaries and testes)	Maturation of ovarian follicles Oestrogen production Sperm production
Luteinizing hormone (LH)	Anterior pituitary gland	Gonads (ovaries and testes)	Triggers ovulation Stimulates production of oestrogen and progesterone Stimulates testosterone production
Prolactin	Anterior pituitary gland	Breasts	Promotes lactation
Melanocyte-stimulating hormone (MSH)	Anterior pituitary gland	Skin	Synthesis of melanin pigment Appetite regulation
Antidiuretic hormone	Hypothalamus (stored in posterior pituitary gland)	Kidneys	Stimulates nephrons (kidney tubules) to reabsorb water
Oxytocin	Hypothalamus (stored in posterior pituitary gland)	Uterus Mammary glands	Stimulates contraction of uterus Initiates the milk ejection ('let-down') reflex
Thyroxine	Thyroid gland	Tissues	Promotes carbohydrate, protein and fat metabolism
Calcitonin	Thyroid gland	Blood	Lowers blood calcium Inhibits bone resorption
Parathyroid hormone	Thyroid gland	Bone	Increases blood calcium by causing bone resorption
Adrenaline	Adrenal medulla	Organs and tissues	Short-term response to stress
Noradrenaline	Adrenal medulla	Organs and tissues	Short-term response to stress
Cortisol	Adrenal cortex	Tissues and body cells	Increases metabolism Depresses immune system
Aldosterone	Adrenal cortex	Kidney tubules	Increases reabsorption of sodium by renal tubules
Angiotensin II	Kidney	Blood vessels	Vasoconstriction
Erythropoietin	Kidney	Red bone marrow	Stimulates red blood cell production
Renin	Kidney	Kidney	Initiates the renin–angiotensin mechanism
Insulin	Pancreas (β-cells)	Organs and tissues	Lowers blood glucose by increasing transport of glucose into cells
Glucagon	Pancreas (α-cells)	Muscle and liver	Promotes glycogen breakdown to increase blood glucose

Hormone	Producing gland or tissue	Target	Major action(s)
Somatostatin	Pancreas (δ-cells)	Pancreas	Inhibits production of insulin, glucagon and pancreatic polypeptide Inhibits exocrine secretions of the pancreas Suppresses release of many gastrointestinal hormones
Pancreatic polypeptide	Pancreas (PP or F-cells)	Pancreas Ileum Large intestine	Moderating and self-regulating role of the functions of the pancreas Inhibits motility Stimulates contraction of the colon
Gastrin	Stomach mucosa	Gastric cells	Increases production of hydrochloric acid
Ghrelin	Stomach wall	Brain	Increases appetite
Somatostatin	Stomach wall and duodenal wall	Gastrointestinal tissues	Inhibits gastric secretions and gastric motility
Cholecystokinin	Duodenal mucosa	Gall bladder	Release of bile by gall bladder
Secretin	Duodenal mucosa	Pancreatic acini	Stimulates secretion of exocrine pancreatic juices Inhibits gastric secretion and motility
Motilin	Duodenal mucosa	Small intestine	Stimulates motility in the small intestine
Vasoactive intestinal peptide	Duodenal mucosa	Stomach Pancreas Small intestine	Inhibits gastric acid secretion Stimulates secretion of exocrine juices Relaxes intestinal smooth muscles
Neuropeptide Y	Hypothalamus	Hypothalamus	Appetite stimulant
Leptin	Adipose tissue	Hypothalamus	Decreases food intake by suppressing the release of neuropeptide Y
Melatonin	Pineal gland	Hypothalamus	Controls day/night rhythms
Atrial natriuretic peptide	Heart	Kidney tubules	Inhibits reabsorption of sodium by the nephron
Oestrogen	Ovaries	Breasts Uterine mucosa (endometrium)	Promotes maturation of reproductive organs Promotes development of sexual characteristics at puberty
Testosterone	Testes	Male reproductive organs	Promotes maturation of male reproductive organs and development of secondary sexual characteristics Required for normal sperm production
Human chorionic gonadotrophin	Trophoblast cells	Placenta	Maintains the corpus luteum
Relaxin	Corpus luteum and placenta	Cervix	Relaxes the cervix
Human placental lactogen	Placenta	Mammary glands	Prepares mammary gland for milk production Promotes growth of fetus

Pineal gland

The pineal gland is located in the posterior part of the roof of the third ventricle of the brain. It contains **pinealocytes**, which are secretory cells that produce the hormone **melatonin**. Melatonin is synthesized from the neurotransmitter serotonin and is involved in the maintenance of **circadian rhythms** (see *Box 5.1*) which are changes in physiological mechanisms that follow a regular pattern on a daily basis, such as the sleep–wake cycle. Circadian rhythms participate in controlling the maturation of gametes (ovum and sperm; see *Chapter 14*) by slowing the process and fine tuning sexual maturation in humans, as well as acting as an antioxidant which protects neurones against damage by free radicals such as nitric oxide.

Melatonin is a drug that is sometimes taken by long haul travellers to prevent or reduce jet lag when crossing time zones, especially when travelling from west to east, because its action adjusts the circadian rhythm, helping to limit the feelings of tiredness.

Hypothalamus

The hypothalamus has a direct neural link to the posterior pituitary gland via the axons of neurosecretory cells, which pass down a stalk connecting the hypothalamus and the pituitary gland, known as the **infundibulum** (see *Figure 5.5*). The hypothalamus has both endocrine function and neurological function with an integrating role between the two communication systems. Many of the functions of the autonomic nervous system and some behavioural mechanisms are controlled by the hypothalamus. The hypothalamus secretes releasing hormones that regulate the production of hormones by the anterior pituitary gland. Releasing hormones secreted by the hypothalamus include growth hormone-releasing hormone (GHRH), thyrotropin-releasing hormone,

---

BOX 5.1

Seasonal affective disorder

Some individuals suffer from seasonal affective disorder (SAD), which is characterized by poor sleeping pattern (insomnia) or tendency to oversleep, changes in mood and depression, little energy and changes in eating behaviour with a tendency to overeat and a craving for carbohydrates. SAD is more prevalent in areas with less sunshine such as the northern temperate regions including the northern USA, Canada and northern Europe, especially the Scandinavian countries. It is suggested that SAD is due to a delay in circadian rhythms, which can be corrected by bright-light therapy. In clinical settings, melatonin capsules can be prescribed to help induce sleep because melatonin helps to adjust the body clock. Only one melatonin product (Circadin) is licensed in the UK as a prescription drug for treating sleep disorders, for a short period of time of up to 3 weeks, in adults aged 55 years and above. Any other use is unlicensed. A prescription is necessary because melatonin should not be taken by individuals with autoimmune, kidney and liver conditions. In addition, melatonin interacts with other medicines and hence it is a prescription-only medication. However, in other countries this drug can be bought without a prescription.

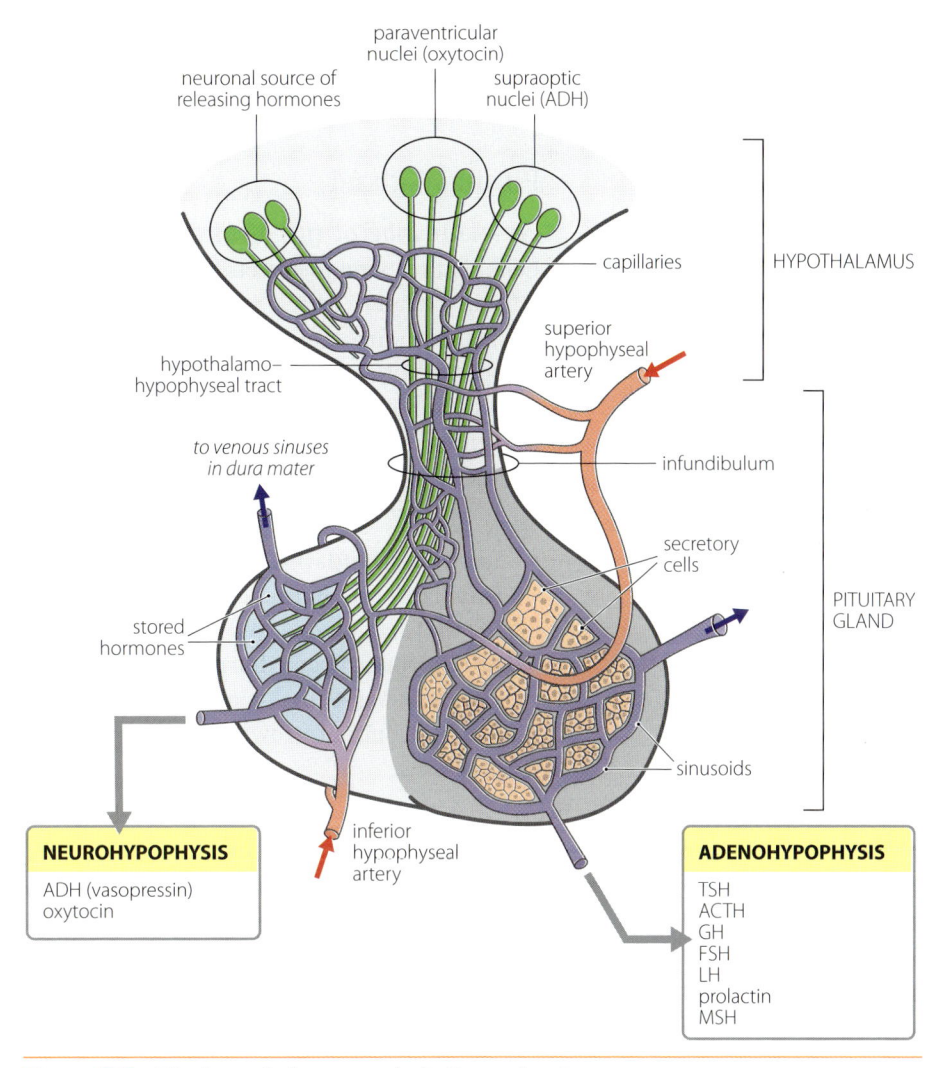

SECTION 5.2 | WHAT YOU NEED TO KNOW – ESSENTIAL ANATOMY AND PHYSIOLOGY

Figure 5.5 – The hypothalamus and pituitary gland.

corticotropin-releasing hormone, gonadotrophin-releasing hormone (GnRH), somatostatin and dopamine. A releasing or **tropic hormone** triggers the release of another hormone by another gland. GHRH stimulates the release of GH by the anterior pituitary gland, thyrotropin-releasing hormone triggers the release of thyroid-stimulating hormone, and corticotropin-releasing hormone stimulates the release of adrenocorticotropic hormone, while GnRH stimulates the release of the anterior pituitary hormones that control activity in the ovaries and testes.

The hypothalamus produces ghrelin, a novel GH-releasing peptide, which is also produced by cells in the wall of the human stomach. Although the functions of ghrelin are not understood completely, it has a role in appetite regulation, energy stores and metabolism. Increasing the concentration of ghrelin levels in both humans and rodents stimulates GH secretion and induces adiposity by increasing food intake and decreasing fat utilization, thus giving us an opportunity to understand some of the factors involved in obesity and in the regulation of appetite.

Pituitary gland

Anterior lobe of the pituitary gland (adenohypophysis)

Cells that respond to secretions from the hypothalamus are found in the anterior pituitary gland, which secretes **tropic** hormones that target other endocrine glands and stimulate them to produce hormones. Some of the hormones of the anterior pituitary gland also have **trophic** effects whereby they stimulate growth of tissue directly, causing **hyperplasia** (increase in cell number) and **hypertrophy** (increase in cell size). Between them, the cells of the anterior pituitary gland produce seven hormones that stimulate secretory activities elsewhere in the body and are called **tropic hormones** or **tropins** (see *Figure 5.6*):

- **Thyroid-stimulating hormone** (TSH), also known as **thyrotropin**, stimulates the thyroid gland. It has both a tropic and a trophic effect on the thyroid gland.
- **Adrenocorticotropic hormone** (ACTH) stimulates the adrenal cortex glands. It has a trophic and tropic effect on the adrenal glands.
- **Somatotropin** or **growth hormone** (GH) controls growth and metabolic processes.

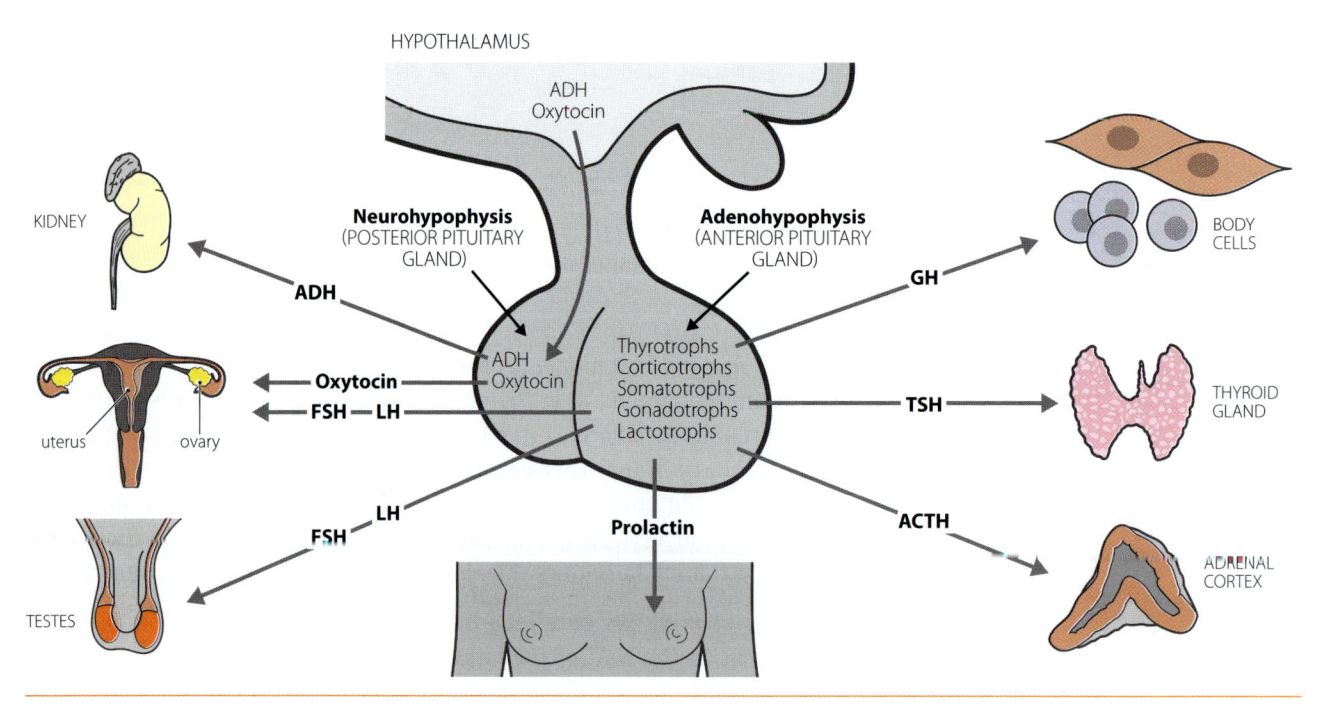

Figure 5.6 – Hormones of the anterior and posterior pituitary glands, showing their target glands, organs and tissue.

- **Follicle-stimulating hormone** (FSH) and **luteinizing hormone** (LH) regulate the function of the gonads (ovaries and testes).
- **Prolactin** stimulates breast development and production of milk.
- **Melanocyte-stimulating hormone** (MSH) controls the production of melanin, which produces different types of skin pigmentation (discussed in *Chapter 12*), and belongs to a group of peptides called melanocortins. The production of MSH is increased in pregnancy, darkening the areola and nipples of the breasts. In humans, melanocortins are involved in energy metabolism through the regulation of appetite, and there is a suggestion that they may be involved in inflammation and in sexual function.

The hypophyseal artery, a branch of the internal carotid artery within the brain, provides an excellent blood supply to the anterior pituitary gland (see *Figure 5.5*). Hormones from the hypothalamus that regulate the anterior pituitary gland are delivered to the pituitary gland by a localized blood supply called the hypophyseal portal system, which forms a network of **sinusoids**. The hypophyseal portal system of blood vessels in the brain connects the hypothalamus with the anterior pituitary gland and ensures that there is good transport of tropic hormones between these two structures. The hormones of the anterior pituitary gland are summarized in *Table 5.1*.

Posterior lobe of the pituitary gland (neurohypophysis)

Tracts of nerve fibres run from the supraoptic nuclei and paraventricular nuclei of the hypothalamus to the posterior lobe of the pituitary gland (neurohypophysis) (see *Figure 5.5*). Neurosecretory cells in these two nuclei of the hypothalamus synthesize two **neurohormones** that are carried by the hypothalamo-hypophyseal neuronal tracts to the posterior pituitary gland. The posterior pituitary gland stores and releases antidiuretic hormone and oxytocin.

Antidiuretic hormone (ADH), which is also called vasopressin, conserves water and minimizes dehydration (see *Chapter 8*). The amount of water and the solute concentration in the body is monitored by osmoreceptors in the hypothalamus. When the osmolality of blood is high (as in dehydration), osmoreceptors send impulses to the supraoptic nuclei of the hypothalamus, stimulating the synthesis of ADH by the hypothalamus and its release from the posterior pituitary gland. In the kidneys, ADH increases the permeability of the distal convoluted tubules and collecting duct of the nephron to water. This allows more water to be reabsorbed from the nephron into blood, decreasing the concentration of blood and resulting in the excretion of concentrated urine. When the osmolality of blood is low (excess body water), ADH release is inhibited. This reduces water reabsorption and increases the loss of water by the nephrons, resulting in the production of dilute urine.

Oxytocin is synthesized by the paraventricular nuclei of the hypothalamus and is released during labour (parturition or childbirth). It increases the strength of uterine smooth muscle contraction as labour continues (see *Chapter 14*). More oxytocin is synthesized by the hypothalamus and released by the posterior pituitary gland as a result of positive feedback from afferent impulses to the hypothalamus in response to the stretching of the uterus and cervix during labour. The increased amount of oxytocin strengthens the contraction of the uterus further, stimulating the release of more oxytocin. As soon as the baby is born, the reduced pressure exerted on the uterine muscle causes the release of oxytocin to be switched off as uterine muscular contraction decreases (negative feedback). The other function of oxytocin is to enhance milk ejection from the mammary glands by the 'let-down' reflex (see *Chapter 14*). Milk 'let-down' is a reflex in which sucking on the mother's nipples causes milk to be released and is reinforced by suckling, reducing when the baby stops.

Thyroid gland

The thyroid gland is located in the anterior part of the neck just below the larynx (see *Figure 5.1*). It has two lobes that are connected by an isthmus lying over the trachea (see *Figure 5.7*). It has a rich blood supply from the superior thyroid artery, which branches off the external carotid artery, and from the inferior thyroid arteries, which branch off the left and right subclavian arteries. Its location is just above the arch of the aorta and between the common carotid arteries. Both its location and its rich blood supply make surgery in this region and of the thyroid gland a very delicate procedure. The thyroid gland has two types of cell, namely follicles and parafollicular cells, also known as C cells. The follicles have walls composed of epithelial cells that produce thyroglobulin

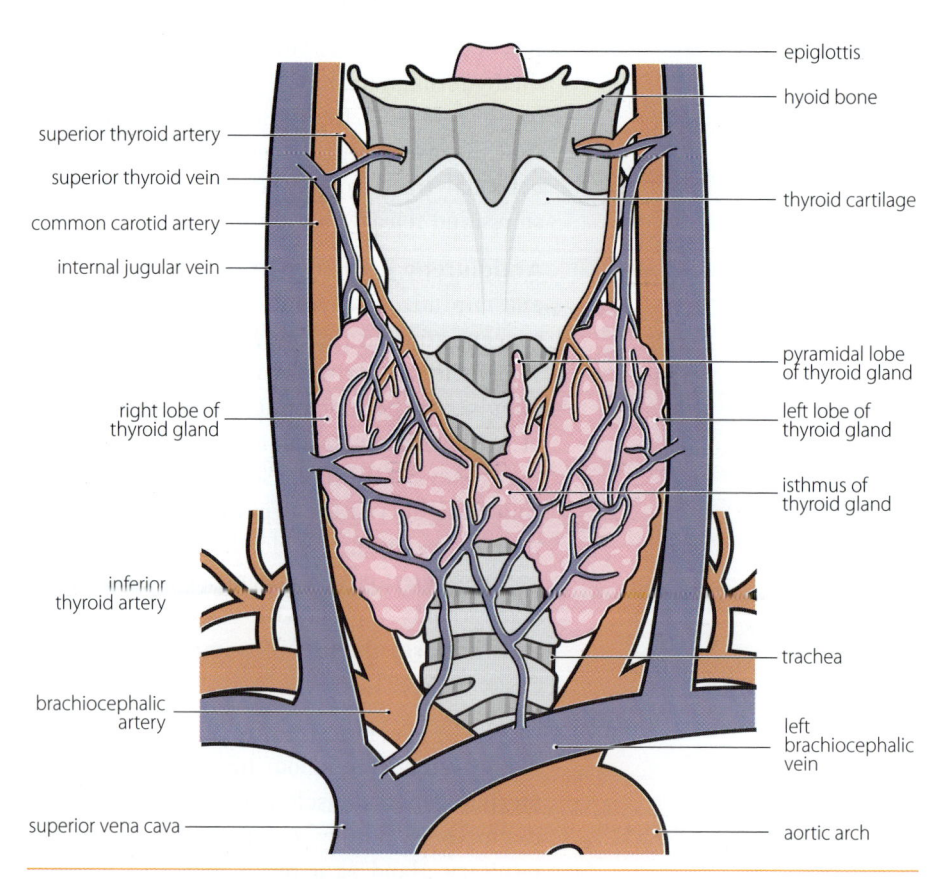

Figure 5.7 – **The thyroid gland.**

molecules from which the hormone thyroxine is produced. The two hormones produced by the thyroid gland are **triidothyronine** (T_3) and **tetraiodothyronine** (T_4), also known as **thyroxine**. Both are protein hormones synthesized from the amino acid tyrosine with the addition of three or four iodine molecules to make T_3 or T_4, respectively. The synthesis of these hormones is stimulated by TSH from the anterior pituitary gland. Both T_3 and T_4 increase the metabolic rate of most cells in the body through the oxidation of glucose via glycolysis and the tricarboxylic acid cycle (see *Chapter 7*). Thyroxine is an important regulator of core body temperature, as the increase in metabolic rate causes body temperature to rise (see *Chapter 1*). An overactive thyroid gland produces excess thyroxine, a condition known as **hyperthyroidism**, which is characterized by a high metabolic rate, heat intolerance, a rapid and irregular heartbeat, sweating, nervousness and weight loss despite increased appetite. The person may also be restless and excitable and may not sleep well; however, these characteristics may be confused with mental illness such as a bipolar state, emphasizing the importance of taking bloods to determine thyroid function.

Inadequate production of thyroxine, known as hypothyroidism, is characterized by a low metabolic rate, cold sensitivity, dry skin, lethargy and mental sluggishness. The lethargic feeling that David (Patient 5.1) was experiencing was in part due to inadequate thyroxine levels in his blood and his inability to metabolize glucose adequately due to impaired insulin sensitivity, such that he was unable to obtain energy from the food he was consuming. The parafollicular cells of the thyroid gland, also known as C (clear) cells because of their failure to stain well, secrete calcitonin. The secretion of calcitonin is not regulated by the hypothalamus or pituitary gland but by the C cells responding to the concentration of calcium ions (Ca^{2+}) in the blood. Calcitonin lowers blood calcium by stimulating the uptake of calcium by skeletal tissue. It also inhibits bone resorption through the inhibition of osteoclast activity (see *Chapter 13*).

Parathyroid glands

Although the number may vary between individuals, typically four parathyroid glands (see *Figure 5.8*) are located on the posterior aspect of the thyroid gland close to the oesophagus. They contain large numbers of small **chief cells** (see *Figure 5.9*) and a few scattered larger, pale **oxyphil cells** whose function is unknown. The chief cells secrete **parathyroid hormone** (PTH), also known as **parathormone**. Low blood calcium levels stimulate the release of PTH by the parathyroid glands. PTH affects calcium homeostasis in three different ways:

1. The release of calcium and phosphate from bone is stimulated by PTH acting on osteoclasts, which digest bone (see *Chapter 13*).
2. PTH activates vitamin D (as calcitriol or D_3), which results in increased absorption of calcium from the small intestines.
3. PTH increases the reabsorption of calcium and excretion of phosphate by the nephrons in the kidneys.

Thymus

The thymus is located behind the sternum, deep within the mediastinum (see *Figure 5.1*). Several polypeptides, one of which is **thymosin**, are produced by the

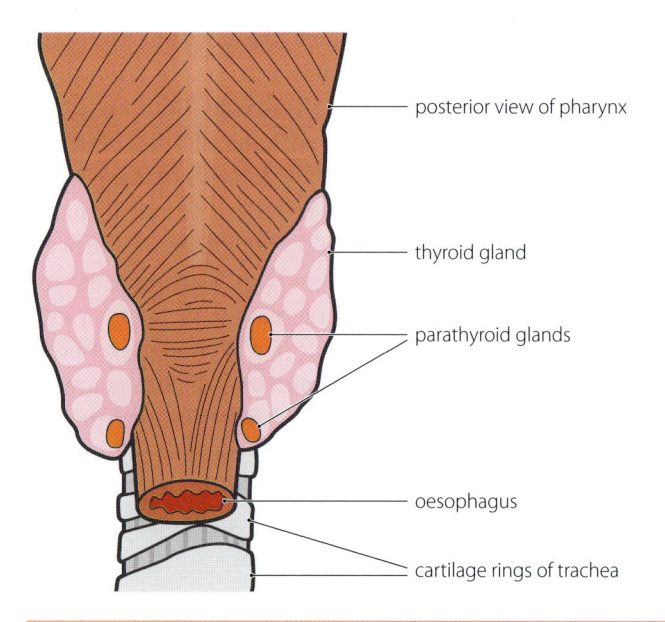

Figure 5.8 – **The parathyroid glands.**

thymus gland. The precise function of these peptides remains poorly understood. The thymus gland is the site of T-lymphocyte development, and thymic hormones regulate T-lymphocyte maturation and other elements of immunity (see *Chapter 11*).

Adrenal glands

The adrenal or suprarenal glands (see *Figure 5.1*) are located on top of the kidneys surrounded by a fibrous capsule and some fat. There are two main regions, an

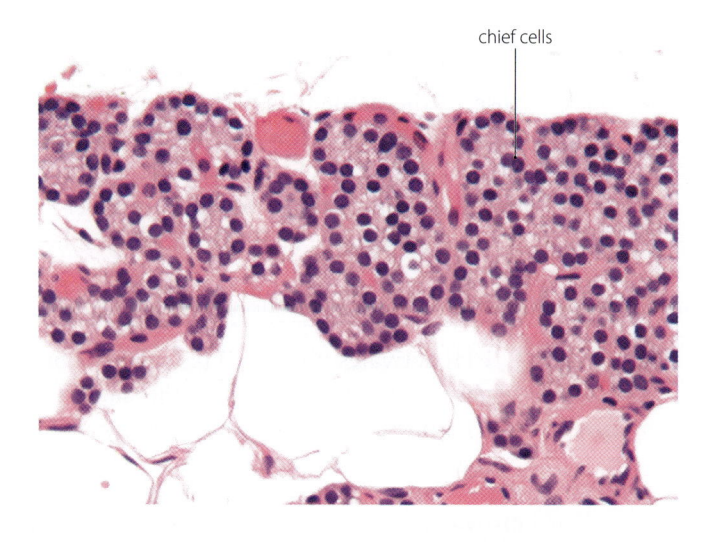

Figure 5.9 – **A micrograph of the chief cells of the parathyroid gland.**
Licensed under a CC BY-SA 3.0 Unported licence. Author: Nephron.

internal medulla and an outer cortex, both of which perform different functions (see *Figure 5.10*).

Adrenal medulla

The adrenal medulla is innervated by sympathetic fibres. It is made up of **chromaffin** tissue, which secretes mainly adrenaline (epinephrine) and some noradrenaline (norepinephrine). These two hormones are known as **catecholamines**. As already highlighted in *Chapter 4*, adrenaline and noradrenaline are also neurotransmitters with a key role in the autonomic nervous system. However, more noradrenaline is released at the synapses than adrenaline, while a great deal more adrenaline is secreted into the circulation by the adrenal medulla than noradrenaline. The effects of both hormones are relatively short lived, and they are involved in the response known as the **fight-or-flight** reaction or the **acute stress response**. Adrenaline and noradrenaline exert their effects on receptors called adrenergic receptors, which are distributed throughout the body. These effects have been described under the autonomic nervous system (see *Chapter 4, Figure 4.21*).

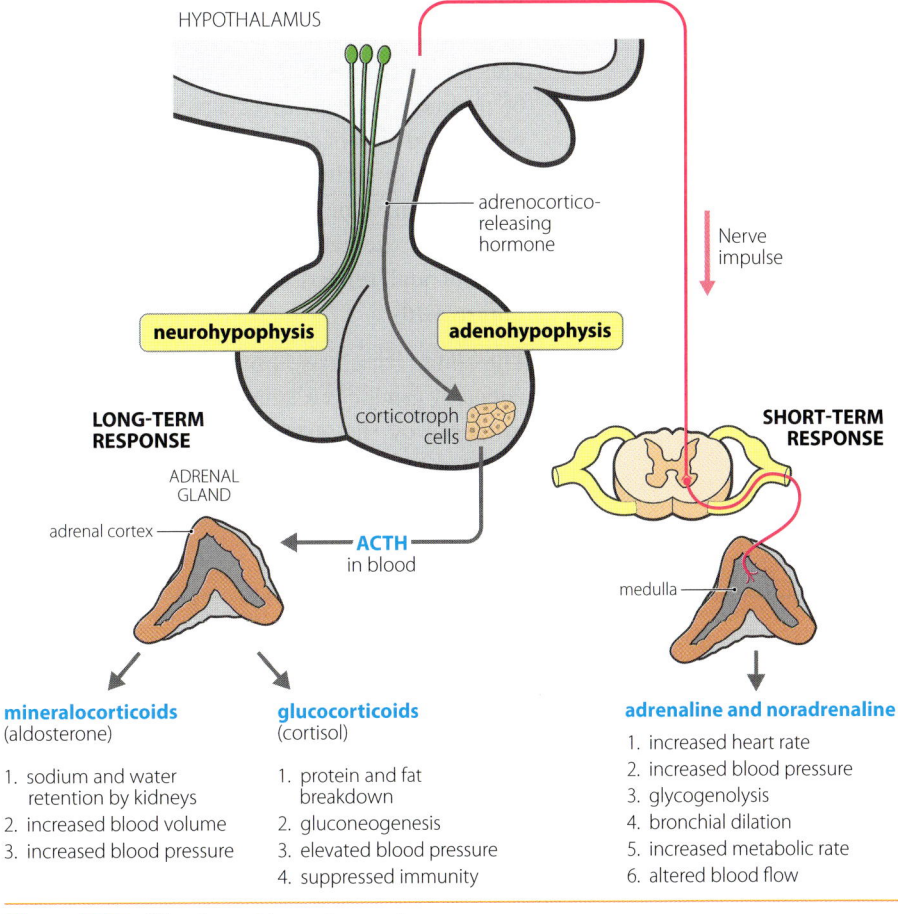

Figure 5.10 – Short- and long-term stress responses.

Adrenal cortex

The adrenal cortex has three layers, each secreting different hormones. The outer layer is called the **zona glomerulosa**, the middle layer is the **zona fasciculata** and the inner layer next to the adrenal medulla is the **zona reticularis**. The adrenal cortex secretes different steroid-based hormones synthesized from cholesterol in response to ACTH. The zona glomerulosa secretes a class of mineralocorticoids including aldosterone, which is involved in sodium and water balance. The production of aldosterone is stimulated by decreased blood volume and low blood pressure, low sodium ion (Na^+) concentration and high potassium ion (K^+) concentration in the blood. Aldosterone increases Na^+ reabsorption from the collecting duct of the nephron, allowing water to follow the Na^+. It also increases secretion and loss of K^+ and hydrogen ions (H^+) from the blood into the nephron (see *Chapter 8*). Thus, aldosterone is important in the regulation of fluid composition and volume.

The zona fasciculata produces most of the corticosteroid hormones that are classified as glucocorticoids. Glucocorticoids, such as cortisol and corticosterone, are stress hormones that affect energy metabolism in the majority of body cells. Cortisol increases blood glucose by stimulating **gluconeogenesis**, a process by which glucose is synthesized from non-carbohydrate sources (see *Chapter 7*), inhibiting the effects of insulin in peripheral tissues and influencing protein and fat metabolism. Prolonged cortisol secretion, which occurs during periods of prolonged stress, affects many physiological mechanisms such as water and electrolyte balance, and bone structure (by reducing calcium absorption from the small intestine), and it reduces cellular immunity. The effects of cortisol complement some of the effects of adrenaline and noradrenaline, the difference being that the catecholamines produce the short-term response to stress, while cortisol and related compounds produce the long-term response to stress (see *Figure 5.10*).

The zona reticularis is much smaller in size when compared with the other two zones. It produces a small amount of androgens and oestrogens similar to those produced by the testes and ovaries, respectively. The androgens and oestrogens secreted by the zona reticularis stimulate the development of secondary sexual characteristics at puberty, such as pubic hair.

Kidney

The kidney produces a number of hormones.

Renin is involved in the renin–angiotensin mechanism, which influences electrolyte and water balance, and blood pressure (discussed in *Chapters 8* and *9*). When blood volume and blood pressure decrease, renin is secreted by the kidney, converting angiotensinogen to angiotensin I. This leads to the production of angiotensin II, a potent stimulator of aldosterone release.

Erythropoietin is a glycoprotein hormone produced by fibroblasts within the renal cortex in the kidney (see *Chapter 8, Figure 8.1*). In the fetus and during the prenatal period, it is produced by liver cells. It stimulates red blood cell (erythrocyte) production by the bone marrow (see *Chapter 9*). The secretion of erythropoietin is stimulated by low oxygen levels in blood (hypoxia) which may be due to a decreased number of circulating erythrocytes as in bleeding, a low haemoglobin level, changes in altitude such as when mountain climbing and chronic lung disorders.

Cholecalciferol is a pro-vitamin D$_3$, which is activated in the kidneys to the active form D$_3$ **(calcitriol)** under the influence of PTH. Calcitriol is a steroid hormone also known as **1,25-dihydroxycholecalciferol** or **1,25-dihydroxyvitamin D$_3$**. Calcitriol raises the amount of calcium in blood by increasing absorption of calcium from the gastrointestinal tract.

Heart

Cardiac myocytes located in the atria and ventricles produce the natriuretic peptides. **Atrial natriuretic peptide** (ANP) is synthesized in atrial myocytes and **B-type natriuretic peptide** (BNP) in ventricular myocytes. Both are released from the heart in response to volume expansion and pressure overload that leads to stretching of the heart muscle. ANP and BNP have similar effects on the kidney. They increase the glomerular filtration rate, decrease the reabsorption of sodium in the distal convoluted tubule and also inhibit the action of the hormones aldosterone and renin. The consequence is an increase in the excretion of sodium (natriuresis) and a fall in blood volume. ANP and BNP also stimulate receptors on the smooth muscle of arterioles to cause vasodilation, resulting in a reduction of peripheral vascular resistance and systemic arterial blood pressure (see *Chapters 8* and *9*).

Pancreas

The pancreas produces four hormones: **insulin, glucagon, somatostatin** and **pancreatic polypeptide**. Insulin and glucagon are involved in the control of blood glucose, while somatostatin and pancreatic polypeptide influence the activities of the pancreas. Located within the pancreas are clusters of endocrine cells called the **islets of Langerhans** in which are found **α-cells**, which secrete **glucagon**, and **β-cells**, which produce **insulin** (see *Figure 5.11*). These two hormones have an antagonistic effect on glucose homeostasis. Both α- and β-cells are sensitive to the concentration of glucose in blood passing through the pancreas. F-cells, which secrete pancreatic polypeptide, are also found as part of the pancreatic islet cells. Approximately 90% of the cells of the pancreas form clusters known as **acini**, which produce digestive enzymes that flow via ducts (see *Chapter 7*).

Insulin has many functions that affect many cells in the body with the exception of the brain, kidneys and liver. These three tissues utilize glucose irrespective of the amount of insulin present. The uptake of glucose by the brain, renal medulla and erythrocytes is mostly independent of plasma concentrations of glucose and insulin. Glucose is transported using a variety of types of transporter protein that mediate the transport of glucose across cell membranes by passive mechanisms. The major transport for glucose in adipose and skeletal muscle tissue, which requires a large amount of glucose, is a transport protein (GLUT-4) that is dependent on insulin for its function. When insulin binds to its receptors on the plasma membrane, a cascade of reactions stimulate the translocation of vesicles containing GLUT-4 transport protein from the cytoplasm of the cell to the plasma membrane. Insertion of GLUT-4 transport protein into the plasma membrane allows

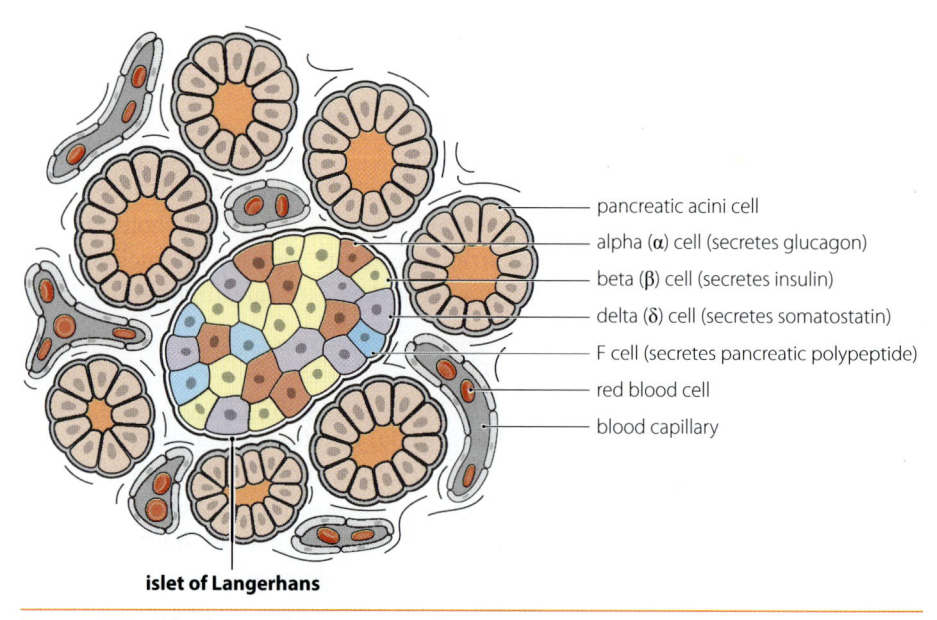

Figure 5.11 – **The islets of Langerhans in the pancreas.**

glucose to enter the cell by facilitated diffusion down its concentration gradient. The glucose is phosphorylated by kinase enzymes (glucokinase in the liver and hexokinase in other tissues) to glucose 6-phosphate, and then metabolized as discussed in *Chapter 7*. The phosphorylation of glucose to glucose 6-phosphate is important because it maintains a diffusion gradient for glucose into the cell. Insulin also stimulates the conversion of excess glucose to glycogen in liver and muscle cells. It increases the uptake of amino acids and promotes the synthesis of protein by muscles. It also inhibits glycogenolysis and gluconeogenesis in the liver and stimulates lipogenesis (fat synthesis) by adipose tissue. Insulin also lowers appetite through its effects on the hypothalamus. Diabetes mellitus is a heterogeneous disease that affects many people all over the world irrespective of race and culture; it can be classified as type 1 and type 2, although there are other forms such as gestational diabetes mellitus. Type 1 diabetes mellitus is due to absolute insulin deficiency as a result of cell-mediated autoimmune destruction of the β-cells in the islets of Langerhans in the pancreas. Type 2 diabetes mellitus is due to insulin resistance and relative insulin deficiency. Typically, most people with type 2 diabetes mellitus are obese and their blood insulin levels are normal or even elevated. However, the blood glucose levels are higher despite the normal or higher insulin levels, hence the use of the term insulin resistance. Race and age are considered risk factors for type 2 diabetes mellitus. When compared with Caucasians, the Pima Indians of North America and people of African–Caribbean and Asian origin are considered to be at a higher risk of developing type 2 diabetes mellitus. People over 65 years old are also considered to be at greater risk than younger people for type 2 diabetes mellitus. Patients with type 1 diabetes mellitus and some with type 2 require insulin administration to maintain stable blood glucose levels. Up until the age of 44, David (Patient 5.1) was able to regulate his blood sugar effectively, indicating that insulin production and activity were normal. However, his development of type 2 diabetes mellitus indicates that he has developed insulin resistance. This means that his cells have become insensitive to the insulin he is producing, and he is no longer able to make efficient use of the glucose in his blood.

In summary, the role of insulin in transporting glucose out of blood and facilitating its entry into cells, as well as enabling the conversion of glucose to other compounds such as glycogen and fats, contributes to the maintenance of glucose homeodynamics.

Glucagon is a hormone that is antagonistic to insulin and increases blood glucose by a cascade of reactions. Its secretion is stimulated by sympathetic nerves to the pancreas. When blood glucose is low, glucagon promotes **glycogenolysis** and **gluconeogenesis** in the liver. Glycogenolysis is the conversion of stored glycogen back to glucose and this occurs to increase blood glucose when levels of blood glucose are low in order to adjust the levels of glucose. Glucagon does not cause glycogenolysis in muscle. Glucagon also promotes lipolysis (fat breakdown), is ketogenic (increases the formation of ketones), and inhibits glycogenesis and lipogenesis. Glucagon exerts its effects via the activation of cyclic AMP (a second messenger), leading to glycogen breakdown in order to increase blood glucose. In clinical settings, glucagon can be given as an injection when patients have low blood glucose (hypoglycaemia), with the effect of raising their blood glucose mobilized from liver glycogen.

Somatostatin is secreted from the **delta cells** (δ-cells) of the pancreas (see *Figure 5.11*). It suppresses the release of many gastrointestinal hormones (discussed later in this chapter) including cholecystokinin, gastrin, gastric inhibitory polypeptide, motilin, pancreatic polypeptide, secretin and vasoactive inhibitory polypeptide. It also suppresses the secretion of insulin and glucagon, as well as the exocrine secretions of the pancreas. The secretion of somatostatin by the pancreas is stimulated by glucose and some amino acids such as leucine and arginine. Thus, somatostatin not only integrates the actions of insulin and glucagon but also regulates the production of a variety of hormones in the gastrointestinal tract (see *Chapter 7*).

Pancreatic polypeptide is secreted by pancreatic polypeptide (PP) cells (also known as F-cells) of the islets of Langerhans in the pancreas. Its secretion is inhibited by somatostatin and stimulated by a protein meal, acute hypoglycaemia, fasting and exercise. It affects other activities of the pancreas such as the production of both endocrine and exocrine secretions (see *Chapter 7*), suggesting that it has a moderating and self-regulatory role on the functions of the pancreas. It has been found to inhibit motility of the small intestine (ileum) and to stimulate contractions of the colon. Its concentration in blood has been found to be raised in anorexia nervosa. The actions of PP and somatostatin highlight the view that the regulation of pancreatic endocrine and exocrine functions is complex, needing both neural and hormonal integration.

Ovaries

Oestrogen and **progesterone** are the main female hormones secreted by the ovaries. Oestrogens are steroid hormones synthesized by the ovaries from cholesterol. The ovaries respond to follicle-stimulating hormone (FSH) and luteinizing hormone

(LH), both of which are produced by the anterior pituitary gland. Oestrogen is responsible for the development of female sexual characteristics such as breasts at puberty and the maturation of Graafian or ovarian follicles (see *Chapter 14*). After release of the ovum from the ovary, the **corpus luteum**, also known as the **yellow body**, is formed in the ovary. The corpus luteum secretes progesterone, the initial function of which is to prepare the uterus for the implantation of the embryo. Following implantation, progesterone maintains the pregnancy by keeping the uterus quiescent, ensuring that there is no synchronized contraction of the smooth muscles of the uterus. As long as the amount of progesterone is high, pregnancy will be maintained. The corpus luteum continues to produce progesterone until this role is taken over by the placenta at about 12 weeks following implantation. Progesterone also prepares the mammary glands for milk production. During the second trimester, the production of progesterone and oestrogen is taken over by the placenta itself, and their production increases exponentially from about 14 weeks until parturition. The role of these hormones is discussed in more detail in *Chapter 14*.

Placental hormones

Approximately 3-4 days after fertilization, the embryo forms into a blastocyst consisting of an outer sphere of cells, known as **trophoblast cells**, and an inner cluster of cells, called the **inner cell mass**. The trophoblast forms two distinct layers: the inner layer is the **cytotrophoblast** and the outer layer is the **syncytiotrophoblast** (also known as **syntiotrophoblast**), the cells of which invade the endometrium of the uterus allowing the blastocyst to embed in the endometrium of the uterus – this is known as implantation. The placenta secretes three hormones in addition to its other important role of supporting development of the fetus: human chorionic gonadotrophin, human placental lactogen and relaxin.

Human chorionic gonadotrophin (hCG) is secreted by the syncytiotrophoblast cells of the trophobast. It maintains the corpus luteum for 3-4 months and stimulates the corpus luteum to continue to produce progesterone and oestrogen. hCG has a role in cellular differentiation and proliferation in the placenta. The concentration of hCG is a marker for pregnancy and can be measured easily in both blood and urine, with an hCG-positive result indicating an implanted blastocyst. This is the basis of urine pregnancy test kits.

Human placental lactogen (hPL) (also known as **human chorionic somatomammotropin**) is produced by the placenta during pregnancy. It helps to prepare the mammary glands for milk production and increases the availability of glucose for the fetus by decreasing maternal insulin sensitivity and maternal glucose utilization. In addition, hPL stimulatory activities are similar to those achieved by GH in other tissues.

Relaxin is a peptide hormone that is secreted by the corpus luteum and by the placenta. It suppresses the release of oxytocin by the hypothalamus, delays labour, softens the cervix, and relaxes pelvic muscles and ligaments, thus allowing the pubic symphysis to expand during labour. This enables the fetus to engage with the vaginal canal during birth (parturition).

Testes

Within the testes (see *Figure 5.12*) are coiled seminiferous tubules surrounded by interstitials cells called **Leydig cells**. **Androgens** such as **testosterone** are produced by the Leydig cells. Testosterone is synthesized from cholesterol and converted to dihydrotestosterone in the prostate gland. Testosterone has a role in the development of male reproductive tissues such as the testis and prostate gland. In addition, it is responsible for the development of secondary sexual characteristics in the male such as enlargement of the larynx, which causes the deepening of the voice, and hair development in the pubic area, axillary pits, chest and face (beard). Other secondary characteristics influenced by testosterone in the male are increased bone density and thickening of the skin. Its anabolic effects lead to the development of muscle and male reproductive organs that include the penis, its ducts and glands. It stimulates spermatogenesis at puberty, the production of semen, erection of the penis and ejaculation, although it is important to say that other factors such as psychological factors and blood flow are also involved in erection and ejaculation (see David, Patient 5.1 in *Chapter 14*).

Gastrointestinal tract

The gastrointestinal tract produces many hormones involved in regulating digestion, motility and appetite including gastrin, cholecystokinin, secretin, ghrelin and motilin; their functions are discussed in *Chapter 7*. Selected hormones will be described briefly in this chapter.

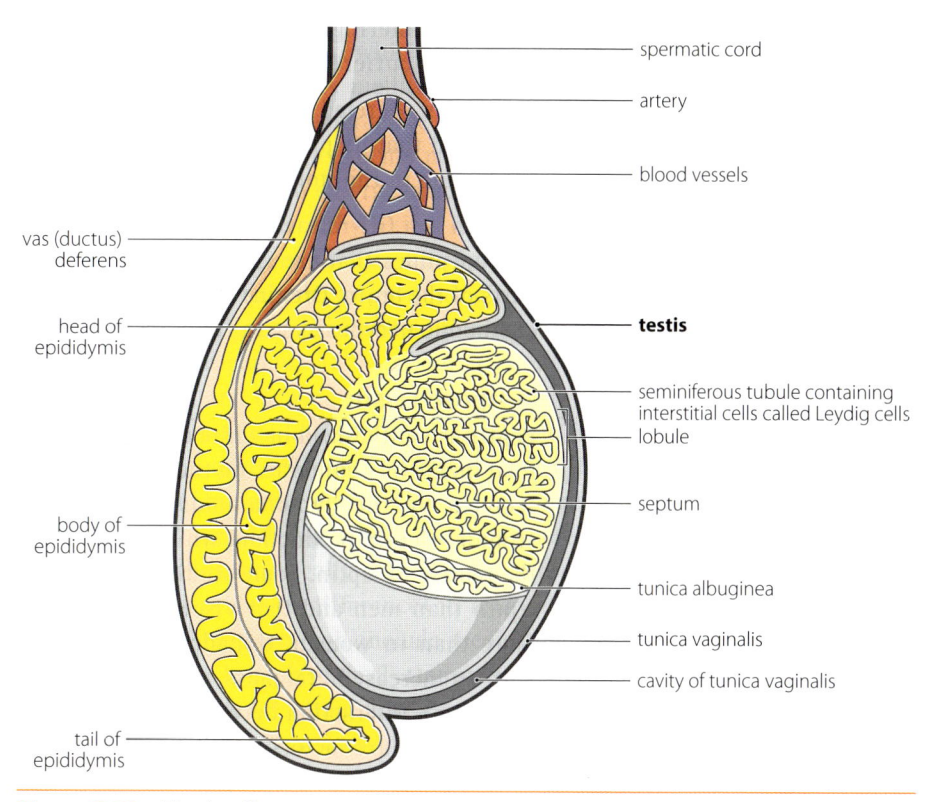

Figure 5.12 – **The testis.**

David has developed type 2 diabetes mellitus, which is associated with obesity. In this type of diabetes mellitus, there is resistance to insulin such that skeletal muscle, liver and fat cells are no longer sensitive to the insulin David is producing and glucose is unable to enter the cells. The pancreas responds to the increased blood glucose by producing more insulin in an attempt to control blood glucose. However, in this context the additional insulin produced by David has minimal effect as his cells are resistant to it. Currently, David's type 2 diabetes mellitus is being managed by diet, which is enabling him to lose weight, and an oral medication called metformin. Metformin is an oral hypoglycaemic drug that works by decreasing gluconeogenesis and by increasing peripheral utilization of glucose. It only works when a person is still producing his or her own insulin, which is still the case for David. Currently, David takes metformin 500 mg three times a day with his breakfast, lunch and evening meal. It is possible that David may require insulin injections in the future. In obese people, losing weight is very important because when they lose weight, their ability to control their blood glucose can improve. In some people with type 2 diabetes mellitus, weight loss is sufficient to enable them to stop taking medication altogether. David is attempting to lose more weight by increasing his exercise and restricting energy intake, especially of foods containing refined sugar and fat. As he loses more weight, the sensitivity of his cells to insulin improves and glucose transport into cells increases. Being treated for hypothyroidism will certainly improve David's chances of losing a significant amount of weight. However, treatment of hypothyroidism can make blood glucose control more difficult because thyroxine is a hormone whose role is to facilitate glucose metabolism. David is likely to benefit from further support from diabetes nurse specialists, in addition to structured educational programmes that are recommended for patients with diabetes mellitus.

Patient 4.2 — Jade and Jordon | 100 | 132 | 138 | **162** | 448 | 473

- 6-year-old boy and 32-year-old mother
- Jade drank alcohol excessively while pregnant
- Jordon has dysmorphic facial features and behavioural issues
- Jordon has fetal alcohol syndrome
- Jordon was small for age and given GH at age 4
- Aged 6 he is up to the 60th percentile on growth charts

The fetal alcohol syndrome that Jordon has is due to Jade, Jordon's mother, drinking excessively when she was pregnant with him. Initially, during standard monitoring of his growth and development, Jordon's health visitor and family doctor noticed that he was not attaining his developmental milestones. This led to Jordon being referred to a paediatrician by his family doctor. Jordon started receiving daily injections of somatotropin (recombinant human growth hormone (GH)) 30 mcg/kg of body weight subcutaneously, when he was 4 years old. The somatotropin injections are making Jordon's bones grow such that his growth has been increasing by approximately 2.5 cm per year over and above the rate of growth that he was achieving without the GH. He reached the 55th percentile of stature for age when he was 5 years old and is now at the 60th percentile of stature for age. Both his mother and his paediatrician are pleased by his growth and physical development. Jordon's limited growth, small body frame and inability to reach developmental milestones at the appropriate time are due to low levels of GH being produced by the pituitary gland caused by the alcohol acting as a teratogen.

In addition to stimulating most of the body cells to increase in size, GH stimulates the skeletal muscles to increase in size, as well as the epiphyseal plates of long bones (see *Chapter 13*), thus enabling the long bones to lengthen. This means that GH has anabolic or tissue-building properties. Jordon will continue with hormonal treatment until his growth and development are much improved and have caught up with those of his peers. It is important that Jade is supported by healthcare professionals. Up to now, Jade has been cooperating with the healthcare professionals by ensuring that Jordon has his daily injection of somatotropin and making sure that he does not miss his appointments with the family doctor and his paediatrician.

The content and patients explored in this chapter have focused on chemical modes of communication, which are essential to integrate the physiology of the body. Hormones have an important role in the integration of many physiological and metabolic processes. Type 2 diabetes mellitus has become one of the most important challenges to healthcare delivery systems, with a significant contribution to morbidity and mortality. As diabetes is a chronic disease, its management with regard to surveillance, prevention, treatment and the minimization of complications is paramount, especially in low- and middle-income countries where up to 80% of resources are taken up by the management of the disease. According to the World Health Organization, the number of people with diabetes mellitus rose almost four-fold, to 422 million, between 1980 and 2014. The World Health Organization has estimated that by 2030 diabetes mellitus will be the seventh leading cause of death.

While this chapter has focused on the role of hormones in integration, it is important to remember that the endocrine system does not achieve integration on its own. Coordination of physiological processes and metabolic activities of the human body is achieved through integration by the nervous and endocrine systems. Activation of the sympathetic nervous system (discussed in *Chapter 4*), together with the hormones adrenaline and noradrenaline, deals with immediate challenges and threats, while integration in chronic stress is achieved by activation of the hypothalamo–pituitary–adrenal axis, resulting in the production of cortisol. Thus, the nervous and endocrine systems enable the human body to adapt to immediate and long-term stress through sympathetic activation and hormone production, respectively.

5.4 Summary

- Homeodynamic regulation of organ systems requires coordination and integration of activity, which is achieved by the endocrine system.
- The endocrine system communicates through autocrines, paracrines and hormones.
- Hormones are secreted into the blood by endocrine glands, organs and tissue (see *Figure 5.1*) and can be protein- or lipid-based molecules.
- Protein hormones have their receptors on the plasma membranes and work via second messengers, while steroid hormones have their receptors in the cytoplasm or cell nucleus (see *Figures 5.3* and *5.4*).

- Some hormones are synthesized in the hypothalamus and stored in the posterior pituitary gland, while others are produced by the anterior pituitary gland and have a tropic effect.
- Hormonal communication is long and slow.
- Pancreatic somatostatin controls both the endocrine and exocrine function of the pancreas and the release of other gastrointestinal hormones.

5.5 Further reading

The National Institute for Health and Care Excellence (NICE) gives advice on the management of type 2 diabetes mellitus that covers many aspects including monitoring of blood glucose, diet, blood lipids, blood pressure and medication: www.nice.org.uk/guidance/conditions-and-diseases/diabetes-and-other-endocrinal--nutritional-and-metabolic-conditions/diabetes

The International Diabetes Federation is an excellent resource that covers issues on the prevention of diabetes, improving diabetes care and management, protecting women's health and education to beat diabetes complications: www.idf.org/

NICE also gives advice on how somatotropin (recombinant human GH, also known as somatropin) can be used for the treatment of growth failure that is due to GH deficiency in children. It highlights the conditions under which somatotropin should be used and reinforces the importance of the discussion that needs to occur between the paediatrician, the patient and their carer(s): www.nice.org.uk/guidance/ta188

The British Thyroid Foundation website gives information on thyroid disorders in both children and adults and supports individuals with such disorders. Guidelines on iodine intake, thyroid function test and thyroid cancer are also available: www.btf-thyroid.org/index.php/thyroid/leaflets/hypothyroidism-guide

5.6 Self-assessment questions

Answers can be found at www.scionpublishing.com/AandP

(5.1) Select the one correct answer. Which of the following hormones is produced by the hypothalamus and stored by the posterior pituitary gland?
 (a) Antidiuretic hormone
 (b) Thyroxine
 (c) Follicle-stimulating hormone
 (d) Prolactin
 (e) Glucagon

(5.2) Select the one correct answer. Which of the following hormones releases calcium from bones?
 (a) Ghrelin
 (b) Melatonin
 (c) Cholecystokinin
 (d) Parathyroid hormone
 (e) Oxytocin

(5.3) Select the one correct answer. Which of the following symptoms describe an underactive thyroid gland?
  (a) Restlessness, excitability and poor sleep
  (b) Tachycardia, palpitations and sweating
  (c) Lethargy, feeling cold and dry skin
  (d) Feeling tired, poor sleep and palpitations
  (e) Increased appetite, feeling cold and weight loss

(5.4) Select the one correct answer. The hormone that stimulates contraction of the gall bladder and relaxation of the hepatopancreatic sphincter is:
  (a) Gastrin
  (b) Motilin
  (c) Secretin
  (d) Cholecystokinin
  (e) Somatostatin

(5.5) Mark each statement either true or false:
  (a) Human chorionic gonadotrophin (hCG) maintains the corpus luteum and is a marker for pregnancy
  (b) The hormone that maintains pregnancy is oestrogen
  (c) Steroid hormones require a second messenger to exert their effect
  (d) Calcitriol is a steroid hormone also known as 1,25-dihydroxyvitamin D_3
  (e) Cortisol is produced by the adrenal medulla of the suprarenal glands

(5.6) Select the one correct answer. Which of the following is not a function of growth hormone?
  (a) It increases the size of cells
  (b) It stimulates muscle growth
  (c) It promotes collagen formation
  (d) It increases glucose utilization
  (e) It increases fat breakdown

(5.7) Explain the differences between autocrine, paracrine and endocrine signal molecules.

(5.8) Describe the production and role of insulin and glucagon in glucose homeostasis.

(5.9) Describe the secretion and role of antidiuretic hormone.

CHAPTER 06 | How the external environment is interpreted

Learning points for this chapter

After working through this chapter, you should be able to:

- Discuss the importance of the special senses
- Name and identify the structures of the eye and ear
- Describe the physiological processes involved in vision and hearing
- Describe the physiological processes involved in the interpretation of taste and smell
- Provide an overview of the physiological response to noxious stimuli that results in the perception of pain

6.1 Introduction and clinical relevance

Each of the cases introduced in this chapter highlights how the integration of sensory information enables us to interpret our environment and its importance for health. These cases are presented to emphasize the knowledge about the sensory nervous system, perception and the impact of impairment of certain major senses on health and the ability to respond to risk and danger that is required for healthcare practice.

Patient 6.1 — Sally — 167 | 188 | 404 | 443

- 50-year-old woman
- Has MS and is now a wheelchair user
- Burning sensation in her hands and double vision
- MRI confirms plaques in her brain consistent with MS

Following a series of investigations, which included lumbar puncture, visual evoked potentials and magnetic resonance imaging (MRI), Sally was diagnosed with multiple sclerosis. Now at the age of 50 years, Sally's mobility has become impaired and she is a wheelchair user. During the long course of her illness, Sally has experienced intense fatigue and various intermittent altered sensations in her body, including burning sensations in her hands and double vision.

Patient 6.2 — Sadia — 167 | 188

- 82-year-old woman
- Mildly hypertensive — on bendroflumethiazide and felodipine

Sadia is 82 years old and, although she has been fit and well for most of her life, she is currently mildly hypertensive, which is controlled by taking the diuretic bendroflumethiazide and the calcium channel blocker felodipine. Due to a family

- Eye tests reveal cataracts but no glaucoma

history, Sadia has undergone regular eye examinations for glaucoma, a group of eye conditions that result in loss of vision and blindness due to damage to the optic nerve from raised intraocular pressure. Screening for glaucoma is recommended for people with a close family history and is aimed at reducing the development of blindness. Sadia has regular screening tests as her mother had glaucoma, and, while Sadia has not developed the condition, over a 3-year period her vision has deteriorated due to the formation of cataracts. Sadia found that her vision was blurred and cloudy, and on a bright day the glare from indirect sunlight meant it was extremely difficult for her to see.

Patient 6.3   Denzel   168   189

- 50-year-old man
- High-pitched ringing in ears for many years
- Conversation now difficult with background noise
- Family doctor refers him to audiologist

Denzel is 50 years old and has been an amateur drummer for many years, playing dance, soul and blues music. He has experienced high-pitched ringing in his ears for a number of years. Recently, his hearing has deteriorated to the point that, when there is a lot of background noise, he misses words and sentences, thus affecting his understanding. While this can be frustrating, Denzel is not distressed by his hearing impairment and it does not significantly impact on his social interaction and relationships. Denzel's family doctor referred him to an audiologist who performed an audiogram, which confirmed Denzel's hearing loss.

In *Chapters 4* and *5*, the nervous and endocrine systems were discussed as the major systems for communication within the body. Making sense of the world in which we live and making appropriate responses to stimuli in our external environment is complemented by the homeodynamic response to stimuli in our internal environment, which together contribute to our protection and safety, for example maintaining our balance to prevent falls, avoiding touching hot materials that will damage the skin, and avoiding ingesting harmful or poisonous food. You may come across individuals with various types of neurological and sensory problems that may affect their ability, to varying degrees, to respond appropriately to changes in the external environment. Sally, Sadia and Denzel, due to sensory impairment, experience a variety of problems affecting their quality of life and maintenance of functional capacity. It is important for healthcare professionals to have appropriate background knowledge about the major senses to help inform the assessment, support, care and rehabilitation provided for individuals with neurological and sensory disorders.

6.2 What you need to know – essential anatomy and physiology

The role of special receptors monitoring the internal environment was discussed in *Chapter 1*. For health and wellbeing, there must be receptors integrated within systems to monitor the condition of the internal environment and to respond to changes. Sensory organs and systems are essential for monitoring and integrating environmental changes as part of homeodynamic adaptation and survival.

Changes in the internal and external environments (stimuli) are detected by sensory receptors, which take many forms. The term **general senses** describes sensitivity to stimuli such as temperature, touch and pressure. For example, thermoreceptors respond to temperature changes and baroreceptors detect changes in pressure and stretch. The term **special senses** refers to vision, hearing, taste and smell. In this chapter, each of the special senses will be discussed, as well as the general sense of touch.

6.2.1 Sensation and perception

Sensation requires **transduction** of the stimulus; for example, temperature, pressure or chemical stimuli are converted into another form (transduced), in this case a nerve impulse (action potential), by a sensory receptor. To hear sounds, fluctuations in air pressure are converted into waves in a fluid in the ear, which ultimately leads to alterations in specific receptors within the inner ear. Waves in the fluid stimulate the production of action potentials that are transmitted to the brain, where hearing is perceived. The sensations of smell and taste require the transduction of chemical stimuli into action potentials, which is achieved through the stimulation of taste and olfactory receptor cells. Similarly, for vision, packets of light energy (photons) stimulate photoreceptors that transduce photons into action potentials, which are transmitted via the optic nerve to the visual cortex of the occipital lobe of the brain where the action potentials are processed.

Sensory receptors may be discrete cells, such as those in the cochlea within the inner ear, or cells that form the retina of the eye. In addition, sensory receptors may be free nerve endings, such as those responsive to pressure or temperature. Free nerve endings may be abundant, as in the fingertips, or less densely packed, for example across the back.

Sensation refers to the immediate, unprocessed effect of stimulation of sensory receptors, while **perception** describes the interpretation of the world through the senses and involves the processing of action potentials from stimulated receptors. The interpretation of sensory impulses (perception) occurs in the cerebral cortex of the brain. Different regions of the cerebral cortex are concerned with specific senses; for example, the visual cortex is located in the occipital lobe. As described in *Chapter 4*, sensory (afferent) impulses, such as those arising from temperature changes, pressure or potentially damaging stimuli (nociception), are conducted to the somatosensory area of the parietal lobe (somatic sensory cortex).

6.2.2 Vision and the eye

For vision, light energy (in the form of photons) from part of the electromagnetic spectrum called visible light, is focused onto specialized photoreceptors that lie within the retina of the eye. These receptors are activated according to the wavelength of the visible light. It is the spectrum of visible light (bands of colours) that we see when visible light is passed through a prism. When light stimulates the photoreceptors, chemical changes occur to create action potentials, which are conducted along sensory pathways to the primary visual cortex in the occipital lobe of each cerebral hemisphere.

The eye is a slightly irregular spherical object divided into two transparent fluid compartments. These are known as the anterior and posterior cavities and are separated by the **lens** and associated structures, including the ciliary body and iris (see *Figure 6.1*). The **anterior cavity**, which has an anterior and posterior chamber, contains a thin watery fluid called **aqueous humour**, which is continuously formed by the **ciliary body**. The formation and circulation of aqueous humour is important as it supplies oxygen and nutrients to the lens and **cornea**, which both lack blood vessels; if blood vessels were present, the passage of light would be obstructed. The constant production, circulation and drainage of aqueous humour maintain a constant intraocular pressure to help support the eye internally. The **posterior cavity**, which lies behind the lens, is filled with **vitreous humour**, a colourless, transparent, jelly-like fluid. Vitreous humour contributes to the intraocular pressure, transmits light and ensures that the two layers of the retina remain attached.

The eye has an outer protective fibrous covering called the **sclera**, and this can be seen as the white part of the eye. The sclera is attached to the orbital bone of the skull by extrinsic muscles, which enable the eye to move and focus on objects. The sclera becomes much thinner and clearer towards the front of the eye, forming the cornea (see *Figure 6.1*). When exposed to air, the sclera and cornea dehydrate quickly and therefore need to be kept constantly moist, and this is achieved by the formation of tears from the lachrymal glands, which are located underneath the top of the eyelid. Keeping the cornea and sclera moist is important to prevent eye infections and damage to the cornea. The importance of the mucus membrane of the eye (the **conjunctiva**), blinking and the production of tears as protective mechanisms to prevent infection is discussed in *Chapter 11*. Some people who suffer from dry eyes can benefit from the use of artificial tears, applied by eye drops, to keep the cornea moist.

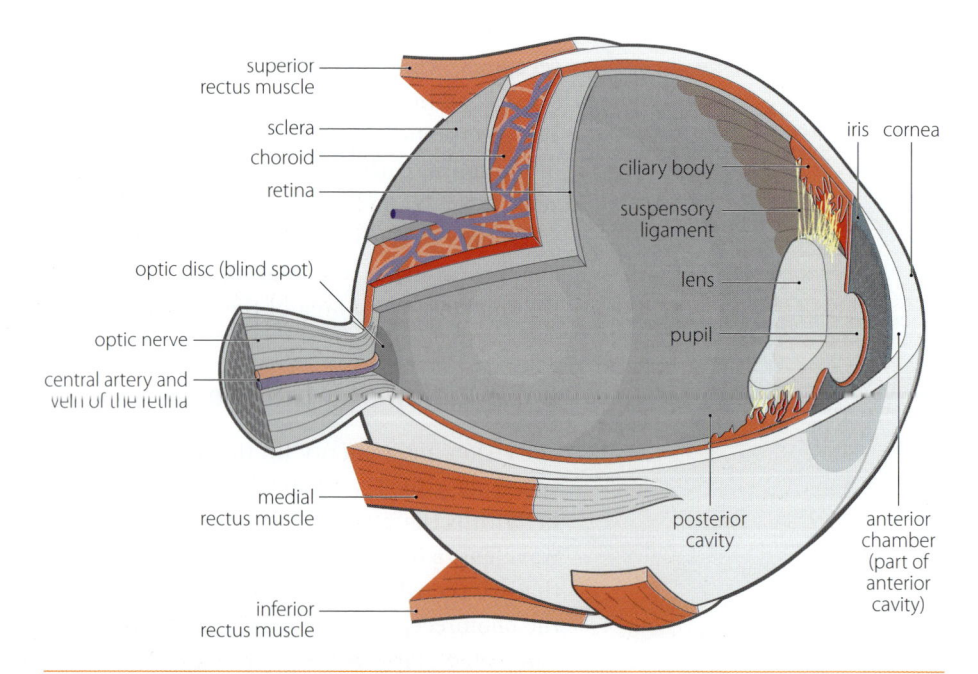

Figure 6.1 – A cross-section of the eye.

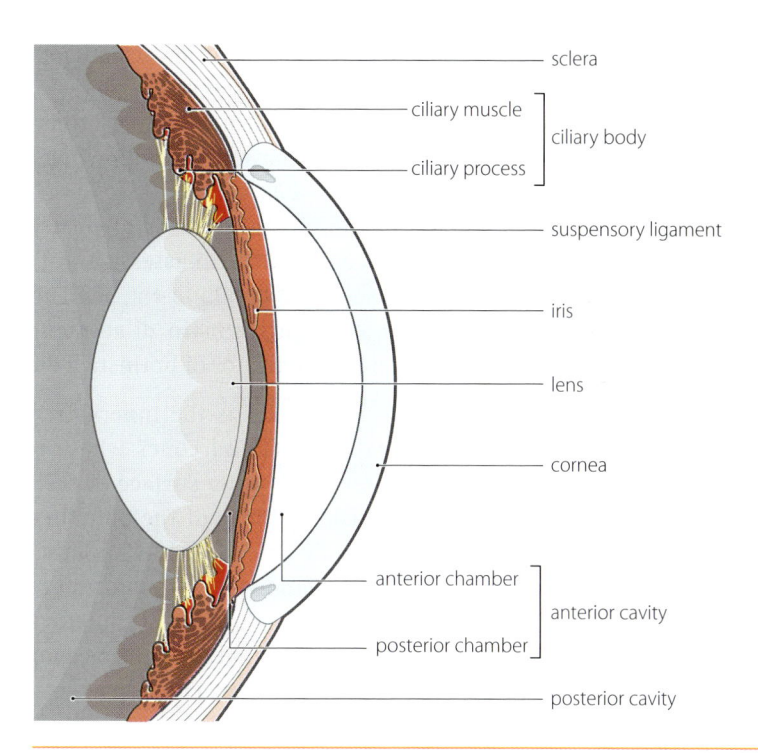

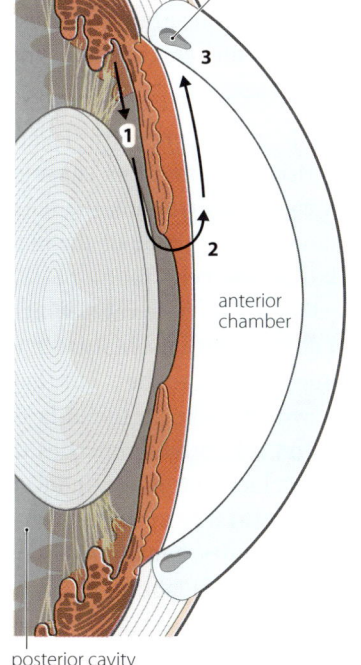

SECTION 6.2 | WHAT YOU NEED TO KNOW – ESSENTIAL ANATOMY AND PHYSIOLOGY 171

Figure 6.2 – The structures supporting the lens.

Figure 6.3 – Circulation of the aqueous humour.
Aqueous humour flows from the ciliary processes filling the posterior chamber (1) through the pupil into the anterior chamber (2) and into the venous system through the canal of Schlemm.

The layer of tissue beneath the sclera is a highly vascular tissue with three regions: the **choroid**, the ciliary body and the **iris**. The choroid forms the posterior part of the vascular tissue, providing nourishment for the retina. The brown pigment of the choroid helps to absorb light, thus preventing light scatter within the eye. Towards the front of the eye, the choroid becomes the ciliary body, which encircles and supports the lens (see *Figure 6.2*). The ciliary body comprises interlacing smooth muscle cells called the ciliary muscle that controls the shape of the lens. Towards the back of the lens, the ciliary body has folds called **ciliary processes** (ciliary trabeculae), which produce the aqueous humour. Aqueous humour flows and drains away continuously (see *Figure 6.3*); it flows from the ciliary processes, filling the **posterior chamber**, through the pupil into the **anterior chamber** in front of the iris. From the anterior chamber, the aqueous humour drains into the venous system through the **canal of Schlemm** (scleral venous sinus). Obstruction to the flow and drainage of aqueous humour can result in an increase in the fluid pressure within the eye, which can be so severe as to compress the retina and optic nerve, resulting in an ophthalmic condition known as **glaucoma** (see Sadia, Patient 6.2).

The lens is situated behind the iris and is held in place by the **suspensory ligaments** (see *Figure 6.2*) which help to support the lens and change the shape of the lens to focus light onto the retina (discussed later in the chapter). The suspensory ligaments are attached to the ciliary processes. The iris of the eye, with its opening, called the pupil, lies between the cornea and the lens. Formed by circular and radial smooth muscle cells and elastic fibres, the iris, under the influence of the autonomic nervous system, can contract or relax, causing constriction or dilation

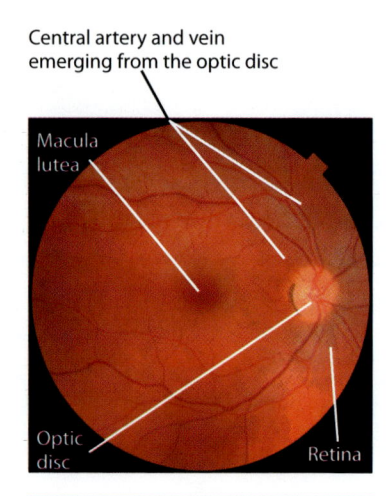

Figure 6.4 – Image of the retina, optic disc and blood vessels, visualized with an ophthalmoscope.
(Häggström, Mikael. "Medical gallery of Mikael Häggström 2014". Wikiversity Journal of Medicine 1 (2). DOI:10.15347/wjm/2014.008. ISSN 20018762. – Own work)

of the pupil and thus regulating accommodation (discussed later). Activation of the sympathetic nervous system causes contraction of radial muscle fibres, resulting in the pupil dilating, whereas constriction of the pupil occurs due to contraction of the circular muscles following stimulation by the parasympathetic nervous system (see *Chapter 4*). Assessing the responsiveness of the eye to light using a pen torch and observing constriction or dilation of the pupil is an important part of a neurological assessment. The normal pupillary reflex is where bright light causes constriction of the pupil. An abnormal pupillary light reflex, where one or both pupils remain dilated and unresponsive to the light, is an important diagnostic indicator of brainstem damage or damage to the optic nerve.

The **retina** (see *Figure 6.1*) is the innermost tissue of the eye, containing light receptor cells called **rods** and **cones** whose response to light will be discussed later in this chapter. The inner surface of the retina contains a network of blood vessels that nourish it. Fibres of the optic nerve exit the eye at a feature of the retina called the optic disc, which is slightly off centre to the incident plane of light that travels through the eye onto the retina. The positioning of the optic disc ensures that the plane of light stimulates light receptors, as the retinal tissue at the optic disc does not contain light receptors; hence, the alternative name for the optic disc is the blind spot. The retina, optic disc and network of blood vessels can be visualized with an ophthalmoscope (see *Figure 6.4*). Retinal vessels are readily visible using an ophthalmoscope, and changes to the appearance of these vessels can be an early indicator of chronic disease such as diabetes mellitus and hypertension.

The lens is a biconvex, transparent, flexible disc made up of concentric layers of highly organized cells. The crystalline lens comprises an outer lens capsule, the lens epithelium and lens fibres. A dense fibrous capsule surrounds the lens. The capsule is highly elastic, contributing to the change in the shape of the lens for focusing. The lens epithelium comprises cuboidal-shaped cells found on the anterior side of the lens. These cells are progenitor cells for lens fibre cells, which are elongated, transparent, tightly packed and found deep in the lens. Mature lens fibre cells are transparent, as they do not contain nuclei or organelles, but they do contain water-soluble proteins called **crystallins,** which make up the bulk of the lens. Crystallins contribute to the transparency and refractive properties of the lens and have a protective function against the development of age-induced deterioration of the lens, delaying the development of **cataracts** until older age (see *Box 6.1*). Lens fibres are added to the lens as ageing occurs, causing the lens to enlarge and become more convex and less flexible. Thus, the ability to focus also becomes impaired with age.

Physiology of vision

Eyes respond to visible light, which is the part of the electromagnetic spectrum that covers wavelengths from 400 to 700 nanometres (see *Figure 6.6a*). When light in the visible range of wavelengths travels through a prism, the light is dispersed to form a visible band of colours (spectrum). Objects have colour because they absorb light rays of certain wavelengths while reflecting other wavelengths. Objects that look white reflect all wavelengths. Colour vision occurs because the cones in the retina respond to different wavelengths of light (see *Figure 6.6b*).

SECTION 6.2 | WHAT YOU NEED TO KNOW – ESSENTIAL ANATOMY AND PHYSIOLOGY 173

> **BOX 6.1**
>
> ### Cataracts
>
> A cataract is an opacity (cloudy area) in the lens (see *Figure 6.5*). According to the World Health Organization, cataracts are the most common cause of blindness worldwide. They can affect one or both eyes and, while more commonly associated with age, can result from other factors such as trauma, reaction to certain drugs and prolonged exposure to ultraviolet light (see the SunSmart guidelines in *Chapter 12*). Cataracts can be classified according to the part of the lens that is affected and whether or not they are congenital (occurring in children from birth), juvenile (occurring in young children) or adult. The presence of the cataract in the lens changes its transparency so an individual with a cataract will experience blurred and cloudy vision, and may find the glare from bright lights and the sun particularly problematic.
>
> **Figure 6.5 – Image of a cataract in the lens.**
> Reproduced from www.sandiegoeyedocs.com.
>
> The lens is a transparent avascular structure with a high refractory index, which is a measure of the extent to which light bends when passing from air into another medium; in this case, it is the extent to which light is refracted when it meets the lens. These properties are achieved by the presence of structural proteins called crystallins within lens fibres. With age, long exposure to bright sunlight and oxidative stress, defective crystallins can accumulate, causing opacity in the lens (cataracts). The development of cataracts is also associated with several other factors including diabetes mellitus and a family history. Mutations in specific genes that encode specific crystallins also make crystallins more sensitive to damage by thermal and chemical stress, leading to the development of cataracts.

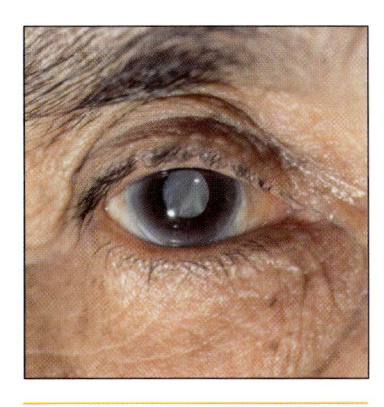

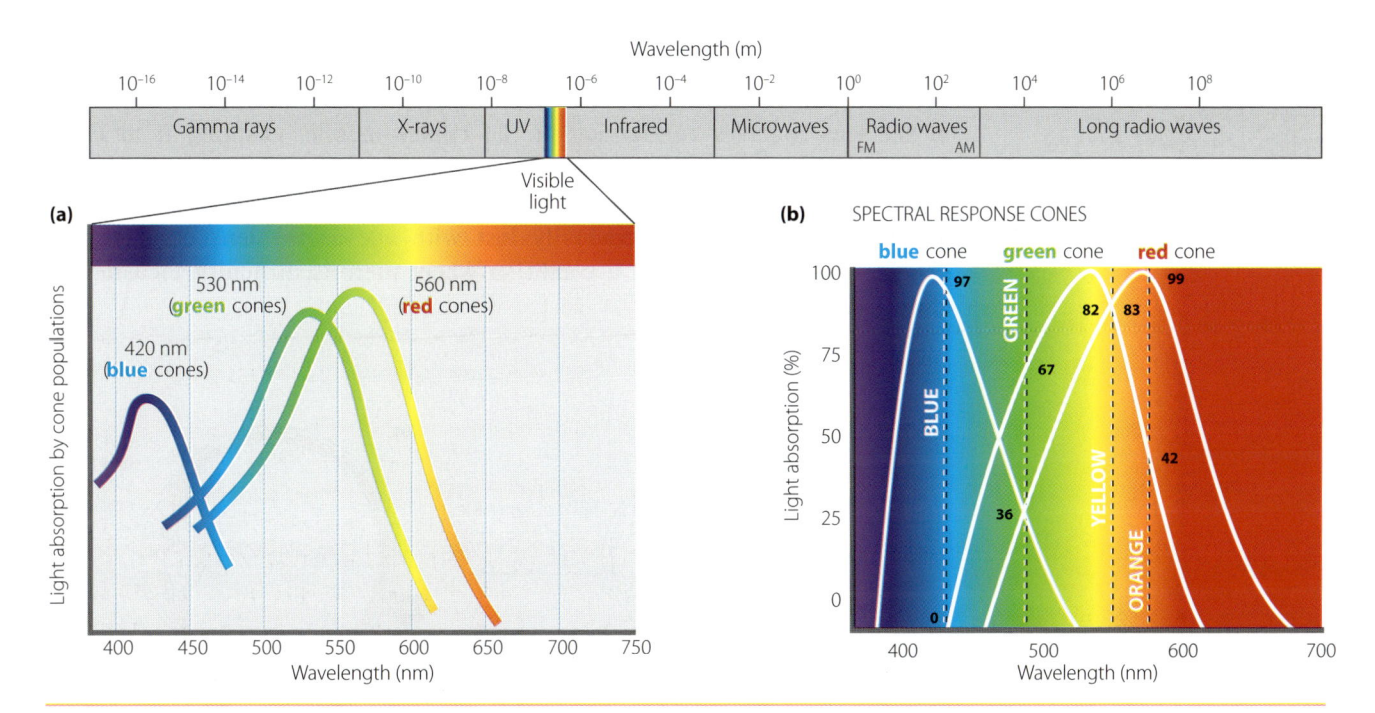

Figure 6.6 – (a) The electromagnetic spectrum and (b) photoreceptor (cone) sensitivities.

Focusing of light onto the retina

When light meets a transparent medium with a different density, its speed changes, and if the light rays meet the surface of the new transparent medium at an angle, the light rays bend. This is called refraction and occurs when light rays in air meet the lens of the eye. When light passes through the eye, it travels through the cornea, the aqueous humour of the anterior segment, the lens, the vitreous humour of the posterior segment and the entire thickness of the retina to stimulate the photoreceptors in the retina. Light is refracted as it passes through the cornea and on entering and leaving the lens. Changing the shape of the lens bends the rays of light so they converge onto the retina. Thus, light from objects at various distances can be focused onto the retina – a process called **accommodation**. If light passing through the cornea and lens is not refracted correctly, the image will appear distorted.

In normal vision, the farthest point of vision beyond which no further change in lens shape is required for focusing is 6 metres (20 feet). This distance is used as a normal standard for visual acuity. The term 20/20 vision is used to express the clarity or sharpness of vision measured at a distance of 20 feet. 20/20 vision means you can see clearly at 20 feet what should normally be seen at that distance. If a person can only see at 20 feet what someone with 'normal vision' could see at 40 feet, then that individual is described as having 20/40 vision. The term 20/20 vision does not mean perfect vision; it only describes the level of clarity or sharpness of vision at a particular distance. During distant vision, the lens is flattened as the ciliary muscle relaxes, producing tension in the suspensory ligaments, which pull the lens, making it stretch and flatten (see *Figure 6.7a*).

When focusing on a close object, light rays are divergent and therefore the lens shape needs to be adjusted to increase refraction (see *Figure 6.7b*). To restore focus, three actions occur: accommodation of the lens, constriction of the pupil and convergence of the eyes (the eyes turn inward). Accommodation of the lens involves contraction of the ciliary muscle, enabling it to move forwards towards the pupil. Tension is then released in the suspensory ligaments so that the elastic fibres of the lens recoil, causing the lens to bulge. Accommodation is gradually lost with age as the lens becomes less elastic, causing **presbyopia**, a condition where there is difficulty focusing on close images.

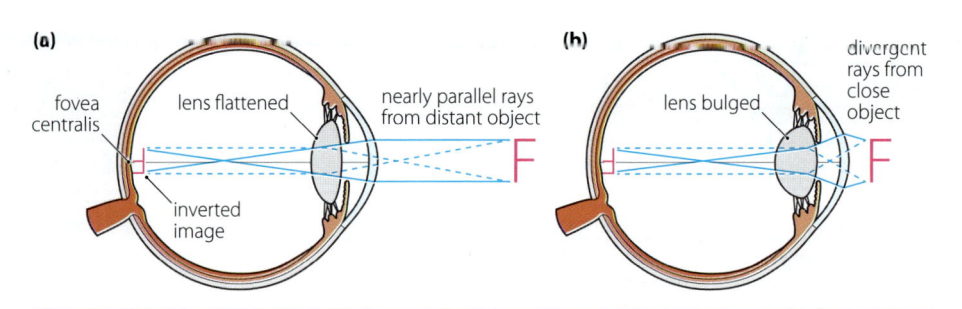

(a) fovea centralis, lens flattened, nearly parallel rays from distant object, inverted image

(b) lens bulged, divergent rays from close object

Figure 6.7 – **Accommodation: focusing for (a) distant vision and (b) close objects.**

The retina and photoreceptors

The retina comprises two layers – an outer pigmented layer that is in contact with the choroid, and a transparent inner layer called the neural layer (see *Figure 6.8*). The pigmented layer absorbs light and prevents light scatter. The neural layer contains the **photoreceptors**, called rods and cones. The junction between the pigmented layer and the neural layer is structurally weak and can separate, resulting in a condition called a detached retina, which is a cause of altered vision.

Photoreceptors (rods and cones) are modified neurones, with an inner segment and an outer segment. The outer segment of photoreceptor is embedded in the pigmented layer of the retina, whereas the inner segment connects to the cell body of the neurone in the neural layer (see *Figure 6.8*). The outer segment is the receptive zone and contains a mass of visual pigments that alter shape as they absorb light. Rods are more numerous, amounting to approximately 110–130 million, and are spread throughout the retina, including the peripheral region. There are fewer cones (approximately 5–7 million), and these are concentrated in an area called the **fovea centralis** of the retina.

Rods and cones contain proteins called **opsins**, which are bound to **retinal**, a light-absorbing molecule derived from vitamin A, to form specific visual photopigments that absorb different wavelengths of light. Rods contain the photopigment **rhodopsin** (a combination of a specific opsin and retinal). Rods contain much more photopigment than cones, and this explains in part their greater sensitivity to light. Cones contain different forms of opsin combined with retinal to form **photopsins**. There are three distinct types of cone, defined by the photopsins present within them, each responsive to a particular wavelength within the visible spectrum. One type of cone is more sensitive to short wavelengths (S cones), one to medium wavelengths (M cones) and the third to medium to long wavelengths (L cones) (see *Figure 6.6b*). They are often called blue cones, green cones and red cones, respectively. The variation in signals from each cone type enables the brain to perceive colour. Cones that are stimulated by wavelengths

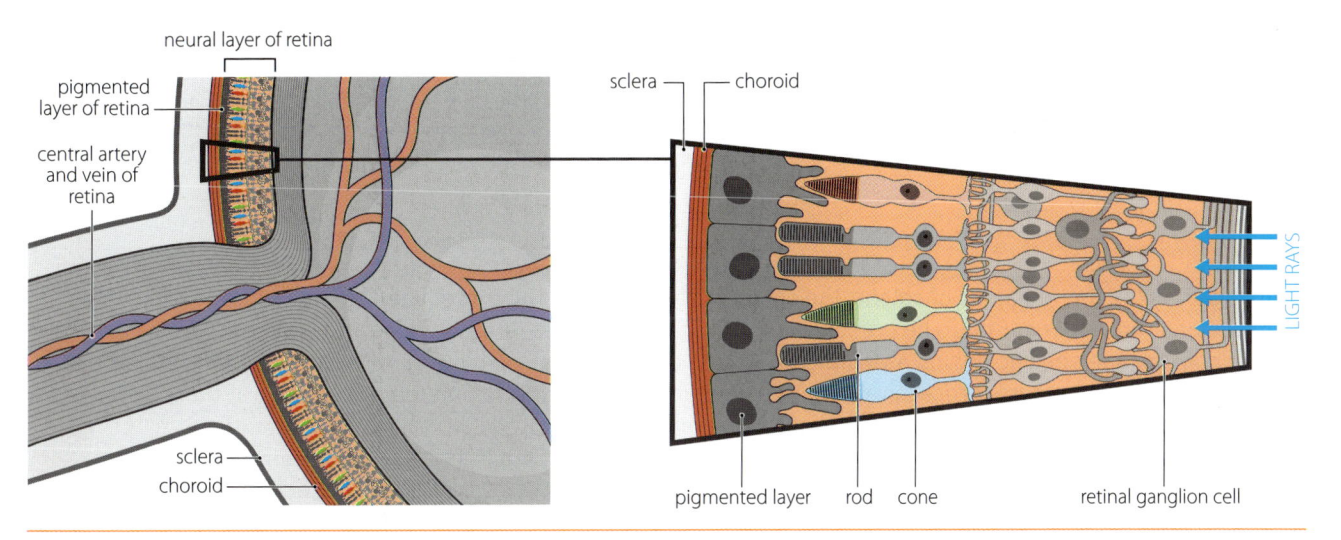

Figure 6.8 – **A simplified diagram of the retina.**

reflecting green and red are particularly located in the fovea centralis onto which light is focused, ensuring greatest visual clarity. Cones that are responsive to light in the blue wavelength, which account for approximately 2% of all of the cones, are more sensitive to light compared with the other cones and therefore they lie outside the fovea centralis. Rods and cones, each via an individual intermediary neurone, connect to retinal ganglion cells in the neural layer of the retina (see *Figure 6.8*). Retinal ganglion cells transmit action potentials from the rods and cones to the brain via the optic nerve.

Rods are very sensitive to dim light and hence ideal for night vision. As they are predominantly located in the peripheral retina, they have an important role in peripheral vision. Rods only contain rhodopsin, and therefore vision is perceived only in grey tones, and because many rods connect with a few retinal ganglion cells, visual acuity is reduced and vision less clearly defined. Cones are activated by bright light and, due to the three different classes of photopsins, vision is perceived in colour. Colour vision depends on the overlap in sensitivity to a range of wavelengths of light across all three receptor types. The activity of one or more types of cone may be impaired, which can lead to colour blindness; this is described in *Box 6.2*. Stimulation of cones produces vision that is sharp and distinct because individual cones connect to individual retinal ganglion cells and therefore perception in the visual cortex is of a higher resolution.

In bright light, rods are inactivated as rhodopsin is bleached by the intensity of the light. Initially, both rods and cones are stimulated, providing a brief glaring effect. As the cones recover following the initial intense stimulation and the rods become deactivated, colour vision and visual acuity improve. This occurs over 5–10 minutes. Moving from areas of light to darkness results in deactivation of cones and the gradual reactivation of rods, as rhodopsin is formed and accumulates slowly. Adaptation from bright sunlight to complete darkness takes approximately 20–30 minutes.

The visual pathway

This involves the conduction of sensory nerve impulses from activated photoreceptors to the brain, where signals are processed in the visual cortex of the occipital lobe. The sensory nerve axons from the retinal ganglion cells are organized into the optic nerve (cranial nerve II) (see *Figure 6.9a*). The arrangement of the axons within the optic nerve means that the activity of the photoreceptor

---

BOX 6.2

Colour blindness

In order to see the full array of colour, the correct proportions of the three types of cone (blue, green and red) are required to be present. Colour blindness is due to mutation of the genes that code for the specific opsins associated with one or more cones. Colour blindness is usually classified as an autosomal recessive X-linked condition (see *Chapter 3*), although mapping of the human genome has identified causative mutations on at least 19 other chromosomes. As the mutations are more commonly linked to the X chromosome, colour blindness is more common in males. The most common form of colour blindness involves the absence of or a reduced number of cones that respond to red or green wavelengths of light.

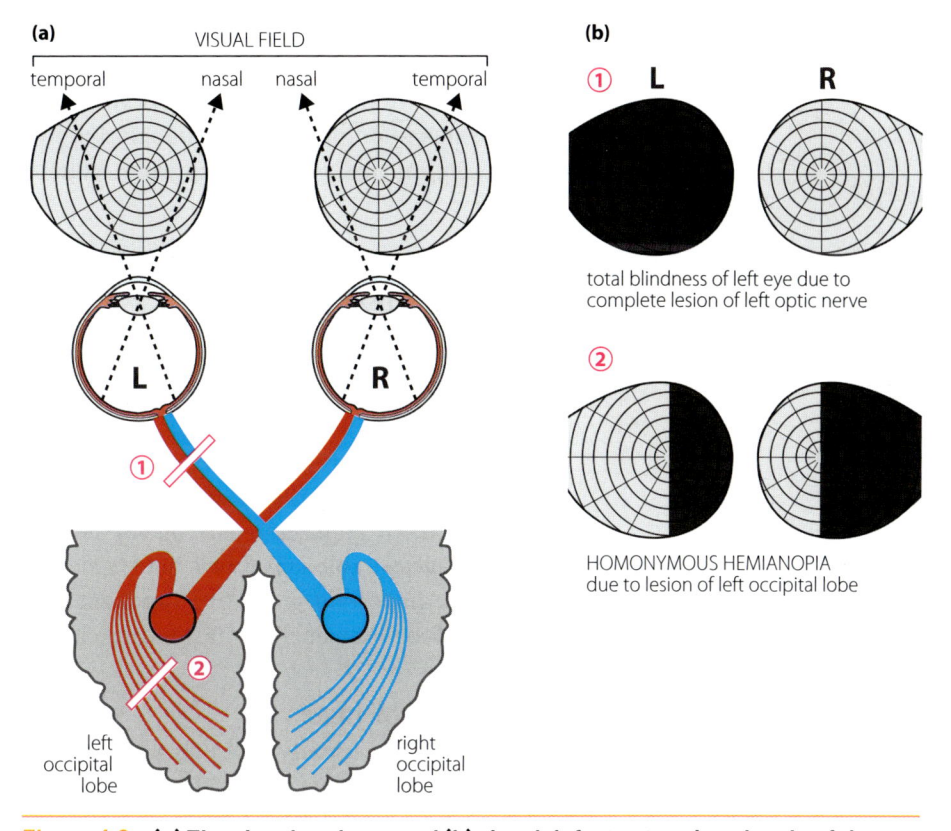

Figure 6.9 – (a) The visual pathway and (b) visual defects at various levels of the visual pathway.

cells of the left side of the retina of each eye is conducted to the left occipital lobe and the activity from the right side of the retina of each eye to the right occipital lobe. In other words, each occipital lobe processes information from the same visual field (see *Figure 6.9a*). Fibres from the medial (nasal) aspect of each eye cross over. The crossing over of the fibres occurs at the **optic chiasma**. Crossing over of the fibres is useful as it helps visual processing by the brain, enabling the perception of depth and three-dimensional images. The relay of sensory impulses to the occipital lobe of the brain and the processing of visual information is complex, involving different parts of the cerebral cortex and areas of the brain including the thalamus. Some people who experience a stroke may have damage to the neural pathways altering vision, such as a **homonymous hemianopia** where there is a loss of vision in either the left or right half of the visual field (see *Figure 6.9b*).

Control of eye movement

Six extrinsic (extraocular) eye muscles control the movement of each eyeball. The eye muscles are attached to the bones that form the eye socket (bony orbit) and to the sclera. The muscles effectively support the eye in the orbit and allow the eye to follow objects. The term **strabismus** (also called a squint) refers to a condition where the eyes deviate (eye turning) when looking at a specific object. This is usually due to a lack of coordination between the extrinsic muscles of the

6.2.3 Taste and smell

The sensations of taste and smell are not mutually exclusive. Taste and smell arise from stimulation of chemoreceptors. In the case of smell, chemicals stimulate chemoreceptors in the nasopharynx and oropharynx, whereas with taste, chemicals within food dissolve in the saliva and activate taste receptors, which are found mainly on the tongue. Activation of receptors involved in the sensation of smell is an important part of our perception of taste. Taste and smell can result in pleasurable sensations, but chemoreceptors involved with taste and smell also have important protective functions; for example, we are less likely to eat harmful food that smells or tastes disgusting.

eyes and can be evident in babies and children. Strabismus can cause **amblyopia**, a condition commonly known as 'lazy eye', where there is reduced vision in one eye and the brain favours signals from the eye with clearer vision. Treatment for strabismus and amblyopia commonly involves glasses with prescriptive lenses, eye exercises and vision therapy, botulinum toxin injections and corrective eye surgery.

The sense of taste

Taste sensation usually involves a combination of qualities. Taste receptors are located in taste buds, the majority of which are located on the tongue. There are five main groups of taste receptors (taste buds) currently recognized. These are sweet, sour, salty, bitter and umami (savoury). Taste is an important aspect governing appetite and nutritional intake, as well as the avoidance of harmful chemicals. Activation of specific taste buds has traditionally been mapped to various parts of the tongue (see *Figure 6.10a*); however, new scientific techniques indicate that different taste qualities can be elicited from all areas of the tongue where there are taste buds. Nevertheless, it is clear that a single taste bud can only respond to a single and specific chemical combination (taste quality).

Most taste buds are located in the papillae of the tongue. Papillae give the tongue a rough appearance and feel. Each taste bud contains numerous taste cells (gustatory cells), with each cell having hair-like projections on the upper surface that project through a taste pore onto the epithelial surface of the tongue (see *Figure 6.10b*). The hairs are the sensitive part of the gustatory cells. Coiled tightly round the gustatory cells are the dendrites of sensory nerves that form the initial part of the taste (gustatory) sensory pathway. When stimulated, taste cells release neurotransmitters that activate sensory neurones. Sensory stimulation of the posterior third of the tongue is conducted to the brainstem along the glossopharyngeal nerve (cranial nerve IX) and that of the remaining two-thirds of the tongue via the facial nerve (cranial nerve VII). Sensory impulses from taste receptors located in the soft palate, pharynx and epiglottis are conducted by the vagus nerve (cranial nerve X). Sensory impulses are conducted through the medulla of the brainstem to a relay station in the thalamus of the brain and then on to the sensory cortex in the insula lobe of the brain (see *Figure 6.11* and *Chapter 4*) and the operculum of the frontal lobe, to produce the conscious perception of taste.

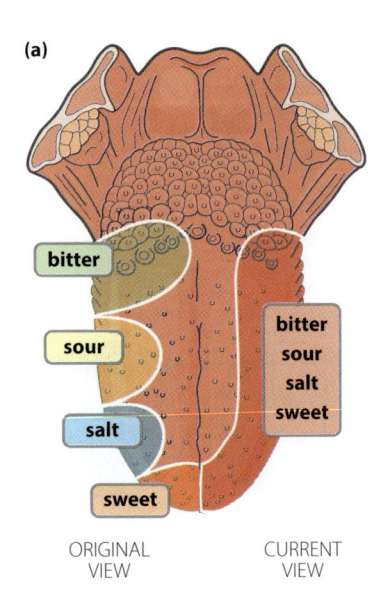

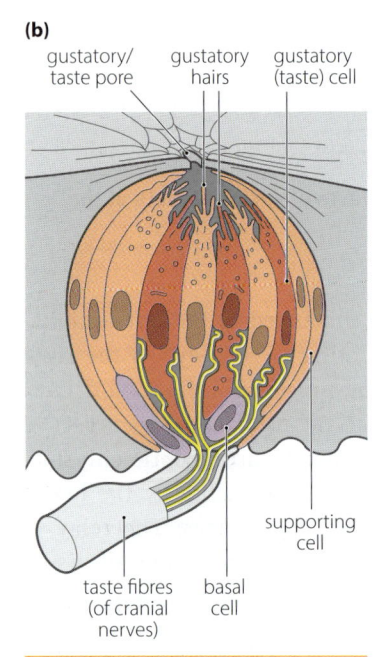

Figure 6.10 – Taste.
The left-hand side of part (a) shows the traditional mapping of the location of receptors on the tongue; this is no longer considered to be entirely accurate. The right-hand side of part (a) shows the current thinking that different taste qualities can be elicited from all areas of the tongue where there are taste buds. Part (b) shows a gustatory receptor.

Alterations in taste, for example the development of a metallic taste, can occur for a variety of reasons, including teeth and gum disease, acid reflux and some drugs.

The sense of smell: olfactory epithelium and neural pathways

The sense of smell depends on activation of **olfactory receptors** (a type of chemoreceptor) present in a region of epithelial tissue (olfactory epithelium) in the roof of the nasal cavity (see *Figure 6.12*). The nasal epithelium contains millions of ciliated olfactory receptor cells coated with a thin mucus produced by olfactory glands. Inhaled chemicals dissolve in the mucus and activate specific receptors located within the membrane of the olfactory receptor cell cilia. When olfactory receptors become saturated, the sense of smell becomes blunted.

Stimulation of olfactory receptors leads to the formation of sensory nerve impulses conducted via axons that collect together to form the filaments of the olfactory nerve (cranial nerve I). These filaments pass through gaps in a section of the ethmoid bone in the roof of the nose called the **cribriform plate** (see *Figure 6.12*). Filaments of the olfactory nerve then synapse with olfactory bulbs overlying the cribriform plate. From the olfactory bulbs, which form the ends of the olfactory tract, sensory nerve impulses are conducted to the olfactory cortex in the base of the temporal lobe and medial aspect of the temporal lobe of the cerebrum. In addition, sensory impulses are also relayed to other parts of the brain such as the hypothalamus and limbic system (see *Chapter 4*), triggering an emotional response, such as pleasure or a sense of danger, or a protective reflex response such as sneezing.

6.2.4 Hearing

Hearing is the perception of sound, which can be described subjectively in terms of loudness and pitch (high or low). Sound consists of fluctuations of pressure, taking the form of waves with alternating high pressure (compression of molecules) and decompressions (rarefactions) that are transmitted in air and, as explained later, also in fluid. In air, a pressure wave produced by a single tone (pure tone) can be illustrated using a sine wave, where positive peaks represent high pressure and negative peaks (troughs) represent decompression (see *Figure 6.13a*). Sound can be regarded as a mixture of pure tones.

The amplitude of the sine wave (see *Figure 6.13b*) is associated with the loudness of the tone. The number of cycles of the wave determines the frequency and is associated with the perception of the pitch of the sound (see *Figure 6.13a*). Frequency is measured in terms of cycles per second or **hertz** (Hz), and one cycle per second is equal to 1 Hz. Typically, young adults can detect sound over a range between 20 and 20 000 Hz where 20 Hz is low frequency and 20 000 Hz is high frequency. With age, the ability to detect higher frequencies deteriorates and the maximum frequency detected by middle-aged adults can fall to 14 000–16 000 Hz.

The magnitude of the pressure wave is referred to as the amplitude. The greater the amplitude, the louder the sound will be perceived. Sound intensity is measured in **decibels** (dB) based on a logarithmic scale from 1 to 140 dB. A decibel is a relative and not an absolute measurement as it expresses how many units one

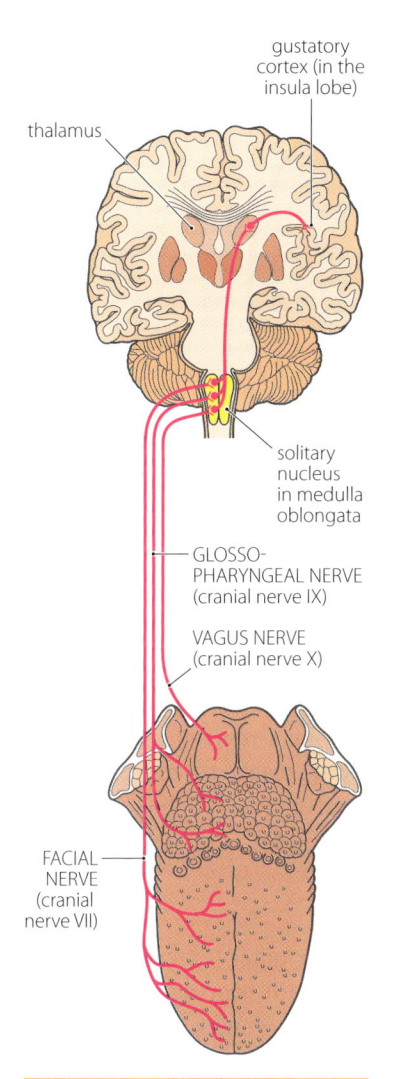

Figure 6.11 – The sensory pathway from the tongue.

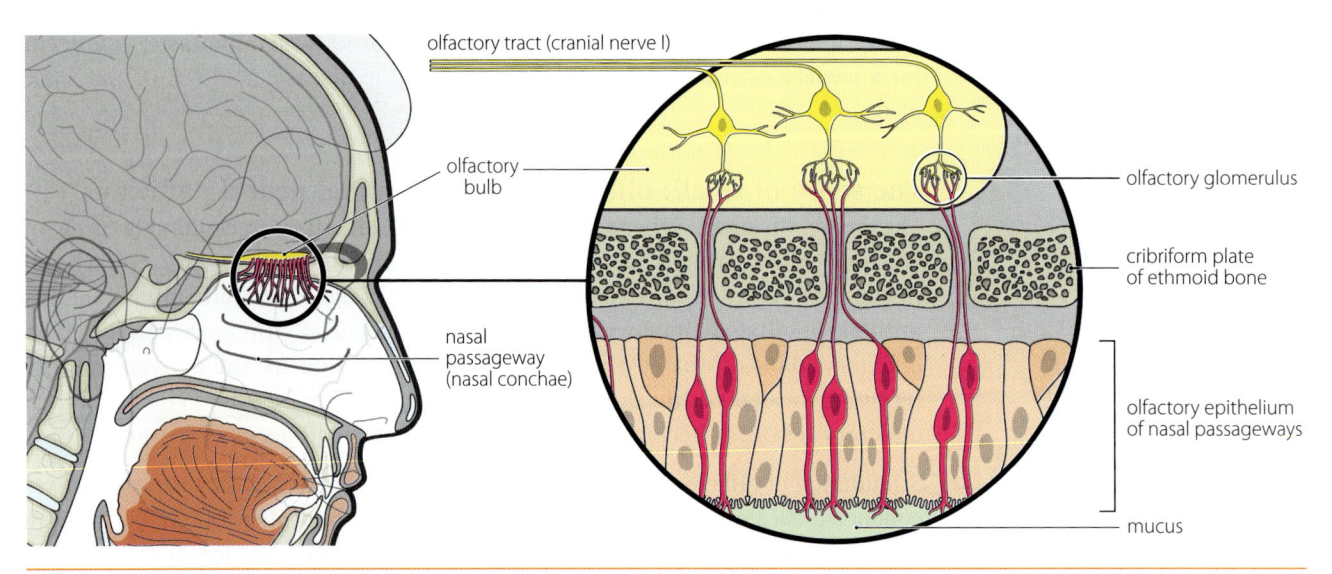

Figure 6.12 – The olfactory epithelium and olfactory tract.

sound intensity is above or below another intensity. In the environment, sound intensity varies considerably. A normal conversation may register as 45–60 dB, while maximum sound through an MP3 player may reach 115 dB. Sustained sound intensity above 85 dB can cause permanent hearing loss. Sudden sounds of 115–120 dB can cause ear pain and disturbance of balance.

Structure of the ear

The ear is divided into three parts (see *Figure 6.14*): the outer (external), middle and inner ear. The outer and middle ear are involved with hearing, whereas the inner ear is concerned with both hearing and balance. The outer and middle ear are referred to as the conductive system, as they conduct sound waves from the environment to the inner ear.

The external ear comprises the pinna, which is also called the auricle, and the external auditory meatus (external auditory canal). The pinna is composed of cartilage covered in skin and is organized into folds, which funnel sound waves into the external auditory meatus. The surface of the auditory meatus comprises skin with hairs and ceruminous glands, which secrete cerumen (ear wax). Cerumen and hairs provide additional protection, preventing infection. Excessive accumulation and impaction of cerumen in the meatus can impede the conduction of sound waves, resulting in deafness. The external auditory meatus meets the tympanic membrane (ear drum), which divides the external and middle ear. The tympanic membrane is a thin, transparent and flexible membrane covered with skin on the external side of the ear, and is able to vibrate. It is shaped like a flattened cone with the apex of the cone pointing into the middle ear. Thinness of the tympanic membrane provides flexibility, allowing the membrane to vibrate when hit by sound waves.

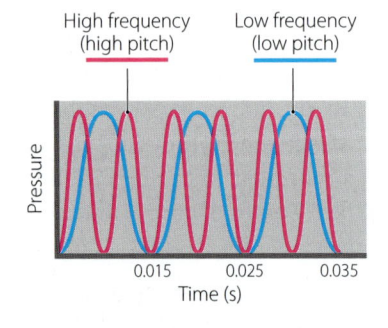

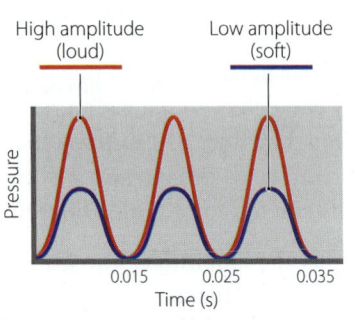

Figure 6.13 – The sine wave: a pure tone sound.

The middle ear is an air-filled cavity, lined by mucosa (mucus-producing epithelial cells), situated within a bony cavity within the temporal bone of the skull. There

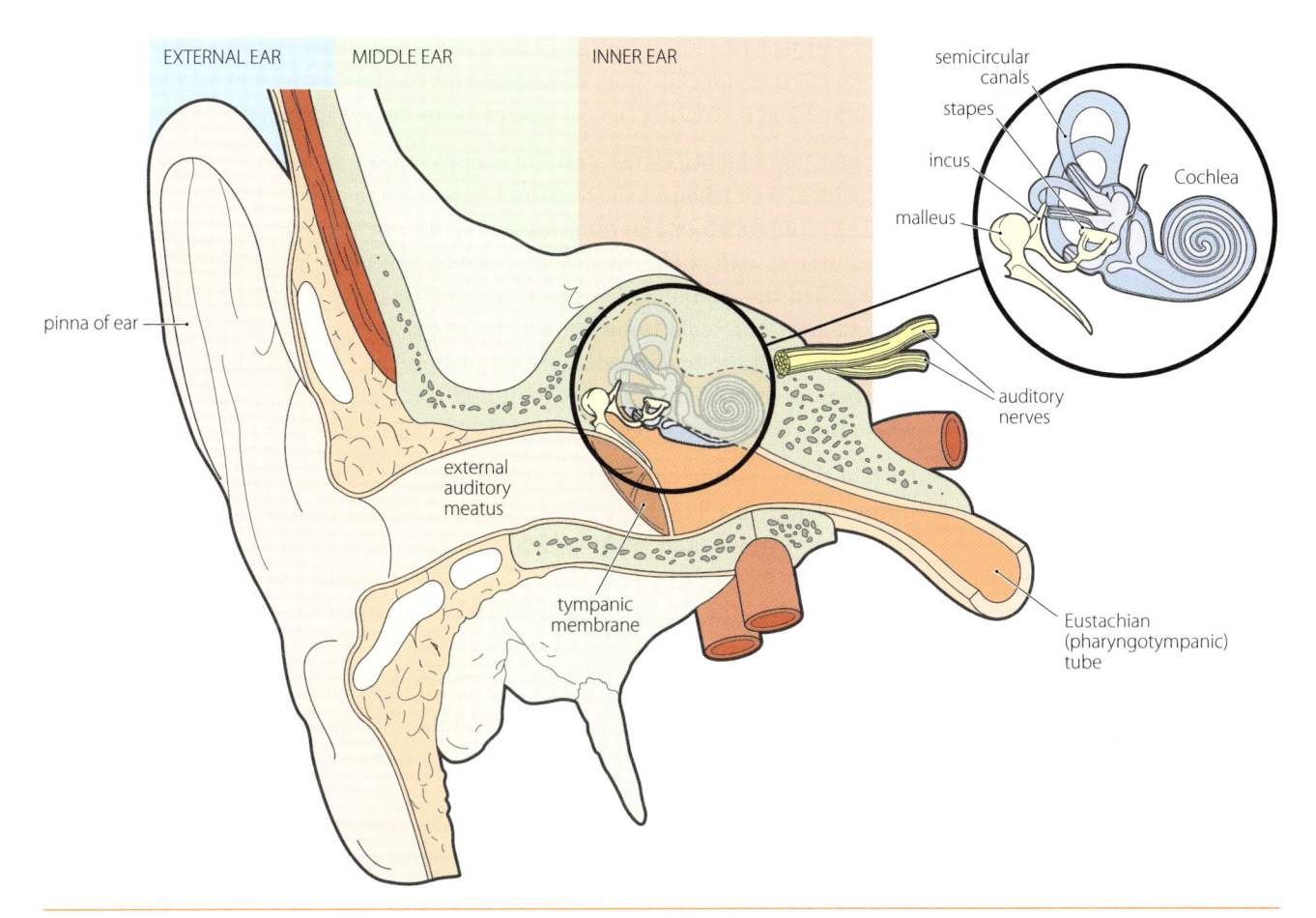

Figure 6.14 – **The structure of the ear.**

are openings in the bony cavity – the oval window, the round window and the **Eustachian tube** (pharyngotympanic tube) (see *Figure 6.14*). This tube runs down to the nasopharynx, linking it with the middle ear, and is responsible for draining mucus produced by cells in the middle ear and for equalizing air pressure in the middle ear, particularly during times of sudden changes in air pressure. For example, when descending in an aeroplane, swallowing and chewing help to keep the tube open. It is not uncommon to have some slight hearing loss when suffering from a cold (an upper respiratory tract infection). This is often because the Eustachian tube becomes blocked due to swelling of the mucosa, leading to a build-up of fluid and air pressure, which impedes vibration of the tympanic membrane. In children, the tube is shorter, narrower and less vertical, increasing the risk of frequent middle ear infections (otitis media).

The middle ear is spanned by the smallest bones in the body (see *Chapter 13*) – the **ossicles**: the malleus (hammer), the incus (anvil) and the stapes (stirrup). The handle of the malleus is attached to the tympanic membrane and the stapes abuts the oval window. Via small synovial joints, the malleus articulates with the incus, which articulates with the stapes, collectively transferring the vibration of the tympanic membrane into vibration of the oval window. A way to remember the order of the ossicles is to think 'the hammer hits the anvil to make the stirrup'. Two very small skeletal muscles are associated with the ossicles and these help to protect the hearing receptor cells from damage during loud noises by tensing the tympanic membrane and restricting the movement of the stapes against the oval window.

The inner ear comprises the vestibular apparatus, concerned with balance, and the cochlea, which houses the hearing receptors, in a structure called the **organ of Corti**. As illustrated in *Figures 6.15a* and *b*, the cochlea is a spiral, bony chamber shaped like a snail shell, composed of three chambers that spiral around a bony pillar called the modiolus. The chambers are the scala vestibule, which abuts the oval window, the scala tympani, which ends at the round window, and a middle chamber called the scala media (also known as the cochlear duct), which houses the organ of Corti. The scala vestibuli and the scala tympani merge at the apex where they connect at a region called the **helicotrema**.

Each of the spiralling chambers is fluid filled. The scala media has a membranous lining filled with a fluid known as endolymph, produced by cells in the membrane. The scala vestibuli and scala tympani contain perilymph, which has a similar composition to cerebrospinal fluid. The floor of the cochlear duct is a flexible structure called the **basilar membrane**, which supports the organ of Corti.

Physiology of hearing

Hearing occurs when the primary auditory cortex in the temporal lobe is stimulated. In the initial stage of hearing, sound waves are conducted down the external auditory meatus, causing the tympanic membrane to vibrate at the same frequency as the sound waves. The greater the amplitude of the sound waves, the greater the displacement of the tympanic membrane. The pressure change against the tympanic membrane is transmitted through the middle ear by articulation of the ossicles, leading to movement of the oval window by the stapes. The action of the ossicles amplifies the motion of the tympanic membrane because the tympanic membrane is much bigger than the oval window and so the pressure exerted on the oval window is about 20 times greater than that exerted on the tympanic membrane. This greater pressure overcomes the resistance in the fluid (perilymph) in the scala vestibuli of the cochlea to the transmission of the pressure wave.

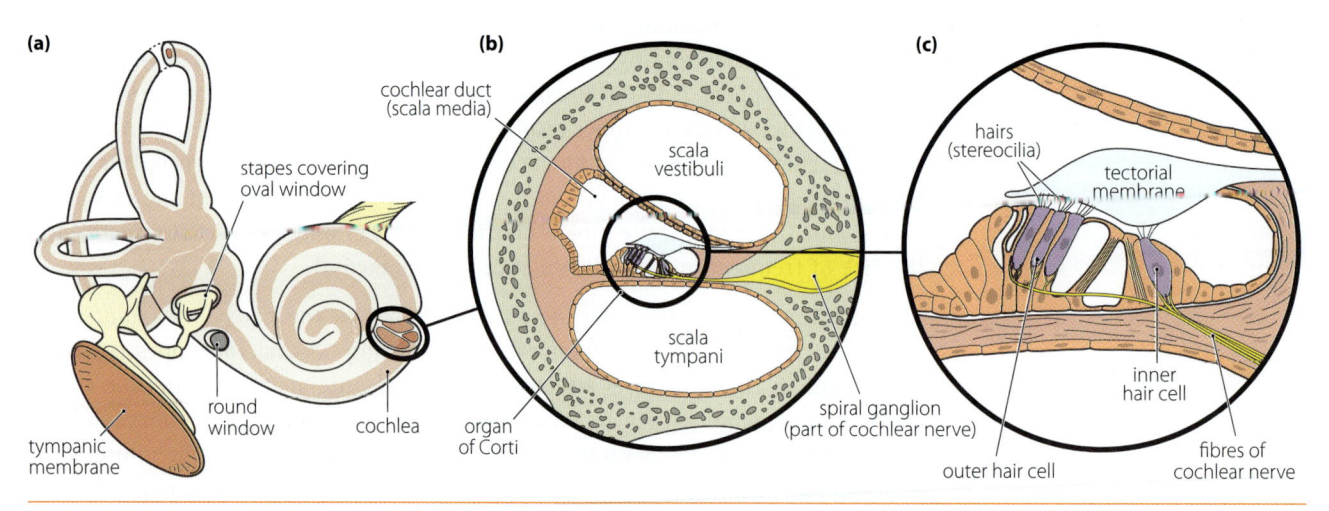

Figure 6.15 – (a) The cochlea, (b) a cross-section of the cochlea and (c) the organ of Corti.

The vibration of the oval window, induced by the motion of the stapes, creates pressure waves through the perilymph from the basal end of the scala vestibuli towards the helicotrema, distorting the basilar membrane at different locations depending on the frequency of the pressure wave. Close to the beginning of the cochlear duct, the basilar membrane is narrow and under tension at its base, and responds best to high-frequency sounds. Towards the helicotrema, at the apex, the basilar membrane becomes wider and under less tension and is therefore adapted to respond to lower-frequency sounds.

The movement of the basilar membrane excites the receptor cells of the organ of Corti. The organ of Corti is located on top of the basilar membrane and comprises supporting cells and cochlear hair cells (receptor cells) (see *Figure 6.15c*). The hair cells typically are arranged as a single row of inner cells and three rows of outer hair cells. Each hair cell has numerous hair-like structures called **stereocilia** that protrude into the endolymph, with the longest stereocilia embedded in an overlying gel-like membrane called the **tectorial membrane**. Sensory fibres from the cochlear nerve (a division of the vestibulocochlear nerve – cranial nerve VIII) are coiled around the base of the hair cells. Localized movement of the basilar membrane, due to the pressure wave in the endolymph, bends the stereocilia (see *Figure 6.16*). Displacement of the stereocilia causes the neurone at the base of the hair cells to generate an action potential that is conducted along the afferent cochlear nerve, which forms part of the vestibulocochlear nerve, to the auditory cortex located in the temporal lobe of the cerebrum for interpretation of the sound. In this way, the hair cells in connection with the basilar membrane transduce mechanical events into neural information. Many factors can influence the transmission of sound waves from the external environment to their eventual transduction and perception as hearing (summarized in *Box 6.3*).

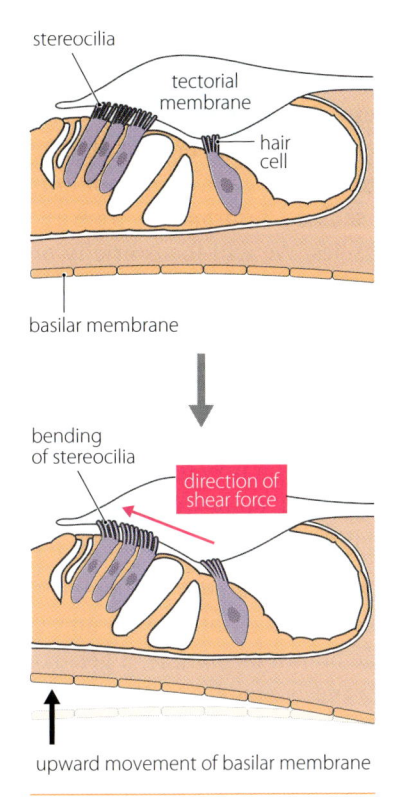

Figure 6.16 – The organ of Corti: excitation of hair cells.

Mechanisms of hearing loss and tinnitus

The mechanisms associated with hearing loss are complex, but essentially hearing loss can arise from a problem with how sound is conducted to the inner ear via the outer and middle ear (conductive hearing loss) and, more commonly, from problems located within the structures of the cochlea (sensorineural hearing loss). There are a number of causes of sensorineural hearing loss, including age-related changes to sensory cells (**presbycusis**), certain types of drugs (e.g. some types of chemotherapy used to treat cancer, or specific antibiotics) and exposure to loud noises.

Persistent exposure to loud noises causes metabolic fatigue and death of cochlear hair cells. Mutations in genes required for the development of hair cells are associated with childhood congenital deafness and age-related hearing loss.

Tinnitus is the perception of noise in the ears without any external auditory stimulus and is often a subjective phenomenon, making it difficult to measure using objective audiological tests. It is often described as a ringing noise, buzzing or high-pitched whining. Tinnitus is caused by a number of factors, the most common of which is noise-induced hearing loss. Various theories have been proposed to explain the cause of tinnitus and most converge on alterations in the processing of neural stimuli in the ear and central nervous system.

BOX 6.3

The vestibular system and the physiology of balance

The vestibular system in the inner ear responds to changes in movement of the head, sending motor signals that stimulate head and eye movements to provide the retina with a stable visual image and to cause adjustments in muscle tone for the maintenance of posture and balance. Maintaining balance involves not only information from the vestibular system but also sensory information from the eyes and proprioceptive receptors in joints and muscles. We will focus briefly on the vestibular system in the inner ear.

The vestibular apparatus

Sensory receptors, located in the semicircular canals and vestibule, respond to changes in head position and are collectively called the vestibular apparatus. The semicircular canals and the vestibule, composed of the utricle and saccule, are illustrated in *Figure 6.17*. Semicircular canals are rigid, bony structures lined with a membranous labyrinth and contain endolymph.

Sensory receptors called maculae detect linear acceleration (changes in movement of the head in a straight line). Each macula, one located in the wall of each utricle and saccule, contains hair cells that project into the otolith membrane, a gel-like mass (see *Figure 6.18a* and *b*). The otilith membrane is studded with calcium carbonate crystals called otoliths. When the head starts or stops moving, the otolith membrane slides forwards or backwards, bending the hair cells, producing sensory nerve impulses that are conducted to the brain via the vestibular nerve (a branch of the vestibulocochlear nerve – cranial nerve VIII).

Rotational movement of the head is detected by a specialized sensory receptor called the crista ampullaris located in the ampulla of each semicircular canal. Each crista is composed of individual hair cells (similar to the hair cells in the

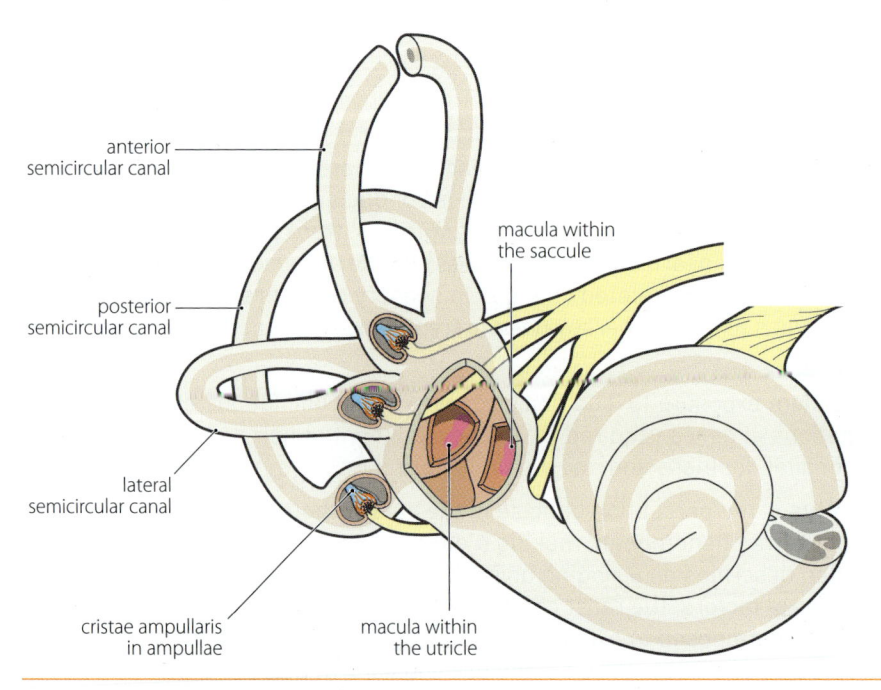

Figure 6.17 – **The vestibular apparatus.**

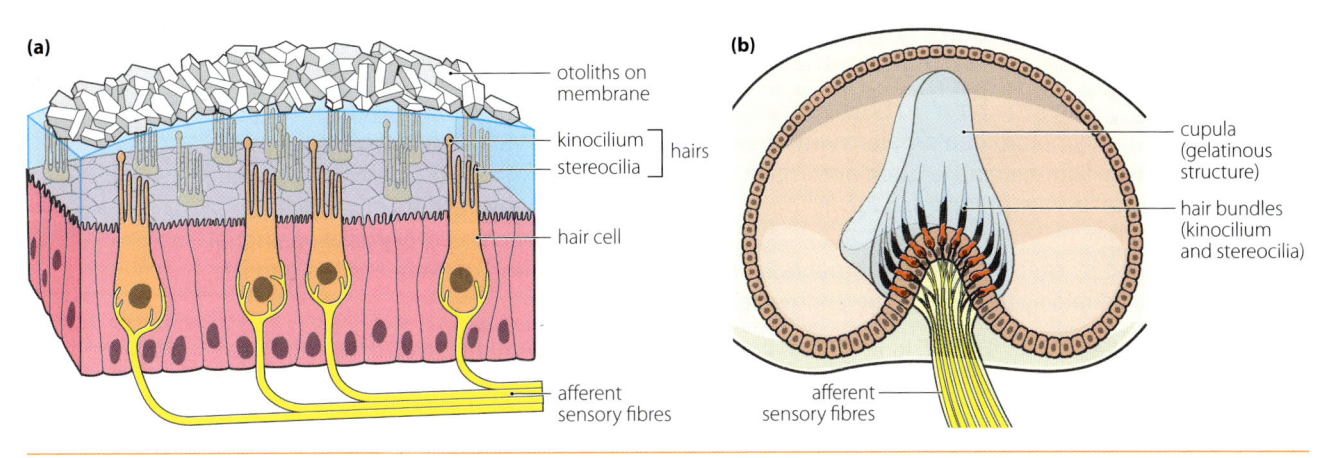

Figure 6.18 – The structure of (a) the macula and otolith membrane, (b) a hair cell and (c) the crista ampullaris.

organ of Corti and the maculae), each with stereocilia and a single kinocilium (a special type of cilium) embedded in a gelled mass called the cupula (see *Figure 6.18c*). When the head rotates in the plane of the semicircular duct, the movement of the endolymph along the length of the duct pushes the crista to one side. Movement of the crista bends the stereocilia. Bending of the stereocilia towards the kinocilium produces an action potential in the hair cell. Movement of the endolymph in the opposite direction, so that the stereocilia bend away from the kinocilium, inhibits the production of an action potential. The cristae in each semicircular duct operate in a complementary way. Depending on the rotational movement of the head and the sudden movement of the endolymph, hair cells in the crista of one semicircular duct will be stimulated, while in another crista the hair cells will not be activated. The positioning of the semicircular canals and ducts is therefore important for determining the position and movement of the head and in achieving equilibrium. Even complex movement can be reduced to three rotational planes. For example, a horizontal motion, as in shaking the head to say no, stimulates the hair cells in the lateral semicircular ducts. Nodding the head stimulates hair cells in the anterior semicircular duct, while tilting the head from side to side excites receptors in the posterior semicircular duct. Sensory impulses from the sensory receptors in the semicircular ducts and vestibule are conducted via the vestibular branch of the vestibulocochlear nerve to the brainstem and cerebellum for processing.

Balance problems and dizziness can be caused by a number of factors, including age, a sudden fall in blood pressure (e.g. postural hypotension) and heart rhythm disturbances, as well as vestibular problems (see *Box 6.4*); falls due to balance problems present a significant health burden.

6.2.5 Touch

Touch receptors are classified as mechanoreceptors. The sensory endings of touch receptors may be free or encapsulated. Touch receptors include the following:

> **BOX 6.4**
>
> **Vestibular problems affecting balance**
>
> **Vertigo** is the feeling you have that the environment, for example a room, is moving or is spinning and is a classic symptom of a problem with the vestibular system. Vertigo is different to feeling light-headed or fainting, and is often accompanied by nausea and vomiting. There are a number of causes of vertigo including infection in the inner ear leading to **labyrinthitis** or reduced blood flow to the inner ear. However, the most common cause is 'benign paroxysmal positional vertigo' caused by specific head movements, due to dislodged otoliths that are carried into the semicircular canals by the flow of the endolymph.
>
> **Ménière's disease** is a disorder of the inner ear affecting hearing and balance. The symptoms vary but typically include rotational vertigo, tinnitus, hearing loss and a feeling of pressure in one or both ears. Attacks are characterized by periods of remission and exacerbation. Ménière's disease is associated with excess endolymph in the membranous labyrinths of the cochlea and vestibular system.

- **Merkel's discs** – these are free nerve endings in contact with cells in the epidermis of the skin.
- **Meissner's corpuscles** – these are located deep within the dermis of the skin and are egg-shaped structures in which nerve endings are encapsulated.
- **Pacinian (lamellar) corpuscles** – these encapsulated receptors are oval structures in the dermis that are sensitive to on and off pressure stimuli. Pacinian corpuscles are also located in the deep subcutaneous tissue, in submucosal tissue, in tissue around joints and in mammary glands.

The sensation of an itch (pruritus) arises from stimulation of itch receptors, located superficially within the basal layer of the epidermis of the skin. They respond to the same range of chemicals (histamine and non-histamine) that are also involved in the perception of pain when noxious chemicals stimulate **nociceptors**.

Nociceptors and the perception of pain

The International Association for the Study of Pain describes pain as 'an unpleasant sensory and emotional experience associated with actual or potential tissue damage, or described in terms of such damage'. The perception of pain is complex and subjective, and is influenced by social and cultural factors, mood and belief systems, as well as neurophysiology. Pain is an unpleasant sensory and emotional phenomenon that can have a significant impact on a person's quality of life, psychological wellbeing, social interactions and economic status. The perception of pain offers protective functions and, in part, limits ongoing damage that may be associated with the sensation of pain. The experience of pain can be categorized as acute or chronic (when the sensation of pain lasts more than 6 months). Acute pain evoked by brief noxious stimuli and the associated sensory transmission is generally well understood, but this is not the case with chronic pain syndromes, which remain to some extent a mystery. This section is not aimed at discussing the perception and management of pain but simply highlights nociception as a major part of sensory function.

The perception of pain starts with the stimulation of **nociceptors**, which are relatively unspecialized nerve endings that respond to various stimuli (chemical, thermal and mechanical). Some nociceptors respond to only one type of noxious stimuli, such as chemical (e.g. histamine, bradykinin and prostaglandins released by damaged cells), while others are polymodal, responding to more than one stimulus. Nociceptors are nerve endings of particular afferent fibres. Nociceptors associated with the perception of sharp pain are connected to small-diameter myelinated A-delta (δ) sensory fibres, which conduct sensory impulses rapidly (5–25 m/second). The perception of an ache, and with that the feeling of nausea, is associated with nociceptors located at the distal end of smaller, unmyelinated C fibres that conduct sensory impulses relatively more slowly at 0.5–2.0 m/second. Nociceptors attached to the fast Aδ fibres are located in the skin and mucous membranes, whereas the C fibre nociceptors are found throughout the skin and body tissues, excluding brain tissue.

Afferent impulses from stimulated nociceptors are conducted to the spinal cord and then travel up the spinal cord to the brain, for example via the major ascending pathway called the spinothalamic tract (see *Chapter 4*). The relay of sensory information and interpretation of the sensory impulses involves various regions in the central nervous system including the brainstem, thalamus and higher centres of the primary sensory cortex of the parietal lobe of the brain.

The transmission of sensory impulses from nociceptors and the perception of pain can be modulated in a number of ways, such as the secretion of naturally occurring opioids (**endorphins**), and through the release of inhibitory neurotransmitters at synapses within the spinal cord as a result of descending influences from the brain. Pain is a subjective experience and therefore difficult to define simply in objective terms. This has given rise to a number of theories of pain perception, the most accepted being the neuromatrix theory of pain, which proposes that pain is a multidimensional experience produced by characteristic patterns of nerve impulses generated by a widely distributed neural network and that transmission of sensory impulses via ascending pathways in the spinal cord is modulated by a gating mechanism in the dorsal horn. Synapses that occur between neurones function as gates. Sensory impulses are transmitted to the brain when the gate is open and are inhibited when the gate is closed. Excitatory neurotransmitters are released at the synapse to 'open the gate' and inhibitory neurotransmitters 'close the gate', preventing the transmission of sensory impulses to the brain and thus the perception of pain. Aβ afferent fibres, when stimulated, release inhibitory neurotransmitters in the spinal cord and can be activated by massage, acupuncture and the use of transcutaneous electrical nerve stimulation (TENS). These techniques are utilized in healthcare to help alleviate pain.

6.3 Clinical application

The special senses and the ability for us to perceive the world are important for responding to others and our environment. Impairment of our senses can leave us exposed to risk, which may result in significant health problems. The cases in this chapter highlight some of the challenges that can occur when one or more of the special senses are impaired.

- **Sally (Patient 6.1)** suffers with multiple sclerosis, a progressive neurological condition affecting sensory and motor function. As a consequence, Sally experienced a number of altered sensations around her body and developed problems with her vision.
- **Sadia (Patient 6.2)** demonstrates how a relatively simple surgical procedure such as cataract removal can make a remarkable improvement to her quality of life, enabling Sadia to retain her independence.
- **Denzel (Patient 6.3)** illustrates some of the problems individuals can experience following exposure to loud noise over time, inducing hearing loss and tinnitus, which can affect the quality of life and awareness of hazards.

Patient 6.1 — Sally | 167 | **188** | 404 | 443

- 50-year-old woman
- Has MS and is now a wheelchair user
- Burning sensation in her hands and double vision
- MRI confirms plaques in her brain consistent with MS

Sally presented to her family doctor with a series of non-specific neurological symptoms that collectively suggested a diagnosis of multiple sclerosis (MS). Sally experienced a burning feeling in her hands, double vision and an inability to focus. Double vision (diplopia) is a common symptom associated with MS due to poor coordination between the eye muscles as a result of impaired nerve conduction to one or more of the eye muscles. Patients sometimes report abnormal sensations including 'pins and needles', stabbing pains, pruritus, burning and numbness (paraesthesia), all of which suggest disordered sensory function. The signs and symptoms are often intermittent and non-specific, making MS difficult to diagnose, especially in the earliest stages of the disease. Sally underwent magnetic resonance imaging (MRI) of the brain, and this demonstrated the presence of lesions called plaques in the white matter of her central nervous system (see *Chapters 4* and *13*), consistent with MS.

Patient 6.2 — Sadia | 167 | **188**

- 82-year-old woman
- Mildly hypertensive – on bendroflumethiazide and felodipine
- Eye tests reveal cataracts but no glaucoma
- Cataract operations on both eyes leave her moving more safely

Over a period of one year, Sadia had successful cataract operations on each eye. On both occasions, the operation and Sadia's recovery were uneventful. Removal of the cataracts and insertion of new intraocular lenses, with appropriate changes in her prescription for her reading glasses, have dramatically improved Sadia's quality of life. With the restoration of her vision, Sadia has a new confidence when walking, shopping and undertaking daily activities. She is more positive in her mood and is once more enjoying reading and knitting, activities that enhance the quality of her life. Importantly, her improved vision also enhances her safety, as she is able to detect and avoid hazards and is less likely to stumble and fracture her hip.

Patient 6.3 — Denzel

- 50-year-old man
- High-pitched ringing in ears for many years
- Conversation now difficult with background noise
- Family doctor refers him to audiologist
- Hearing loss is confirmed
- Loss is at high frequency so hearing aid not required

Following band gigs over a number of years, Denzel experienced ringing in his ears and some hearing loss. Denzel is able to identify key moments when he felt the damaging effects of loud noise while playing in the band. Denzel wore ear plugs for monitoring purposes and not as ear protection. At points when the music was very loud, he experienced sudden discomfort in his ears and felt the room spin. Unfortunately, over the years Denzel did not wear ear defenders developed for musicians when playing in the band and has consequently developed symptoms associated with acoustic trauma – tinnitus (persistent ringing and hissing in the ears) and hearing loss. Fortunately, Denzel is able to cope with the tinnitus and has not needed specific therapy such as counselling and sound therapy. Denzel underwent an audiogram, and a similar audiogram to Denzel's, associated with acoustic trauma, is illustrated in *Figure 6.19*. The circles and crosses on the audiogram indicate the intensity level at which the person just starts to hear a sound at different frequencies (Hz), represented as the hearing level in decibels (dB HL). If a person can only just hear the sound at 20 dB HL or higher, he or she is judged to have a hearing impairment. The audiogram illustrates that hearing loss increases progressively as the higher frequencies are tested. For example, at 3000 Hz the hearing level for the right ear is 40 dB HL, which is at a level regarded as abnormal. In Denzel's case, his hearing loss was most noticeable at 3000 Hz and above. With a hearing loss at high frequencies, a hearing aid is not always required. Denzel is able to hear others talk in most conversations, he can engage fully in work and social interactions, and he is not at risk, for example by not hearing traffic approach, so he does not require a hearing aid.

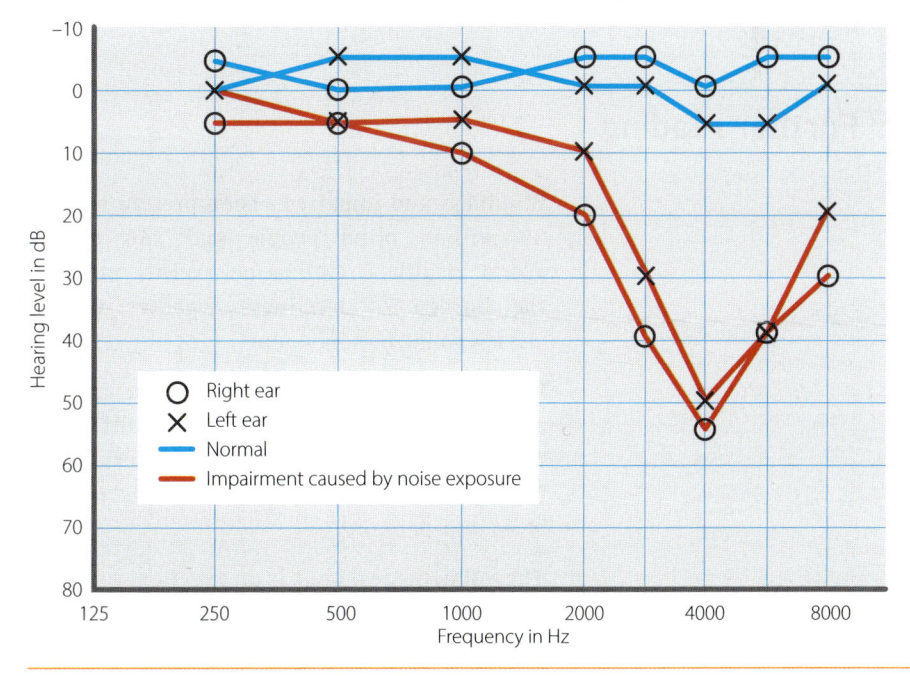

Figure 6.19 – Audiogram demonstrating the effects of noise exposure, showing the results of a normal hearing test and an impaired-hearing test.

6.4 Summary

- Sensation refers to the immediate, unprocessed stimulation of sensory receptors, and perception describes the interpretation of the world through the processing of sensory information. Both are essential for responding to the environment to ensure survival.
- Vision involves the processing of stimuli from light-sensitive receptors (rods and cones) contained in the retina of the eye (see *Figure 6.8*).
- Taste and smell result from stimulation of chemoreceptors primarily on the tongue (taste) and nasal cavities (smell) (see *Figures 6.10, 6.11* and *6.12*).
- Hearing involves the conduction of pressure waves through the external, middle and inner ear, resulting in the displacement of the hair cells of the organ of Corti (see *Figure 6.16*) and the production of action potentials, which are conducted via the acoustic nerve to the temporal lobe of the brain.
- Balance is maintained through the integration within the central nervous system of complex sensory information involving stimulation of sensory receptors located in the vestibular apparatus of the inner ear caused by changes in the position of the head, initiating motor responses to maintain balance (see *Figure 6.17*).
- Touch involves the activation of specialized mechanoreceptors located throughout the body such as in the skin, subcutaneous tissue and joints.
- The perception of pain commences with the stimulation of nociceptors, which respond to various noxious stimuli. Nociceptors may either be specific for one chemical or polymodal, whereby they respond to a variety of stimuli (chemical, thermal and mechanical).

6.5 Further reading

Blindness and impaired vision present a huge global burden with approximately 39 million blind people and 246 million people with low vision. The World Health Organization (WHO) provides a useful resource highlighting the burden of blindness together with strategies to prevent blindness: www.who.int/blindness/en/

Understanding the cause, assessment and management of pain is an important aspect of healthcare but pain can be difficult to describe and sometimes difficult to manage. The web pages for the International Association for the Study of Pain (IASP) contain a wealth of valuable resources to guide health professionals: www.iasp-pain.org/

The following textbook is an excellent reference source, covering a comprehensive range of topics, including basic aspects, clinical states, therapeutic aspects, neurophysiology, psychology and the measurement of a variety of pain syndromes: McMahon, S.B., Koltzenburg, M., Tracey, I. and Turk, D. (2013) *Wall and Melzack's Textbook of Pain*. 6th edn. Elsevier Churchill Livingstone, Philadelphia, USA.

6.6 Self-assessment questions

Answers can be found at www.scionpublishing.com/AandP

(6.1) Select the one correct response. Conduction of sound from the middle ear to the inner ear involves the movement of:
(a) the malleus against the oval window
(b) the incus against the tympanic membrane
(c) hair cells in the organ of Corti
(d) air along the external auditory canal
(e) the stapes against the oval window

(6.2) Select the one correct answer. The impairment of drainage of aqueous humour can result in which one of the following conditions?
(a) Conduction deafness
(b) Glaucoma
(c) Colour blindness
(d) Cataracts
(e) Compaction of wax in the external auditory canal

(6.3) Select the one correct response. The perception of smell occurs in the olfactory cortex in the:
(a) occipital lobe
(b) frontal and temporal lobe
(c) insula
(d) parietal lobe
(e) brainstem

(6.4) Select the one correct response. Polymodal nociceptors are stimulated by:
(a) light rays
(b) only chemical stimuli
(c) fluid waves
(d) only thermal changes
(e) noxious chemical, thermal and mechanical stimuli

(6.5) Identify the type of receptor involved in each sensory activity by indicating the appropriate letter from the key (each receptor type may be used once, more than once, or not at all).

Sensory activity	*Receptor type key*
(i) You have just scalded yourself with hot water	A. Chemoreceptor
(ii) You feel uncomfortable after a very large meal	B. Photoreceptor
(iii) You have bumped your arm and it is sore	C. Nociceptor
(iv) You enjoy the smell of newly cut grass	D. Thermoreceptor
(v) You react quickly to the glare of bright sunlight	E. Mechanoreceptor

(6.6) Outline how rods are involved in the adjustment from light to dark environments.

(6.7) Outline why it is good to check for compacted ear wax if a person starts to complain of hearing loss.

CHAPTER 07 | Why food is needed: the chemical basis of health

Learning points for this chapter

After working through this chapter, you should be able to:

- Name and describe the different food components necessary for health
- Describe the structures that form the digestive (gastrointestinal) system
- Describe how food is digested
- Describe how end products of digestion are absorbed
- Describe metabolism and how cells use end products of digestion to maintain health
- Describe the importance of monitoring food intake

7.1 Introduction and clinical relevance

Food plays an important role in our lives:

- Social – as shown by group eating.
- Cultural – as shown by the value put on certain food items.
- Psychological – in terms of the wellbeing experienced.
- Physiological – by meeting the needs of the body for nutrients.
- Biochemical – through its participation in metabolic pathways.
- Immunological – by providing nutrients that contribute to protecting the body.

Knowledge of nutrition is essential in gaining an understanding of the role of nutrition in physiology, health and wellbeing. It is necessary to explore how the food that is consumed is used to sustain life and maintain health. Food provides the chemical resources and the energy that the body needs to function. It is important to have a knowledge and understanding of the nutritional basis of health and the metabolic processes involved in utilizing food. Insufficient food is sometimes associated with feelings of nausea and light-headedness. An unbalanced diet, in terms of both intake and proportions, results in malnutrition leading to a poor state of health, while the inability to digest food, absorb and metabolize it interferes with homeodynamic processes. Each of the patient cases discussed in this chapter emphasizes the importance of adequate nutrition and good dietary intake, and indicates how diseases of the gastrointestinal tract can compromise nutritional status and cause malnutrition.

Patient 1.1 — Amy | 1 | 20 | **194** | 235 | 447 | 473

- 18-year-old woman
- BMI 16.3
- Downy hair on face and arms
- Referred to eating disorder clinic
- Eating under supervision to increase intake and also getting psychological support
- Also anaemic

Amy, who is 18 years old and attends a further education college, has lost body weight, looks emaciated and has developed lanugo-like hair on her arms and legs, and she had a body mass index (BMI) of 16.3 kg/m² when she was admitted to hospital. Amy's low BMI was due to fear of gaining body weight and food restriction as a result of her distorted body image. During assessment at the hospital by a nurse specialist, Amy admitted to purging behaviour by self-induced vomiting and to misuse of laxatives after meals she ate at home. When Amy looked in the mirror, she thought she looked larger than she really was (dysmorphia) and she thought she was heavier than she really was. A protocol to manage Amy was agreed, which included Amy eating under strict supervision with the aim of increasing her energy and protein intake slowly, together with vitamin and mineral supplements. Amy received psychological support from a clinical psychologist to help her change her view and perception of food. Amy was encouraged to eat foods she liked and to take liquid supplements. Amy was supervised by clinical staff for 1 hour after eating a meal or drinking a supplement to stop her from purging. Further assessment while in hospital indicated that her levels of growth hormone and cortisol were higher than normal. She was anaemic and hypotensive (see *Chapter 9*). When her body weight returned to normal, she was discharged from hospital and now regularly attends an eating-disorder unit as an outpatient, where she continues to receive monitoring, counselling and support.

Patient 1.3 — Francine | 2 | 21 | **194** | 235 | 338 | 371

- 40-year-old woman
- Crohn's disease – on steroids
- Presents with inflamed bowel and anaemia
- MRSA screen ahead of potential surgery

Francine is a 40-year-old lady who works as a financial management executive and has Crohn's disease, an inflammatory bowel condition. Years ago, Francine noticed that when she ate bread, oatmeal and creamed soups she experienced dyspepsia and abdominal pain with some distension, and her visits to the toilet to open her bowels increased. Her other symptoms included pale and foamy stools, diarrhoea (sometimes with blood) and occasional nausea and vomiting. She has had periods of relapses and remissions over the years, but she has learned to live with her condition by avoiding eating certain foods that she knows trigger her condition, such as spicy foods, milk and caffeine. She has been treated with steroid medication that included prednisolone and budesonide, and antibiotics such as metronidazole and ciprofloxacin, as well as nutritional supplements during relapses. Recently, her condition has become worse and she has been admitted to hospital with diarrhoea, blood in her stools, fatigue, pallor and weight loss. It is envisaged that Francine might require surgery as her family doctor has been unable to control her symptoms. Her current BMI is 21 kg/m² and her blood test results show that she is anaemic. As a new admission and candidate for potential surgery, Francine is screened to see if she is colonized with meticillin-resistant *Staphylococcus aureus* (MRSA).

Patient 3.1 — Sarah — 60 | 94 | **195** | 237 | 311 | 333

- 17-year-old girl
- CF diagnosis at age of 1 year via a sweat test
- Frequent admissions for chest infections affecting breathing
- PERT added to meals to help digest her food

Sarah, who is now 17 years old, was diagnosed at the age of 1 year with cystic fibrosis. Ryan and Sophie, Sarah's parents, noticed that she had problems eating her food as she often had no appetite to eat. They also noticed that when she did eat, she was unable to digest the food properly, indicated by her stools being greasy, pale or clay-coloured with an offensive smell – a symptom known as steatorrhoea. Sarah's parents also noticed that she had problems with breathing, with a productive cough of thick purulent mucus, and that her nostrils always appeared to be blocked. A sweat test showed that she had high concentrations of chloride in her sweat with levels of up to 65 millimoles/L confirming a diagnosis of cystic fibrosis. Sarah has learned to live with her condition and she takes all her meals and snacks supplemented with pancreatin enzyme replacement therapy (PERT). PERT consists of enteric coated microspheres or capsules known as pancreatin (Creon). When Sarah eats a meal, she takes a capsule before, during and towards the end of a meal and she makes sure that she swallows the whole capsule without chewing it; the capsule needs to remain intact until it arrives in the duodenum where it releases the enzymes that digest the food she eats.

Patient 5.1 — David — 138 | 161 | **195** | 237 | 448 | 474

- 44-year-old man
- Increased urine output; thirsty and hungry
- Blood test: low thyroxine and raised blood glucose
- Has hypothyroidism and the start of a goitre
- Given levothyroxine; dose adjusted until thyroxine levels stabilise
- Has diabetes associated with obesity – diet modified and given metformin

David is a 44-year-old manager of a very successful restaurant with a BMI of 35.92 kg/m^2. David is a very sociable person, and when diners come to his restaurant, he is very welcoming and excellent at making them feel at ease. Recently, David noticed that he was passing a lot of urine and was becoming more thirsty and feeling more hungry, which meant that he ate more food. Despite eating more food, David noticed that he was feeling more lethargic. When David visited his family doctor, blood samples were taken for a full blood count and tests were taken for liver and thyroid function and for random and fasting blood glucose. The results showed that David has an underactive thyroid gland, and both his random glucose and fasting blood glucose levels are high.

The cases of each of the patients discussed in this chapter illustrate how the inability of the body to utilize food can affect homeodynamics and lead to numerous health problems. Amy (Patient 1.1) is emaciated with a low BMI of 16.3 kg/m^2 due to inadequate nutrition and dietary intake, made worse by purging behaviour that includes self-induced vomiting and misuse of laxatives. Psychologically, Amy thinks she is heavier than she really is when she looks in the mirror, even though this is not the case. The symptoms of dyspepsia, abdominal pain and distension experienced by Francine (Patient 1.3) were associated with her body's reaction to the foods in her diet. Her symptoms were managed with steroid and antibiotic therapy. Although Sarah (Patient 3.1) was diagnosed at the age of 1 year with cystic fibrosis, she has learned to live with her condition by taking pancreatin capsules with her food whenever she eats, whether this is a main meal or a snack. David (Patient 5.1) noticed the symptoms of feeling hungry, becoming thirsty, passing excessive amounts of urine and being lethargic later on in his middle

(a)

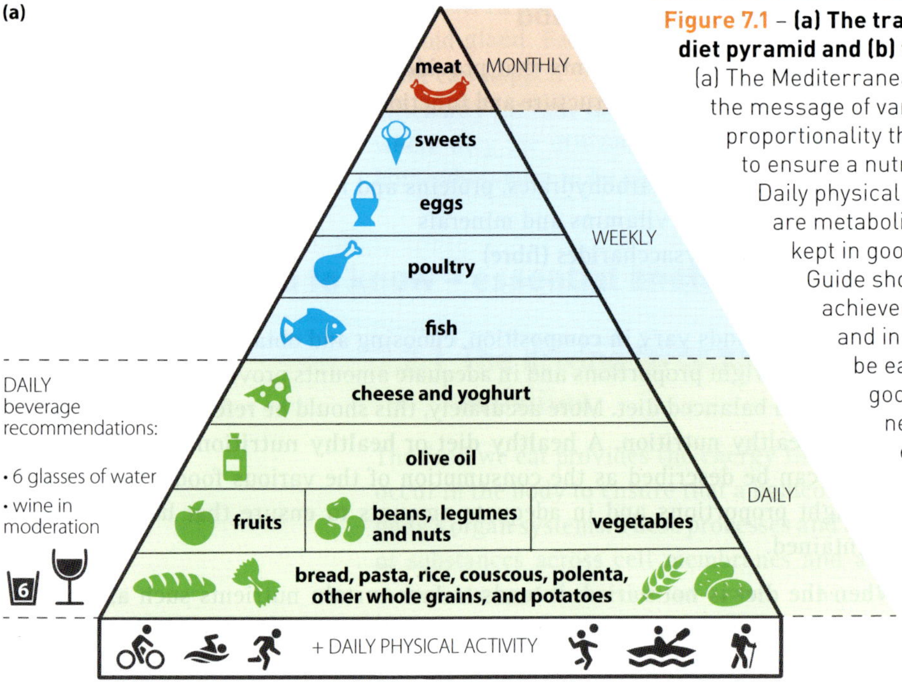
meat
MONTHLY
sweets
eggs
poultry
WEEKLY
fish
DAILY
beverage
recommendations:
• 6 glasses of water
• wine in
moderation
6
cheese and yoghurt
olive oil
DAILY
fruits
beans, legumes
and nuts
vegetables
bread, pasta, rice, couscous, polenta,
other whole grains, and potatoes
+ DAILY PHYSICAL ACTIVITY

(b)

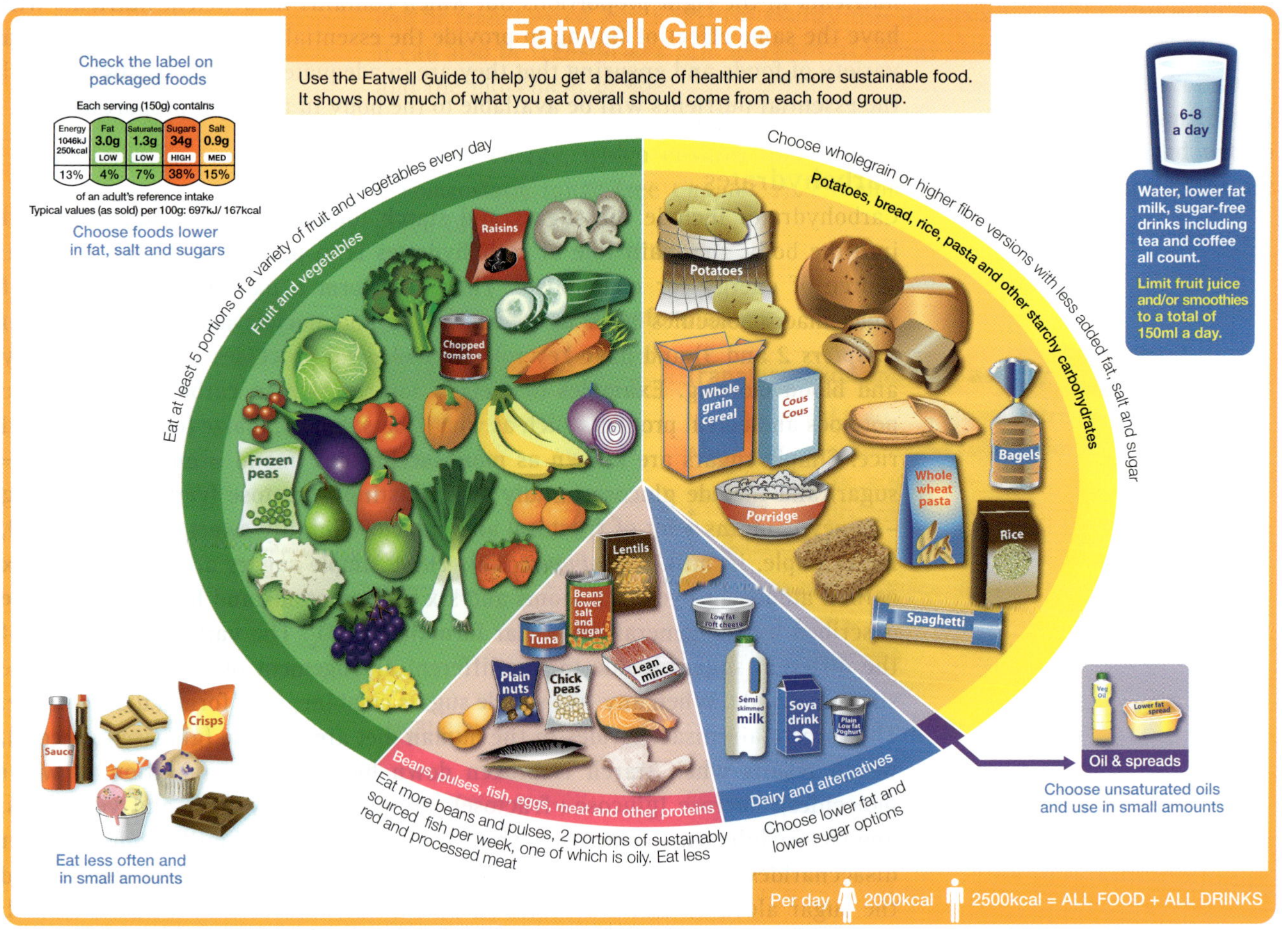
Eatwell Guide
Use the Eatwell Guide to help you get a balance of healthier and more sustainable food.
It shows how much of what you eat overall should come from each food group.
Check the label on
packaged foods
Each serving (150g) contains
Energy 1046kJ 250kcal 13%
Fat 3.0g LOW 4%
Saturates 1.3g LOW 7%
Sugars 34g HIGH 38%
Salt 0.9g MED 15%
of an adult's reference intake
Typical values (as sold) per 100g: 697kJ/ 167kcal
Choose foods lower
in fat, salt and sugars
Eat at least 5 portions of a variety of fruit and vegetables every day
Fruit and vegetables
Raisins
Chopped tomatoes
Frozen peas
Choose wholegrain or higher fibre versions with less added fat, salt and sugar
Potatoes, bread, rice, pasta and other starchy carbohydrates
Potatoes
Whole grain cereal
Cous Cous
Porridge
Bagels
Whole wheat pasta
Rice
Spaghetti
Lentils
Beans lower salt and sugar
Tuna
Plain nuts
Chick peas
Lean mince
Beans, pulses, fish, eggs, meat and other proteins
Eat more beans and pulses, 2 portions of sustainably sourced fish per week, one of which is oily. Eat less red and processed meat
Semi skimmed milk
Soya drink
Plain low fat yoghurt
Dairy and alternatives
Choose lower fat and lower sugar options
6-8 a day
Water, lower fat milk, sugar-free drinks including tea and coffee all count.
Limit fruit juice and/or smoothies to a total of 150ml a day.
Oil & spreads
Choose unsaturated oils and use in small amounts
Sauce
Crisps
Eat less often and
in small amounts
Per day 2000kcal 2500kcal = ALL FOOD + ALL DRINKS

Figure 7.1 – (a) The traditional healthy Mediterranean diet pyramid and (b) the Eatwell Guide.
(a) The Mediterranean diet pyramid demonstrates the message of variety, adequacy, moderation and proportionality that needs to be adhered to in order to ensure a nutritional balance of good health. Daily physical exercise ensures that nutrients are metabolized appropriately and organs are kept in good shape and healthy. (b)The Eatwell Guide shows how variety in one's diet can be achieved by eating different types of food and in what proportions these foods can be eaten in order to achieve a balance of good health. There are some foods that need to be eaten daily, while others can be eaten weekly and/or monthly with no adverse effect to health. Reproduced with permission from Public Health England in association with the Welsh government, the Scottish government and the Food Standards Agency in Northern Ireland.

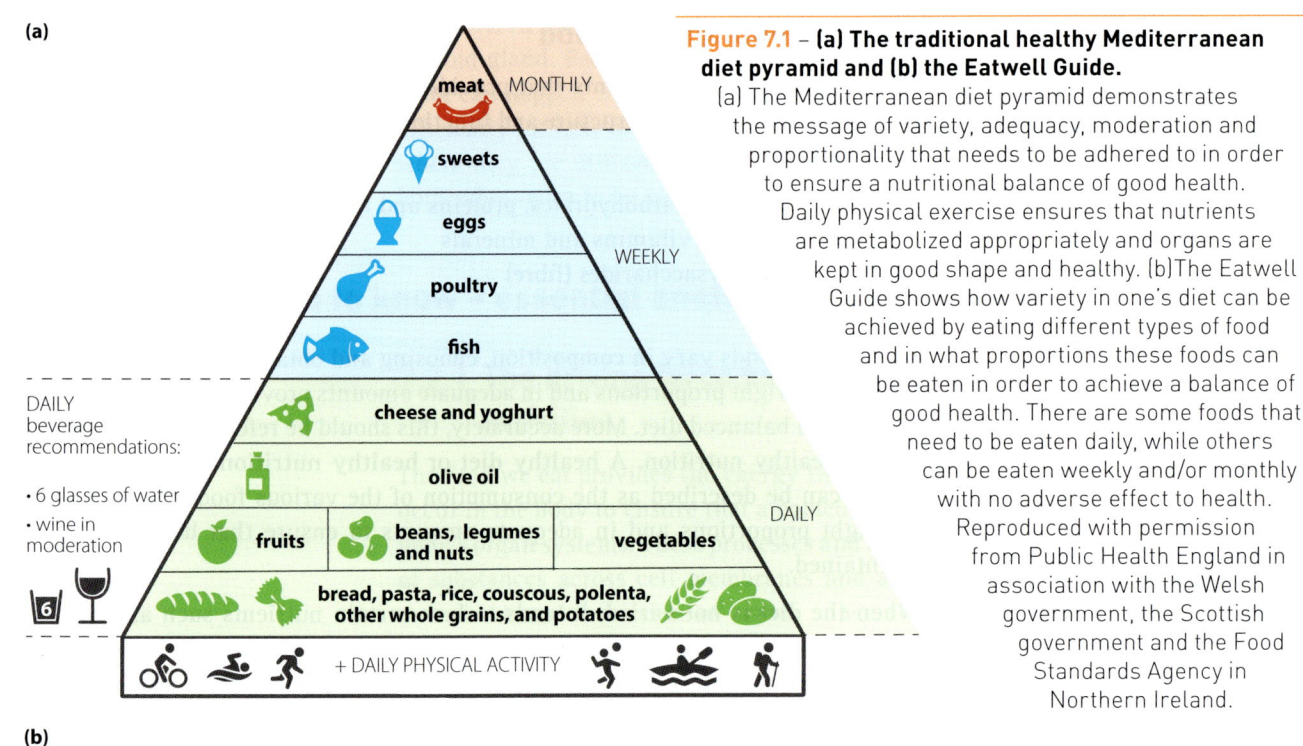

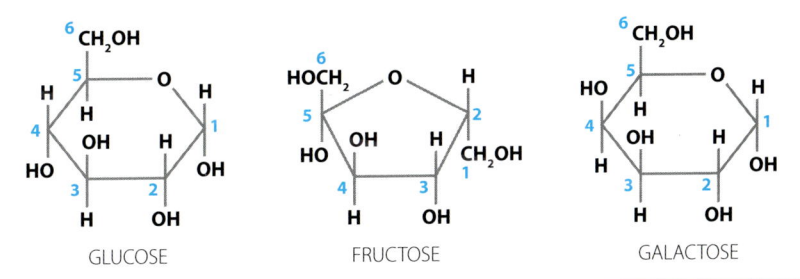

Figure 7.2 – Simple sugars and end products of carbohydrate digestion.
Simple sugars are known as monosaccharides and are found in carbohydrate foods. They have a backbone of between three and eight carbon atoms, with those containing five or six carbon atoms being the most common. The consumption of foods high in sugar is implicated in the increase in the obesity epidemic all over the world.

sorbitol and xylitol. Humans possess the specific enzyme trehalase, which enables the digestion of the disaccharide trehalose. Inositol is present in many foods including the bran of cereals, while isomalt, a derivative of sucrose, is found in baked products, ice creams and chewing gum. Lactitol is produced when the sugar component of the disaccharide lactose is reduced and is found in chocolate, ice cream and chewing gum. Sorbitol is found in some fruits such as cherries; it is a very stable sugar alcohol at high temperatures and is used as a sweetener during food manufacturing. Xylitol is found naturally in many fruits and vegetables; it is an approved food additive used as a sweetener in medicines such as throat lozenges and cough syrups, in toothpaste and mouthwashes, and in chewing gum.

Short-chain carbohydrates are a diverse group that include naturally occurring **oligosaccharides** such as raffinose, stachyose and verbascose found in beans, broccoli, Brussels sprouts, cabbage and peas, as well as fructans such as inulin found in asparagus, garlic and onions. The short-chain carbohydrates are not hydrolysed by digestive enzymes but can be fermented by bacteria in the large intestine to yield methane, carbon dioxide and hydrogen sulphide, a source of flatulence that is often experienced after consuming beans, a rich source of short-chain fatty acids.

Complex carbohydrates are formed when many monosaccharide units are linked together to form starch and fibres known as **polysaccharides**. Within the body, the simple sugar glucose is converted into a branched-chain polysaccharide called glycogen. Glycogen is structured in a way that allows more energy contained in the glucose molecule to be stored within cells (especially in liver and large muscle cells) and so represents a compact energy store. Starch and sugars are described as available carbohydrates because they can be digested quite easily in the human gastrointestinal tract, while non-starch polysaccharide (fibre) is not readily available because it is not digested easily; both are discussed later in this chapter.

Proteins
Proteins are made up of **amino acids** containing the elements carbon, hydrogen, oxygen and nitrogen. The synthesis of proteins from amino acids is determined by the genetic code (discussed in *Chapter 3*). There are 20 amino acids that

commonly occur in protein-rich foods (see *Table 7.2* and *Figure 7.3*). In adult humans, eight of the 20 amino acids are known as *essential amino acids*, whereas in children, nine amino acids are known by this term. In children, another amino acid, histidine, is essential because children are unable to synthesize this amino acid in sufficient amounts to meet the demand for greater rates of growth and

Non-polar amino acids

GLYCINE — Gly — G
ALANINE — Ala — A
VALINE — Val — V
LEUCINE — Leu — L
ISOLEUCINE — Ile — I — FULL NAME / Abbreviation / Single-letter code

Branched chain

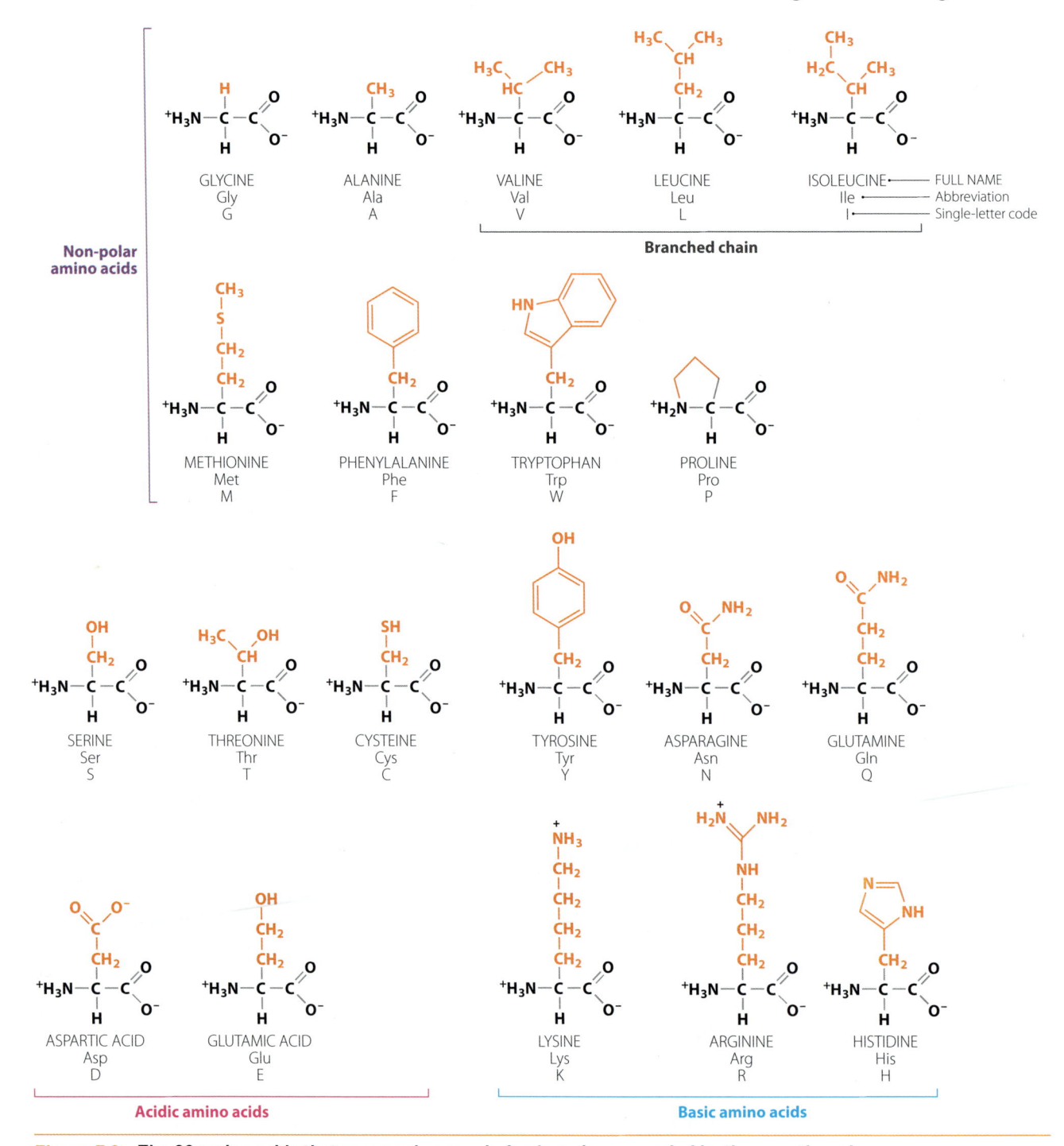

METHIONINE — Met — M
PHENYLALANINE — Phe — F
TRYPTOPHAN — Trp — W
PROLINE — Pro — P

SERINE — Ser — S
THREONINE — Thr — T
CYSTEINE — Cys — C
TYROSINE — Tyr — Y
ASPARAGINE — Asn — N
GLUTAMINE — Gln — Q

ASPARTIC ACID — Asp — D
GLUTAMIC ACID — Glu — E
LYSINE — Lys — K
ARGININE — Arg — R
HISTIDINE — His — H

Acidic amino acids

Basic amino acids

Figure 7.3 – **The 20 amino acids that commonly occur in foods and are encoded by the genetic code.**
When one of the essential amino acids is in small amounts in a protein, it is known as a limiting amino acid.

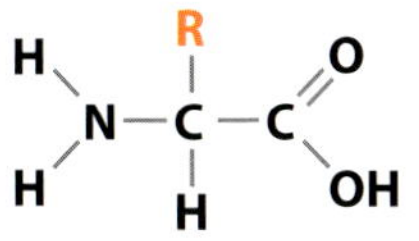

R = side chain

Figure 7.4 – The structure of an amino acid (un-ionized form). In the dipolar form of an amino acid, the amine group is protonated (–NH₃).
The structure shows an amine group (NH₂), a carboxylic acid group (COOH), a hydrogen and a variable side-chain, which is specific for each amino acid. The amine and carboxylic acid groups are referred to as functional groups.

development. The other eight essential amino acids are the same in adults and in children. However, on some occasions, a non-essential amino acid becomes a conditionally essential amino acid. For example, in a condition known as **phenylketonuria**, tyrosine (a non-essential amino acid) becomes essential because the body is unable to convert phenylalanine to tyrosine due to the absence of the enzyme **phenylalanine hydroxylase**, which is responsible for this conversion. Thus, adequate levels of tyrosine must be obtained in the diet. Essential amino acids are not more important than the others, but it is *essential* that they are obtained from the diet because they cannot be synthesized in the body. The remaining amino acids are *non-essential* (see *Table 7.2*). The non-essential amino acids, although available from the diet, can also be made in the body by a process called **transamination**. Structurally, all amino acids contain an amino group (NH₂), a carboxylic acid (COOH) group and a third group, known as an R group or side-chain, which is chemically different for each of the 20 amino acids that commonly occur to make up proteins. The R groups affect both protein structure and function. The general structure of an amino acid is shown in *Figure 7.4*. Two amino acids can link together by a peptide bond to form a molecule called a dipeptide, and when several amino acids link together they form polypeptides. How peptide bonds are formed by the loss of water molecules is shown in *Figure 7.5*. Water is formed when a hydroxyl (OH⁻) group from the carboxyl group of one amino acid bonds with a hydrogen (H⁺) atom from the amino group of the next amino acid. The two amino acids then form a covalent peptide bond. Covalent bonding is a strong stable chemical bond in which atoms share a pair of electrons.

Table 7.2 – Essential and non-essential amino acids

Essential amino acids	Non-essential amino acids
Leucine (branched chain)	Alanine
Isoleucine (branched chain)	Serine
Valine (branched chain)	Proline
Lysine	Tyrosine
Tryptophan	Glutamine
Threonine	Asparagine
Methionine	Aspartic acid
Phenylalanine	Glutamic acid
Histidine (children only)	Cysteine
	Arginine
	Glycine

Proteins do not exist as long, straight polypeptide chains but rather as one or more chains folded into three-dimensional structures. Proteins are described as having four levels of structure. Each level represents greater complexity in the structure of the protein:

- Primary structure is determined by the order of amino acids that make up a polypeptide chain.
- Secondary structure represents the interaction between amino acids (mostly via weak hydrogen bonds) within a polypeptide chain and provides a two-dimensional structure – typical forms that arise are represented by α-helices and β-sheets.

Figure 7.5 – The formation of peptide bonds.
The covalent bonds that hold amino acids together are called peptide bonds. These bonds are formed by a dehydration synthesis reaction in which water is formed by the removal of a hydroxyl group (OH⁻) from the carboxylic acid group and a hydrogen atom (H⁺) from the amine group.

- Tertiary structure represents further interaction between amino acids involving a variety of chemical bonds and interactions with chemicals in the local environment.
- Quaternary structure results when tertiary structures of multiple polypeptide chains interact, and sometimes when post-translational modification (introduced in *Chapter 3*) forms subunits to form a functional protein. The activity of the protein may also be influenced by other chemical groups such as cofactors. Haemoglobin is an example of a complex protein that has a quaternary structure (see *Figure 7.6*).

The three main classes of proteins that fulfil many different functions in the body are membrane proteins, fibrous proteins and globular proteins. *Membrane proteins* are found in cell membranes and in cell organelles (see *Chapter 2*). Membrane proteins function as receptors that transmit signal molecules (see *Chapter 5*), as transport proteins that allow the movement of molecules and ions across cell membranes, as enzymes, and as adhesion molecules that enable cell-to-cell recognition. *Fibrous proteins* such as **collagen** play a role in mechanical support, giving tensile strength to organs such as bone and skin, while **keratin** is the structural protein of hair and nails. *Globular proteins* such as haemoglobin in erythrocytes transport oxygen, a role achieved by myoglobin in muscle, while transferrin in blood plasma carries iron, which eventually gets stored as ferritin in the liver.

Figure 7.6 – The quaternary structure of haemoglobin.
An example of the quaternary structure of proteins is shown by haemoglobin in which two α-globulin chains and the two β-globulin chains in the polypeptide chain fold round each other.

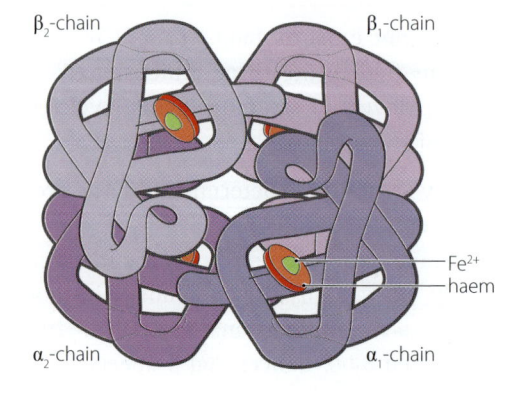

Fats

Fats are also composed of carbon, hydrogen and oxygen, but their arrangement is different to that of carbohydrates, and it is important to emphasize that fats have less oxygen, consisting almost exclusively of carbon and hydrogen. The unique ability of carbon atoms to form strong carbon–carbon bonds and long chains on their own makes it possible for both short- and long-chain molecules of carbon to be formed with hydrogen atoms attached to them. Hydrogen does not have the ability to form chains of hydrogen–hydrogen molecules.

The lack of oxygen in fats makes them hydrophobic ('water-hating'), thus preventing them from mixing with water (see *Chapter 2*). However, like carbohydrates, fats exist in different forms. *Oil* refers to fats that are liquid at room temperature, while the term fat usually refers to those fats that are solid at room temperature. The term *lipid* refers to both liquid and solid fats. Glycerol (see *Figure 7.7a*) and fatty acids (see *Figure 7.7b*) are components of lipids. Fatty acids comprise chains of carbon atoms. The combination of glycerol with three fatty acids forms a **triglyceride**, the main form of fat in the body, as shown in *Figure 7.8*, and may contain a variety of types of fatty acid. The three fatty acid chains can be different lengths as well as being a mixture of *saturated* and *unsaturated fatty acids*. Fatty acids have a carboxylic acid (COOH) end and a methyl end (CH_3) (see *Figure 7.4b*). Glycerol contains three hydroxyl molecules and each hydroxyl group can make a bond with a carboxyl group of a fatty acid to form what is known as an ester bond. An unsaturated fatty acid is one where some of the hydrogen atoms have been eliminated or removed from the chain of carbon atoms linked together, resulting in double bonds being present between the carbon atoms, while a saturated fatty acid has all the hydrogen atoms present to make bonds with the carbon atoms and has no double bonds. The significance of saturated and unsaturated fatty acids to health is discussed later in this chapter.

Oils and fats can be modified by a process known as **interesterification**, whereby there is a rearrangement of the fatty acids on the glycerol molecule. For example, when the three fatty acids are separated from the glycerol molecule and the triglyceride molecule is reformed, the fatty acids may not return to their original position but may bond at a different position on the glycerol molecule. Modification by interesterification affects the properties of oils and fats. These properties include consistency or hardness of fats, stability at high temperature,

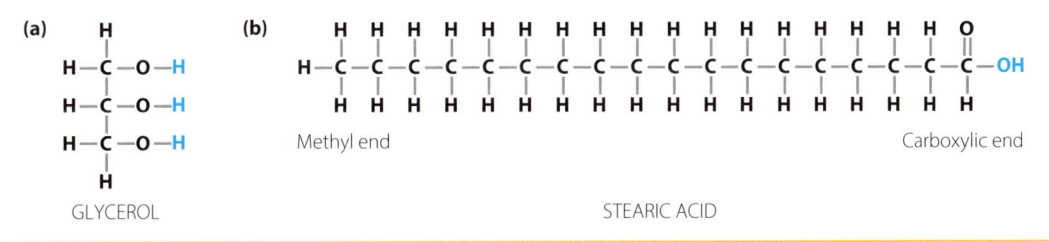

Figure 7.7 – The structure of (a) glycerol and (b) a fatty acid.
(a) The structure of a glycerol molecule, with three hydroxyl (OH⁻) groups that represent the positions where fatty acids are attached during the formation of triglycerides. (b) The structure of a saturated fatty acid (stearic acid) showing an even number of carbon atoms in an unbranched chain and with no double bonds.

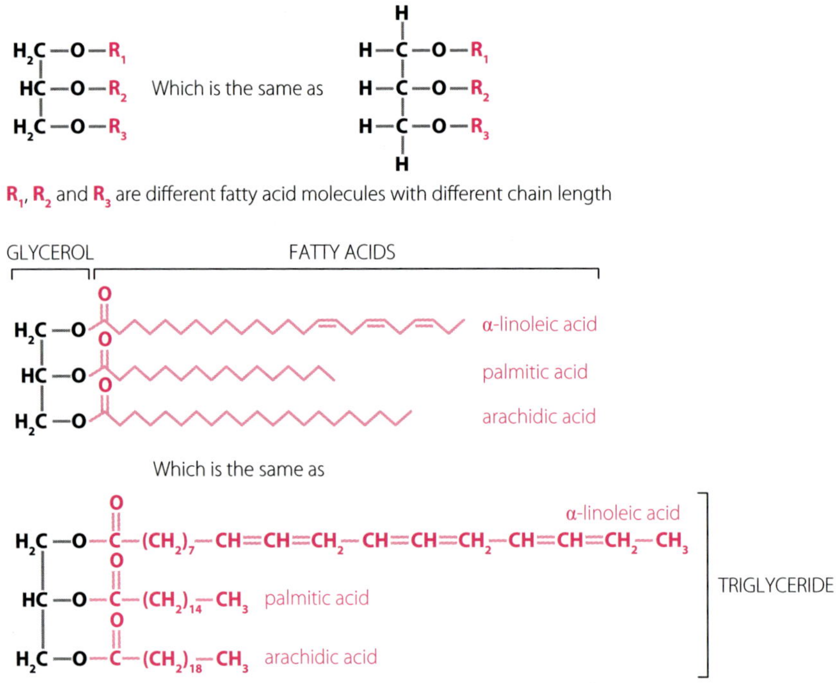

Figure 7.8 – The structure of a triglyceride.
A triglyceride is composed of a glycerol molecule attached to three fatty acids, which may or may not be identical.

lowering of the melting point, spreadability or soft texture, and good eating qualities such as rapidly melting in the mouth, as seen in chocolate. The health consequences of consuming foods high in fat include obesity, hypertension and some cancers.

A fat is described as saturated if its fatty acids contain the maximum number of hydrogen atoms, and unsaturated when there are fewer hydrogen atoms resulting in double bonds, as described above. The absence of hydrogen atoms ensures that one or more bonds in that fat are double. Fats with one double bond are known as monounsaturated fats, while those with many double bonds are known as polyunsaturated fats. There are different types of fat depending on structural differences and chain length of the fatty acids. Monounsaturated fats have one double bond due to the absence of two hydrogen atoms, while polyunsaturated fats have more than one double bond with four or more hydrogen atoms that have been removed. Two examples of polyunsaturated fats are those containing *linoleic acid*, an omega-6 (ω-6) fatty acid, and *α-linolenic acid*, an ω-3 fatty acid. The double bonds of monounsaturated and polyunsaturated fatty acids can be converted to single bonds by passing hydrogen through the fat, a process known as hydrogenation. Hydrogenation alters the physical properties of fats, increasing their shelf life, providing a soft consistency and making them easier to spread. Palmitic acid (a chain of 16 carbon atoms) and stearic acid (a chain of 18 carbon atoms) are examples of saturated fatty acids.

Phospholipids (described in *Chapter 2*) have an important role in the formation of plasma membranes, and the most common phospholipids are lecithins. Like triglycerides, lecithins have a backbone of glycerol with two fatty acids, a phosphate group and choline. The structure of phospholipids makes them soluble in both fat and water because the phosphate-containing group enables them to dissolve in water; this property is exploited in industry where they are used as emulsifiers in foods such as mayonnaise.

Dietary fats give texture to foods, enhance flavour and taste, and increase palatability. Nutritionally, like carbohydrates, fats provide the body with energy but they are *energy dense*, providing twice as much energy (9.1 kcal/g) when compared with carbohydrates (4.1 kcal/g) and proteins (4.1 kcal/g). The typical diet of Western industrialized nations, and increasingly some less industrialized nations too, has become very energy dense due to increased levels of saturated fats and sugar. This represents one of the two most important factors for the increased prevalence of obesity and cardiovascular disease, especially in the Western world, the other being sedentary behaviour.

Cis *and* trans *fats*

Monounsaturated fats and polyunsaturated fats can exist in two different forms (isomers) as *cis* and *trans*. The two hydrogen atoms adjacent to a double bond in *cis* fatty acids are on the same side of the double bond, resulting in a kink in the molecule and making the fatty acids more difficult to pack together. This makes most of these fats liquid (oils) at room temperature. *Trans* fatty acids (TFAs) have the hydrogen atoms adjacent to a double bond on the opposite sides of the double bond, which makes them easier to pack closely together and so they behave like saturated fats: they are solid at room temperature. Naturally occurring TFAs are found in animal protein such as beef and milk because the *cis* form can be converted into the *trans* form in the stomach of ruminant animals such as cows, sheep and goats.

During the industrial manufacture of margarines, polyunsaturated fats are hydrogenated in a process known as 'shortening', which results in most of the fatty acids being in the *trans* form instead of the *cis* form (see *Figures 7.9a and b*). Manufactured foods that contain TFAs are biscuits, buns, cakes, crackers, pastries

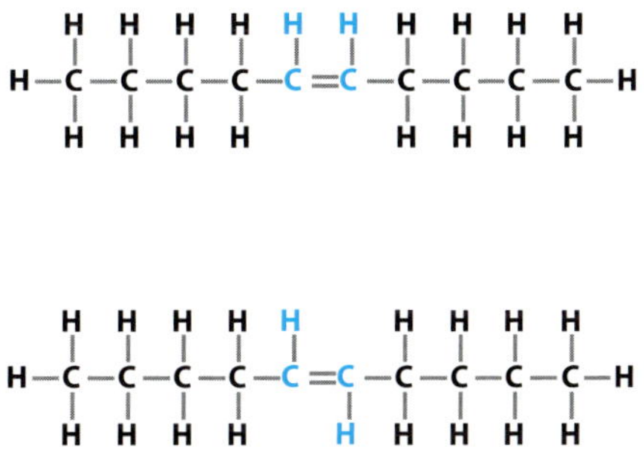

Figure 7.9 – **Fatty acids in (a) the *cis* form and (b) the *trans* form.**
Cis and *trans* refer to the arrangement of hydrogen atoms around the double bonds. In *cis* fatty acids, the hydrogen atoms are on the same side of the double bond, while in *trans* fatty acids, the hydrogen atoms are on opposite sides.

and snack foods such as crisps and chocolates. TFAs are associated with the development of coronary heart disease, and the consumption of foods containing *trans* fats in high amounts should be avoided.

Essential fatty acids

Polyunsaturated fatty acids such as linoleic acid, an ω-6 fatty acid, and α-linolenic acid, an ω-3 fatty acid, are essential fatty acids because they need to be taken in the diet as they are not synthesized in the body. Dietary sources of essential fatty acids are vegetables such as leafy vegetables, pumpkin seeds, soybean, nuts such as walnuts, and oils from fish. The presence of an unsaturated bond within the last seven carbon atoms of a fatty acid closest to the methyl end (the **omega end**) makes it an essential fatty acid. Essential fatty acids are needed for proper development and functioning of the brain and retina. Essential fatty acids also form eicosanoids, which are important compounds involved in cell signalling, especially inflammatory responses (see *Chapter 11*). The other important role of ω-3 fatty acids, especially eicosapentaenoic acid and docosahexaenoic acid, is their anti-thrombotic effect, meaning that they prevent the clotting of blood, thereby conferring protection against coronary heart disease (discussed in *Chapter 9*). Increased consumption of oily fish, nuts and plant oils helps to protect against heart disease, and it is thought that the reduction in fish consumption that may have occurred in the last century may be contributory to the increase in coronary heart disease.

Cholesterol

Cholesterol is synthesized by the liver and is also consumed in the diet; sources rich in dietary cholesterol include egg yolk, meat and full-fat dairy products. Plants do not contain cholesterol; the approximate amount of cholesterol in animal products does vary. Dietary cholesterol has only a small influence on the levels of cholesterol in the blood, except in situations where diets high in saturated fats are consumed. This is because consuming foods high in saturated fats raises the amount of low-density lipoprotein cholesterol in blood. Thus, limiting the intake of saturated fats is more effective in lowering blood cholesterol than limiting cholesterol intake.

Cholesterol levels in the body are regulated by the enterohepatic circulation between the blood and the gut and are influenced by many factors including cholesterol synthesis by the liver, the amount of bile production by the liver, dietary factors and the hormone insulin, which, in addition to regulating blood glucose levels (see *Chapter 5*), also increases cholesterol synthesis. More cholesterol is synthesized when there is a greater secretion of insulin. The structure of cholesterol is shown in *Figure 7.10*. Cholesterol is the most common sterol, made up of four hydrocarbon rings linked together with a hydrocarbon tail at one end of the structure and a hydroxyl (OH⁻) group at the other end. There are a few side-chains attached to the molecule. Its structure makes it an important substance that serves as a precursor molecule (starting point) for vitamin D, a variety of bile acids (discussed later in this chapter) and steroid hormones such as cortisol, oestrogen, progesterone and testosterone (see *Chapter 5*). Cholesterol in the plasma membrane functions to increase membrane stability and to decrease membrane

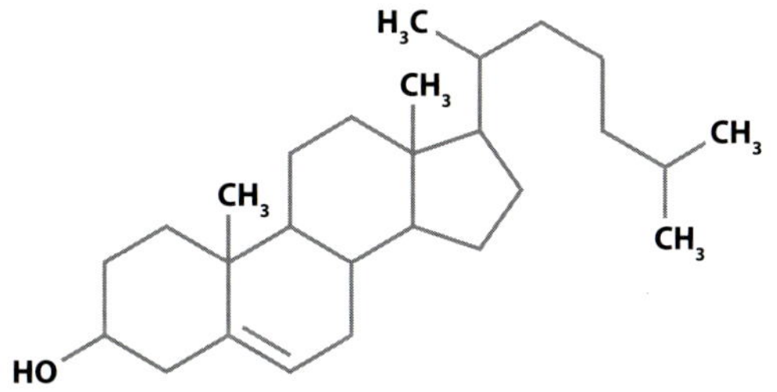

Figure 7.10 – The structure of cholesterol.
Four hydrocarbon rings are linked together with a hydrocarbon tail at one end of the structure and a hydroxyl group at the other end. There are a few side-chains attached to the molecule.

permeability (discussed in *Chapter 2*). Cholesterol is found in the brain, nervous tissue and blood. However, excess cholesterol can lead to health problems when it accumulates in the arterial wall, a disease called atherosclerosis, which can lead to the development of vascular disease. Measurement of cholesterol levels in the blood can be a useful guide for assessing the risk of coronary heart disease, and the recommended upper limit is 5.2 millimoles/L.

In addition to cholesterol synthesis, liver cells make molecules known as lipoproteins (lipid and protein molecules) that are used to transport fats in the body. Very-low-density lipoproteins (VLDLs) transport triglycerides from the liver to other tissues in the body. As the triglycerides are given to other tissues, VLDLs gather cholesterol from other lipoproteins in the blood and become low-density lipoproteins (LDLs). LDLs transport cholesterol from the liver to cells of all tissues. High-density lipoproteins (HDLs) carry cholesterol and phospholipids from the cells to the liver where they are metabolized and destroyed. Based on these differences in roles, LDL is referred to as 'bad' cholesterol while HDL is referred to as 'good' cholesterol because HDL has a protective effect. The ratio of HDL:LDL and the overall lipid profile are important when reviewing the health status of an individual.

Minerals

The body requires 17 minerals, of which seven are macro- (major) elements and ten are micro- (trace) elements (see *Table 7.3*). Although minerals make up a small percentage (approximately 3%) of the body by weight, they are vitally important to health. Minerals provide structure to bones, teeth and soft tissue such as cartilage and connective tissue. Physiologically, minerals have a role in the transmission of nerve impulses, movement, blood clotting and the activity of hormones. Minerals form part of pH buffering systems (solutions containing a weak acid and a weak base that ensure that the pH remains stable) and their presence, in tiny amounts in enzymes, serves to regulate metabolism.

Macroelements are present in the body in relatively high amounts, the most abundant being calcium, followed by phosphorus, sulphur and potassium. A 70 kg adult human contains approximately 1200 g of calcium, 660 g of phosphorus, 200 g of sulphur, 149 g of potassium, 99 g sodium and 26 g of magnesium. The recommended daily allowance for calcium in the UK for adult males and females

Table 7.3 – Macro- (major) and micro- (trace) elements

Macro- (major) elements	Micro- (trace) elements
Sodium (Na)	Chromium (Cr)
Potassium (K)	Cobalt (Co)
Calcium (Ca)	Copper (Cu)
Magnesium (Mg)	Iodine (I)
Phosphorus (P)	Iron (Fe)
Sulphur (S)	Manganese (Mn)
Chloride (C)	Molybdenum (Mo)
	Selenium (Se)
	Zinc (Zn)
	Fluoride (F)

aged 19 years and above is 700 mg/day. In the UK, the recommended daily allowance for calcium varies in children, ranging from 350 mg/day between the ages of 1 and 3 years to 1000 mg/day at 18 years of age. The majority of calcium is deposited in bones and teeth, providing their strength (see *Chapter 13*). Loss of calcium from bones causes them to become fragile, increasing the risk of fractures, a condition called **osteoporosis**. Calcium, sodium and chloride, present in blood and extracellular fluid in relatively large amounts, form extracellular ions, whereas magnesium, potassium and phosphorus are relatively more abundant within cells, forming intracellular ions. Sulphur, the third most abundant element in the body, is an essential component of some amino acids such as methionine, cysteine and taurine. Taurine is important in enzyme function and formation of connective tissue, and is also required for the synthesis of glutathione, an important intracellular antioxidant (see *Chapter 2*).

Microelements (trace elements), while required in minute quantities of less than 100 mg/day, are essential for good health. Trace elements, such as selenium and copper, are essential because they are often cofactors required for enzyme function.

Selenium is included in some proteins to form selenoproteins, which are mostly antioxidant enzymes. One such enzyme is **glutathione peroxidase**, which is widely distributed in tissues and has a collaborative role with vitamin E in the detoxification of peroxides and free radicals, which damage cell membranes. High concentrations are found in red blood cells, heart, liver, nails, spleen and tooth enamel. Selenium has a role in thyroid function and in the immune system, acting as an antioxidant that helps to fight the damaging effects of free radicals. Selenium deficiency can occur in infants who are fed on artificial formula feeds and in adults fed with parenteral nutrition (directly into a vein). Dietary selenium intake, reflecting levels of selenium available in the soil, has been observed to correlate with the risk of a variety of cancers and heart disease. However, the exact relationship between dietary selenium and health remains unclear.

In the human body, high concentrations of copper are found in the kidneys, liver, brain, heart and bone. Copper is associated with cytochrome oxidase enzymes involved in the electron transport chain during **adenosine triphosphate (ATP)** synthesis within mitochondria, and in superoxide dismutase and **ceruloplasmin**, two enzymes involved in the scavenging and disposal of oxygen free radicals that damage cells (see *Chapter 11*). The copper-containing ceruloplasmin enzyme has a role in the oxidation of Fe^{2+} (the ferrous form of iron) to Fe^{3+} (the ferric form), which enables its attachment to transferrin, the protein that transports iron in the blood. High levels of free Fe^{2+} in the blood react with peroxides producing free radicals that damage proteins, DNA and lipids. Iron is transported in the blood attached to transferrin and is stored in tissues as a protein complex called ferritin. Copper is essential in the process by which iron is changed from the ferrous form to the ferric form to enable its transport and storage. Iron toxicity occurs when there is inadequate transferrin to bind to Fe^{2+} ions. Copper is also a component of dopamine β-hydroxylase required for the synthesis of catecholamines in the brain and in the adrenal medulla (see *Chapters 4* and *5*).

Iodine is needed for normal thyroid function and for the production of the thyroid hormone, thyroxine (see *Chapter 5*). Deficiency in some of the trace elements such as iodine and iron causes significant health problems. Disorders associated with iodine deficiency sometimes begin during pregnancy leading to spontaneous abortion, stillbirth, congenital abnormalities, impaired cognitive development, impaired intellectual capacity and mental health problems in children. The hormone thyroxine (discussed in *Chapter 5*) requires the trace element iodine. Iodine deficiency is responsible for causing goitre (swelling of the thyroid gland) and conditions of hypothyroidism (underactive thyroid gland) as seen in David (Patient 5.1). A diet deficient in iodine can result in an underactive thyroid gland.

Iron is found in two forms in food: as haem iron (this is incorporated into haemoglobin) and non-haem iron. Haem iron is found in meat, poultry and fish, while non-haem iron is found in both plant and animal foods such as vegetables, grains, fruit, eggs, fish, meat and poultry. Vegetarian diets tend to be low in iron, especially a vegan diet where no animal products are consumed. The amount of iron that is absorbed depends on iron stores in the body as well as other factors such as vitamin C intake. Ferrous (Fe^{2+}) iron is more readily absorbed than ferric (Fe^{3+}) iron. Vitamin C improves the absorption of iron from the small intestine. This is because vitamin C increases the conversion of non-haem iron in food, the ferric form, to the ferrous form by hydrochloric acid in the stomach. The conversion from Fe^{3+} to Fe^{2+} increases iron absorption in the duodenum. Iron serves as a cofactor for enzymes involved in energy metabolism and occurs in the proteins haemoglobin, found in the red blood cells, and myoglobin, found in the muscle cells. The molecular structures of haem and haemoglobin are shown in *Figures 7.11a* and *b* (for discussion of haemoglobin in the transport of oxygen, see *Chapters 9* and *10*).

Zinc is well distributed in human tissue, with the highest amounts in skin and hair followed by nails, the retina, bone and the male reproductive organs. A significant amount is found in the liver, kidney, muscle and pancreas. Zinc is required for the activity of more than 100 different enzymes associated with carbohydrate metabolism, protein synthesis and degradation, nucleic acid synthesis and red blood cell transport of carbon dioxide (carbonic anhydrase). Within the pancreas, zinc is associated with the secretion of proteases in exocrine pancreatic juices required for protein digestion. In males, zinc affects the development of the male reproductive tract, testosterone production and spermatogenesis (see *Chapter 14*).

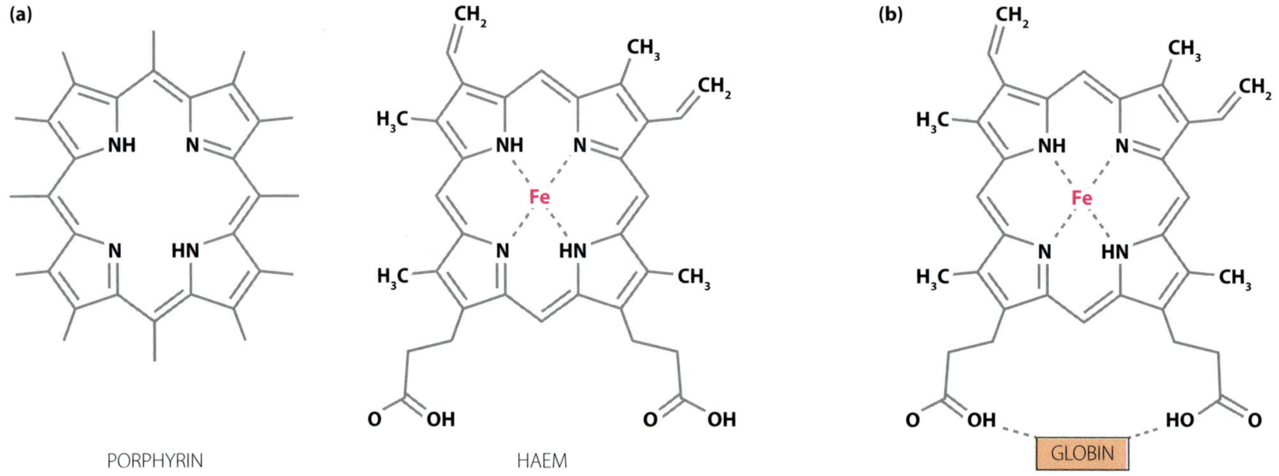

Figure 7.11 – (a) The porphyrin ring and structure of haem and (b) the structure of haemoglobin showing how haem is attached to the protein globin to form haemoglobin.
(a) A haem group consists of an Fe ion as iron II (Fe^{2+}) held at its centre in a heterocyclic ring known as porphyrin. A heterocyclic ring is a ring of atoms of more than one kind that form a closed loop. (b) It is the ferrous (Fe^{2+}) atom that gives haemoglobin its red colour. The Fe^{2+} atom is converted to Fe^{3+} when haemoglobin combines with oxygen.

It is required for the synthesis of retinol-binding protein in the liver, for vitamin A metabolism and alcohol detoxification. Zinc is a cofactor in **collagenase** and indirectly promotes epithelial cell differentiation and wound healing. Zinc deficiency results in reduced growth due to its role in all cells.

Vitamins

Vitamins are also micronutrients. They are organic molecules required in minute quantities that are essential for many physiological, metabolic and biochemical functions. Vitamins have to be obtained directly from the diet because humans are unable to synthesize them in sufficient amounts. Like other nutrients, deficiency, excess or imbalance lead to poor health. Vitamins are grouped into fat-soluble and water-soluble vitamins (see *Table 7.4*).

Fat-soluble vitamins

The fat-soluble vitamins are vitamins A, D, E and K (see *Table 7.4*). These vitamins are absorbed together with fat, and therefore conditions that interfere with either the digestion or absorption of fat can result in deficiencies of the fat-soluble vitamins. Fat-soluble vitamins are stored in the liver and fatty tissue, and are eliminated from the body slowly. They become toxic if consumed in large amounts, especially vitamin A, which can cause teratogenic effects (malformation of organs resulting in birth defects) when taken in large doses during pregnancy.

Vitamin A is known by different names depending on its form: as retinol in the alcohol form, as retinal in the aldehyde form, and as retinoic acid, the acid form of vitamin A; all of these different forms are active in the body. Sources of retinol include butter, cheese, eggs, liver and fortified milk. The orange pigment known

Table 7.4 – Fat- and water-soluble vitamins

Fat-soluble vitamins	Water-soluble vitamins
A – retinol/retinal and retinoic acid	Thiamine (B_1)
D – ergocalciferol (D_2) and cholecalciferol (D_3)	Riboflavine (B_2)
E – tocopherol: α-tocopherol and γ-tocopherol	Niacin (B_3) – nicotinic acid and nicotinamide
K – phylloquinone	Cobalamin (B_{12}) – hydroxycobalamin, cyanocobalamin and methylcobalamin
	Pyridoxine (B6) – pyridoxal and pyridoxamine
	Biotin
	Ascorbic acid (C)
	Folic acid (pteroylglutamic acid)
	Pantothenic acid

as β-carotene found in plants is a precursor of vitamin A and can be split in the intestines and liver to form retinol. Good sources of β-carotene are apricots, carrots, sweet potatoes, pumpkins, some dark green vegetables and broccoli. Both vitamin A and β-carotene act as antioxidants. Vitamin A has a role in preventing night blindness, in cell differentiation, in promoting growth and bone remodelling, and in boosting the immune system. Retinol-binding protein transports vitamin A in blood. Vitamin A is stored in the liver. Excess consumption of liver by pregnant women can lead to toxicity in the fetus, while taking supplements such as cod liver oil can also lead to toxicity. The signs of toxicity include blurred vision, nausea, vomiting, headache, dizziness, irritability and skin changes such as oily skin and peeling skin. Globally, vitamin A deficiency is the leading cause of preventable blindness in children.

Vitamin D (in the form of D_3 or cholecalciferol) can be synthesized in the body by utilizing sunlight and 7-dehydrocholesterol, a precursor made in the liver from cholesterol (sun exposure and vitamin D are discussed in *Chapter 12*). In the liver, hydroxylation (the addition of a hydroxyl (OH) group) occurs to form 25-hydroxyvitamin D_3 (25-hydroxycholecalciferol), the main circulating form of the vitamin in plasma. Further hydroxylation occurs in the kidneys resulting in 1,25-dihydroxyvitamin D_3 (1,25-dihydroxycholecalciferol) or calcitriol, the active form of the vitamin, which acts like a steroid hormone. Vitamin D acts like a hormone and can cross cell membranes, including the nuclear membrane, entering the nucleus where it attaches to specific receptors on DNA, thus affecting cell differentiation. Vitamin D increases the absorption of calcium from the gastrointestinal tract by promoting the elongation of intestinal villi, and deficiency can result in rickets in children and osteomalacia in adults, but the vitamin is also now believed to have other roles important in the regulation of immunity, the nervous system and reproduction. Foods of animal origin such as oily fish, egg yolk, liver and fortified milk are good sources of vitamin D. Studies have suggested that vitamin D deficiency may lead to the development of breast, colorectal and prostate cancers, although there is no firm evidence that vitamin D supplements reduce specific cancers. Within the immune system, vitamin D has a role in reducing the severity of asthma and allergic conditions. In pregnancy, vitamin D deficiency is linked to **pre-eclampsia**, insulin resistance and gestational diabetes mellitus.

Vitamin E represents various forms of compounds formed from tocopherols and tocotrienol compounds. α-Tocopherol is the most abundant and most biologically active. Vitamin E can be found associated with the plasma membrane acting as an antioxidant (see *Box 7.1*) to protect the membrane from free radical damage by limiting the oxidation of polyunsaturated fatty acids. Vitamin E modulates gene expression and activity of the immune system, and protects erythrocytes from haemolysis. Sources of vitamin E include whole grains, green leafy vegetables, nuts, seeds, liver and egg yolk. Although very rare, deficiency of vitamin E can result in haemolysis and neuromuscular dysfunction such as loss of muscle coordination, severe pain in the calf muscles, muscle weakness and muscle atrophy.

Antioxidants

An antioxidant can be defined as *'any substance that delays or inhibits oxidative damage to a target molecule'*. This means that antioxidants function in the body to protect tissues of the body from chemical damage. This is particularly important for the nucleic acid DNA, for proteins and for polyunsaturated fatty acids such as those associated with the plasma membrane. Oxidative damage to tissues occurs when highly reactive chemical groups known as free radicals are formed.

A free radical can be defined as *'any substance capable of independent existence that contains an unpaired electron'*. Free radicals are always unstable, highly reactive compounds involving oxides of oxygen or nitrogen, and are often referred to as reactive oxygen or reactive nitrogen species (ROS/RNS).

Antioxidant systems in the body include a variety of non-enzymatic defences against ROS/RNS chemistry, such as the antioxidant vitamins A, C and E and glutathione, and also enzymatic defences such as the enzyme superoxide dismutase. Superoxide dismutase is so important that it is found in all organisms that rely on oxygen for respiration, as oxygen itself can be a source of free radicals when it gains one electron instead of two (which it does when it reacts with hydrogen to form water).

Free radical activity or a deficiency in antioxidant defences is associated with many disease states, including chronic inflammation, cancer and heart disease. It is important to recognize that the formation of free radical compounds is a normal part of biochemistry and that sometimes the body generates high levels of free radicals (this is discussed further in *Chapter 11*).

BOX 7.1

Vitamin K has a number of forms; the form phylloquinone (K_1) is synthesized by green leafy vegetables and is found in high amounts in green leafy vegetables, cruciferous (cabbage-type) vegetables, liver and milk. A small amount of a form of vitamin K known as menaquinone (K_2) is synthesized by colonic bacteria in the gastrointestinal tract, but bacterial synthesis alone does not produce amounts adequate for the needs of the body. Vitamin K is essential for the synthesis of some plasma proteins such as prothrombin and is involved in the blood clotting process (see *Chapter 9*). Vitamin K deficiency is seldom seen, although it may occur when fat absorption is impaired, for example due to impaired bile production and in malabsorption syndromes such as coeliac disease. Babies are born with a sterile gastrointestinal tract and for several weeks following birth, they lack the bacteria that synthesize vitamin K, making them susceptible to haemorrhage soon after birth, especially when premature. For this reason, parents are routinely offered a prophylactic injection of vitamin K for their baby shortly after birth, in order to minimize haemorrhagic reactions.

Water-soluble vitamins

Water-soluble vitamins comprise the B complex, biotin, pantothenic acid, vitamin C and folic acid (see *Table 7.4*). Excess water-soluble vitamins are excreted in urine and therefore tend not to be stored in the liver; toxicity is rarely seen for this reason. However, abdominal cramps, nausea and diarrhoea have been reported after taking large amounts of vitamin C as supplements, and excess vitamin C can reduce the effectiveness of anticoagulant medication. Vitamin C can be synthesized from glucose by most plants and animal tissue, but humans and other primates, guinea pigs and some birds lack the ability to synthesize the vitamin, making dietary intake of the preformed vitamin essential. It is a powerful reducing agent and reduces ferric (Fe^{3+}) iron to the more stable ferrous (Fe^{2+}) iron. It increases the absorption of non-haem iron from the gastrointestinal tract, has a role in the synthesis of collagen and is required for the structural integrity of blood vessels, cartilage and connective tissue. Together with vitamin E, vitamin C has another important role as an antioxidant (see *Box 7.1*). Deficiency of vitamin C results in the condition known as scurvy, characterized by bleeding and swollen gums, subcutaneous haemorrhages, painful joints and poor healing of wounds. Rich sources of vitamin C are fresh fruit and vegetables. The vitamin can be lost during cooking and storage. There is an increased requirement for vitamin C following surgery to promote the formation of new connective tissue and minimize spontaneous breakdown of surgical wounds, and also in people who smoke, because smoking generates free radicals that damage cells.

Some of the B group vitamins participate in metabolic processes that generate ATP. For example, thiamine has a role in energy metabolism and thiamine deficiency results in beriberi, a condition in which there is inflammation of the peripheral nerves (peripheral neuritis) resulting in a tingling sensation in the extremities. Other water-soluble vitamins are involved in energy metabolism including riboflavin and niacin. Deficiency in niacin results in pellagra, which is characterized by gastrointestinal tract problems, dermatitis, diarrhoea and dementia. Vitamin B_6 has a role as a **cofactor** or **coenzyme** in protein metabolism. A coenzyme or cofactor is a non-protein substance that is attached to a protein and is essential for the biological activity of the protein. Vitamin B_6 (also known as pyridoxine) occurs in three different forms, namely pyridoxine, pyridoxal and pyridoxamine. All forms of vitamin B_6 can be converted to a coenzyme called **pyridoxal phosphate**, which enables the synthesis of some non-essential amino acids from other amino acids when these are in short supply during protein metabolism. Vitamin B_6 is widely distributed in foods, making deficiency rare, but when it does occur it can cause convulsions. Vitamin B_{12} (cobalamin) is required for the formation of normal red blood cells, for the formation of the myelin sheath that surrounds some neurones and in protein metabolism. In adults, deficiency symptoms include pernicious anaemia, glossitis (red inflamed tongue), fatigue, mouth lesions and dermatitis.

Non-starch polysaccharides (fibre)

Fibre includes cellulose, hemicelluloses, pectins (present in fruit and vegetables), gums and lignin (the woody part of some vegetables).

Fibre can be divided into **soluble fibre** and **insoluble fibre**. Gums and pectins are classified as soluble fibre because they dissolve in water to form gels. Fruit and vegetables, in particular legumes and grains such as oats and barley, are rich in soluble fibre. Gums are made of various monosaccharides such as glucose and rhamnose, while all pectins contain the sugar rhamnose and have a variety of monosaccharide side-chains such as glucose, arabinose and xylose, and form gels with water very easily. Pectins are found in many vegetables and fruit such as apples and citrus fruit. Soluble fibre slows both stomach emptying and the absorption of glucose into blood. This helps to limit the **post-prandial sugar spike** – peak concentrations of both glucose and insulin observed in the blood after a carbohydrate-rich meal that cause tiredness. Soluble fibre also decreases both plasma cholesterol and the concentration of LDLs in blood by binding to bile acids formed from cholesterol; this reduces their absorption from the gastrointestinal tract back into the blood, increasing their excretion (see enterohepatic circulation of cholesterol, discussed earlier in this chapter).

Insoluble fibre, found in leafy vegetables such as cabbages and sprouts and in the bran component of grains, is made from **cellulose**, a polysaccharide that forms the cell wall of plants. **Hemicelluloses** are the main component of cereal fibres, which possess branching side-chains of monosaccharides and are made up of several sugars such as mannose, rhamnose and xylose. Hemicelluloses are sparingly soluble. **Lignin** forms the woody material in plants. Dietary insoluble fibre regulates transit time in the gastrointestinal tract by increasing bulk, thus minimizing constipation. Fibre provides a feeling of fullness (satiety), which helps to reduce the overconsumption of calories, thereby helping to reduce obesity. A high-fibre diet is thought to be protective against colon and rectal cancer, possibly by binding to irritants and carcinogens, in addition to speeding up the transit of these along the gut and thus limiting their absorption. Bacterial fermentation of fibre yields short-chain fatty acids such as propionate and butyrate that provide energy needs for cells lining the colon. In addition, short-chain fatty acids increase fluid and mineral absorption from the colon, have an immunomodulatory function by reducing inflammation and promote natural killer cell activity (see *Chapter 11*). The dietary reference value (DRV) for non-starch polysaccharides or fibre is 18 g/day, although levels of consumption of fibre are estimated to be lower than the DRV for most people in the Western world.

Water

All food contains some water, even if the food appears dry to the naked eye. Water itself is an important component of the diet because it is the universal solvent, providing the transport medium for nutrients dissolved in plasma (discussed in *Chapter 8*). Water is an essential component in the process of digestion and all other metabolic processes. The main source of water is beverages, although most fruit and vegetables contain up to 95% water, while meat may contain as much as 50%. Some water is generated during metabolism when carbon and hydrogen combine with oxygen to form carbon dioxide and water, especially during fat metabolism. Water deprivation or excessive loss of water from the body leads to dehydration. The importance of water in the body is discussed in *Chapter 8*.

7.2.3 Making nutrients in food available

We need to process the food we have consumed so that the nutrients become available for use by tissues. Digestion and absorption occur in the gastrointestinal tract or digestive system. The gastrointestinal tract has been structurally and functionally adapted to fulfil this role. It is important to emphasize that, due to the complexity of multi-cellular organisms (see *Chapter 1*), in order for tissues to obtain nutrients, they must be well perfused with blood and this blood must be intimate with the absorptive surface of the gut. The thin mucosal surface of the

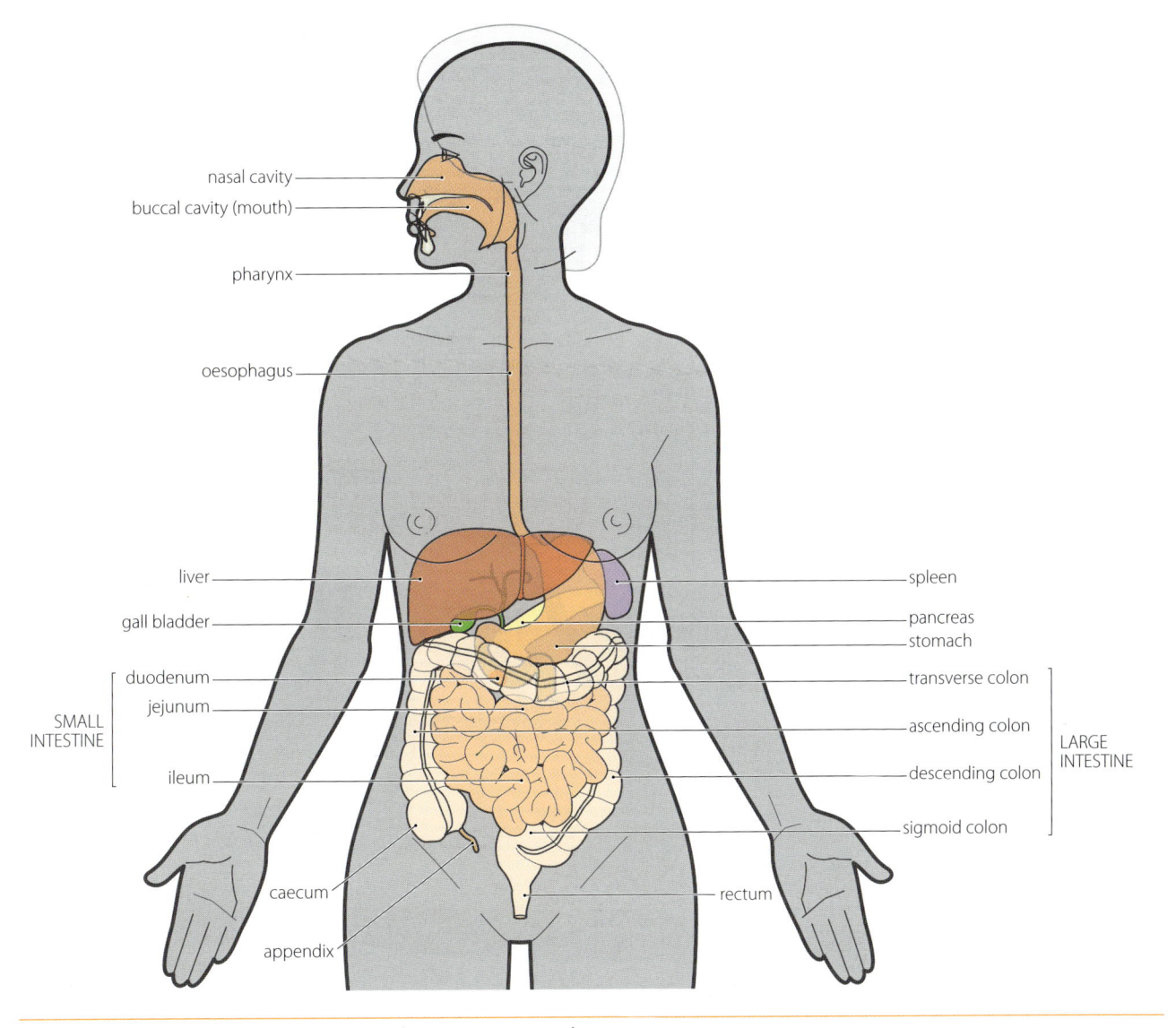

Figure 7.12 – **The gastrointestinal tract (digestive system).**
The structures of the gastrointestinal tract are shown, together with its accessory organs, without which digestion would be incomplete.

gut has been estimated to have a large surface area of approximately 400 m², thus providing a large surface area for absorption.

Role of the gastrointestinal tract

The gastrointestinal tract (see *Figure 7.12*) is a tube running from the mouth or oral cavity to the anus. When viewed as a cross-section (see *Figure 7.13*), the whole of the gastrointestinal tract, from the oesophagus to the colon, has a similar structure comprising four layers: the mucosa, submucosa, muscularis and serosa.

- The **mucosa** is the innermost layer surrounding a hollow cavity known as the lumen. The mucosal layer is made up of stratified squamous epithelial cells in the oesophagus (this is an area subject to wear and tear, and cells are rubbed away constantly during swallowing) and simple columnar cells in the rest of the gastrointestinal tract. Acid-resistant bacteria called

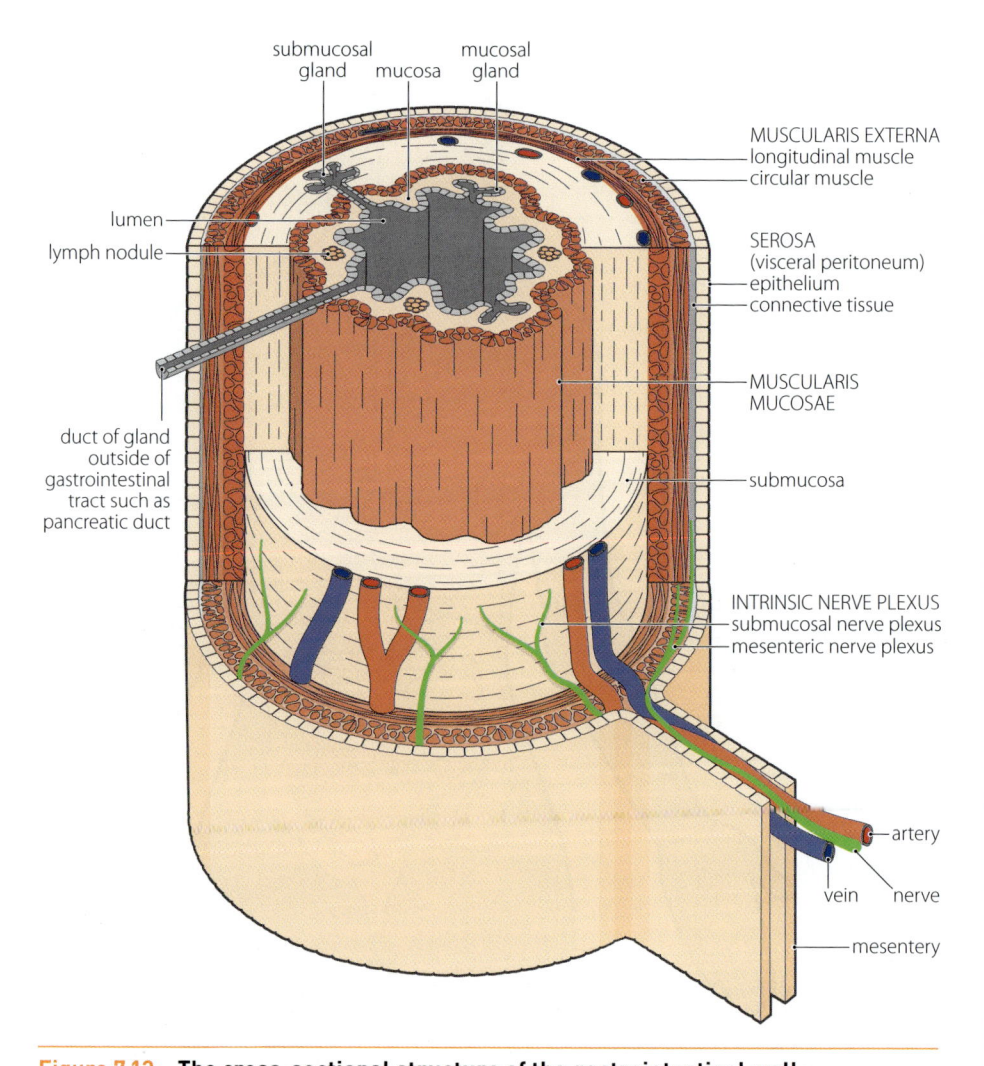

Figure 7.13 – **The cross-sectional structure of the gastrointestinal wall.**
The four main structures comprising the mucosa, submucosa, muscularis externa (circular and longitudinal) and serosa are shown.

Helicobacter pylori, which colonize the stomach mucosa, are associated with an increased risk of development of peptic ulcers.
- The **submucosa** is the next layer to the mucosa. It consists of connective tissue (lamina propria), blood vessels, nerve endings, lymphatic nodules and lymphatic vessels. At the end of the ileum, furthest away from the stomach, within the submucosa are found **Peyer's patches**, which are collections of lymphoid tissue that minimize the entry of microorganisms such as bacteria into the blood.
- A smooth muscle layer called the **muscularis externa** consisting of an inner circular muscle and an outer longitudinal muscle covers the submucosa. A third oblique layer of smooth muscle is found in the stomach wall only. This extra layer helps to strengthen the stomach wall, as well as causing churning and mixing of food in the stomach. The smooth muscle layer is highly innervated by an interconnected network of nerve fibres known as the **myenteric nerve plexus**, which lies between the circular muscles and longitudinal muscles. The nerve plexus within the gastrointestinal tract is linked to the central nervous system by afferent (sensory) fibres and by sympathetic and parasympathetic branches of motor fibres, thus signifying the important link between the brain and the role of the gastrointestinal tract. This coordinated activity ensures that gut motility occurs, as well as production of relevant secretions to facilitate digestion.
- The **serosa** is the outermost layer, as illustrated in *Figure 7.13*. It is a double-folded membrane with an inner visceral peritoneum and an outer parietal peritoneum that separates the internal environment from the external environment by lining organs within the abdominal and pelvic regions. The serosa below the diaphragm is called the peritoneum.

Processes of food digestion

Digestion is the breakdown of food into small molecules within the gastrointestinal tract. There are two processes involved in the digestion of food: mechanical and chemical digestion.

Mechanical digestion is the physical breakdown of food and begins in the mouth. Food is broken down by mastication (chewing), a process that breaks food into smaller pieces to increase the surface area of the food available to digestive enzymes. Saliva is released in anticipation of food, as well as during mastication, by the parotid, sublingual and submandibular glands. Saliva lubricates the food and makes swallowing easier. The movement of food in the mouth, enabled by the tongue, eventually results in the formation of a bolus, which is swallowed. The early stage of swallowing is a voluntary process coordinated by the brain, but the second stage is an involuntary process coordinated from the swallowing centre in the **medulla oblongata**, a specific part of the brainstem. Following a stroke, a person may have difficulties in swallowing; therefore, it is important that the swallowing reflexes of a patient who has had a stroke, such as Bessie (Patient 4.1), are assessed (usually by a speech and language therapist) before introducing fluids. The swallowed bolus of food is propelled down the oesophagus by a process known as **peristalsis** (see *Figure 7.14*), which is the movement of food

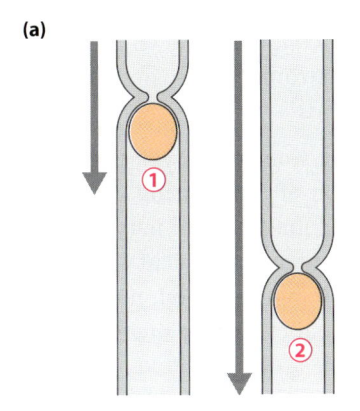

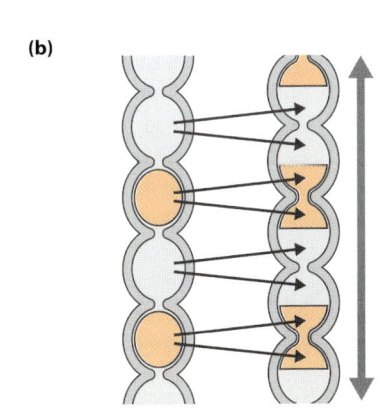

Figure 7.14 – (a) Peristalsis and (b) segmentation.
Peristalsis refers to wave-like contractions of the longitudinal smooth muscles in the gastrointestinal tract (GIT), which propels the food being digested down the GIT. Segmentation involves relaxation of the longitudinal muscles and contractions of the circular muscles at alternating sections, resulting in back and forth movement of the food in a confined area of the GIT, allowing the food to mix with enzymes; non-adjacent segments of the GIT contract and relax alternately.

in one direction from the mouth to the anal canal. Peristalsis is the involuntary contraction and relaxation of the smooth muscles of the gastrointestinal wall, resulting in unidirectional wave-like movements of the contents within the lumen. The swallowed food enters the stomach via the oesophageal–gastric (or cardiac) sphincter. The integrity of this sphincter is important, as weakness of the cardiac sphincter can result in the regurgitation of gastric contents into the oesophagus and mouth, causing symptoms of dyspepsia or heartburn. Weakness of the muscular diaphragm around the lower oesophageal sphincter can lead to part of the stomach sliding into the thoracic cavity, a condition known as hiatus hernia, which is associated with chronic reflux of gastrointestinal contents into the oesophagus called gastro-oesophageal reflux disease.

Within the stomach, food is mechanically digested by stomach movements, in a process known as churning. The mechanical digestion of food during churning is achieved by contraction of the circular, oblique and longitudinal muscles that form part of the stomach wall and is helped by the presence of leaf-like folds called **rugae** in the stomach (see *Figure 7.15*). Partially digested food, now called **chyme**, leaves the stomach via the pyloric sphincter and enters the duodenum of the small intestine.

Another mechanical process that aids digestion is **segmentation** (see *Figure 7.14*), which refers to the *back and forth* movement of food in a confined region of the gastrointestinal tract, especially within the small intestine. During segmentation, longitudinal muscles relax while circular muscles contract at alternating sections of the confined area. Segmentation allows thorough mixing of food with

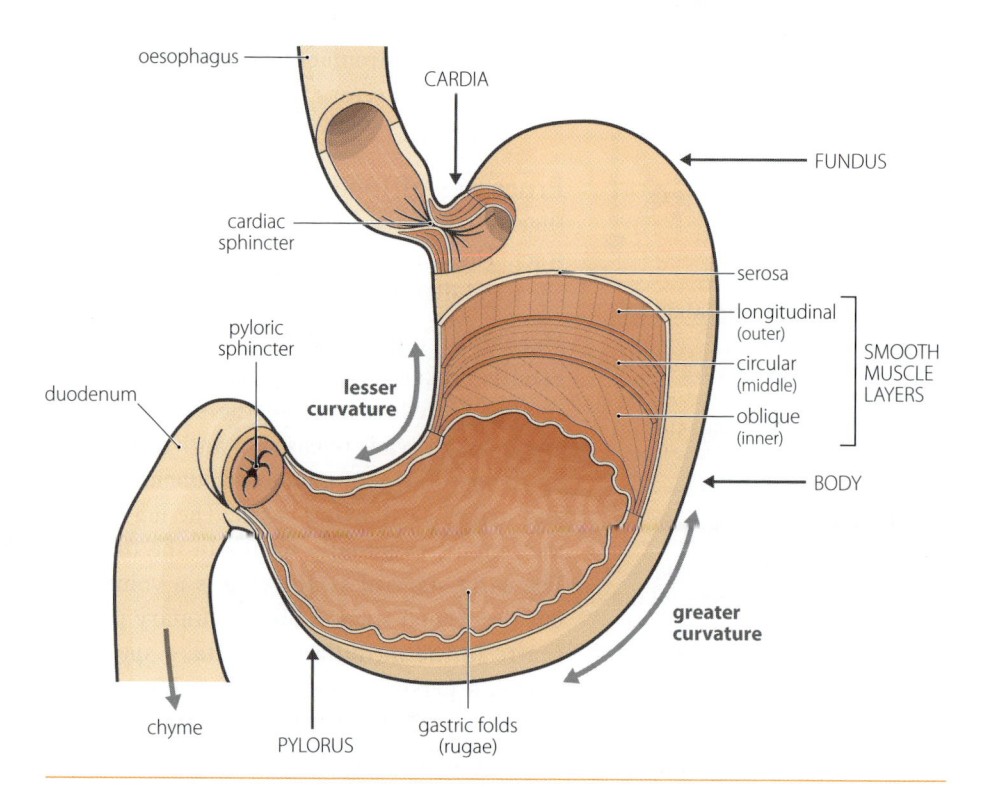

Figure 7.15 – **Diagram of the stomach showing the gross anatomy and rugae (leaf-like folds) that assist with digestion of food in the stomach.**

enzymes and maximizes the potential for absorption. Within the small intestine, bile facilitates digestion by breaking down large fat globules entering the small intestine into smaller droplets (a process called emulsification) to create a larger surface area for digestive enzymes to work on. The action of bile on fatty chyme is a physical process rather than a chemical process because the fat droplets are simply made smaller and are not chemically altered.

Chemical digestion is the breaking down of the chemical bonds in food by the action of digestive enzymes. Three main groups of enzymes break down the chemical bonds:

- **Amylases**, which break down carbohydrates.
- **Proteases**, which break down proteins.
- **Lipases**, which break down fats.

Chemical digestion of food commences in the mouth with the action of salivary amylase, which begins the digestion of carbohydrates or starch. Saliva also contains lingual lipase, which starts the digestion of fat. However, food is not in the mouth long enough for the action of either salivary amylase or lingual lipase to be very significant. There are no protein-digesting enzymes in saliva.

The action of salivary amylase is stopped by the low pH of the stomach as soon as the food enters the stomach. The presence of hydrochloric acid (HCl) secreted by **parietal cells** located in the gastric pits of the stomach in response to food in the stomach results in an acidic environment (see *Figure 7.16*). The process of HCl formation is complex, involving stimulation by the hormone gastrin and the pumping of hydrogen ions (H⁺) from the parietal cells into the stomach lumen.

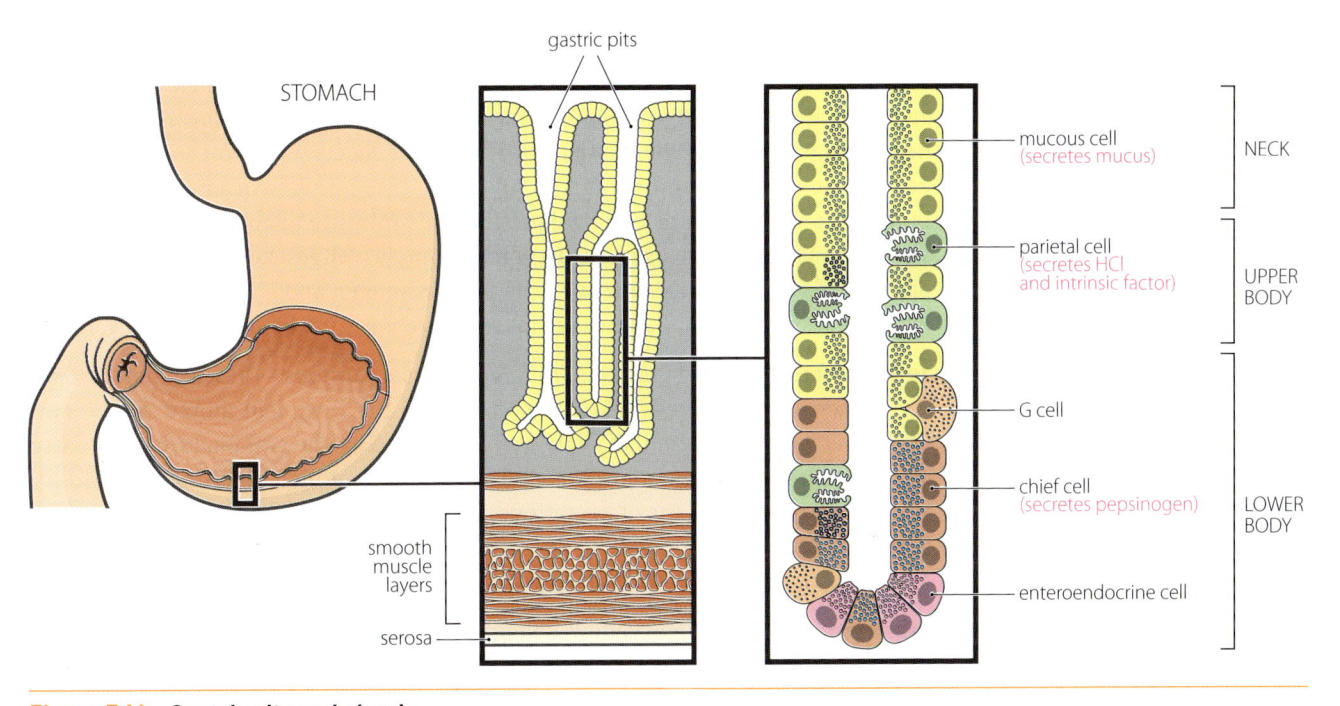

Figure 7.16 – Gastric pits and glands.
The locations of parietal cells, which secrete hydrochloric acid (HCl) and intrinsic factor, and the chief cells, which secrete pepsinogen, are shown.

For this to happen, the parietal cells contain proton pumps within the plasma membrane (see *Chapter 2*). Drugs known as proton pump inhibitors reduce gastric acid (HCl) secretion by interfering with the proton pump system in the membrane of the parietal cells. Proton pump inhibitors are used as short-term treatment for gastric and duodenal ulcers, and in the eradication of *Helicobacter pylori*. The acidic environment is essential for optimal functioning of stomach enzymes. One enzyme found in the stomach that digests protein is rennin (chymosin), which is found in large amounts in the stomach of infants and curdles milk. The other enzyme is **pepsin**, which converts proteins to **peptones**. Peptones are water-soluble molecules that result from the partial breakdown of proteins by acid and enzymes in the stomach. Pepsin is secreted in an inactive form as pepsinogen by **chief cells** (see *Figure 7.16*) located in the gastric pits and is activated by HCl. It is important for the pepsinogen to be inactive until it encounters the HCl so that the gastric mucosa is not digested. The stomach wall is protected from corrosion by gastric acid because it secretes significant amounts of mucus. The stomach mucosa is also protected by bicarbonate production and a highly adaptable blood supply. Gastric lipase is an acidic lipase that works at low pH (optimum pH 3–6) and is secreted by the chief cells of the gastric pits. The acidic lipases are more important in neonates, where as much as 50% of fat in the diet of the neonates is digested in the stomach by these two lipases. Food stays in the stomach for about 2–4 hours depending on the volume and type of food ingested, and enters the duodenum as **chyme**. Following further digestion of fats in the small intestine, a milky fluid of emulsified fats called **chyle** is produced that eventually leaves the gastrointestinal tract and enters the lymphatic vessels.

Digestion in the small intestine

The first part of the small intestine is the duodenum, the second part is the jejunum, and the third and longest part is the ileum (see *Figure 7.12*). When relaxed, the approximate length of the duodenum is 25 cm, the jejunum is 2.5 m and the ileum is 3.6 m. Within the duodenum, the chyme meets with exocrine pancreatic juices that contain bicarbonate and all of the three groups of enzymes that are required to digest the various food groups. This mixture of chyme and pancreatic secretions is referred to as chyle. Pancreatic amylase digests carbohydrates, while protease is secreted in an inactive form as trypsinogen and is activated to trypsin, which digests proteins. Pancreatic lipase actively begins the digestion of fats.

To digest fats, secretory products from the accessory organs – the liver, gall bladder and pancreas – are required. Bile secreted by the liver and stored in the gall bladder is required to emulsify fats and is released by the gall bladder when fatty chyme enters the duodenum. The hepatopancreatic sphincter (**sphincter of Oddi**), which controls the entry of secretions within the pancreatic duct and common bile duct into the duodenum, relaxes and allows bile to enter the duodenum (see *Figure 7.17*).

Bile is a dark greenish/yellow-coloured substance that contains water, bile pigments such as bilirubin and biliverdin, and primary bile acids and their salts – principally cholic acid and chenodeoxycholic acid. A variety of electrolytes, neutral fats and phospholipids are also present. The bile acids are conjugated (joined to other compounds) in the liver with the amino acids glycine and

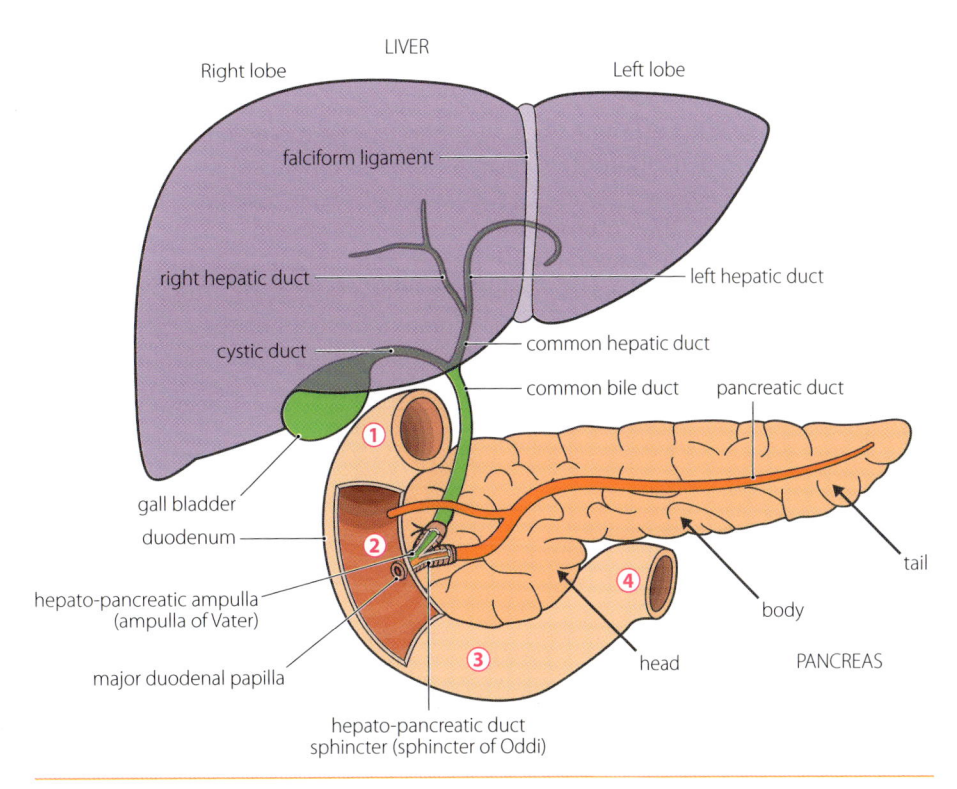

SECTION 7.2 | WHAT YOU NEED TO KNOW – ESSENTIAL ANATOMY AND PHYSIOLOGY

Figure 7.17 – **The accessory organs of the gastrointestinal tract.**
The stomach has not been shown in order for the pancreas to be seen. Although short, the duodenum can be divided into the four parts shown in this diagram.

taurine, forming glycocholic acid and taurocholic acid, respectively. These acids eventually form salts with sodium and potassium. Bile is alkaline and, together with pancreatic juices, helps to neutralize acidic chyme in the duodenum, providing a pH environment suitable for the digestive enzymes to work. Bile also gives colour to and deodorizes faeces.

Bile salts are amphiphilic molecules with two distinct surfaces: a hydrophilic surface and a hydrophobic surface. Bile salts are useful in allowing fats and water – which do not normally mix – to emulsify. Thus, the presence of bile salts changes the physical properties of the fatty chyme by emulsifying fats. Emulsification is a physical process that facilitates the formation of small droplets known as **micelles** (see *Box 7.2* and *Figure 7.18*) in which the hydrophilic heads of bile salts are on the outside of the droplet and hydrophobic tails are on the inside of the droplet. The bile salts act as a **surfactant** (surface acting agent) that stabilizes the interface between the fat and water molecules, allowing the fat material to be suspended in water as tiny stable droplets with a greatly increased surface area. This allows lipase enzymes to digest the fatty chyme more effectively and increase the rate of absorption of digested fat into the body.

Role of the accessory organs
The digestion of food would not be complete without the activity of accessory organs that secrete substances into the gastrointestinal tract to assist digestion. The accessory organs are the liver, gall bladder and pancreas (see *Figure 7.17*).

> **BOX 7.2**
>
> ### Micelles
>
> Micelles are small aggregates or tiny spheres of fat molecules less than 10 nm in diameter that form as a result of bile salts (see *Chapter 2*, *Figure 2.5c*). Bile salts have hydrophilic (water-loving) polar heads that interact with the watery chyme in the small intestine, and hydrophobic (water-hating) tails that interact with the monoglycerides and long-chain fatty acids. The micelles migrate to the brush border region of the epithelial cells and establish contact. The micelles then release their contents into the epithelial cells of the intestinal wall.
>
> **Figure 7.18.** – **Structure of a micelle.**

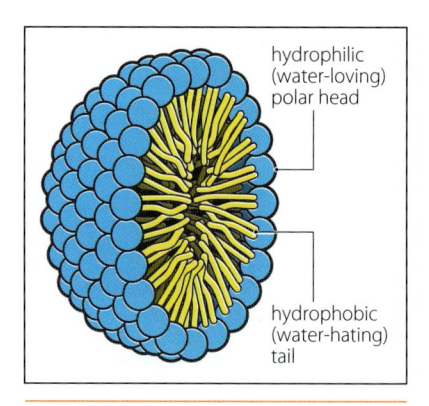

Liver

The liver is the largest abdominal organ and lies mainly in the right upper abdominal quadrant. It extends into the epigastric region and lies inferior to the diaphragm and anterior to the stomach. It is almost entirely enclosed by the visceral peritoneum with the exception of a bare area at the top.

The liver has two main lobes, the anterior left and right lobes, and two small posterior lobes known as the caudate and quadrate lobes. These two posterior lobes are considered as part of the left lobe. The left and right lobes are joined together by the **falciform ligament**, which is part of the mesentery (doubled-layer membranes and extensions of the peritoneum), which also anchors the liver to the anterior abdominal wall and to the diaphragm, lying above it. Liver cells (**hepatocytes**) form single layers (hepatocyte plates) between which are **sinusoids**, through which blood from the portal vein and its branches flows. Blood reaches the hepatocytes via the **portal venules**. This means that there is very good contact between the hepatocytes and blood. The portal vein brings blood that is rich in nutrients collected from the gastrointestinal tract. Blood flowing via the sinusoids eventually reaches the central veins, which join together to form the hepatic veins from which the blood is taken to the **inferior vena cava**. Oxygenated blood is carried to the liver by the hepatic artery, which divides to form **portal arterioles** that supply the hepatocytic plates with oxygenated blood. **Kupffer cells**, which project into the lumen of the sinusoids, are found anchored in the endothelium of the sinusoids. Kupffer cells are macrophages that have a phagocytic function. They remove worn-out red blood cells, bacteria and other debris. Several bile **canaliculi** lie next to each liver cell; these are channels or canals that drain bile into the **intralobular bile ducts**. The portal arteriole, portal venule and intralobular bile ducts form what is referred to as the **portal triad** (see *Figure 7.19*). The intralobular bile ducts join to form the left and right hepatic ducts, which eventually unite to form the common hepatic duct; this then unites with the cystic duct from the gall bladder to form the common bile duct. The hepatocytes secrete bile, which is stored in the gall bladder. The functions of the liver are summarized in *Table 7.5*.

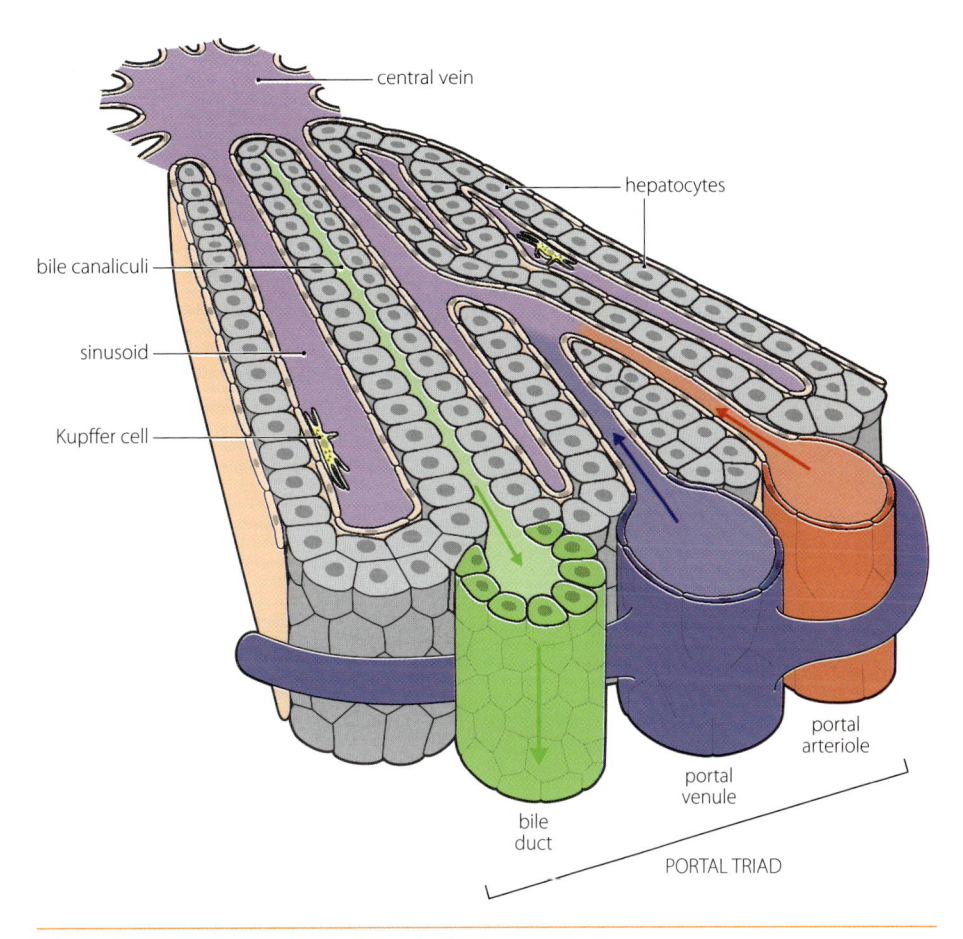

SECTION **7.2** | **WHAT YOU NEED TO KNOW – ESSENTIAL ANATOMY AND PHYSIOLOGY** 223

Figure 7.19 – Microscopic anatomy of the liver.
The central vein, portal triad, liver sinusoids, bile canaliculi and Kupffer cells are shown. The direction of flow is indicated by the arrows.

The enterohepatic circulation is involved in the recycling of cholesterol and bile from the liver via the gall bladder, through the small intestine and back to the liver again. Bile is synthesized in the liver from cholesterol. Following its synthesis, bile is stored in the gall bladder and released when fatty chyme arrives in the duodenum. From the small intestine, bile salts are recycled back into the blood and taken to the liver where they replenish the supply of bile. It has been suggested that the enterohepatic circulation occurs twice per meal and several times a day. It is important to remember that the absorption of bile acids and fats is more efficient in the ileum than in the duodenum and jejunum. This means that resection of the ileum results in inefficient absorption of fats and can lead to diarrhoea due to unabsorbed bile salts entering the large intestine.

Gall bladder
The gall bladder is a small, thin-walled sac located on the inferior surface of the right lobe. The bile formed in the liver travels along the hepatic duct to the gall bladder where it is stored. Bile is released into the cystic duct, which carries it to the common bile duct, which transports it to the duodenum. The release of bile by the gall bladder is stimulated by the hormone cholecystokinin (see *Chapter 5*)

Table 7.5 – Functions of the liver

Category	Function
Metabolic	Carbohydrate metabolism: • Glycogenesis • Glycogenolysis • Gluconeogenesis • Conversion of fructose and galactose to glucose • Conversion of glucose to fat Fat metabolism: • β-Oxidation • Ketogenesis • Synthesis of lipoproteins • Synthesis of cholesterol and phospholipids • Breakdown of cholesterol Protein metabolism: • Synthesis of plasma proteins • Production of heparin • Deamination of amino acids • Conversion of ammonia to urea Transamination reactions
Detoxification	Removal of worn-out blood cells Destruction of poisons Destruction of drugs Deamination of proteins Secretion of bile
Storage	Storage of glycogen Storage of iron Storage of fat-soluble vitamins Storage of blood

when fatty chyme arrives in the duodenum. Bile enters the duodenum to meet the fatty chyme via the hepatopancreatic sphincter (see *Figure 7.17*).

Pancreas

The pancreas is an elongated glandular organ, with a head, neck, body and tail. It lies behind the peritoneum, posterior to the stomach, and stretches transversely across the posterior abdominal wall. The head of the pancreas is expanded and lies in a C-shaped area close to the duodenum. The tail extends to lie next to the spleen in the upper left quadrant. The pancreas has both endocrine functions (see *Chapter 5*) and exocrine functions. Within the pancreas are found exocrine acinar cells (see *Figure 7.20*) containing zymogen granules, which contain the precursors of digestive enzymes, and rough endoplasmic reticulum where protein synthesis occurs. The acinar cells secrete pancreatic juices containing digestive enzymes, water, bicarbonate and other electrolytes into small ducts that connect with the main pancreatic duct to carry pancreatic juices to the duodenum. Bicarbonate is needed to neutralize the acid chyme from the stomach because pancreatic enzymes can only work at a much higher pH (more alkaline) than that found in the stomach. The pancreas produces a variety of enzymes including **amylase**, which

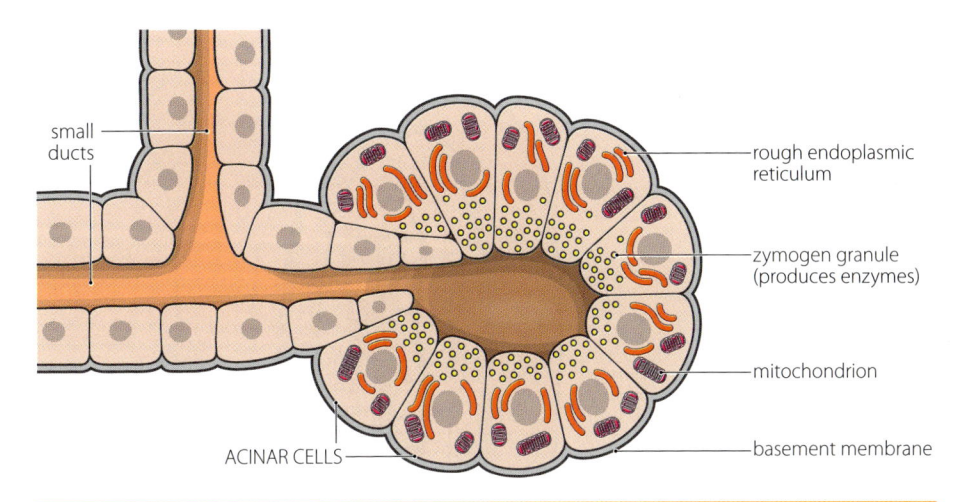

Figure 7.20 – The structure of pancreatic acinar cells showing the enzyme-producing inclusions.
Production of the enzymes that are stored in the zymogen granules occurs on the rough endoplasmic reticulum.

digests carbohydrates, lipases, which digest fats, and proteases such as **trypsin** and **chymotrypsin**, which digest protein. Amylase and lipases are secreted in an active form, while trypsin and chymotrypsin are secreted in an inactive form as trypsinogen and chymotrypsinogen, respectively, and are activated by **enteropeptidase** (also called enterokinase), a brush border enzyme produced by the cells in the walls of the duodenum. A brush border enzyme is one that is not within the intestinal lumen but is an integral protein in the plasma membrane of **enterocytes** (cells in the wall of the small intestine). Another pancreatic protease, also secreted in an inactive form, is procarboxypeptidase, which is activated by trypsin to carboxypeptidase. The secretion of pancreatic juice is regulated by the hormones secretin and cholecystokinin. Secretin stimulates the production of bicarbonate-rich juice and cholecystokinin increases the secretion of digestive enzymes. The normal end products of the digestion of carbohydrates, proteins and fats are: the simple sugars glucose, fructose and galactose; amino acids; and glycerol and fatty acids, respectively (see *Table 7.6*), and these are absorbed into the body by a variety of transport mechanisms.

Absorption of food

Small intestine

Absorption occurs throughout the small intestine, starting in the duodenum. The wall of the small intestine is structured to facilitate absorption by increasing its surface area due to the presence of circular folds (**plicae circulares**), villi and microvilli. Plicae circulares are deep folds found in mucosa and submucosa. Villi are finger-like projections of the mucosa, approximately 1 mm high, containing a rich blood supply from capillaries and lacteals (part of lymphatic drainage) (see *Figure 7.21*), while microvilli are tiny projections of the mucosal membranes that increase the absorptive surface area. Loss of microvilli increases malabsorption from the small intestine. Microvilli produce brush border enzymes such as

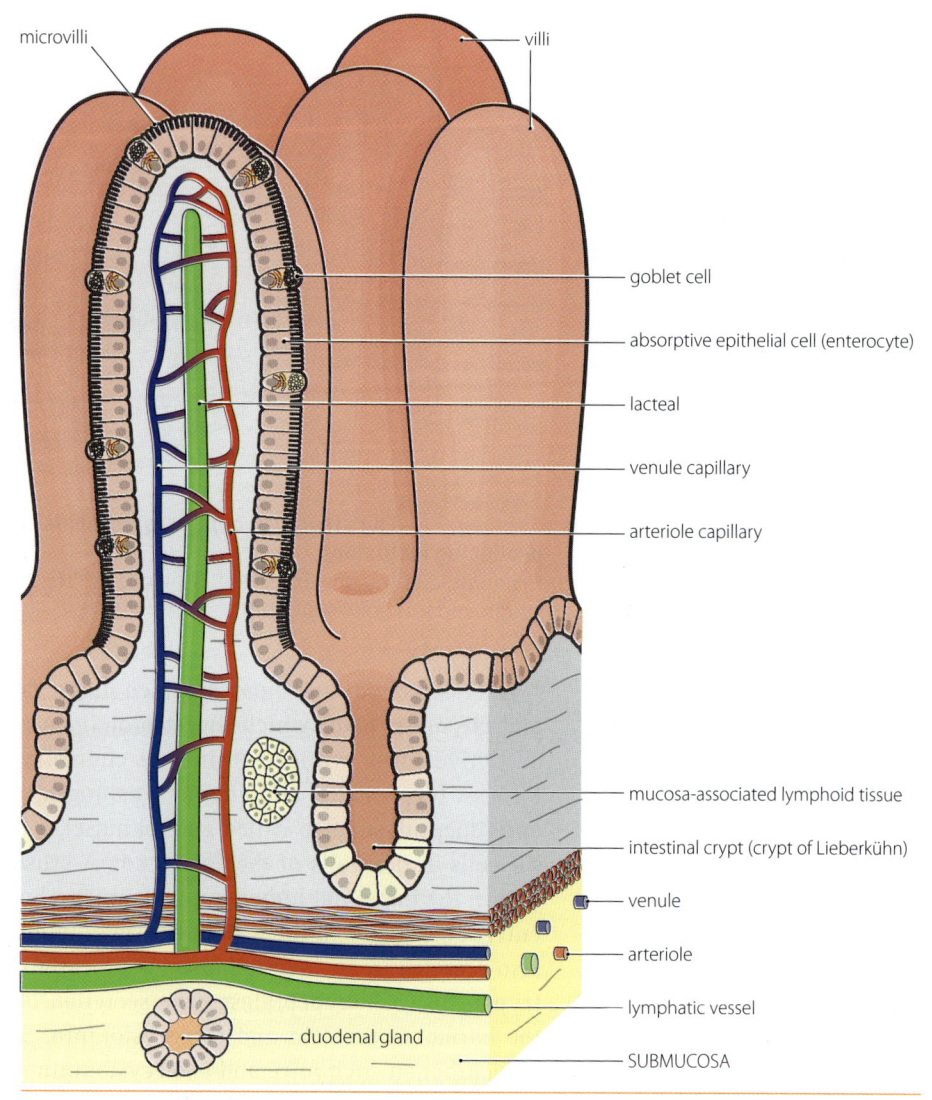

Figure 7.21 – The structure of villi.
Villi are finger-like projections found on the mucosa of the small intestine. They are about 1 mm in height and give the intestinal mucosa a velvety appearance. Each villus is densely packed with microvilli that increase the surface area and secrete brush border enzymes that complete the digestion of carbohydrates and proteins.

aminopeptidase, **carboxypeptidase** and **dipeptidase** from their membranes, which complete the digestion of proteins. They also produce **maltase**, **sucrase** and **lactase**, which complete the digestion of disaccharides, as well as **glucoamylase and dextrinase**, which complete the digestion of oligosaccharides (see *Table 7.6*).

The end products of the digestion of carbohydrates, proteins and fats, together with minerals and vitamins, are absorbed and taken to the liver for metabolism via the portal vein. Different molecules are absorbed from different parts of the small intestine by various mechanisms such as passive diffusion, facilitated diffusion and active transport (each of these mechanisms is discussed in *Chapter 2*).

Table 7.6 – End products of digestion

Food group	Enzyme group	Intermediate products	End products
Carbohydrates (polysaccharides and oligosaccharides)	Amylases • Salivary amylase • Pancreatic amylase Brush border enzymes (small intestine): • Maltase • Sucrase • Lactase • Glucoamylase • Dextrinase	Disaccharides Maltose Sucrose Lactose Oligosaccharides Oligosaccharides	Glucose Fructose Galactose
Proteins (polypeptides)	Proteases: • Rennin • Pepsin • Trypsin Brush border enzymes: • Aminopeptidase • Carboxypeptidase	Dipeptides Dipeptidases	Amino acids
Fats (triglycerides)	Lipases: • Lingual lipase • Pancreatic lipase	Diglycerides	Fatty acids Glycerol

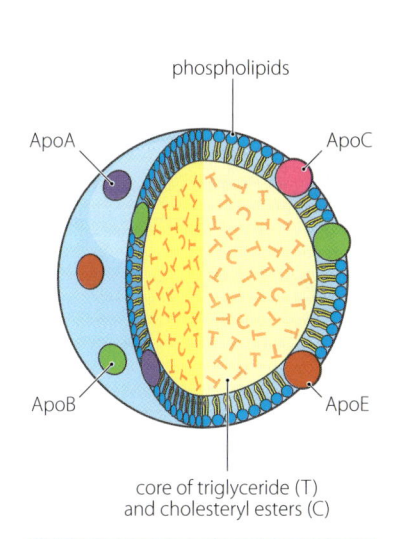

Figure 7.22 – The structure of a chylomicron.
Apolipoproteins (ApoA, ApoB, ApoC and ApoE), triacyglycerol (T), cholesterol (C) and phospholipids are shown.

Glucose and galactose are absorbed into absorptive epithelial cells (enterocytes) by co-transport with sodium ions and then transported out of the epithelial cell by facilitated diffusion, while fructose is absorbed by facilitated diffusion only. Amino acids are absorbed into enterocytes by active transport and enter the blood capillaries from the villus epithelial cell by facilitated diffusion. Approximately 90% of ingested water and 80% of electrolytes are absorbed by the small intestine.

Fats and fat-soluble vitamins are incorporated into **micelles** (see *Box 7.2* and *Chapter 2*) and diffuse into the cell by passive diffusion. Short-chain fatty acids (12 carbon atoms or fewer) dissolve in water and are absorbed into the epithelial cell of the intestinal wall by simple diffusion. They then enter capillaries and the portal vein with amino acids, glucose and other end products of digestion and are transported to the liver. Long-chain fatty acids and monoglycerides have a different fate – they become part of micelles. They then leave the micelle and enter the epithelial cell by simple diffusion once the micelle reaches the epithelial cell.

Triglycerides are reformed within enterocytes from glycerol, free fatty acids and monoglycerides. They combine with cholesterol, lecithin and phospholipids to form larger water-soluble globules called **chylomicrons** (see *Figure 7.22*) that can be excreted from the enterocytes by exocytosis (see *Chapter 2*) into lacteals (modified lymphatic capillaries within each villus). The triglycerides are then taken by lymphatic vessels to the thoracic duct. The thoracic duct delivers its contents into the neck veins (left subclavian and left jugular veins) where they enter the general circulation and are eventually taken to the liver.

Large intestine (colon)

The first part of the large intestine or colon (see *Figure 7.23*) is the *ascending colon*, which is connected to the ileum at the ileocaecal valve. A small proximal section of the ascending colon leading from the ileum forms the caecum from which protrudes the vermiform (worm-like) appendix, a vestigial structure with no apparent physiological function. The ascending colon continues upwards on the right side of the abdominal cavity until it reaches the area of the right kidney where it turns to form the hepatic flexure, which continues into the transverse colon, which travels across the abdominopelvic cavity until it reaches the left side of the abdomen where it turns to form the splenic flexure and then continues downwards as the descending colon followed by the sigmoid colon (an S-shaped part of the colon), rectum, anal canal, anal sphincters and anus. The colon has a wider diameter than the ileum. It is shortened by smooth muscles to provide pouch-like structures called **haustra** that hold the segments of remaining indigestible material that will form the faeces.

The colon does not digest food, as most of the absorption has already occurred in the small intestine. The colon does absorb water, electrolytes and some vitamins synthesized by bacteria resident in the colon, but its main function is to hold faeces.

A large variety of microorganisms are found in the colon, such as *Escherichia coli* (*E. coli*). These microorganisms, called 'normal flora' (see *Chapter 11*), are

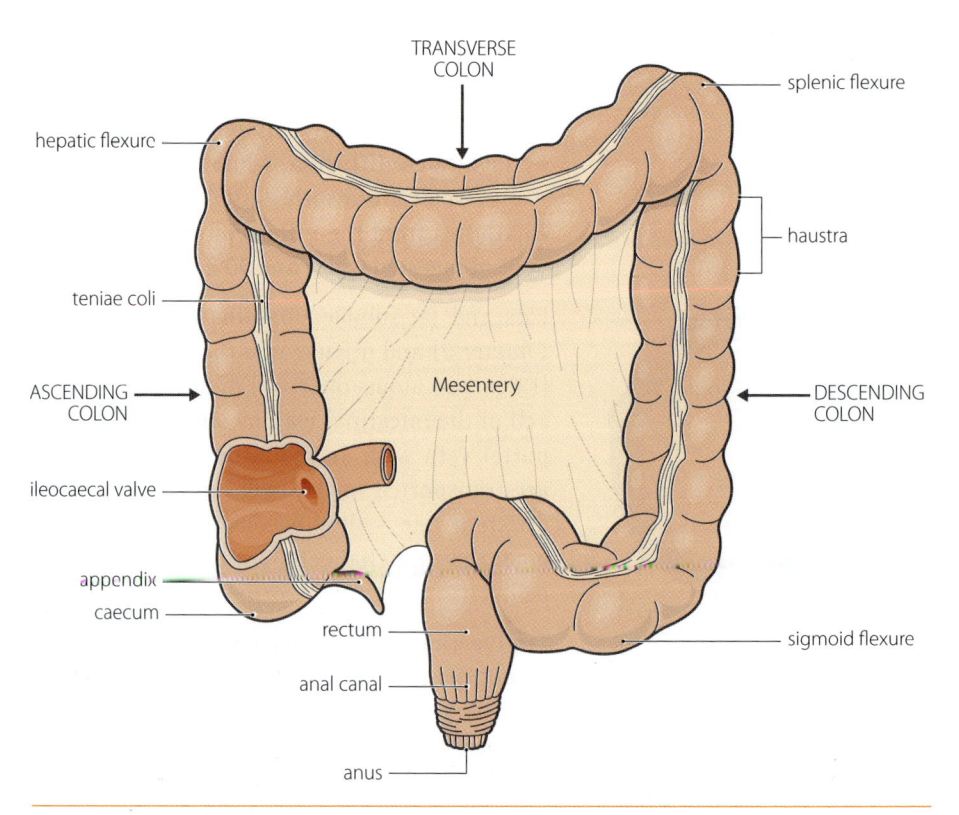

Figure 7.23 – **The large intestine.**
The mesentery and the positions of the ileocaecal valve and hepatic and splenic flexures are shown.

normally present and do not cause infection as long as they remain in the colon. Colonic bacteria digest non-starch polysaccharides (fibre), producing short-chain fatty acids such as acetic, propionic and butyric acids, which are absorbed and used as a source of energy. In addition, colonic bacteria have an immunological role by excluding pathogens from the gastrointestinal tract (see *Chapter 11*); they also synthesize small amounts of vitamin B_6 and some vitamin K (as K_2, also known as menaquinone) required by the body, and these are absorbed into the blood. Enterohepatic circulation of bile acids is facilitated by deconjugation (the removal of glycine and taurine) and conversion of primary bile acids into secondary bile acids (discussed earlier), which can be absorbed from the gut into the blood. The majority of water (approximately 90%) is absorbed from the small intestine, with the remaining 10% being absorbed from the colon. Water and fibre are important components of diet involved in avoiding constipation (see *Box 7.3*).

BOX 7.3

Constipation

Constipation is common with increasing age. Bowel movement is highly variable between individuals in that, for example, three bowel movements per day and three bowel movements per week can both be regarded as normal. Constipation can be due to either primary causes associated with diet, fluid intake and physical activity, or to secondary causes associated with diseases and drug side-effects. When smooth muscle tone decreases, peristaltic contractions become weaker and motility in the gastrointestinal tract decreases, resulting in a slow rate of faecal movement and consequently in constipation. Inadequate dietary fibre intake due to consumption of refined foods, common in the Western world, and reduced fluid intake result in constipation. This is because dietary fibre increases the bulk of faeces, while water keeps the faeces soft, so dehydration results in hard, pellet-like faeces. A daily intake of at least 18 g of insoluble fibre is recommended and all healthy adults are recommended to drink 1.5–2 L of water per day.

Gastrocolic reflex and defecation

Indigestible food residue in the colon, now called faeces, is moved along the colon by haustral contractions, which force the residue to move from one **haustrum** to another. Haustral contractions result from contractions of the smooth muscles in the wall of the colon and occur approximately every 30 minutes. Peristalsis is also involved in the movement of faeces from one **haustrum** to another towards the anus. During or following a meal, faeces in the colon move en masse due to peristalsis, a phenomenon known as **mass movement**, whereby the contents of the colon are propelled towards the rectum. The texture of the faeces and the presence of insoluble fibre, which adds bulk to the faeces, stimulate contractions of the colon. The presence of food in the stomach initiates mass movement via the **gastrocolic reflex**. Food in the stomach during or following a meal stimulates stretch receptors and chemoreceptors in the stomach wall. Enteroendocrine cells in the gastric glands within the stomach wall produce the hormone gastrin, which is transported by blood to the ileocaecal valve, causing it to open. Intestinal contents pass from the ileum into the colon, and this action leads to mass movement with haustral contractions propelling the contents of the colon from one haustrum to another. Long, slow peristaltic contractions push the indigestible material along the colon and it eventually enters the rectum.

Defecation

The end result of the gastrocolic reflex is defecation (the reflex of which is illustrated in *Figure 7.24*). Ascending pathways from the rectum to the cerebral cortex bring about conscious awareness of distension in the rectum. Rectal contractions and relaxation of the internal anal sphincter by parasympathetic motor stimulation, together with voluntary relaxation of the external sphincter, bring about **defecation**. This is facilitated by the contraction of the **levator ani** muscle, which raises the anal canal, and by the **Valsalva manoeuvre**. The Valsalva manoeuvre is when the abdominal muscles contract while the glottis in the throat closes to prevent exhalation. This increases the intra-abdominal

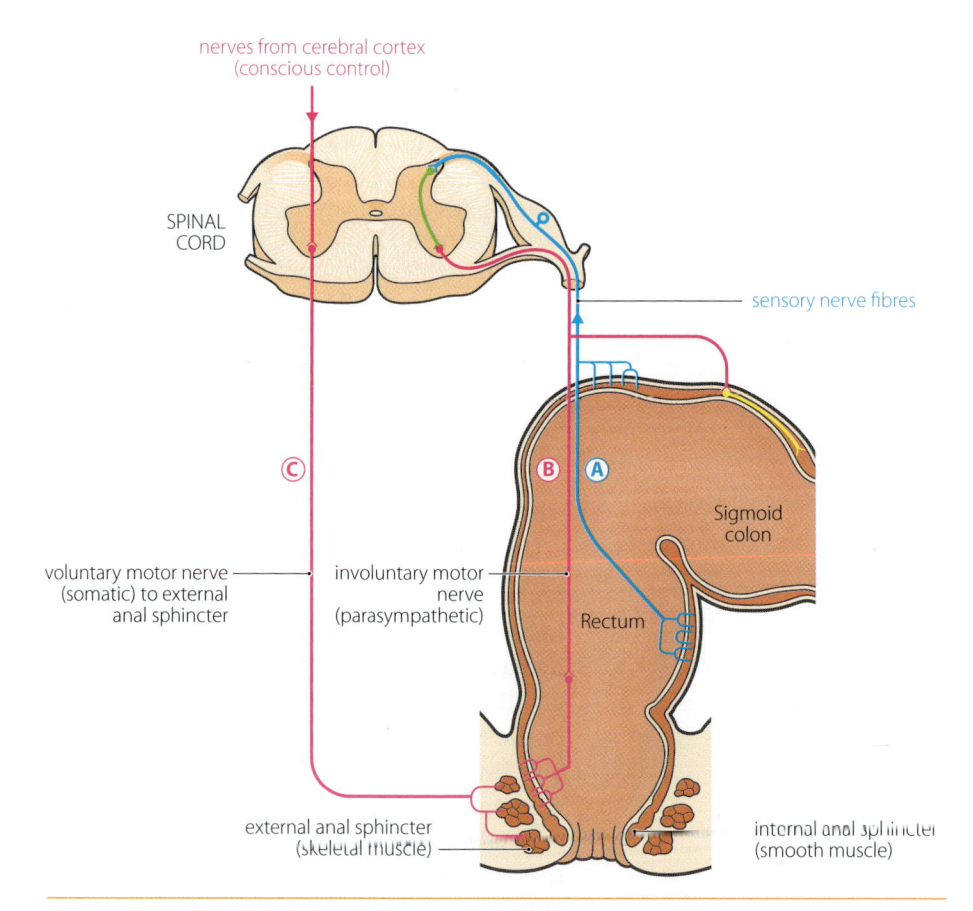

Figure 7.24 – The defecation reflex.
Mass movement of faeces into the rectum distends the rectal walls stimulating stretch receptors and initiating an involuntary parasympathetic spinal reflex that stimulates contraction of the rectal walls and relaxation of the internal anal sphincter. A, Ascending pathways from the rectum to the cerebral cortex bring about conscious awareness of distension. B, Parasympathetic motor stimulation to the anal sphincter causes rectal contraction and relaxation of the internal anal sphincter. C, The voluntary motor nerve causes voluntary relaxation of the external sphincter bringing about defecation.

pressure. Voluntary defecation is influenced by psychological and social factors and is generally regarded as a private activity; voluntary constriction of the external sphincter for the control of defecation is learned in childhood.

Metabolism of food

Metabolism represents the sum of all anabolic and catabolic processes that occur in the body (see *Figures 7.25a* and *b*). In anabolic processes, macromolecules are synthesized from simple ones utilizing energy from **adenosine triphosphate** (ATP). For example, at the cellular level, glucose molecules are joined to form glycogen in liver and muscle cells, while glycerol and fatty acids combine to form triglycerides and proteins are formed from amino acids. Anabolism is a building-up process whereas catabolism refers to the processes where macromolecules are broken down to simple ones, usually resulting in the capture of energy in the form of ATP. For example, glycogen, a storage form of glucose, is broken down to provide glucose, and this reaction produces ATP (see *Figure 7.25b*), which is used to drive the functions of all the various organs and systems of the body. ATP releases its energy when one of its bonds is broken to form **adenosine diphosphate** (ADP), which is split further to form **cyclic adenosine monophosphate** (cyclic AMP). Metabolic processes take place in many organelles of the cell (see *Chapter 2*).

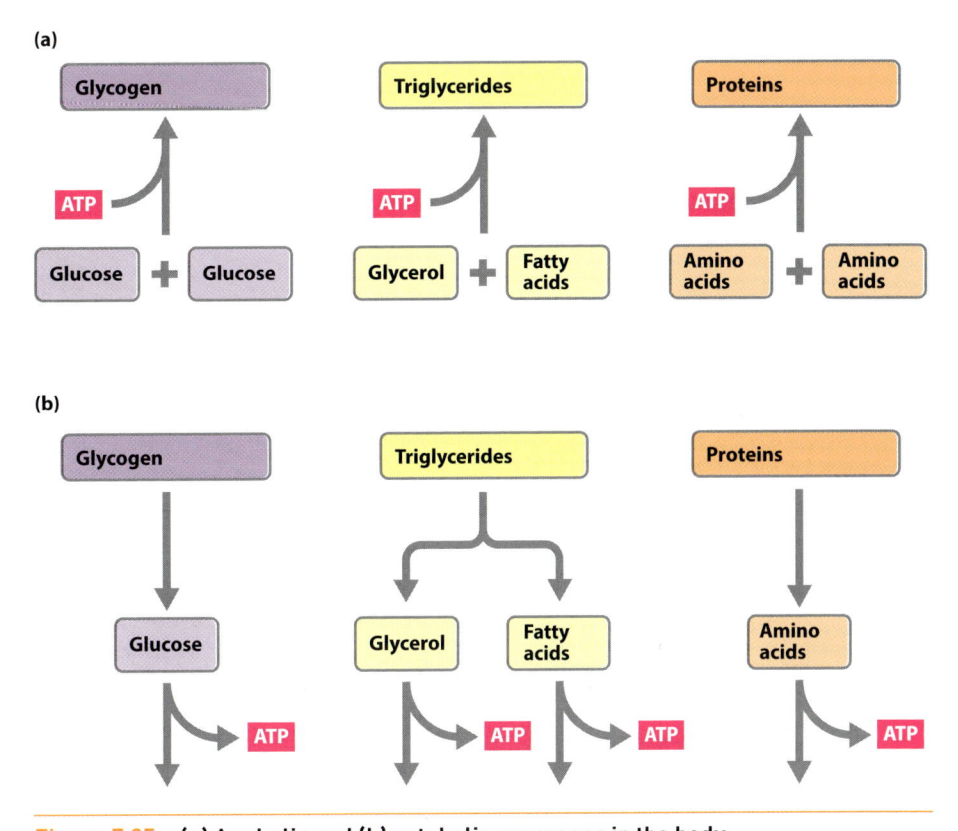

Figure 7.25 – (a) Anabolic and (b) catabolic processes in the body.
In anabolic processes, large molecules are synthesized from simple ones, while in catabolic processes, large molecules are broken down to simple ones. Anabolic processes utilize energy in the form of ATP, while catabolic processes release energy.

ATP synthesis

Glucose is the nutrient that is required to synthesize ATP. The breakdown of glucose involves three steps. First, glucose is broken down in the cytoplasm of the cell, a process called **glycolysis**. The final product of glycolysis, pyruvic acid, then enters the **tricarboxylic acid cycle (TCA cycle)**, also known as the **citric**

GLYCOLYSIS
Occurs in cytosol (cytoplasm)
Anaerobic (no oxygen)
Yields 2 ATP molecules

Glucose 6C
↓
Glucose-6-phosphate 6C
↓
Fructose-1,6-bisphosphate 6C
↓
Dihydroxyacetone phosphate 3C ⇌ Glyceraldehyde phosphate 3C
↓ Via several intermediate steps
Pyruvic acid 3C → Lactic acid (dead end) NO OXYGEN
↓
Acetyl CoA 2C
→ Citric acid 6C
→ Isocitric acid 5C
→ α-ketoglutaric acid 5C
→ Succinyl CoA 4C
→ Succinic acid 4C
→ Fumaric acid 4C
→ Malic acid 4C
→ Oxaolacetic acid 4C

TRICARBOXYLIC ACID CYCLE
Occurs in mitochondria
Aerobic (requires oxygen)
Yields 34 ATP molecules

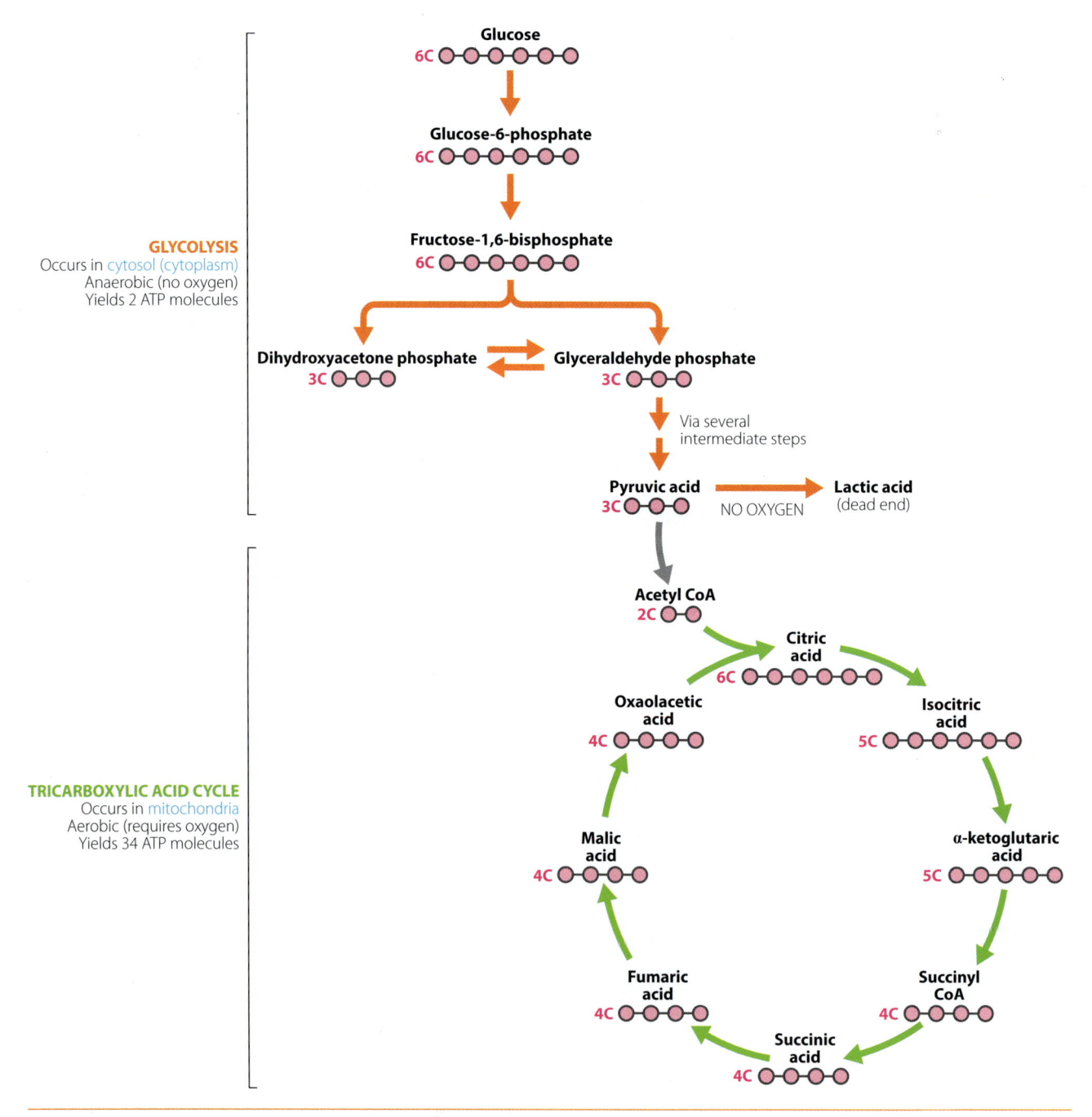

Figure 7.26 – Glycolysis and the tricarboxylic acid cycle.
Glycolysis is an anaerobic process in which each glucose molecule is broken down to two pyruvic molecules in the cytoplasm of the cell. The pyruvic acid synthesized in glycolysis enters the tricarboxylic acid cycle (Krebs cycle) in which aerobic reactions occur in mitochondria with the synthesis of ATP.

acid cycle or **Krebs cycle** (see *Figure 7.26*). The pyruvic acid is converted to acetyl coenzyme A, a process referred to as intermediary metabolism, catalysed by thiamine pyrophosphate and lipoic acid. Finally, the acetyl coenzyme A, a two-carbon compound, combines with oxaloacetate, a four-carbon compound, to form citric acid. Citric acid goes through a series of reactions, yielding ATP in the process, until it forms oxaloacetate, and the cycle repeats itself; hence the name citric acid cycle.

The final catabolic reactions that produce ATP take place in the **electron transport chain**, which is located on the mitochondrial cristae. Glycolysis is an anaerobic and inefficient process that yields a net two ATP molecules. The tricarboxylic acid cycle and the electron transport chain are, on the other hand, very efficient, yielding a net 34 ATP molecules. The metabolism of glucose in which energy is produced with water and carbon dioxide as waste products is represented by the following equation:

$$C_6H_{12}O_6 + 6O_2 \rightarrow 6H_2O + 6CO_2 + \text{Energy (ATP)}$$

It is an absolute requirement that there is enough glucose available in blood to synthesize ATP in cells. The metabolism of glucose is a good example of a catabolic reaction, as it is broken down into carbon dioxide and water during ATP synthesis. Excess glucose is stored as glycogen in the liver and muscles, while excess fats are stored as triglycerides in adipose tissue. The hormone insulin (see *Chapter 5*) is used in the anabolic processes in which both glycogen and triglycerides are synthesized. During fasting, glycogen is converted to glucose for immediate use, a process facilitated by the hormone glucagon. However, the amount of stored glycogen only lasts for approximately 12 hours, and after this time other sources of stored fuel are used. Triglycerides are broken down to glycerol and fatty acids, both of which can be converted to glucose, which is utilized by the normal processes to form ATP. In prolonged starvation when fat reserves are depleted, protein stored in muscle is used to provide glucose. The protein is catabolized to amino acids and the carbon skeletons of the amino acids are used to synthesize glucose by a process known as **gluconeogenesis**. Gluconeogenesis is a process by which glucose is synthesized from non-carbohydrate sources such as amino acids and fatty acids. Malnutrition results in patients utilizing their fat reserves and if malnutrition persists, lean (muscle) tissue is broken down to amino acids, resulting in weight loss. This can be a problem in hospitals if patients do not eat properly.

7.3 Clinical application

Food plays an important role in healthy living, and the act of eating fulfils social, cultural, psychological and biological roles, while the nutrients consumed ensure that the physiological, immunological and biochemical needs of the human body are met (see *Figure 7.27*). A varied, adequate diet in the right proportions ensures that these needs are met. However, what is often forgotten is the important relationship between healthy nutrition and a well-functioning gastrointestinal tract. Disorders of the gastrointestinal tract that result in poor digestion of food and malabsorption of nutrients can affect health significantly due to malnutrition,

234 CHAPTER 07 | WHY FOOD IS NEEDED: THE CHEMICAL BASIS OF HEALTH

while loss of integrity of the epithelial barrier of the lower gastrointestinal tract causes diarrhoea (see Sumina, Patient 2.2) and dehydration.

- Amy (Patient 1.1) has an eating disorder that has led to inadequate consumption of food and inappropriate behaviours; this has resulted in significant weight loss and a low BMI. Amy needs help to enable her to change her behaviours in relation to how she views her body, so that she can adopt appropriate eating behaviours and gain weight to reach a healthy BMI.

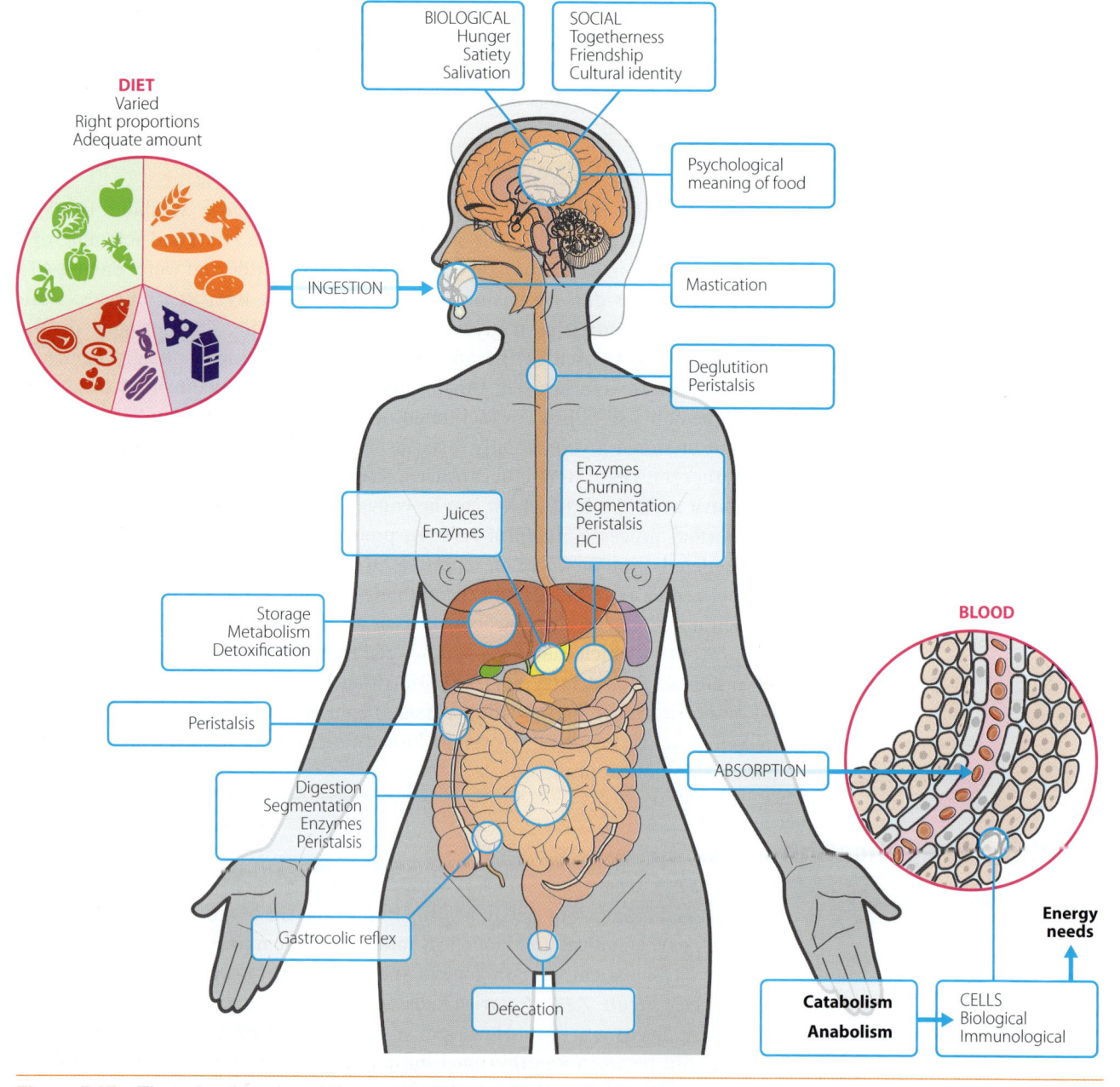

Figure 7.27 – The role of food, and the mechanisms and processes involved.
The biopsychosocial uses of food and the processes involved in making food available to cells are indicated.

- **Francine (Patient 1.3)** suffers from Crohn's disease, which can result in diarrhoea, abdominal pain and scarring in the small intestine and colon. Crohn's disease leads to malabsorption of nutrients.
- **Sarah (Patient 3.1)** has cystic fibrosis, which has affected the production of exocrine pancreatic juices that contain the enzymes she needs to digest the food she eats. Sarah will have to take capsules that help her digest food with every meal she eats for the rest of her life.
- **David (Patient 5.1)** is obese and has type 2 diabetes mellitus. Obesity is a risk factor for other health conditions. David needs to change his eating habits so that he can reduce his energy intake and lose weight. David also has an underactive thyroid gland for which he is receiving treatment.

Patient 1.1 — Amy — 1 | 20 | 194 | **235** | 447 | 473

- 18-year-old woman
- BMI 16.3
- Downy hair on face and arms
- Referred to eating disorder clinic
- Eating under supervision to increase intake and also getting psychological support
- Also anaemic

Amy's story illustrates the need for adequate energy provision in the diet. Inadequate food consumption and energy intake due to eating reduced quantities of food followed by purging behaviour and abuse of laxatives have resulted in Amy breaking down her own fat mass and lean tissue to provide her with energy. Inadequate consumption of food is likely to affect the proportion of nutrients consumed by Amy, and her purging behaviour and use of laxatives limit the absorption of nutrients. Laxatives reduce transit time, resulting in food being in the gastrointestinal tract for a very limited amount of time, insufficient for nutrients to be absorbed from the small intestine. Prolonged starvation has resulted in the breakdown of the fat that Amy needed to give her energy. It is also possible that Amy is breaking down some of her muscle in order to provide her with energy. Breaking down fat and then muscle protein is what happens when a person has been starving for some time. The fatty acids are converted to ketones, while the glycerol is converted to glucose by gluconeogenesis. Both the ketones and the glucose are used by the brain and red blood cells, two tissues that have priority for energy in the body. Amy's body is undergoing an adaptive process in order to conserve energy (similar to **hibernation**) due to weight loss, emaciation, slowed metabolism and low body temperature. As described in *Chapter 1*, the loss of body fat resulted in Amy developing lanugo-like body hair and caused her cortisol levels to rise due to the stress her body was experiencing. Amy has been helped by being encouraged to eat the foods she likes and to take liquid supplements so that she can gain weight. Supervising Amy after meals ensures that the food she has eaten has sufficient time to be digested and absorbed, while psychological support enables discussions that have been making her view her relationship with food and her body image differently.

Patient 1.3 — Francine — 2 | 21 | 194 | **235** | 338 | 371

- 40-year-old woman
- Crohn's disease – on steroids
- Presents with inflamed bowel and anaemia
- MRSA screen ahead of potential surgery

Francine suffers from Crohn's disease, which affects different parts of the small intestine and colon, especially the ileum and ascending colon. When Francine has relapses, she suffers from diarrhoea (sometimes with blood) and abdominal pain, with nausea and vomiting on occasions. Due to the relapses, Francine is

- TPN given IV to recovery during relapse
- Positive MRSA screen – decolonized over 5 days

likely to have protein energy malnutrition and may have deficiencies in calcium, magnesium, iron, zinc, folate, vitamin B_{12}, vitamin C and fat-soluble vitamins. In the long term, Crohn's disease can result in scarring leading to strictures of the ileum; this may result in resection of the ileum as an intervention. Both the disease process and resection of the ileum lead to malabsorption, especially of bile, fatty acids and fat-soluble vitamins that are part of micelles. Resection of the ileum causes more malabsorption than resection of a similar length of the jejunum. When the unabsorbed bile salts reach the colon, they minimize the absorption of sodium and water, resulting in diarrhoea. Diarrhoea is the abnormal passage of loose or liquid stools with increased frequency of three or more times a day. Diarrhoea can occur at any age, and the consequences can be very severe, especially in children and vulnerable older adults. Loss of fluid leads to dehydration and loss of electrolytes can lead to death if these are not replaced. It is important to recognize that there are many causes of diarrhoea (see *Box 7.4*) that include infections (see *Chapter 1*), gastrointestinal diseases, hereditary conditions (see *Chapter 3*), endocrine conditions (see *Chapter 5*) and some drugs such as laxatives. Francine finds that during periods of relapse, taking steroid medication, such as prednisolone and budesonide, as well as antibiotics (metronidazole and ciprofloxacin) helps. Francine's last relapse has resulted in her admission to hospital. Her anaemia is being treated and she is receiving total parenteral nutrition (TPN) to enable her intestines to rest. Although enteral nutrition is the preferred feeding route, Francine is being given all the nutrients she needs via a central catheter inserted in the right subclavian vein and threaded into the right superior vena cava, with the tip of the catheter lying close to the heart. She is receiving approximately 2500 kilocalories per day from intravenous solutions of dextrose and lipid emulsions, amino acids, vitamins, macro and trace elements. Lipid emulsions will provide Francine with half her energy needs but it is important to remember that it is difficult to maintain energy needs via TPN for long periods. Francine will remain on TPN until a decision is made whether she needs surgery or not. Should a decision be made for her to have surgery, small bowel resection may be done.

Causes of diarrhoea

- Infections, e.g. bacteria (*Campylobacter*, cholera, *Escherichia coli*, *Salmonella*, *Staphylococcus* and *Shigella*), viruses, protozoa and worms
- Diseases, e.g. diverticular disease, cystic fibrosis (exocrine pancreatic failure), inflammatory bowel disease, lactase deficiency, malabsorption
- Drugs, e.g. laxatives
- Iatrogenic
- Surgery (small bowel resection)

BOX 7.4

Patient 3.1 | Sarah | 60 | 94 | 195 | **237** | 311 | 333

- 17-year-old girl
- CF diagnosis at age of 1 year via a sweat test
- Frequent admissions for chest infections affecting breathing
- PERT added to meals to help digest her food

Sarah is 17 years old and has cystic fibrosis. One of the consequences of cystic fibrosis is the production of thick, sticky secretions that block pancreatic juices containing the three enzymes needed to digest food in the duodenum. Sarah has no protease, amylase and lipase (PAL) enzymes to help her digest the food she eats, and as a result, she takes capsules of Creon, which contain pancreatin, a mixture of protease, amylase and lipase. PAL enzymes complete the digestion of food to produce the end products of digestion. Without Creon, Sarah would not be able to benefit nutritionally from the food she eats, which would result in semi-digested food and clay-coloured stools with a very offensive smell. The production of such stools containing semi-digested food is known as **steatorrhoea**.

Patient 5.1 | David | 138 | 161 | 195 | **237** | 448 | 474

- 44-year-old man
- Increased urine output; thirsty and hungry
- Blood test: low thyroxine and raised blood glucose
- Has hypothyroidism and the start of a goitre
- Given levothyroxine; dose adjusted until thyroxine levels stabilise
- Has diabetes associated with obesity – diet modified and given metformin
- The levothyroxine helps him to metabolize food better

David is an example of excess energy intake, while Amy (Patient 1.1) is an example of insufficient energy intake. David works in an environment where food is plentiful. Availability increases voluntary food intake. David's energy intake has been much higher than his energy expenditure for a long period, resulting in weight gain and obesity (BMI of 35.92 kg/m^2) (see *Table 7.7*) with the development of type 2 diabetes mellitus (see *Chapter 5*). Obesity is a risk factor for the development of a variety of chronic health problems including cardiovascular disease, high blood cholesterol, atherosclerosis, high blood pressure, joint problems, infertility and cancer. The current increase in childhood and adult obesity due to the consumption of foods high in saturated fats and decreased activity is a cause of concern. If obesity rates in children continue to increase at current rates, the number of people suffering from the chronic health problems described will be much higher, leading to problems in meeting the health needs of the population and strained health services. As David is receiving treatment for his underactive thyroid, this will help him to metabolize food more efficiently, which should help him with weight management.

Table 7.7 – BMI in adults according to the World Health Organization (WHO) and National Institute for Health and Care Excellence (NICE) Classification

BMI (kg/m^2)	Classification
<18.5	Underweight
18.5–24.9	Normal
25–29.9	Overweight
>30	Obese
>40	Morbidly obese

This chapter has explained the reasons why food is needed in the human body. Many nutrients enable the formation of body structures such as the skeleton that forms the framework of the body, and the soft tissues that attach to the skeleton.

In addition, food provides the energy that powers the many physiological and biochemical activities of the body at cellular level, including body defence, in order to maintain homeodynamics. However, for the nutrients to be available, the food has to be digested to simpler forms that can be absorbed from the lumen of the small intestine into the blood, which transports the nutrients to cells where they are metabolized. It is important that the food consumed in the diet is varied, in the right proportions and in adequate amounts. Failure to do this means that the diet will be deficient in some nutrients, resulting in malnutrition, as indicated by the four patients discussed in this chapter. Both weight loss and weight gain, resulting in anorexia nervosa and obesity, respectively, are forms of malnutrition in relation to energy intake supplied by the macronutrients, and both lead to ill health. Deficiencies in micronutrient intake result in many deficiency diseases as well as a variety of other diseases and conditions. Thus, the importance of food in the homeodynamics of body processes should not be underestimated.

7.4 Summary

- Food is at the centre of life because it is biologically essential; it also has important social and psychological roles (see *Figure 7.27*).
- The food that is consumed in the diet needs to be varied, in the right proportions and in adequate amounts for health (see *Figure 7.1a*).
- Energy cannot be created or destroyed but can be transformed from one form into another (see *Table 7.1*).
- Once consumed, food provides chemical energy in the form of ATP, which drives all the activities in the body (see *Figures 7.25* and *7.26*).
- Inadequate consumption of food results in weight loss and body wasting, as in anorexia nervosa (Amy, Patient 1.1), while excessive consumption of food results in obesity, as is the case for David (Patient 5.1).
- For food to be useful to the body, it has to be digested and absorbed into the blood in order for the nutrients to become available at the cellular level.
- Absorption of food occurs in the small intestine and is facilitated by the presence of structures known as villi (see *Figure 7.21*), which increase the surface area for absorption, and by bile, which helps to break down fats.

7.5 Further reading

The British Nutrition Foundation website gives information on the basics of nutrition that have been covered in this chapter, including all the components of foods; it also gives tips on healthy eating and how to achieve a healthy, varied diet. It participates in nutrition health programmes such as nutrition in schools: www.nutrition.org.uk/

The National Diet and Nutrition Survey (NDNS) is a cross-sectional survey that assesses the diet, nutrient intake and nutritional status of the general population from 18 months upwards, living in private households. It uses interviews, a 4-day dietary diary, bloods and urine samples to make the assessment:
http://tinyurl.com/AandP7a *(takes you to* https://www.gov.uk/government/statistics/national-diet-and-nutrition-survey-results-from-years-1-to-4-combined-of-the-rolling-programme-for-2008-and-2009-to-2011-and-2012)

This World Health Organization (WHO) document gives indicators and a Framework for the Global Monitoring of Maternal, Infant and Young Child Nutrition:
www.who.int/nutrition/topics/en/

The Cystic Fibrosis Trust website gives information on the disease and offers support to families who have children recently diagnosed with cystic fibrosis. It explains the causes of cystic fibrosis, what it is like to live with the illness and how care is delivered in the UK:
www.cysticfibrosis.org.uk/

7.6 Self-assessment questions

Answers can be found at www.scionpublishing.com/AandP

(7.1) Select the one correct answer. Which of the following is not a function of proteins?
- (a) To act as catalyst
- (b) To act as coenzymes
- (c) To function as hormones
- (d) To defend the body against pathogens
- (e) To act as carrier molecules

(7.2) Select the one correct answer. An essential amino acid is:
- (a) one that is needed to synthesize proteins
- (b) one that is needed to make enzymes
- (c) one that is synthesized in the body
- (d) one that has to be taken in the diet
- (e) one that comes from animal proteins

(7.3) Select the one correct answer. Which monosaccharides make up the disaccharide sucrose?
- (a) Glucose and galactose
- (b) Galactose and fructose
- (c) Glucose and glucose
- (d) Glucose and lactose
- (e) Glucose and fructose

(7.4) Select the one correct answer. Which fats are implicated in the causation of diseases such as coronary heart disease and diabetes mellitus?
- (a) Monounsaturated fats and high-density lipoproteins
- (b) *Cis* fats and polyunsaturated fats
- (c) *Trans* fats and saturated fats
- (d) *Trans* fats and monounsaturated fats
- (e) *Cis* fats and monounsaturated fats

(7.5) Mark each statement either true or false:
- (a) The chief cells in the gastric pits secrete hydrochloric acid.
- (b) Trypsinogen and chymotrypsinogen are activated by enteropeptidase.
- (c) The synthesis of glucose from non-carbohydrate sources is called glycolysis.
- (d) The falciform ligament joins the left and right side of the liver lobes.
- (e) Bile is synthesized in the gall bladder.

normal range. Indeed, on one occasion the level of urea in Marcus's blood was 16 mmol/L (normal range: 2.5–7.5 mmol/L) and the level of creatinine was 200 μmol/L (normal range: 60–125 μmol/L). Marcus's treatment is managed through regular visits to a hospital department specializing in renal medicine. Chronic kidney disease is a condition that is typically asymptomatic in the early stages. Marcus is prescribed medication for his kidney disease and receives advice from a renal dietician about how he can manage his diet to best control his condition.

As a healthcare professional, you may come across people like Marcus who have a health problem affecting the ability to preserve equilibrium between fluid compartments and to maintain fluid and electrolyte balance. Knowledge of the behaviour of water and electrolytes in the body is important to help you understand the significance of body water volume and alterations in the solute concentration in the blood, and the resulting risks to health.

8.2 What you need to know – essential anatomy and physiology

8.2.1 Water and electrolytes

Cells of the body both contain and are surrounded by water (see *Chapter 1*). Water molecules are composed of hydrogen and oxygen atoms. A water molecule is described as a polar molecule because the protons within the nucleus of the oxygen atom exert a greater pull on the electrons of the two hydrogen atoms, resulting in a slight positive charge on one side of the molecule and a slight negative charge on the other (see *Chapter 2, Box 2.2*). It is this fact that provides water with its unique properties, making it absolutely essential for life (discussed in *Chapter 2*); these are summarized as follows:

- Water is a universal solvent – a huge variety of solutes necessary for life dissolve in it. The type of substances that can dissolve are determined by the polar nature of water.
- Water is a good transport medium and takes part in a number of different chemical reactions.
- Water molecules move across the plasma membrane via osmosis (see *Chapter 2*).

Water molecules hold themselves together weakly through the attraction of adjacent positive and negative charges. These weak bonds are constantly being broken and reformed; this dynamic property enables water to remain a fluid at physiological temperatures and makes it an ideal medium in which substances can dissolve. Chemical substances such as salts, acids and bases dissolve in water to form **ions** in solution (atoms or molecules with either a positive or a negative charge), and because these are able to conduct electricity, they are also called **electrolytes**. Electrolytes with a positive or a negative charge are termed **cations** and **anions**, respectively. Ions have a number of roles in the body. One example is the movement of sodium (Na^+) and potassium (K^+) ions across plasma membranes to produce action potentials, which lead to nerve impulse generation and muscular contraction (see *Chapter 4*). Some specific roles for individual electrolytes are given in *Table 8.1*.

Table 8.1 – Examples of electrolytes and their roles within the body

Electrolyte	Role within the body
Sodium (Na^+) (the main extracellular and most abundant ion)	The main contributor to the osmotic potential of extracellular fluid and thus important in the movement of water between fluid compartments by osmosis. Active transport across the cell membrane via the Na^+/K^+ pump ensures polarization of nerve cell membranes and hence the potential propagation of an action potential (see *Chapter 4*). Contributes to fluid balance and blood pressure regulation through the renin–angiotensin–aldosterone system (RAAS).
Chloride (Cl^-)	A key contributor, along with sodium, to the osmotic potential of extracellular fluid and thus important in the movement of water between fluid compartments. Involved in adjusting the pH of body fluids together with other ions, for example HCO_3^- exchange, known as the 'chloride shift' (see *Chapter 10*). Constituent of hydrochloric acid in the stomach.
Potassium (K^+) (the main intracellular ion)	Active transport across the cell membrane via the Na^+/K^+ pump ensures polarization of nerve cell membranes and hence the potential propagation of an action potential (see *Chapter 4*). This is particularly important in cardiac and skeletal muscles.
Calcium (Ca^{2+})	Combines with phosphate ions to form calcium phosphate, one of the main constituents of bone and teeth. Movement of calcium ions across muscle and nerve cell membranes is associated with muscle contraction and nerve conduction, respectively. Required in the clotting cascade, which culminates in the formation of fibrin.
Phosphate (PO_4^{3-})	Combines with calcium ions to form calcium phosphate, one of the main constituents of bone and teeth. Acts as a buffer in body fluids by binding to hydrogen ions, thus maintaining the pH of body fluids. Essential in the formation of adenosine triphosphate (ATP).
Hydrogen (H^+)	Determines the acidity or pH of body fluids. Hydrogen ions have a major effect on cellular enzyme activity. The concentration of hydrogen ions must be precisely regulated and the pH of extracellular fluid is maintained in the range 7.35–7.45.
Bicarbonate (HCO_3^-)	Acts as the main chemical buffer in extracellular fluid, with the aim of resisting changes in pH when acid is added. Bicarbonate ions bind to hydrogen ions released from a strong acid to form a weaker acid, thus maintaining the optimal pH of body fluids.

The levels of substances dissolved and transported in body fluids, such as electrolytes, are affected by sources of gain, storage and loss. Electrolytes such as sodium, which is the most abundant extracellular cation, are gained through ingested food. Another abundant mineral, calcium, is stored as calcium salts in the matrix of bone and teeth. Calcium is required within cells and in extracellular fluid, as well as in bone. To enable its movement and to regulate the levels of these compounds between the body compartments, it is essential that calcium and all other substances are carried in solution. Excess electrolytes are excreted, especially via the kidneys.

The amount of water in the body is increased by the ingestion of fluids and food containing water. Water is also generated via cell metabolism. Water is lost from the body via urine and faeces, sweat and insensible losses, which are defined as losses that cannot easily be measured such as water vapour in expired air.

The balance between water and solute concentration in the body is very important for health, as this affects the volume of cells in all tissues (*discussed later in this chapter*). Osmosis is the movement of solvent (usually water) from an area of high solvent concentration, across a semi-permeable membrane, to an area of low solvent concentration. This has been described fully in *Chapter 2*. The solvent concentration of a solution is determined by its solute concentration – as the amount of solute increases, there is a necessary and corresponding decrease in solvent concentration. Traditionally, the concentration of a solution is described in terms of its solute concentration, which is determined by the number of particles dissolved in the solution. The number of particles is measured in moles. A mole contains a specific quantity of particles (6.022×10^{23}, otherwise known as the Avogadro constant), which is useful as it provides a standard measure that can be used to compare concentrations of different solutions; for example, a 1 molar solution contains 6.022×10^{23} particles in 1 L, which would be written as 1 mol/L or 1 M. Molar concentrations (known as the molarity) are used in healthcare when describing the concentrations of different solutes in the body (see *Chapter 1, Table 1.1*). For example, the normal range of fasting glucose concentration in the blood is between 4.0 and 5.9 mmol/L (there are 1000 millimoles in 1 mole).

The molar concentration, however, is not always sufficient to describe the process of osmosis. Whereas a 1 M solution of glucose contains 1 mole of particles, a 1 M solution of sodium chloride will dissociate into 1 mole of Na^+ and 1 mole of Cl^-, effectively doubling the concentration of particles. This is because sodium chloride is an electrolyte and glucose is a non-electrolyte. As a result, we use a different unit of concentration, the **osmole**:

Number of osmoles in a solution =
number of moles × number of particles into which the solute dissociates

The number of osmoles in a solution is important in terms of describing the process of osmosis, and the number of osmoles in 1 L of solution is the **osmolarity** of that solution. Sometimes the term **osmolality** is used instead of osmolarity. Osmolality is the number of osmoles in 1 kg of solution rather than in 1 L.

Note that one term refers to the *volume* of a solution and the other to the *weight* of the *solvent* that substances are dissolved in. In clinical settings, the term osmolarity is usually used. Osmolality is commonly used in laboratory settings, when reporting clinical investigations and in physiology texts. Osmolality is expressed as milliosmoles (mOsm) per kg of water. Normal plasma osmolality ranges from 285 to 295 mOsm/kg of water. The kidneys have an important role in maintaining the osmolality and overall volume of body fluids by regulating the excretion of water (solvent) and solutes.

The concentration of the fluid inside the cell (intracellular fluid) is the same as the concentration of the fluid outside the cell (extracellular fluid). These fluids are **isotonic**, which means that, although solute and solvent are exchanged across the cell membrane, there is no net movement between the two. When patients receive intravenous fluids as part of their care, these are typically isotonic, which is very important as they mix with plasma, which contains blood cells. Thus, isotonic fluids can be added to blood without influencing the movement of fluid by osmosis. If **hypertonic** (more concentrated) fluid was given intravenously, then water would move out of the blood cells by osmosis and the cells would shrink, develop a notched surface and become crenated. If **hypotonic** (less concentrated) fluid was given intravenously, then water would move into the blood cells by osmosis, causing them to swell and burst (see *Chapter 2, Figure 2.10*). It is therefore vital that patients are given isotonic intravenous fluids, such as 0.9% sodium chloride (also known as normal saline).

8.2.2 Functions of the kidney

Fundamentally, the role of the kidney is to accept solutes from the plasma and produce urine to maintain plasma osmolality within a normal range. Every day in healthy adults, the kidneys filter as much as 180 L of plasma, enabling the removal of waste products and ensuring that water balance is maintained. In fact, the kidneys have a number of major functions including:

- regulation of body fluid osmolality within the range 285–295 mOsm/kg of water
- regulation of blood pressure
- regulation of electrolyte balance
- regulation of the acid–base balance of extracellular fluid within the range pH 7.35–7.45
- excretion of metabolic waste products and harmful substances such as urea
- production and secretion of hormones including renin and erythropoietin
- contribution to vitamin D metabolism.

To enable these functions to take place, both kidneys have an excellent blood supply, receiving approximately 25% of the output of blood from the heart (approximately 1.25 L/minute).

Gross anatomy of the kidney

A section of a kidney is shown in *Figure 8.1*. The outer surface of the kidney is covered in a capsule made of connective tissue. Below this lies the **renal cortex**, which is a red colour; lying deeper to this, where the colour changes to a more reddish brown, is the **renal medulla**. The medulla contains discrete cone-shaped structures called renal pyramids. The apex of each pyramid, the papilla, points internally towards the centre of the kidney. The renal pyramids have a striped appearance because they are formed by bundles of urine-collecting ducts. The outer cortex extends inwards between the pyramids, forming areas called renal columns. The renal **nephron** – the functional unit of the kidney that makes urine – spans the renal cortex and medulla, and the tubules of many nephrons pass, a number of times, between the two. Beyond the cortex and medulla lies a cavity called the renal sinus in which are found the renal artery and vein, renal lymphatic vessels, renal nerves and also a flat funnel-shaped structure called the renal pelvis, which directs urine into the ureter. Urine reaches the renal pelvis

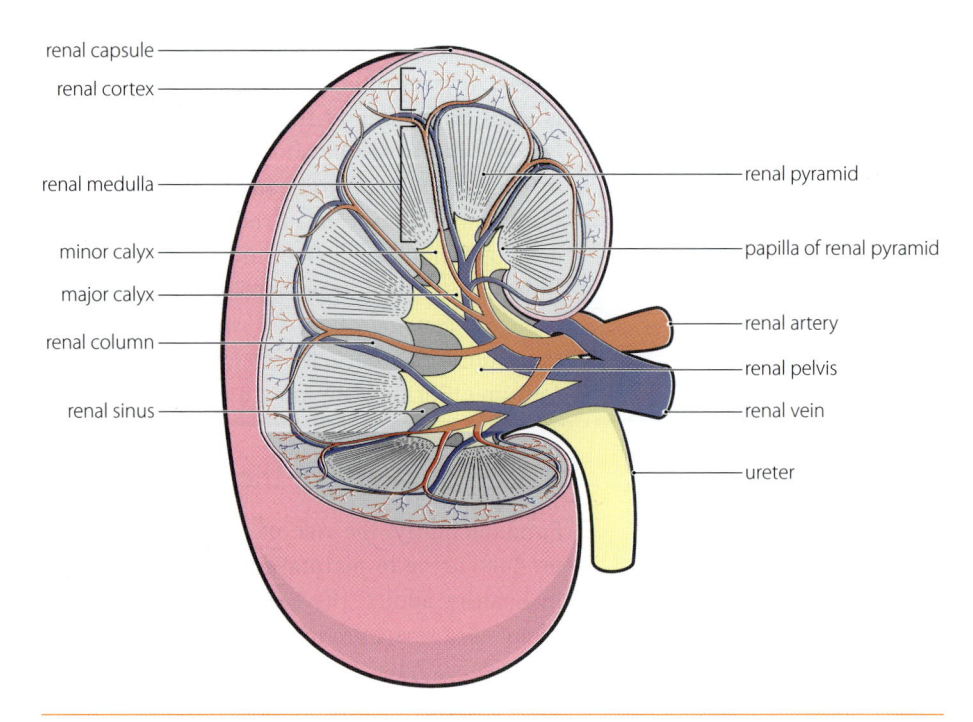

Figure 8.1 – **The gross anatomy of the kidney (sagittal view).**

from the collecting ducts of the nephron by first draining through ducts in the papilla of the renal pyramids and then through a set of ducts called calyces. Urine then drains from the renal pelvis into the ureter from where it flows to the bladder due to the squeezing peristaltic contractions of the muscle wall of the ureter.

Ureters and urinary bladder

The **ureter** from each kidney drains urine into the bladder (see *Figure 8.2*). The inner mucosal layer of the ureter, comprising transitional epithelium, produces mucus to protect the epithelial cells from the variable solute and pH concentrations that exist in urine. The middle muscularis layer contains longitudinal and circular smooth muscles responsible for peristalsis. The final outer layer or adventitia consists of fibrous connective tissue. Each ureter is approximately 25–30 cm long, entering the bladder at an oblique angle to create a physiological valve. Thus, as urine fills the bladder and bladder pressure increases, the opening to the ureter is compressed, preventing the backflow of urine upwards towards the kidney.

The **urinary bladder** itself is composed of four layers – the mucosa, submucosa, muscularis and adventitia (serosa). The inner mucosal layer is important because the arrangement of the transitional epithelium allows the cells to slide over each other as the bladder distends, therefore preventing disruption of the internal mucosa. When the bladder empties, the mucosa becomes arranged in folds called rugae; these disappear as the bladder fills. There is a triangular area of the mucosa at the base of the bladder called the trigone that has no rugae and is relatively fixed in its position (see *Figure 8.2*). This area lies between the openings of the two ureters and the urethra and contains a large number of stretch receptors. The bladder trigone is very sensitive to being stretched as the bladder fills, and

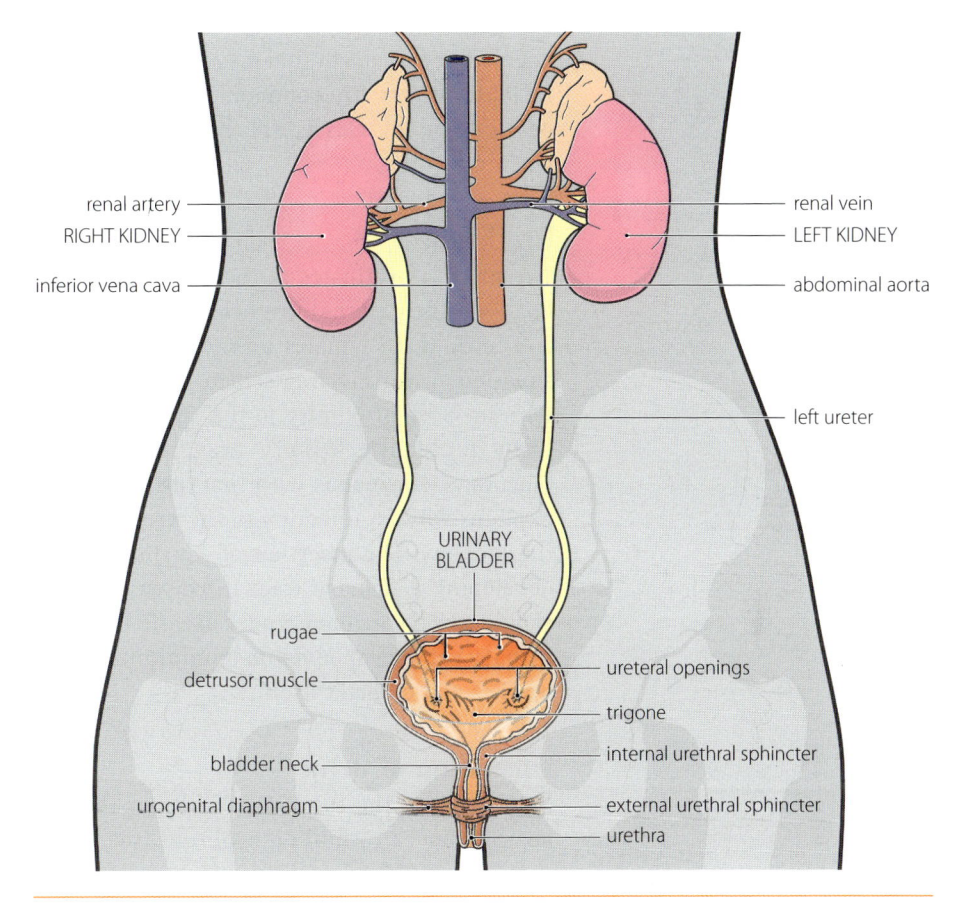

Figure 8.2 – **The female urinary system (anterior view).**

inflammation of this region can cause the symptoms of **cystitis**. The muscularis layer of the bladder, called the **detrusor muscle**, is composed of longitudinal and circular muscle fibres, with the circular muscle layer sandwiched between inner and outer longitudinal muscle fibres. The bladder is therefore able to shorten both its length and diameter when contracting, which facilitates its complete emptying. The sandwiched middle layer of circular smooth muscle also forms the internal urethral sphincter at the base of the bladder (see *Figure 8.2*). This acts as a valve, allowing urine to either leave or remain in the bladder. Contraction of the detrusor muscle mechanically pulls the sphincter open, allowing urine to leave the bladder and enter the urethra, whereas relaxation of the detrusor muscle keeps the sphincter closed and urine within the bladder. The outer layer of the bladder, the adventitia (serosa) is a fibrous connective tissue layer.

The internal urethral sphincter is made of smooth muscle and lies at the bladder–urethral junction, and below this, continuous with the urogenital diaphragm, is the external urethral sphincter. The urogenital diaphragm is a triangular sheet made up of three layers: a middle layer of skeletal muscle sandwiched between two layers of fascia. The external sphincter is thus made of skeletal muscle and is under voluntary motor control. The levator ani muscles of the pelvic diaphragm or pelvic floor, when contracted, also maintain closure of the external sphincter. The pelvic floor supports the positions of the pelvic organs and helps to resist any downward movement that may occur as a result of increasing intrapelvic pressure. Intrapelvic pressure commonly increases during coughing, and weakness of the pelvic floor muscles is associated with the development of stress incontinence when coughing.

Urethra

The urethra originates at the neck of the bladder and conveys urine out of the body via the external urethral opening or meatus. The urethra is approximately 3–4 cm long in females and 20 cm long in males, where it has the additional function of transporting semen. The short length of the female urethra combined with its close proximity to the opening of the anus means that women are more likely to acquire urinary tract infections compared with men. The urethral mucosa is continuous with that of the bladder, ureters and renal pelvis, and this explains why an infection in the urethra can ascend the urinary tract and affect the kidneys. The insertion of a urinary catheter increases the risk of a person developing a urinary tract infection; therefore, insertion of a urinary catheter should always be done under aseptic conditions and the care of a person with a urinary catheter should aim to minimize the risks of microorganisms entering the urethra and catheter itself.

Formation of urine

Nephrons are the functional units of the kidney, with each kidney containing approximately 1.2 million nephrons (see *Figure 8.3*). Nephrons consist of two key components: blood vessels, which deliver blood, and tubules, which receive the fluid portion of blood and then process this into urine. The arrangement of the blood vessels and tubules is very close to one another in order to facilitate the movement of water and solutes between them, thus maximizing the efficiency of urine formation.

Urine formation involves three major processes:

- glomerular filtration
- tubular reabsorption
- tubular secretion.

Glomerular filtration occurs within a mass or 'tuft' of capillaries called a glomerulus, enclosed in a cup-like structure called the **Bowman's (glomerular) capsule** (see *Figures 8.3* and *8.4*). Filtration occurs across the endothelial cells that make up the glomerulus and the epithelial cells of the Bowman's capsule. Only a portion of the blood arriving at the glomerulus is actually filtered; the remainder continues to circulate. If all the blood was filtered, it would become too viscous to move along the blood vessels.

The pressure for filtration is provided by the hydrostatic pressure of the blood arriving at the glomerulus (see *Figure 8.4*). The arrangement of cells between the glomerulus and the Bowman's capsule form the filtration membrane, comprising pores and slits that allow the filtration of the fluid portion of blood. The pores are found between the endothelial cells of the glomerular capillary wall and are

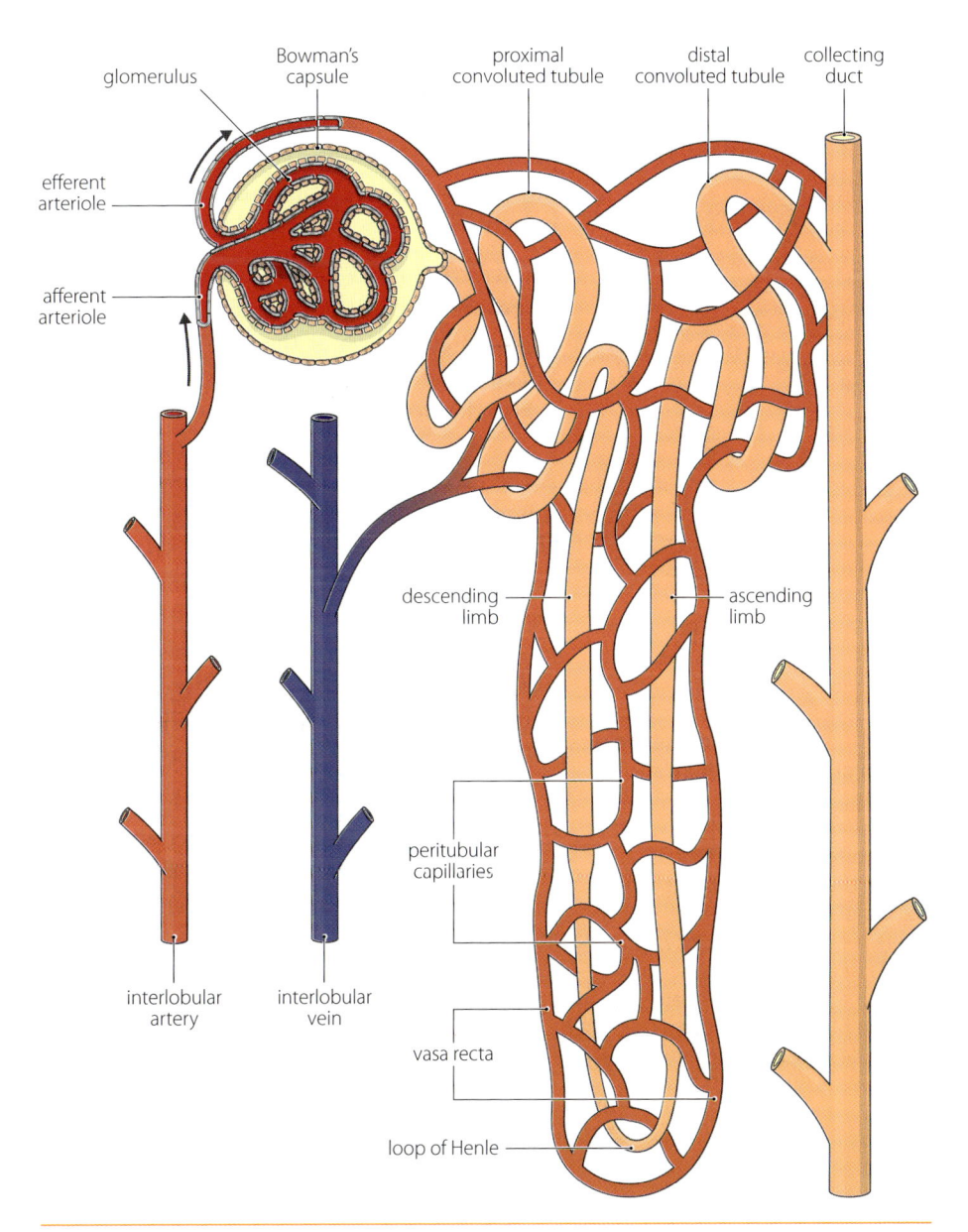

Figure 8.3 – **The nephron.**

also known as fenestrations; the slits are found between the cells (podocytes) of the inner layer of the Bowman's capsule. Sandwiched between the two layers is a basement membrane, also containing pores. Thus, the filtration membrane is composed of three layers, which solutes have to cross to access the lumen of the Bowman's capsule. The structure of the filtration membrane, with its pores and slits, ensures that only solutes below a fixed size are able to pass across the membrane. This means that small molecules such as water, electrolytes and glucose pass readily into the Bowman's capsule, while larger molecules such as plasma proteins, with a high molecular mass, and blood cells do not. Keeping the plasma proteins within the blood is useful because it ensures that not all water is lost from the blood, as the plasma proteins contribute to the **oncotic pressure** (the

Afferent arteriole
Efferent arteriole
Bowman's capsule
Proximal convoluted tubule

→ Glomerular hydrostatic pressure
→ Blood colloid osmotic pressure
→ Filtrate hydrostatic pressure

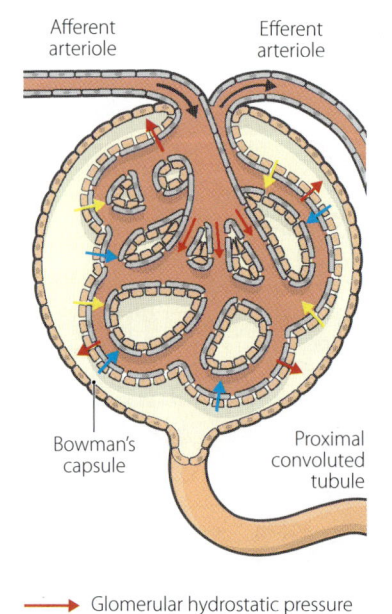

Figure 8.4 – Forces across the glomerular and Bowman's capsule.
The driving force pushing water and solutes from the blood across the filtration membrane is glomerular hydrostatic pressure. Significant opposing forces are the hydrostatic pressure of the ultrafiltrate and the blood colloid osmotic pressure. The net filtration pressure is 10 mmHg.

osmotic pressure achieved by plasma proteins alone) and the retention of water by osmosis. In healthy kidneys, blood cells and proteins should never appear in the urine. Blood in the urine (called haematuria) and protein in the urine (called proteinuria) are indicative of possible urogenital disease. The fluid that enters the Bowman's capsule, containing only low-molecular-weight solutes, is called an **ultrafiltrate**.

An effective renal blood pressure and optimal renal blood flow are necessary to ensure that filtration and urine production occur. As the kidneys receive approximately 25% of the cardiac output, disruption to renal blood flow and a fall in blood pressure (hypotension) can lead to impairment of renal function. (It is also the case that chronic hypertension can impair renal function – see *Box 8.3* and Marcus, Patient 8.1). Hydrostatic pressure generated by the blood pressure is the driving force behind the movement of substances out of capillaries, and this also applies to capillary beds in other parts of the body (discussed under capillary fluid exchange in *Chapter 9*). In addition to hydrostatic pressure, osmotic pressure also influences the movement of water molecules between the capillaries and tissue spaces (called oncotic pressure in this context). The physiological relationship between these two pressures in regulating the movement of fluid to and from circulating blood is discussed further in *Chapter 9* (*Figure 9.18*). The balance of opposing forces in the glomerulus and Bowman's capsule limits the volume of water and solutes that becomes the ultrafiltrate.

It is important to remember that when taking into account the effects of all of the pressures on the movement of water and solutes, the net result is water and solutes being forced across the filtration membrane into the Bowman's capsule. This is called the net filtration pressure, which when measured equates to approximately 10 mmHg (illustrated in *Figure 8.4*). This is achieved by the fact that the hydrostatic pressure is largely maintained along the glomerular capillaries with only a relatively small reduction in pressure. The high hydrostatic pressure is maintained by renal blood pressure and blood flow, and by the pressures maintained in the afferent and efferent arterioles entering and leaving the glomerulus, respectively. The afferent arteriole supplies the glomerulus with blood and the efferent arteriole receives blood leaving the glomerulus (see *Figure 8.4*). The efferent arteriole has a smaller lumen compared with the afferent arteriole, effectively resisting the flow of blood out of the glomerulus and therefore maintaining the hydrostatic pressure within the glomerulus.

The **glomerular filtration rate (GFR)** is the rate of ultrafiltrate formation. GFR represents the amount of fluid filtered from the plasma into the Bowman's capsule per unit of time and is equal to the sum of the filtration rates of all functioning nephrons. GFR is determined by the surface area of glomeruli over which filtration can take place (this is approximately 1.73 m^2), the permeability of the filtration membranes and the net filtration pressure. Typically, the surface area of the glomeruli and permeability of the filtration membranes are both constant, but the net filtration pressure can vary depending on a person's hydration status, blood pressure and age. As an example, a high blood pressure will result in an increase in GFR, whereas a low blood pressure will reduce it. Also, after the age of 30 years, GFR typically declines. However, this decline usually does not adversely affect either the kidneys' excretory function or the ability to maintain osmolality or electrolyte and acid–base balance. The typical GFR adjusted for body size is similar in men and women, varying between 100 and 130 ml/minute/1.73 m². Significant alterations in the GFR can be a useful indicator of kidney disease.

Tubular reabsorption represents the movement of solutes from the filtrate back into the plasma and is an essential step following filtration that allows the composition (volume and concentration) of plasma to be adjusted and remain within the optimal range. The first site for this is the **proximal convoluted tubule** (PCT) (see *Figure 8.3*). The PCT is surrounded by an intimate network of peritubular capillaries that receive blood from the efferent arteriole of the glomerulus (remember that the blood within this arteriole has been filtered and depleted of some of its water and so has an increased osmolality). The capillary network and convoluted arrangement of the tubule together with microvilli on cells of the tubule increase the surface area available for efficient reabsorption to occur.

In the normal kidney, the PCT reabsorbs approximately 67–80% of the filtered water, most of the Na⁺, Cl⁻, K⁺ and bicarbonate ions (HCO_3^-) and all of the glucose and amino acids. The driving force for the reabsorption of water is the osmotic gradient across the tubular cells, created by blood with an increased osmolality (hyperosmolar) flowing into the peritubular capillaries from the efferent arteriole. Passive movement of a variety of solutes and water back into the blood also occurs by diffusion and osmosis, because the PCT is highly permeable to water and a variety of solutes. Fluid in the PCT and in the capillaries is separated by the cells of the PCT, the interstitial fluid between those cells and the capillary walls. As illustrated in *Figure 8.5*, tubule cells are described as having a luminal membrane, which is in contact with the filtrate in the PCT lumen, and a basolateral membrane, which is in direct contact with the interstitial fluid. Using the movement of Na⁺ as an example, Na⁺ passes across the luminal membrane of the tubule cell, usually coupled to the transport of other solutes such as glucose. This is facilitated by a co-transport protein located in the plasma membrane and is referred to as secondary active transport. Na⁺ is then actively pumped out of the tubule cell into the interstitial fluid, against the concentration gradient, by a Na⁺/K⁺ pump, resulting in a higher concentration of sodium within the interstitial fluid than in the blood of the peritubular capillaries. Na⁺ then diffuses out of the interstitial fluid into the capillary. The movement of Na⁺ creates an electrochemical gradient, which causes negatively charged Cl⁻ to follow the Na⁺. The overall effect is to add to the osmotic gradient between the plasma in the peritubular capillaries and the filtrate, so that water molecules follow the solutes into the capillaries by osmosis. As water is obliged to follow the solutes, this form of water reabsorption is often referred to as obligatory water reabsorption (see *Figure 8.5*). The efferent arteriole receives hyperosmotic blood (following filtration from the glomerulus to the Bowman's capsule) and then forms the peritubular capillaries. This then provides an osmotic pressure difference, which facilitates the reabsorption of water back into the blood, described in more detail later in this chapter.

Both glucose and amino acids are reabsorbed with Na⁺ via secondary active transport mechanisms. Secondary active transport, or co-transport, is where substances move across the membrane as an indirect result of primary active transport. The active transport of Na⁺ out of the cells of the PCT produces a

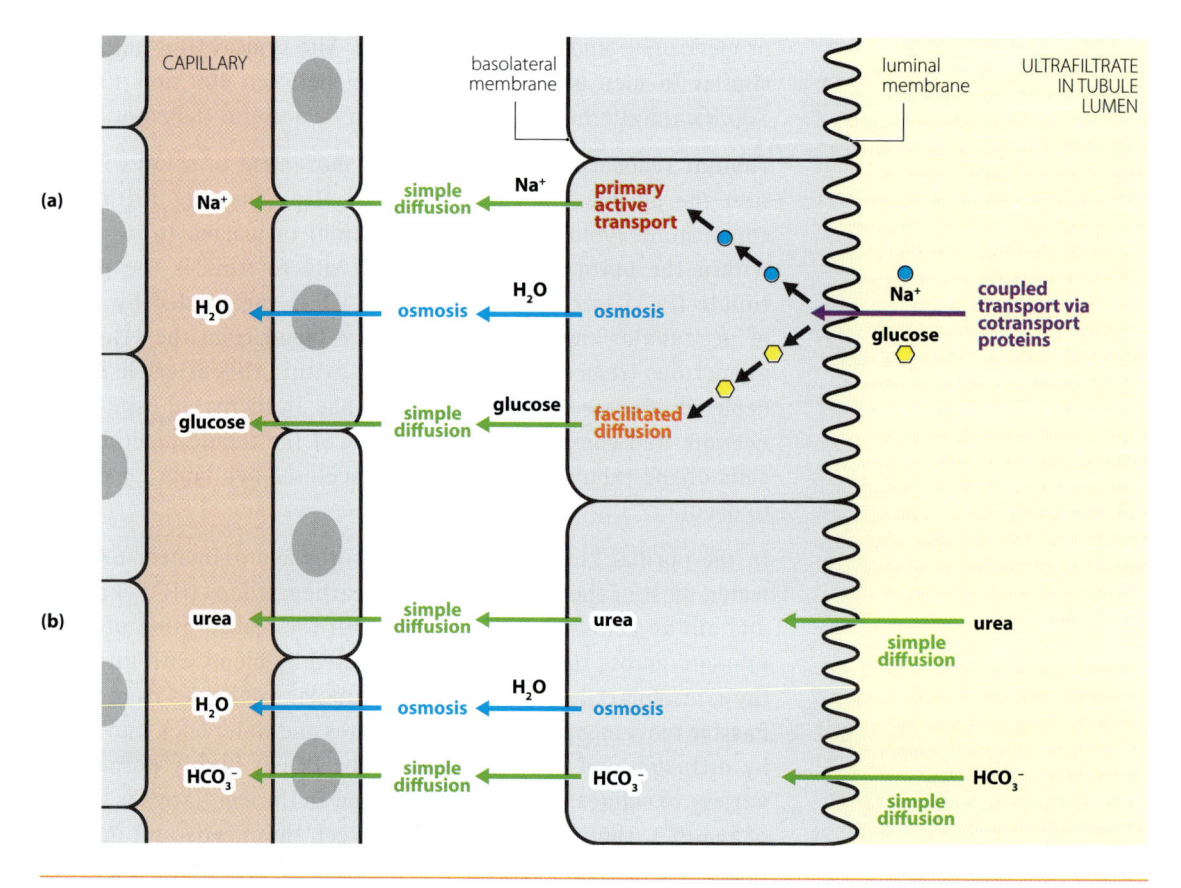

Figure 8.5 – **Reabsorption of (a) sodium, glucose and water and (b) urea and bicarbonate ions in the proximal convoluted tubule.**
Note the luminal and basolateral membranes of the tubule cells, which substances need to cross before passing into the capillary via osmosis and simple diffusion.

gradient of Na+ across the plasma membrane. This electrochemical gradient is used to co-transport another molecule.

With regard to the reabsorption of glucose, there are a finite number of co-transporter proteins in the PCT cell membranes, and once they are saturated with glucose and Na+ their ability to increase the rate of transport reaches a maximum. In optimal health, these proteins are never saturated because the level of glucose in the plasma entering the nephron is kept within the normal range by the action of the hormones insulin and glucagon (discussed in *Chapter 5*). The number of co-transporter proteins present on the luminal membrane is optimal to cope with the load of filtered glucose that enters the PCT. If the level of glucose in the filtrate exceeds the capacity of the finite number of co-transporter proteins to transport glucose, then they will become saturated. Excess glucose will remain in the filtrate and will be excreted in urine. This is detected as **glycosuria** on urinalysis (urine testing). In this case, the amount of glucose in the filtrate will have exceeded the **renal threshold** for glucose. This occurs in uncontrolled diabetes mellitus, when a high level of blood glucose is filtered into the PCT. Elevated glucose in the filtrate has a secondary consequence in that it increases the solute concentration of the filtrate, effectively lowering its water concentration; as a result water moves, via osmosis, from the plasma into the filtrate, causing the production of large volumes of dilute urine (**polyuria**) and *increased* osmolality of plasma, resulting in a feeling of thirst (**polydipsia**). Polyuria and polydipsia are two of the clinical features classically associated with the disease diabetes mellitus (see David, Patient 5.1).

The **loop of Henle** consists of the straight part of the PCT – the descending thin limb, which ends in a tight bend or 'loop', and the ascending thin limb, which becomes the thick limb as it approaches the distal tubule (see *Figures 8.3* and *8.6*). Nephrons are classified as cortical and juxta-medullary nephrons; with the latter type, the loop of Henle dips into the medulla of the kidney (see *Figure 8.6*). This is important as these nephrons are able to produce urine of varying concentration because they penetrate the medulla, which has an increasing osmolality with depth. The excretion of dilute and concentrated urine requires normal function of the loop of Henle. Under normal circumstances, the excretion of water is regulated separately from the excretion of solutes. This occurs in the loop of Henle and in particular in the thick ascending limb. The permeability of the tubule cells to water and solutes varies along the loop of Henle and in the **collecting duct** (see *Figure 8.3*), and the concentration of solutes (Na^+, Cl^- and urea) in the interstitial fluid surrounding the loop of Henle and peritubular capillaries in the medulla is maintained at a high level. In other words, the intramedullary interstitial fluid has an increased osmolality and this is maintained by **countercurrent mechanisms**, which are based on the anatomical arrangement of the loop of Henle and the associated capillaries called the **vasa recta** (see *Figures 8.3 and 8.6*).

The descending thin limb is highly permeable to water, which is reabsorbed by diffusion, so that when the filtrate reaches the ascending limb it is highly concentrated. The filtrate remains concentrated as it passes up the thick ascending limb, which is *completely impermeable to water* and urea, but Cl^- is actively transported from the filtrate into the interstitial fluid (see *Figure 8.6*). Na^+ follows passively by diffusion and the filtrate becomes more diluted. This is because the removal of Na^+ and Cl^- (solutes) from the tubule fluid increases the water (solvent) concentration *relative* to the solute within the tubule fluid. This process can occur because the high osmotic gradient in the renal medulla is maintained by the movement of Na^+ and Cl^- and also by the presence of urea in the intramedullary fluid, having moved by diffusion from the collecting ducts.

As illustrated in *Figure 8.6*, the descending loop of Henle carries filtrate down from the cortex of the kidney to the medulla, while the parallel ascending loop of Henle carries filtrate upwards from deep in the medulla to the cortex. The flow of filtrate in one limb is counter (or opposite) to the flow of filtrate in the other limb and this is the basis of the countercurrent mechanism. The vasa recta also consists of a descending portion and ascending portion. Blood flows in opposite directions in the descending and ascending vessels. This again is countercurrent flow and contributes to the maintenance of the increased osmolality of the intramedullary interstitial fluid. As the blood flow descends into the medulla, Na^+, Cl^- and urea diffuse into the blood, increasing the osmolality of the blood, but as blood flows up the ascending vessel to the cortex, Na^+, Cl^- and urea move into the interstitial fluid of the medulla to maintain the high solute concentration. The impermeable

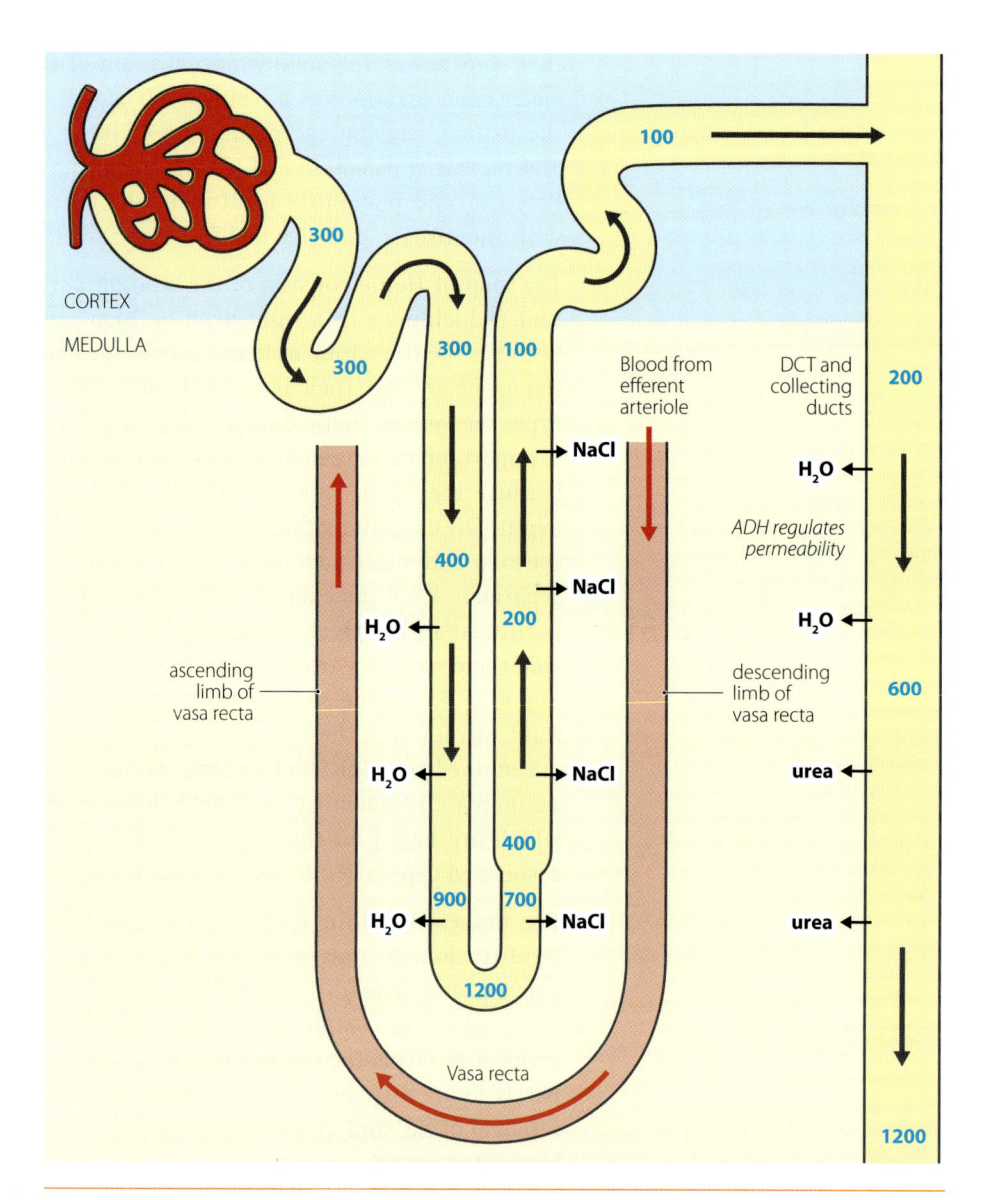

Figure 8.6 – The countercurrent mechanism in the loop of Henle.
The numbers reflect the osmolality of the tubule fluid in mOsm.

ascending limb of the nephron, together with the function of the vasa recta, enables water to be conserved and to produce urine that is more concentrated than plasma.

As the ascending limb of the nephron rises towards the renal cortex, it forms the **distal convoluted tubule (DCT)**; by this time, only about 10% of the Na⁺ and Cl⁻ and 25% of water originally filtered remain within the tubule. As the filtrate flows through the DCT, it is further modified according to physiological needs. Na⁺ and water are selectively reabsorbed under the influence of the hormones aldosterone and antidiuretic hormone, respectively; this is called **selective reabsorption**. In the absence of regulatory hormones, the DCT and **collecting ducts** are relatively impermeable to Na⁺ and water. The actions of the regulatory hormones on the selective reabsorption of water and solutes such as Na⁺ will be discussed in more detail following discussion of the third stage of urine formation, tubular secretion.

Tubular secretion is the movement of substances from the plasma to the filtrate via active transport mechanisms. It is necessary for a number of reasons:

- To eliminate waste products that have been reabsorbed by passive processes, such as urea. This also applies to K$^+$ as most is reabsorbed in the PCT.
- To eliminate substances not filtered through the Bowman's capsule, such as drugs.
- To regulate the secretion of hydrogen ions (H$^+$), which provides exquisite control of blood pH.

Secretion of potassium ions
The hormone aldosterone (discussed later in this chapter) causes Na$^+$ to be reabsorbed from the DCT and collecting ducts of the nephron into the blood. Aldosterone also stimulates the secretion of K$^+$ into the DCT and collecting ducts. A rise in plasma K$^+$ levels, which might occur, for example, following a potassium-rich meal, stimulates the secretion of aldosterone, resulting in K$^+$ secretion into the DCT and collecting ducts of the nephron. Additionally, a rise in plasma K$^+$ causes K$^+$ channels to be synthesized and inserted into the membrane of the collecting ducts, which then increase the tubular secretion of K$^+$.

Secretion of hydrogen ions
The kidney has an important role in maintaining the plasma acid–base balance (pH). The normal range of H$^+$ in the plasma is very narrow, providing a pH of 7.35–7.45. H$^+$ ions are generated continuously during cell metabolism, and in order to maintain optimum plasma acid–base balance, they need either to be bound to chemical buffers in the blood or excreted in the urine. When the H$^+$ concentration increases and pH falls, the tubules of the nephron are able to regulate the H$^+$ concentration by:

- reabsorbing more bicarbonate (HCO$_3^-$) and phosphate (PO$_4^{3-}$) ions from the filtrate into blood, which will bind to the excess H$^+$ in the blood
- producing more HCO$_3^-$ to bind to the excess H$^+$ in the blood
- secreting the excess H$^+$ from the blood.

H$^+$ ions are actively secreted into the PCT and collecting ducts of the nephron. In order to excrete the level of H$^+$ required to maintain the optimal acid–base balance, much of the H$^+$ binds to ammonia and phosphate buffers present in the urine. HCO$_3^-$ is mostly reabsorbed during urine formation and so tends to buffer the plasma pH rather than urine pH.

Composition of urine
Urine is a medium through which the human body can eliminate waste produced from cell metabolism, such as **urea**, a nitrogenous waste arising from protein metabolism, and **creatinine**, which is generated in muscle cells during the metabolism of **creatine phosphate** to create **adenosine triphosphate** (ATP). Blood levels of urea and creatinine are easily measured and are often used clinically as

markers of kidney function. When there is renal failure, blood levels of urea and creatinine increase above the normal range (see Marcus, Patient 8.1).

Many other substances including ions (for example Na^+, K^+ and Cl^-) are eliminated in urine. The excretion or retention of various ions is regulated through a homeodynamic control mechanism (see *Chapter 1*). The homeodynamic control mechanism also applies to the regulation of body water to maintain plasma osmolality within a normal range. The volume of urine produced varies significantly, as it is dependent on how much water is gained (from food/drink) and lost (in urine and faeces, sweat and insensible losses). It is also affected by the concentration of solutes in plasma and is ultimately determined by how much water is required to maintain optimum plasma osmolality.

The approximate composition of urine is 95% water and 5% solutes. The normal characteristics of urine are presented in *Table 8.2*. Urine testing (urinalysis) is a common procedure performed in the healthcare setting. Factors to consider when undertaking this procedure are presented in *Box 8.1*. As discussed earlier in this chapter, blood cells and large proteins should not pass across the glomerular membrane. The presence of red blood cells, proteins and white blood cells in urine indicates damage to kidney structures such as the glomeruli and other parts of the urinary tract such as the bladder and urethra.

Table 8.2 – Characteristics of urine in health

Characteristic	Optimal result
Colour	Amber ('straw')
Turbidity (the cloudiness of a fluid due to the presence of suspended particles)	Clear or slightly opaque
Specific gravity (a measure of urine concentration. The higher the value, the more concentrated the urine)	1.010–1.025
pH (this varies with dietary acid intake)	4.6–8
Glucose	Negative
Ketones (strong organic acids produced from fatty acid metabolism)	Negative
Blood	Negative
Protein	Negative
Urobilinogen (a colourless, water-soluble compound formed in the intestines following the breakdown of bilirubin by bacteria)	0.1–1 mg/dl
Nitrite	Negative
Leukocytes	Negative

Homeodynamic regulation of water and sodium concentration

Role of antidiuretic hormone

Antidiuretic hormone (ADH), also known as vasopressin, is a potent vasoconstrictor and acts on the kidneys to regulate the volume of urine and the plasma osmolality. ADH is synthesized by neuroendocrine cells situated in the

BOX 8.1

Factors to consider when undertaking urinalysis

Reagent strips, which change colour when exposed to abnormal constituents, are commonly used. The colour change is then compared to a standard colour chart, typically on the reagent strip bottle (see *Figure 8.7*). Timings are given for when individual reagents on the strip react and change colour; these should be followed to avoid false results. Urinalysis should be undertaken with urine collected in a clean, dry and preservative-free container. The first morning specimen is usually the best, as urine is likely to be more concentrated and fewer false negative results will be obtained. This is particularly true when testing for nitrite, as the enzyme produced by the bacteria needs to be in contact with the urine for at least 3 hours. Freshly voided urine should be tested, if possible, as bilirubin and urobilinogen are degraded when exposed to light and room temperature.

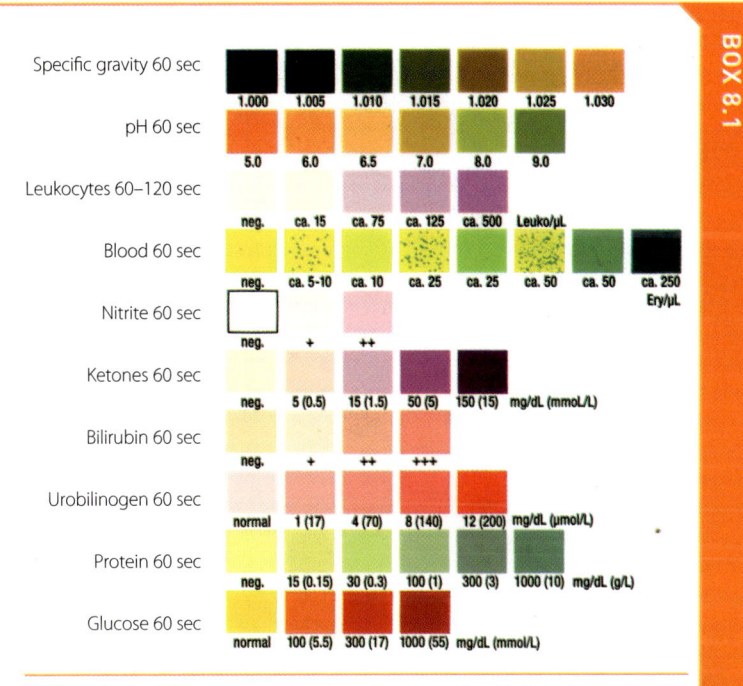

Figure 8.7 – The colour chart on a urine dipstick bottle.

---

hypothalamus (see *Chapter 5*). The hormone is packaged into vesicles and stored in the nerve terminals in the posterior pituitary gland, from where the hormone is released. As the name suggests, ADH exerts an antidiuretic effect, reducing the amount of urine produced by increasing the amount of water reabsorbed from the DCT and collecting duct, and thus increasing the concentration of urine. Normally, it is expected that ADH is secreted when the body needs to conserve water, for example when a person is dehydrated.

Osmoreceptors located in the hypothalamus respond to changes in the osmolality of the plasma as it flows through the hypothalamus (see *Figure 8.8*). Osmolality increases, for example during dehydration, and this activates osmoreceptors, leading to activation of the thirst centre in the hypothalamus. This in turn encourages the ingestion of oral fluids. In addition, activation of osmoreceptors triggers the synthesis of ADH in the hypothalamus and release of ADH from the posterior pituitary gland into the blood, where it reaches the tubule cells of the DCT and collecting ducts. Here, ADH binds to its specific receptor, which leads to a sequence of intracellular events resulting in the insertion of water channels (aquaporins) into the membrane of the tubular cells. This increases the permeability of the tubules to water, and therefore more water is reabsorbed and the urine concentration is increased. Abnormalities in ADH secretion have profound implications for health; these are commonly caused by head trauma or brain neoplasms (see *Box 8.2*).

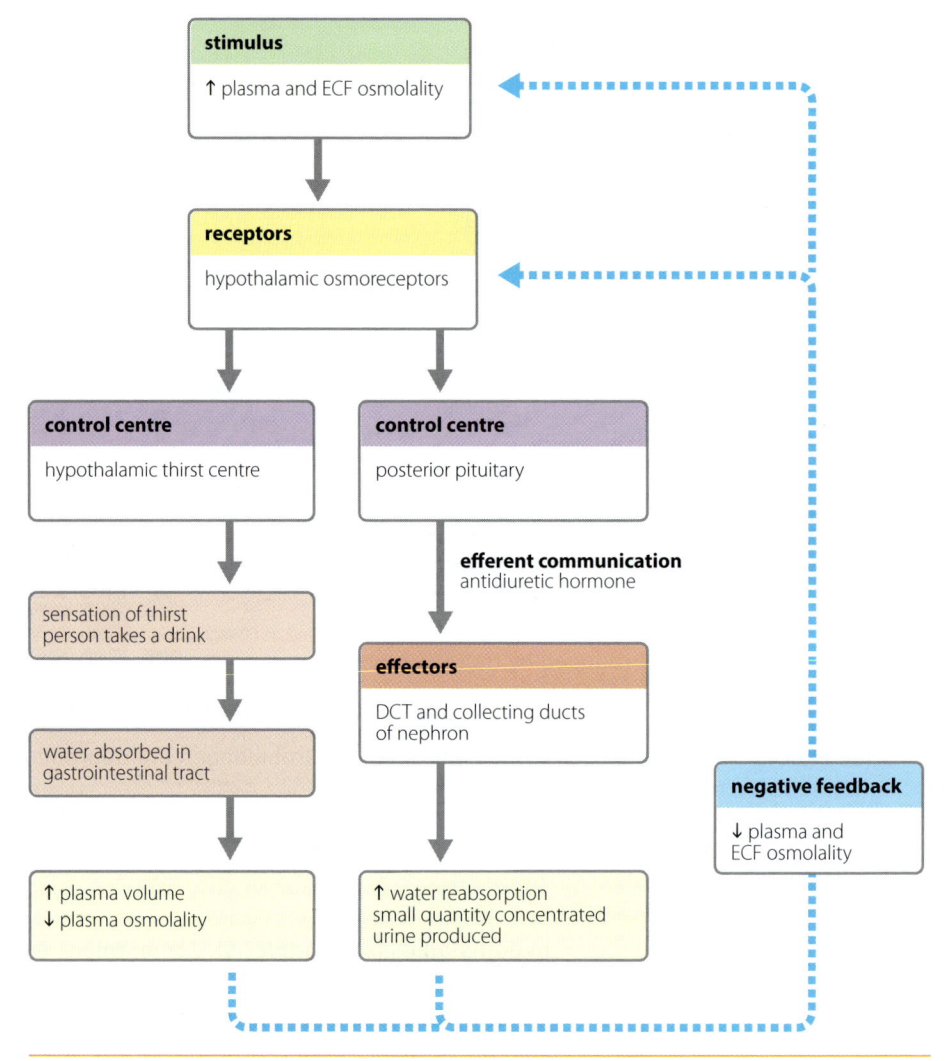

Figure 8.8 – The homeodynamic regulation of water via ADH.

stimulus
↑ plasma and ECF osmolality

↓

receptors
hypothalamic osmoreceptors

↓

control centre
hypothalamic thirst centre

↓

sensation of thirst
person takes a drink

↓

water absorbed in gastrointestinal tract

↓

↑ plasma volume
↓ plasma osmolality

control centre
posterior pituitary

efferent communication
antidiuretic hormone

↓

effectors
DCT and collecting ducts of nephron

↓

↑ water reabsorption
small quantity concentrated urine produced

negative feedback
↓ plasma and ECF osmolality

The release of ADH is increased when the arterial blood pressure or blood volume falls markedly, as might occur following a severe haemorrhage. ADH raises blood pressure by both constricting blood vessels and increasing blood volume by the retention of water in the blood. This is a good example of how physiological systems (cardiovascular and renal) are integrated to maintain homeodynamics. The regulation of arterial blood pressure is discussed further in *Chapter 9*.

As outlined previously, the osmolality of plasma is constantly monitored to determine the level of water in the plasma. Osmolality is determined by both the volume of water and the concentration of solutes that are effective osmoles (i.e. solutes that stimulate osmoreceptors). Na^+, the most abundant cation in plasma, is an effective osmole and is a significant determinant in the regulation of plasma osmolality. As Na^+ moves from one fluid compartment to another, water tends to follows by osmosis. The movement of Na^+ into a particular compartment increases the Na^+ concentration and thus the relative water concentration decreases, causing

> **BOX 8.2**
>
> **Consequences of a lack of ADH**
>
> Damage to the posterior pituitary gland may follow a head injury or a brain neoplasm and can result in a lack of ADH production. In this situation the patient will be unable to concentrate his or her urine sufficiently and will produce large amounts of dilute urine. The reduced ability to reabsorb water also makes the patient constantly thirsty, as drinking is the only way to make up for the increased fluid loss. This condition is called *central diabetes insipidus*. The underlying problem can be corrected by the administration of ADH via a nasal inhaler.

water to diffuse into that compartment by osmosis, in an attempt to maintain a dynamic equilibrium of water concentration (discussed in *Chapter 2*). Thus, the regulation of plasma osmolality by adjusting body water reabsorption also involves the regulation of the concentration of Na^+ in the plasma. A well-known saying that summarizes this is: '*Where salt goes, water follows.*'

Role of aldosterone

Aldosterone is a hormone produced by the cortex of the adrenal gland (see *Chapter 5*) acting on the DCT and collecting ducts of the nephron, making them more permeable to Na^+. The result is that more Na^+ moves from the tubules into the capillaries, which reduces the amount of Na^+ lost in urine by increasing its reabsorption into plasma. Secretion of aldosterone is primarily stimulated by an increase in plasma K^+ and a fall in extracellular volume, as well as low plasma Na^+. Typically, a lowered concentration of Na^+ in plasma leads to a fall in extracellular volume, and the effect of this on the secretion of aldosterone is mediated through the **renin–angiotensin–aldosterone system** (RAAS) (this is discussed further in *Chapter 9* as the RAAS has a key role in the long-term regulation of arterial blood pressure).

The RAAS is activated when a fall in extracellular fluid volume and renal blood pressure arriving at the afferent arteriole to the glomerulus is detected by the **juxtaglomerular apparatus** in the nephron (see *Chapter 9, Figure 9.15*). This stimulates the release of **renin** from specialized cells located next to the glomerulus. Renin is an enzyme that breaks down the plasma protein angiotensinogen into a smaller protein called **angiotensin I**. Angiotensin I circulates in the blood and is exposed to a converting enzyme called **angiotensin-converting enzyme** (ACE), located on vascular endothelial cells, particularly in the lungs and kidneys. This enzyme converts angiotensin I into the active form and potent vasoconstrictor called **angiotensin II**. It is angiotensin II that stimulates the release of aldosterone from the adrenal cortex of the adrenal glands (see *Chapter 9, Figure 9.15*). Angiotensin II also stimulates the thirst centre in the hypothalamus, encouraging the ingestion of oral fluids, which helps to expand plasma volume and maintain blood pressure. The juxtaglomerular apparatus comprises cells in the DCT that lie close to the afferent arteriole (and sometimes the efferent arteriole), and this means that any changes to blood pressure and blood flow that will affect the GFR will be detected and corrected. If blood pressure and renal blood flow fall, nephrons can become damaged and the excretory function of the kidneys compromised, leading to renal failure.

Role of atrial natriuretic peptide and B-type natriuretic peptide

Atrial natriuretic peptide (ANP) and B-type natriuretic peptide (BNP) are peptide hormones synthesized and stored in cardiac muscle cells. ANP is synthesized in atrial myocytes and BNP in ventricular myocytes. Expansion of the heart muscle caused by increased volume and pressure causes the release of ANP from atrial myocytes and the release of BNP from the ventricular myocytes. ANP and BNP have similar effects: with regard to the activity of the kidney, they increase the GFR, decrease the reabsorption of Na^+ in the DCT and also inhibit the action of the hormones aldosterone and renin. The consequence is an increase in the excretion of Na^+ (natriuresis) and a fall in blood volume. ANP and BNP also bind to receptors on the arteriolar smooth muscle cells, causing vasodilation, resulting in a reduction of peripheral vascular resistance and systemic arterial blood pressure. The measurement of BNP is used to assess the severity of heart failure and evaluate the progress of patients with this condition.

The micturition reflex

Micturition, also known as urination or voiding, is the act of emptying the bladder with the passage of urine out of the body. Micturition occurs involuntarily in babies and infants because their central nervous system is not fully mature. Typically, between the ages of 3 and 5 years, micturition becomes regulated voluntarily, influenced by social factors. The sensory and motor neural pathways that coordinate micturition are complex, involving many levels of the brain, and spinal cord and the peripheral nervous system. The storage and periodic elimination of urine depends on the coordination of smooth and skeletal muscle in the lower urinary tract, namely the bladder, which is the reservoir, and outlet structures comprising the bladder neck, urethra and the internal and external sphincters. For voiding to be controlled, an intact spinal cord is required.

In babies and infants, micturition is regulated by a primitive spinal reflex pathway. As urine fills the bladder, it becomes distended and the rugae become smooth. A small amount of urine is sufficient to activate stretch receptors in the bladder trigone and bladder wall. Sensory impulses are sent via afferent pathways to the sacral spinal cord. As this is a reflex, an efferent motor response via parasympathetic neurones is initiated, leading to contraction of the detrusor muscle of the bladder and the consequential opening of the internal urethral sphincter; thus, the baby passes urine. However, with developmental changes that occur in the maturing nervous system, control moves away from the level of the spinal cord, and supraspinal control centres located in the pons area of the brainstem (pontine micturition centre) dominate.

Bladder filling and the guarding reflex

Voluntary control of micturition is achieved in adults as follows (illustrated in *Figure 8.9*): for the bladder to fill, the detrusor muscle needs to be relaxed and the internal sphincter closed. This is achieved by *sympathetic* stimulation of the bladder through hypogastric and pelvic nerves, coupled with the inhibition of parasympathetic nerves that supply the bladder. Continence is maintained through

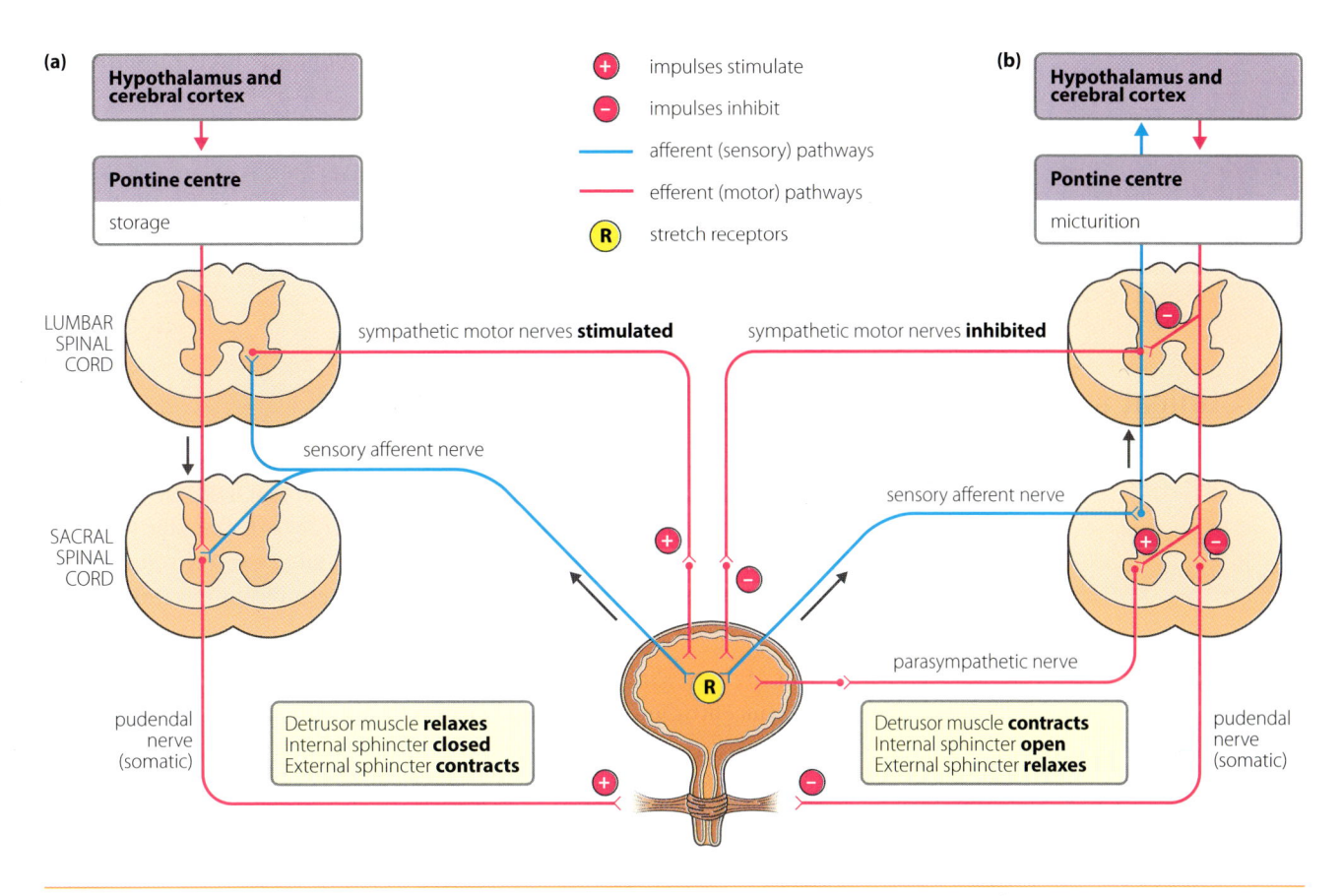

SECTION 8.2 | WHAT YOU NEED TO KNOW – ESSENTIAL ANATOMY AND PHYSIOLOGY 261

Figure 8.9 – Control of micturition: (a) bladder filling (storage) and (b) micturition.

the somatic stimulation of the external sphincter muscle, via the pudendal nerve. Somatic motor impulses are generated by the **pontine micturition centre (PMC)**, and these travel down the spinal cord, via descending pathways, to stimulate the pudendal nerve. The overall process is sometimes described as the guarding reflex.

The PMC has connections to many regions of the brain including the hypothalamus and the cortex, especially that of the frontal lobe. The frontal lobes play an important part in the perception of the need to void urine and in determining the socially learned appropriateness of voiding urine.

During the voiding of urine, sensory nerve impulses from stretch receptors in the bladder wall travel up ascending pathways to the hypothalamus and the PMC cortex, which coordinate parasympathetic motor impulses down descending pathways to the sacral spinal cord (see *Figure 8.9*). Activation of the parasympathetic system leads to contraction of the detrusor muscle, relaxation of the internal sphincter and inhibition of sympathetic activity on the bladder. In addition, voluntary nerve impulses to the muscle of the external sphincter (voluntary control) are inhibited, enabling relaxation of the external sphincter (*see Figure 8.9*). The flow of urine from the bladder along the urethra reinforces activity from the PMC.

If voiding does not occur, the perceived desire to micturate subsides until further filling of the bladder with approximately 200–300 ml of urine stimulates the micturition reflex again and the perceived need to void urine returns. Typically, this stimulus can be avoided again, if the time and place is not convenient. Should the volume of urine in the bladder reach approximately 500–600 ml, micturition can no longer be resisted and urine will be voided.

8.3 Clinical application

Water is a universal solvent and, as such, a huge variety of solutes necessary for life dissolve in it. The amounts of water and solute are regulated by homeodynamic processes, and the nephrons of the kidney act as important effectors for this. The ability to produce both concentrated and dilute urine, and to excrete solutes from the body, is vital to ensure that the composition of the internal environment is kept stable.

- The case of Marcus (Patient 8.1) illustrates how body water volume and the solute concentration of the blood have a significant impact on health.

Patient 8.1 — Marcus — 241 **262**

- 62-year-old Afro-Caribbean man
- Long-standing hypertension
- High urea and creatinine levels suggest kidney disease – classed as stage 3
- Hypertension managed with ACE inhibitor

Marcus is 62 years old and has stage 3 chronic kidney disease. Some common conditions that can lead to chronic kidney disease are identified in *Box 8.3*. His care is complex and requires input from a variety of healthcare professionals from within the multidisciplinary team, including doctors and nurses who are renal specialists, and a renal dietician.

Assessment of the glomerular filtration rate (GFR) is an important measure in the diagnosis and assessment of kidney disease. Marcus's estimated GFR (eGFR) has been calculated to be 50 ml/minute/1.73 m². This calculation is derived from his creatinine level, and also from his age, sex and ethnicity. Age, sex and ethnicity are all factors that differ among individuals and provide a good illustration that the balance of fluid and electrolytes is a homeodynamic process. As he is in

BCX 8.3

Chronic kidney disease

Arteriosclerosis, hypertension and the vascular damage associated with diabetes mellitus can seriously compromise the structure and function of the blood vessels surrounding the nephron, which can lead to chronic kidney disease. As a result, nephrons are progressively destroyed, the quantity of destruction being directly proportional to the observed glomerular filtration rate (GFR), which gradually falls. The ability of the kidney to excrete Na^+ and water becomes impaired, which reduces the amount of urine produced and also raises the patient's blood pressure. The ability to excrete urea, K^+ and H^+ is also reduced and levels of these substances increase in the plasma. Damage to the glomerulus can also cause proteinuria.

stage 3 of chronic kidney disease, Marcus's condition is managed by monitoring his serum creatinine, urea and electrolyte levels and by ensuring that his blood pressure is well controlled (ideally it should be no higher than 140/90 mmHg). A GFR of only 50 ml/minute/1.73 m² markedly limits the ability of his kidneys to excrete solutes, and consequently their levels can rise significantly in his plasma.

In addition, Marcus is also regularly assessed for the presence of anaemia (a deficiency in the number of red blood cells or the haemoglobin content). Chronic kidney disease can reduce the ability of the kidney to produce the hormone **erythropoietin**, which stimulates the formation of erythrocytes (red blood cells) in the bone marrow (discussed in *Chapter 5*).

Marcus's medical care is complex and involves a multidisciplinary approach. He is prescribed an angiotensin-converting enzyme (ACE) inhibitor drug to manage his hypertension, which lowers the amount of active angiotensin II available to cause vasoconstriction of his blood vessels and so lowers his blood pressure. Dietary management of chronic kidney disease is also important, and Marcus receives advice from a renal dietician. As the metabolism of protein generates urea, it is therefore logical to limit the amount of protein obtained from the diet. However, this has to be balanced against ensuring that protein intake is sufficient to prevent the breakdown of muscle tissue. A low-sodium diet is also recommended. Marcus already follows this diet in an attempt to reduce his hypertension. The inability to excrete Na⁺ is likely to worsen as Marcus's kidney disease progresses, and limiting the intake of Na⁺ will, to some extent, combat this. The retention of Na⁺ and water can cause swollen oedematous ankles to develop. This can be a sign that the kidney disease is deteriorating and is something Marcus needs to take note of and inform his family doctor about, as it may mean that he needs renal dialysis.

Understanding how the fluid composition of the internal environment is maintained is important for healthcare professionals caring for all patients. Marcus illustrates how one condition, hypertension, can influence the development of another, chronic kidney disease. Vascular damage in the kidney is associated with arteriosclerosis, hypertension, obesity and type 2 diabetes, the prevalences of which are increasing in the world, largely due to the adoption of an unhealthy lifestyle. Healthcare professionals need to understand the factors that influence lifestyle choices and work with patients to enable them to make healthier choices.

8.4 Summary

- Water is a polar molecule, which accounts for many of its properties, such as being the 'universal solvent'.
- Chemical substances such as salts, acids and bases dissolve in water, forming ions, which are also called electrolytes. Electrolytes are found in all body fluids.
- Urine is a medium through which metabolic wastes, drugs, hormones and water are excreted.

CHAPTER 09 | Organs need to be perfused

Learning points for this chapter

After working through this chapter, you should be able to:

- Describe the importance of the heart and circulatory system in maintaining health
- Describe the structures and functions of the cardiovascular system that contribute to the flow of blood through the heart and body and that maintain blood pressure
- Describe the major factors that influence the movement of tissue fluid (capillary fluid dynamics)
- Outline the major components of blood and describe how blood cells are formed
- Describe the major blood groups and their specific roles in maintaining health
- Outline the major events that occur during haemostasis and blood clotting

9.1 Introduction and clinical relevance

Each of the patients discussed in this chapter highlight the importance of the cardiovascular system and blood for health. The patient stories are common, emphasizing the knowledge required by healthcare practitioners to effectively assess and support patients with cardiac and haematological problems. For example, Sheila (Patient 2.3) and Katherine (Patient 3.3) highlight the integration of physiological systems and how this is essential for health, and illustrate the extent of knowledge healthcare practitioners need to apply in their practice.

| Patient 2.3 | Sheila | 30 | 54 | 59 | 93 | **267** | 304 | 448 | 473 |

- 47-year-old woman
- Recent diagnosis of breast cancer
- Biological therapy with trastuzumab (Herceptin) to block HER2 action an option
- Is still offered surgery, chemotherapy and radiotherapy
- Adds trastuzumab to chemotherapy plan

Sheila has breast cancer. Sheila is very anxious about her diagnosis and the fact that she requires a wide local excision of her breast to remove the cancer. To help allay her anxiety, Sheila has access to support from a named breast care nurse. Sheila has been informed that there is the potential for the surgery to alter the circulation of fluid through her tissues.

Patient 3.3 — Katherine — 61 95 **268** 305

- 41-year-old woman
- Recent diagnosis of hypertrophic cardiomyopathy
- ECG shows arrhythmia and USS shows thickened left ventricle
- Given warfarin and anti-arrhythmic drugs
- Genetic tests on one daughter

Katherine is reviewed regularly for her heart condition (hypertrophic cardiomyopathy). She is coping well with this and is leading a full and active life. However, the nature of her heart problem and the associated disturbance to her heart rhythm increase her risk of developing blood clots in her heart chambers, which could dislodge and cause a stroke. For this reason, she takes warfarin tablets, an anticoagulant, to prevent clot formation.

Patient 3.4 — Yasmeen — 61 95 **268** 306

- 17-year-old girl
- Has sickle cell disease but no long-term organ damage
- Discussed option of bone marrow transplant
- Referred to clinical geneticist to find out more

Yasmeen is an active 17 year old, managing her sickle cell disease, an inherited blood disorder. She has had repeated admissions to hospital to help her deal with episodes of acute pain, including pains in her chest and abdomen associated with sickle cell crisis, and experiences swollen hands and feet. She has required repeated blood transfusions to improve the oxygenation of her blood and tissues.

Patient 9.1 — Robert — **268** 305 448 474

- 56-year-old man with family history of CVD
- First MI at 38, stent at 45, and coronary artery bypass graft at 49
- ECG shows changes consistent with another MI; confirmed by biochemical marker tests

Robert has a history of chest pain and cardiovascular problems, including experiencing a myocardial infarction (MI) while on holiday when he was aged 38. At the age of 56, Robert presented at the local emergency department with severe retrosternal chest pain associated with sweating. An electrocardiogram (ECG) indicated changes in the inferior part of the left ventricle consistent with an MI. Subsequent blood tests for biochemical markers confirmed the presence of myocardial **necrosis** (cell death) consistent with the diagnosis of acute myocardial infarction. At the time, Robert's serum total cholesterol and serum triglyceride were on the upper range of normal at 5.7 and 1.9 millimoles/L, respectively. There is a history of cardiovascular disease in Robert's family, as his father also had an MI at the age of 64. Robert continued to have intermittent chest pain after his first MI, and 7 years later he underwent angioplasty with the insertion of a stent to correct a stenosis in one of the branches of his left coronary artery. However, Robert's heart problems continued, and he had further episodes of severe cardiac chest pain. Robert had a coronary artery bypass graft inserted when he was aged 49. Robert has mild chronic heart failure, which was confirmed by a cardiac echocardiogram, which demonstrated that the function of his left ventricle was impaired.

Patient 9.2 — Jane — **268** 306

- 28-year-old woman pregnant with second child
- Blood group O Rh −ve
- Given anti-D Ig at 28 weeks

Jane is a 28-year-old married woman expecting her second baby. Following her first antenatal appointment, blood samples taken at 8 weeks' gestation identified her blood group as 'O rhesus negative'. There is concern that if her baby has rhesus-positive blood, Jane might develop antibodies that could destroy her baby's red blood cells. At 28 weeks of pregnancy, Jane attended an appointment for prophylactic anti-D immunoglobulin at a hospital maternity unit. It is the policy of the hospital to give prophylactic anti-D immunoglobulin to all pregnant women who are rhesus negative. Jane had no particular past medical history and no history of a previous blood transfusion. Jane has a healthy 3-year-old daughter, delivered vaginally at 40 weeks' gestation following a normal pregnancy.

Cells and tissues require chemical energy gained from oxidative phosphorylation (see *Chapter 2*). This requires an effective circulatory system, primarily to deliver oxygen and nutrients to the cells and tissues. Some of the major functions of the circulatory system, including blood, can be summarized as follows:

- Transportation of hormones, respiratory gases, drugs and nutrients.
- Removal of waste products, which are transported to excretory organs, such as the kidney, for removal (see *Chapter 8*).
- Thermoregulation and distribution of heat (see *Chapter 1*).
- Maintenance of acid–base balance and pH.
- Blood clotting (haemostasis).
- Immunity (see *Chapter 11*).

You are likely to meet people such as Sheila, Katherine and Yasmeen, Robert and Jane with a range of problems related to their circulatory system. It is important for you to have a clear understanding about the circulatory system and how tissues are perfused effectively. This knowledge underpins the diagnostic investigations, advice and approaches to management used in the support of people with cardiovascular problems.

9.2 What you need to know – essential anatomy and physiology

The cardiovascular system, comprising the heart and blood vessels, keeps blood continuously circulating to ensure that cells receive the required nutrients, hormones and oxygen; it also ensures that waste products such as carbon dioxide are constantly removed. In addition, it is involved in distributing heat throughout the body and in regulating core body temperature. The cardiovascular system and blood flow are carefully regulated to enable these functions to occur.

The term **perfusion** is used to describe the flow of blood through the vascular bed of tissues. You may be aware that when an area of skin is inflamed, it appears red and hot. This is called **hyperaemia** and is due to an increase in blood flow (discussed in *Chapter 11*). In contrast, the skin of patients who are critically ill following a major haemorrhage is often cold, clammy and pale. In this example, as a response to the loss of blood, blood flow is diverted away from the skin towards the vital organs; the skin consequently receives less blood flow and becomes poorly perfused. Assessment of skin can be very informative about a patient's state of health; its appearance and how it feels can indicate the state of the cardiovascular system, providing an important indicator of whether a patient is acutely or critically ill.

9.2.1 Structure and function of blood vessels

Although blood vessels vary in terms of size, distribution and function, they do share common structural features. All blood vessels except capillaries have the same basic structure comprising the main three layers of tissue: the tunica intima (inner), tunica media and tunica adventitia (outer) layers (see *Figure 9.1*). The tunica intima consists of flattened endothelial cells supported by a connective tissue matrix called the basement membrane. The tunica media comprises smooth

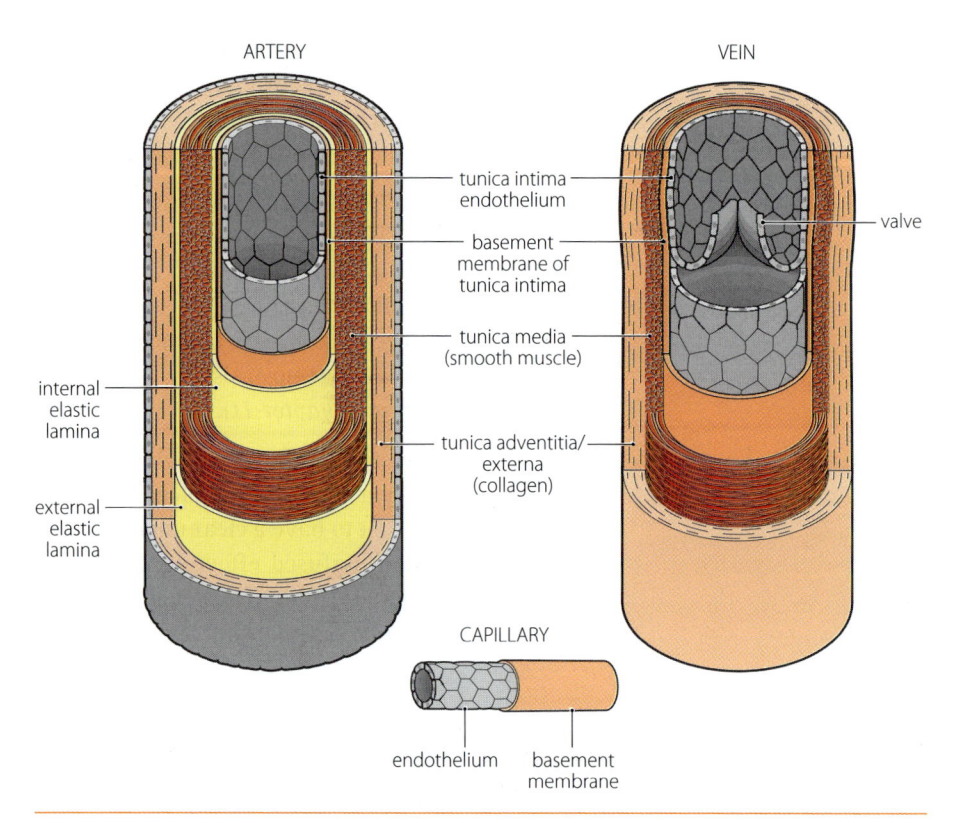

Figure 9.1 – **The structure of (a) an artery, (b) a vein and (c) a capillary.**

muscle cells with elastin and collagen fibres. The outer layer, the tunica adventitia, is a protective sheath made from loose collagen and elastin fibres and serves to anchor the blood vessel to the surrounding tissue.

The circulation of blood throughout the body is termed the **systemic circulation** (see *Figure 9.2*) and requires the ejection of blood from the left side of the heart into the aorta, which distends and then recoils, pushing blood into the arteries. This is possible because the aorta has a relatively thin and highly elastic wall. In contrast, the other arteries have a thicker wall, with a thick smooth muscle layer and fewer elastic fibres.

Due to the thick smooth muscle wall, arteries distribute blood over long distances without the blood pressure falling. Indeed, a thick muscular wall is required to withstand the high blood pressure present within the arterial system. While arteries take blood away from the heart, veins return blood back to the heart. Veins have much larger diameter lumens compared with arteries but they have very thin walls with minimal smooth muscle. Consequently, veins are highly distensible and collapse easily. The veins in the extremities of the body, such as the legs and arms, contain valves that contribute to the return of blood back to the heart against the effects of gravity. Veins can be described as capacitance vessels because they hold 60–70% of the blood volume, and this blood is at a lower pressure compared with that in the arterial system.

The smooth muscle layer in the arteries and particularly arterioles contracts to constrict the lumen (vasoconstriction) and then relaxes causing vasodilation.

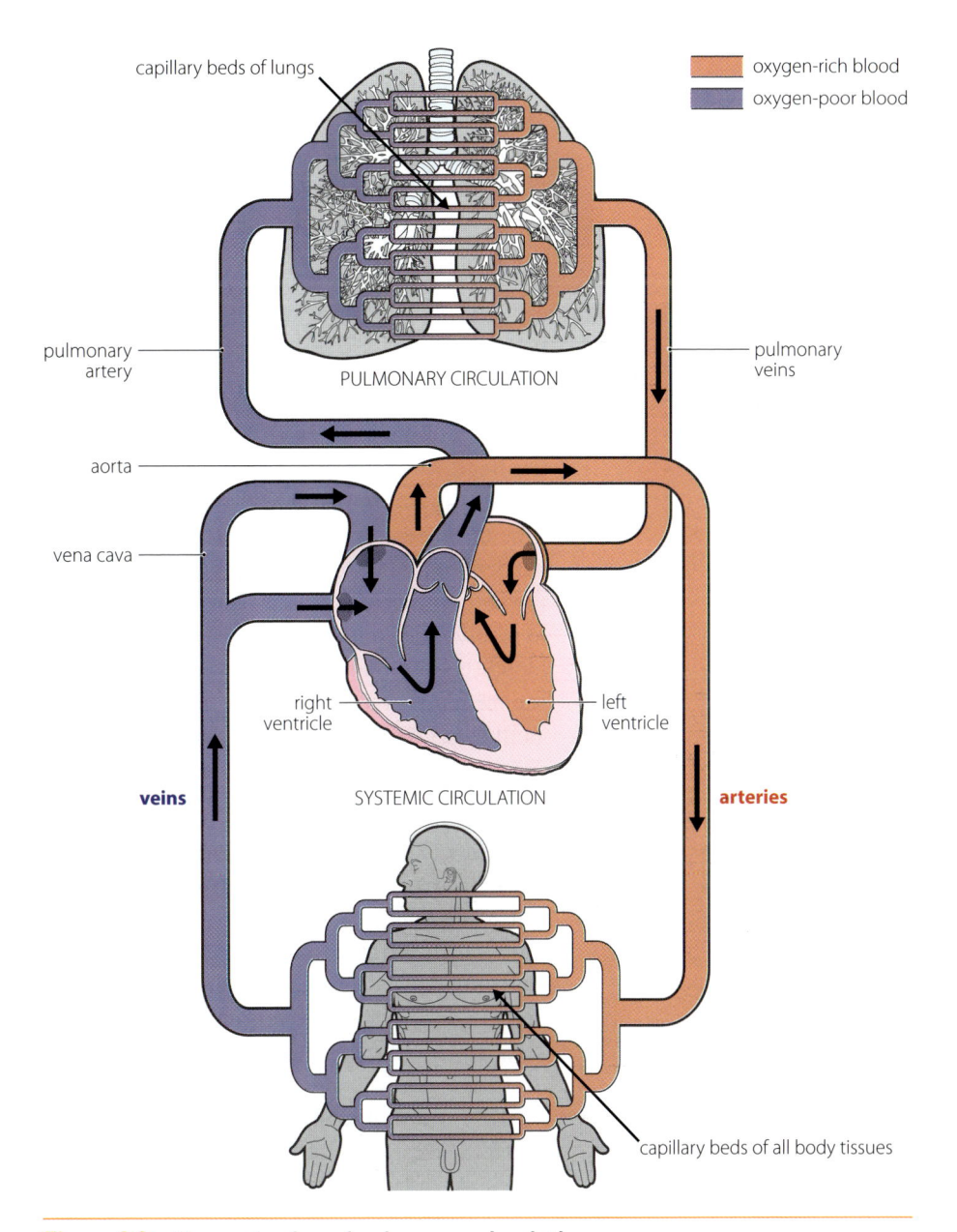

Figure 9.2 – **The systemic and pulmonary circulation.**

In this way, blood flow can be regulated, in particular the flow of blood from arterioles to the capillaries. Regulation of smooth muscle contraction is through the autonomic nervous system via the selective action of neurotransmitters such as noradrenaline (norepinephrine), or via specific hormones from the endocrine system such as adrenaline (epinephrine) and antidiuretic hormone (vasopressin). As will be discussed later in this chapter, arterioles are called resistance vessels because they have an important role in regulating blood pressure by altering the resistance to blood flow.

Capillaries are the conduit between the arterial and venous circulation; these are organized into capillary beds, forming a large surface area for the exchange of water and solutes. Capillaries comprise a single layer of cells and basement membrane, allowing the effective and rapid exchange of water and solutes between the blood and tissue cells. Capillaries contain pores in the endothelial cell membrane, which enhance the movement of water and solutes. For these reasons, capillaries have an important role in maintaining homeostasis through the exchange of fluid and solutes between capillaries and the tissue cells.

9.2.2 Blood flow and perfusion

Perfusion refers to the amount of blood that flows through a tissue or organ. The flow of blood, as with the movement of any fluid, is promoted by a pressure gradient, where the blood flows from a region of higher pressure towards a region of lower pressure (i.e. down the pressure gradient). The driving pressure for the flow of blood is produced by the pumping action of the heart, which raises the aortic blood pressure and increases the pressure gradient between the aorta and the veins. The elastic aorta contributes to the flow of blood as it initially stretches to receive the blood ejected from the left ventricle and then recoils. The volume of blood that circulates through the tissue capillary beds is closely matched to meet the metabolic requirements of the tissues for oxygen and other substrates, such as glucose. This is a good example of the fine regulation of the cardiovascular system to maintain homeostasis.

Cells require oxygen in order to generate energy (in the form of ATP) (described in *Chapter 7*). If blood flow to the cells becomes impaired, and *insufficient* oxygen reaches the tissues to meet metabolic requirements, then **ischaemia** occurs, which causes the normal metabolic activity of cells to be disrupted. For example, a switch from aerobic to **anaerobic processes** occurs and the pH of the intracellular environment falls, causing impairment of the normal plasma membrane transport process responsible for the movement of solutes and water. Ischaemia leads to impairment in cell function, which is restored only when there is resumption of an adequate blood flow and delivery of oxygen. Unless this occurs within a limited time period, the biochemical changes in the tissue lead to rapid cell death (**necrosis**). A localized area of **necrotic tissue** resulting from **ischaemia** is called an **infarction**; for example, an obstruction in a coronary blood vessel of the heart causing infarction of heart muscle is called a **myocardial infarction**. The urgent priority when treating an individual experiencing an acute coronary event such as this is to confirm the obstruction to blood flow to the cardiac muscle and to restore blood flow. If there is evidence of myocardial cell injury and necrosis, reperfusion is achieved ideally via primary percutaneous coronary intervention. A brief summary of coronary heart disease and the management of acute coronary syndrome is presented in *Box 9.1*.

Blood flow to the tissues is regulated by a number of factors, including ambient temperature and a reduction in tissue oxygen, and by the release of chemical mediators from the endothelium; these include nitric oxide (a vasodilator) and endothelins, which are vasoconstrictors. The autonomic nervous system, particularly the sympathetic nervous system, and the endocrine system also regulate blood flow (described later in this chapter).

SECTION 9.2 | WHAT YOU NEED TO KNOW – ESSENTIAL ANATOMY AND PHYSIOLOGY 273

> **BOX 9.1**
>
> ## Coronary heart disease
>
> The term 'coronary heart disease' refers to a spectrum of heart diseases arising from impairment of blood flow through the coronary arteries. Depending on the severity of the obstruction to the blood flow, an individual may experience chest pain that occurs on exercise and is relieved on rest or after the self-administration of glyceryl trinitrate spray – this provides nitric oxide, which causes vasodilation. This condition is commonly called angina. However, the obstruction to blood flow can become more severe when the cardiac muscle cells move from being ischaemic to becoming infarcted, culminating in a myocardial infarction (MI). In the majority of cases, the impairment of blood flow is due to a narrowing in the coronary artery arising from the presence of atherosclerosis. Less commonly, the impaired blood flow is due to spasm of the coronary artery. 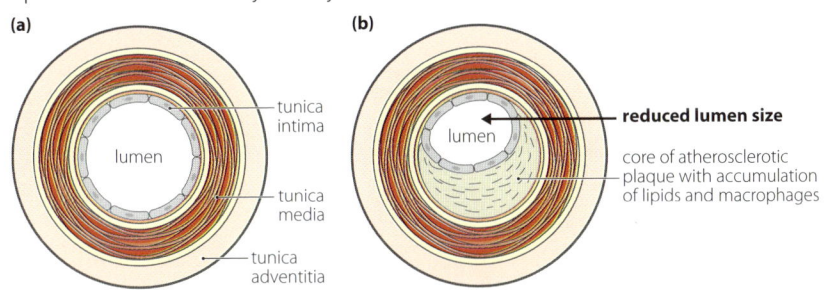
>
> **Figure 9.3** – The major tissue layers that form the wall of (a) a normal artery and (b) an artery where there is atherosclerosis.
>
> Atherosclerosis is a disease of the arterial wall that occurs at susceptible sites, in this case within the coronary artery circulation. It involves injury to the endothelial cells of the artery, provoking an inflammatory response and the accumulation of lipid within the intima of the arterial wall, followed by a repeating cycle of inflammation and repair, leading to the development of an atherosclerotic plaque (see *Figure 9.3*). This plaque leads to narrowing (stenosis) of the artery lumen (*see Figure 9.4a*), reducing blood flow. Thinning and fissuring (splitting) of the outer covering of the atherosclerotic plaque (called the cap) increases the likelihood of a blood clot (thrombus) forming at the site of the stenosis. It is the rapid aggregation of platelets to form a thrombus at the site of the stenosis that leads to the development of acute coronary syndromes and the possibility of an MI. 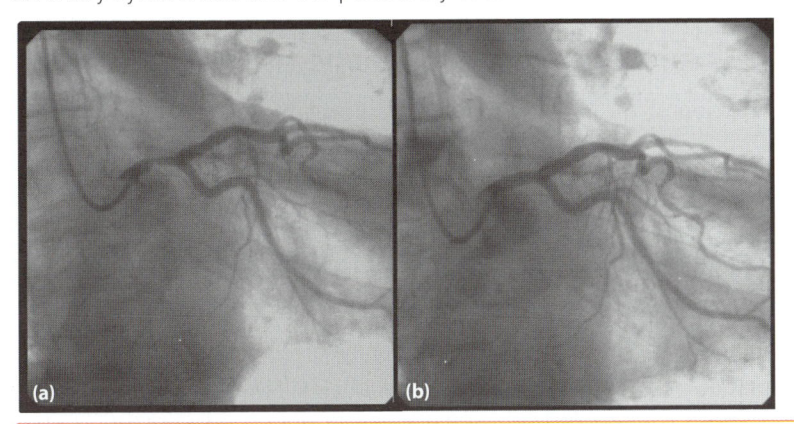
>
> **Figure 9.4** – Digital angiogram of a coronary artery (a) before and (b) after primary percutaneous coronary intervention and insertion of a stent.
> Reproduced from Fajadet, J and Chieffo, A. Current management of left main coronary artery disease. *European Heart Journal*, 2012, 33(1): 36–50, by permission of the European Society of Cardiology.

To manage the acute event, the treatment of choice is primary percutaneous coronary intervention (PCI), where a balloon catheter is inserted via the femoral or radial artery into the coronary artery to reach the site of the stenosis. The balloon, when inflated, dilates the narrowed (also called stenosed) artery and a metal stent is positioned at the newly dilated site to ensure the artery lumen remains open (see *Figure 9.5*). Where primary PCI is not available and assuming there are no contraindications, clot-busting (thrombolytic) drugs such as tenecteplase and alteplase can be given to break down the thrombus (thrombolysis). It is imperative that careful clinical decisions are made when selecting patients to receive thrombolytic drugs because this therapy carries its own risks to the patient, such as causing bleeding into the brain, leading to a stroke, and bleeding from the gastrointestinal tract. Not all patients are eligible to receive thrombolysis. The aim with both approaches is to restore blood flow to the injured myocardium. The restoration of good blood flow in the previously stenosed coronary artery following PCI and insertion of a stent is illustrated in *Figure 9.4b*.

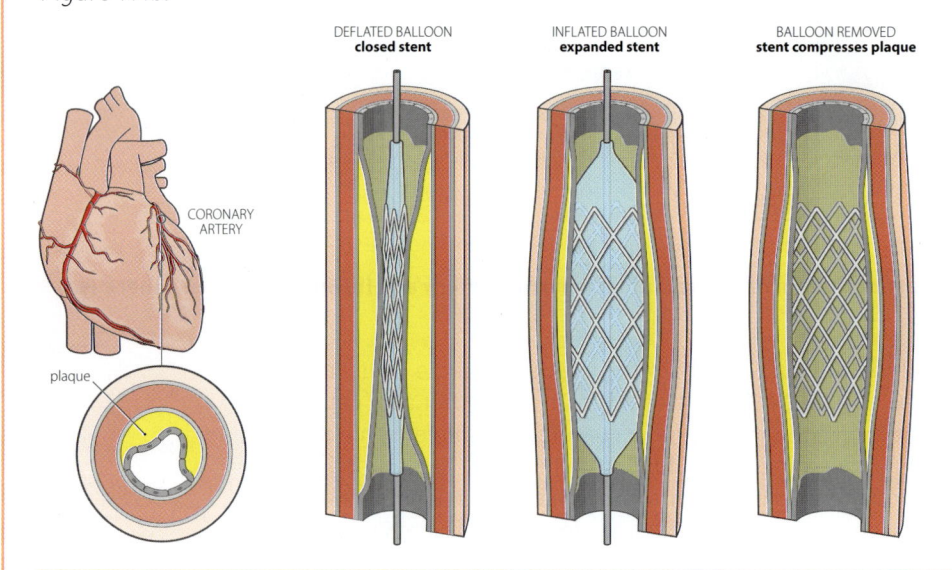

Figure 9.5 – **PCI and insertion of a stent.**

9.2.3 The heart: structure and function

A major function of the heart is to generate pressure to cause blood to flow and this is maintained throughout life to meet the metabolic needs of the body. The pumping of the heart is adjusted rapidly in response to changing internal and external factors, such as the increased demand for oxygen when exercising.

Anatomy of the heart

The heart is essentially a muscular pump that can be considered to be shaped like an upside-down cone. It is located in the thoracic cavity between the lungs and posterior to the sternum, in an area of the thorax called the **mediastinum**. The heart is divided into four chambers (atria and ventricles) and is separated into the left and right sides by the septum. The major structures of the heart and the associated blood vessels are illustrated in *Figure 9.6*. The top of the heart, called the base, comprises the left and right atria, while the lower chambers are the right and left ventricles,

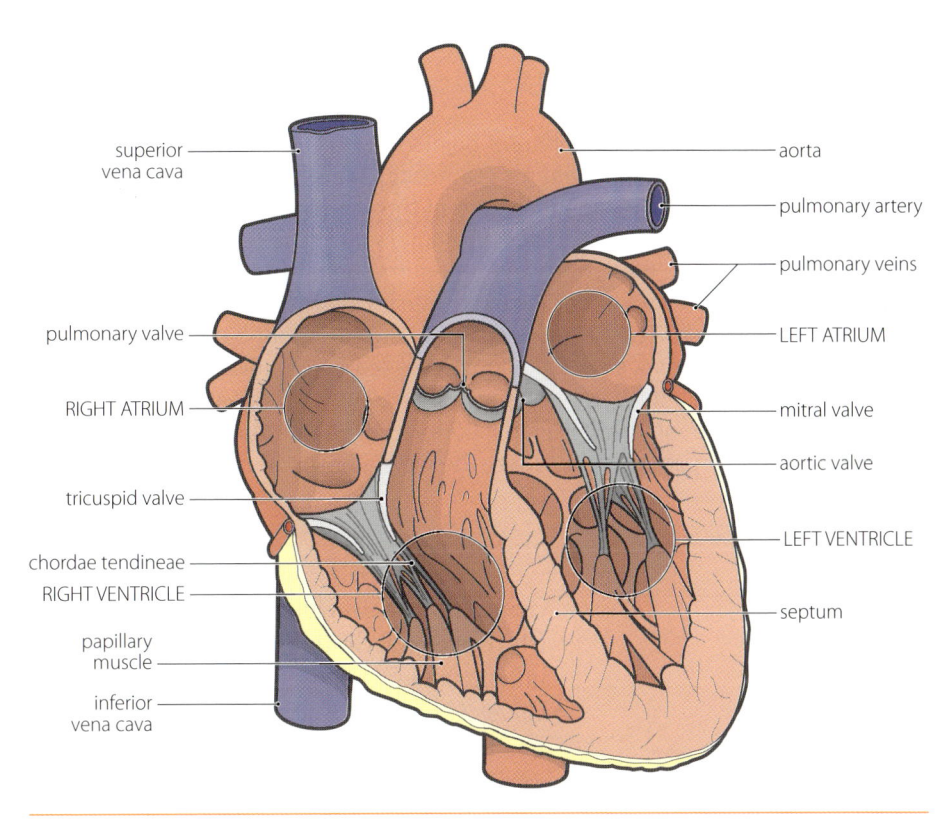

Figure 9.6 – **The major structures of the heart.**

with the left ventricle forming the apex of the heart. The heart is positioned on a slight angle, so that the apex points towards the left hip. The atria are separated from the ventricles by a ring of fibrous tissue that supports the **atrioventricular valves** (the **tricuspid** and **mitral** (**bicuspid**) valves) and the semilunar **aortic** and **pulmonary** valves. The exit routes for blood from the right and left ventricles are through the pulmonary and aortic valves, situated at the entrance to the pulmonary artery and aorta, respectively. The valves open and close in sequence during each heartbeat to ensure that blood flows in only one direction through the heart. The opening and closing of the valves produces the heart sounds, which can be heard by cardiac auscultation with a stethoscope (see *Box 9.2*).

While the heart is principally a muscular pump made up of specialized cardiac muscle called the myocardium, two other tissue structures make up the wall of the heart (see *Figure 9.7*). These are a resistant outer layer of fibrous connective tissue called the **pericardium**, which provides the heart with some resistance to pressures produced during muscular contraction, and an inner layer called the **endocardium**, comprising a layer of flattened squamous endothelial cells sitting on a thin layer of connective tissue that ensure an incredibly smooth surface for blood to flow against.

The endocardium is continuous with the endothelial cells that form the tunica intima of blood vessels and covers the entire inner surface of the heart chambers and valves. As a smooth covering, the endocardium helps to prevent the development of **thrombi** (blood clots) on the valves and wall of the heart

> **BOX 9.2**
>
> **Heart sounds and cardiac valves**
>
> The closing of the valves at different points during the heartbeat explains the 'lub dub' heart sound, which can be heard when a stethoscope is applied to the chest wall (auscultation). The first heart sound (lub) is due to closure of the mitral and tricuspid valves as the ventricular muscle starts to contract and pressure builds up in the left and right ventricles. The second heart sound (dub) is when the aortic valve and pulmonary valve close after blood has been ejected from the ventricles. Abnormal heart sounds (murmurs) may be detected when auscultating the heart with a stethoscope. Heart murmurs are due to turbulent blood flow passing through the valves. Murmurs may be innocent, related to increased blood flow rather than any cardiac disease, or may occur when the valve is stenosed (narrowed) or does not close effectively, allowing blood to leak through the valve (an incompetent valve). Murmurs are described by a number of characteristics such as the location, the timing of the murmur during the cardiac cycle and the intensity.

chambers. The development of blood clots can occur as a result of endocarditis, where the endocardium becomes damaged and roughened due to infection and inflammation; this leads to the development of thrombi and destruction of the valve. Thrombi can break off the valves and pass through the circulation into smaller arteries in the cerebral circulation to obstruct blood flow to the brain, causing a **stroke**. Alternatively, they can move into the pulmonary circulation, obstructing blood follow to lung tissue and causing a **pulmonary embolism**.

The **myocardium** is the greatest contributor to the mass of the heart and is formed from specialized cardiac muscle cells, which are organized in parallel lines with branching and connecting cells. Each cell is connected to other cardiac cells at specialized sites called intercalated discs, ensuring that heart muscle cells work as an integrated functional unit (see *Figure 9.8*). For this reason, the myocardium is described as a functional syncytium (the term syncytium refers to a large cell-like structure with many nuclei and no internal cell boundaries). Effective

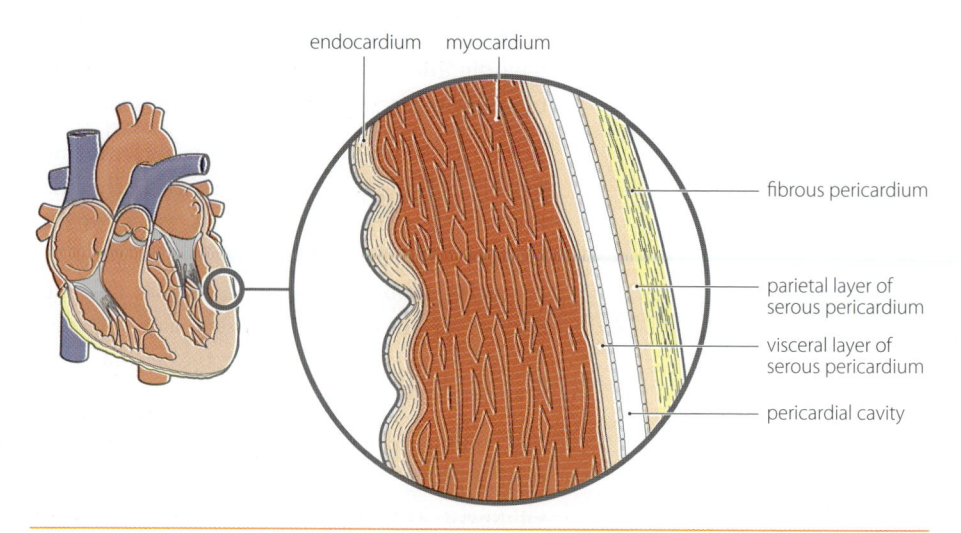

Figure 9.7 – **The major tissues that form the wall of the heart.**

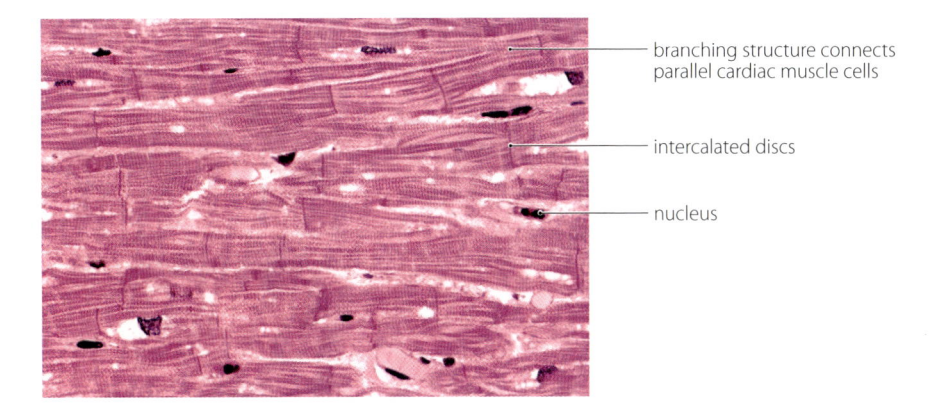

Figure 9.8 – A histology slide of myocardium.
Image by Dr Gladden Willis, reproduced with permission from Science Photo Library.

contraction of the cardiac muscle fibres provides force, pushing blood through the heart and ultimately ejecting blood from each ventricle.

The **pericardium** is a membranous sac made of two main layers (see *Figure 9.7*). The outer layer, called the fibrous pericardium, is made of dense connective tissue that protects the heart and secures it to the diaphragm, sternum and great vessels. The inner layer, called the serous pericardium, is composed of two layers (the parietal and visceral layers) arranged with a space between them that contains pericardial fluid. This fluid works as a lubricant to enable the surfaces to move across each other with minimal friction when the heart relaxes and contracts. The parietal layer lines the fibrous pericardium, while the inner layer covers the heart and great vessels and is often described as the **epicardium**.

Blood flow through the heart

The blood flow through the heart, starting with the right atrium to eventual ejection from the aorta, is illustrated in *Figure 9.9*. This can be summarized as follows:

- Blood from the venous circulation, which has a reduced oxygen content and enriched carbon dioxide content, flows into the right atrium via the superior and inferior vena cava. The superior vena cava returns blood from the head, neck and arms, while the inferior vena cava returns blood from regions of the body lying below the heart. Venous blood from the vessels that perfuse the heart wall (coronary arteries, capillaries and coronary veins) collects in a structure on the posterior aspect of the heart called the **coronary sinus**, from which blood flows into the right atrium.
- From the right atrium, blood flows into the right ventricle via the opened tricuspid valve.
- Filling of the right ventricle is aided by contraction of the right atrium.
- Blood is then ejected from the right ventricle through the opened pulmonary valve into the pulmonary artery. Immediately prior to this, as the right ventricle contracts, the build-up of pressure closes the tricuspid valve. This prevents the backflow of blood into the right atrium and ensures the flow of blood is forwards along the pressure gradient into the

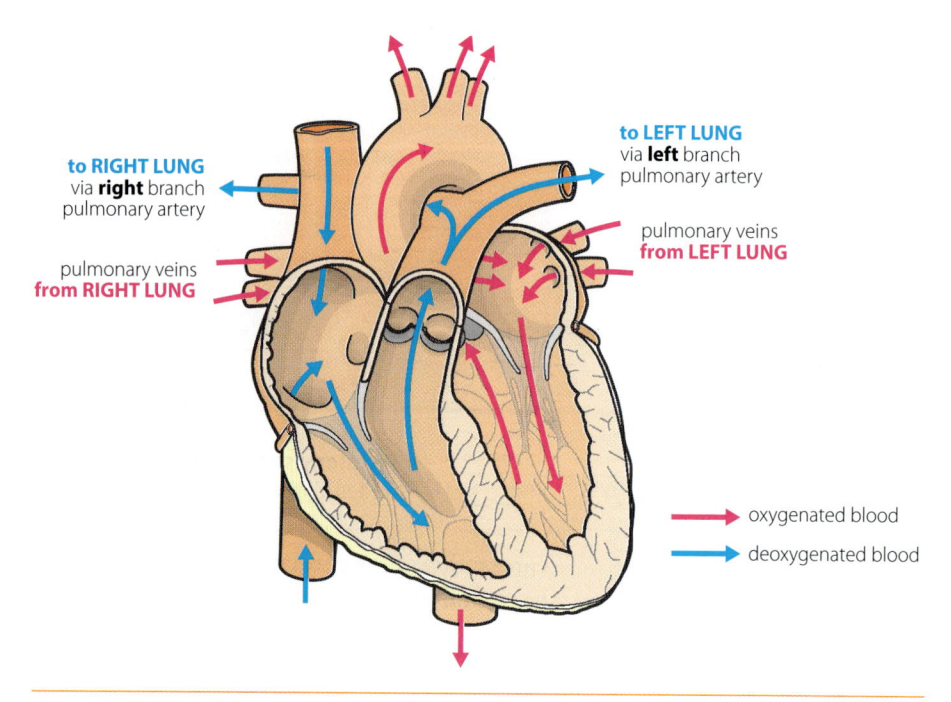

Figure 9.9 – **Blood flow through the heart.**

right and left branches of the pulmonary artery (illustrated in *Figure 9.9*). This is a unique situation, where blood with a reduced oxygen content and enriched carbon dioxide content flows along an artery. Arteries typically transport oxygenated blood but here the definition of an artery is fulfilled as the pulmonary arteries take blood away from the heart to the lungs.

- Blood from the right side of the heart then flows through the pulmonary circulation where some carbon dioxide is removed and oxygen added (this is discussed in more detail in *Chapter 10*).
- Oxygenated blood from the lungs flows to the left atrium via four pulmonary veins (two from the right lung and two from the left lung). The use of the term vein is appropriate as they return blood to the heart.
- Blood in the left atrium passes through the mitral valve, filling the left ventricle. The filling of the left ventricle is aided by contraction of the left atrium.
- The left ventricle then contracts, producing the pressure required to close the mitral valve (ensuring backflow of blood does not occur) and to open the aortic valve to eject oxygenated blood into the aorta and systemic circulation. As mentioned earlier in the chapter, the aorta has a relatively large lumen and highly elastic walls, enabling it to distend to accommodate the blood ejected from the left ventricle. Subsequent recoiling of the elastic wall helps to push the blood through the systemic circulation vasculature.

Heart valves have an important role in ensuring that blood follows the correct path. The structure of the atrioventricular valves is different from that of the semilunar aortic and pulmonary valves. The valve located between the right atrium and right ventricle has three leaflets (cusps). The mitral valve on the left side of the heart normally has only two leaflets and the name mitral valve arose from the fact that the shape produced by the two leaflets resembles a bishop's hat (a mitre). The leaflets are made of fibrous connective tissue covered with endocardium. Most notably, attached to the leaflets of the tricuspid and mitral valves are white collagen fibres called **chordae tendineae** (see *Figures 9.6* and *9.10*) and these are attached to specific muscle fibres called papillary muscles. The chordae tendineae are of a fixed length, which, together with the contraction of the papillary muscles, prevents the leaflets of the atrioventricular valves flipping back into the atria when the pressure builds up in the ventricles as the ventricles contract (see *Figure 9.10*). The combination of the chordae tendineae and papillary muscles ensures that the valve leaflets remain in close approximation and so prevent blood flowing back into the atria from the ventricles. Some of the problems arising from damage to the heart valves, which in some cases require correction by valve replacement cardiac surgery, are outlined in *Box 9.3*.

The heart as a pump

It is important to note that the volume of blood pumped out of the heart is affected by the volume of blood that returns to the heart. In other words, the heart must adequately fill with blood returning from the body into the right ventricle and from the lungs into the left ventricle. The filling of the ventricles and the degree to which they are stretched prior to their contraction directly influence the strength of contraction of the myocardium. The relationship between the degree of stretch of the myocardial cell fibres produced by ventricular filling and the volume of blood ejected with each ventricular contraction (**stroke volume**) is known as **Starling's Law of the Heart**, where stretching of the myocardial cells during diastole (see below), prior to contraction, enhances the subsequent contraction. It is important that the volume of blood within the circulating fluid compartment is

(a) Chordae tendineae relaxed, mitral valve open

(b) Chordae tendineae stretched to fixed length prevent mitral valve prolapsing

BLOOD FLOW

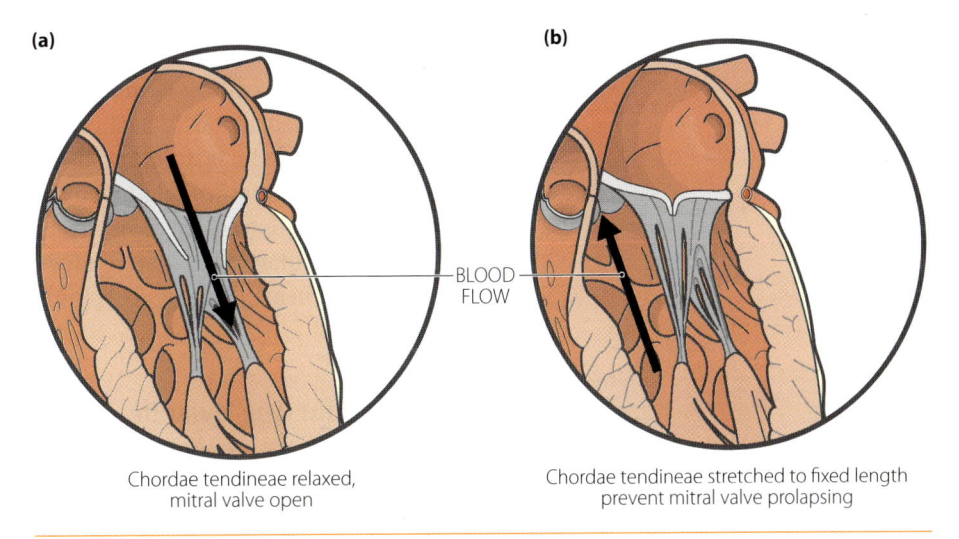

Figure 9.10 – The action of the chordae tendineae.
The mitral valve is open in (a) and closed in (b).

> **BOX 9.3**
>
> **Heart valve abnormalities**
>
> Impairment of the normal functioning of the valves can occur where there is damage to the valves, leading to abnormal blood flow through the heart. The valve opening may become smaller (valve stenosis) or the cusps may not close together effectively, resulting in blood leaking through the valve (valve incompetence). In both instances, the efficiency of the heart as a pump becomes compromised and more work is needed to pump blood. In the longer term, this can lead to the heart muscle failing and becoming less effective, leading to the build-up of extracellular fluid in the interstitial spaces of lung tissue (called pulmonary oedema) and peripheral tissues (called peripheral oedema). Valve dysfunction can lead to the development of chronic heart failure.

maintained within normal limits in order to ensure that an optimal stroke volume is produced, thus ensuring that tissues and organs receive the optimum amount of blood to meet the metabolic needs of the cells. A reduction in blood volume can lead to a fall in the stroke volume and the flow of blood to tissues and organs. For this reason, it is vital to replace fluids when a patient suffers significant fluid loss, such as following a haemorrhage, in order to restore and maintain blood volume.

Two key terms are used when considering the pumping action of the heart:

- *Cardiac output*: this is the volume of blood ejected from either ventricle per minute. At rest for an adult man this is around 5.0 L/minute. Cardiac output is determined by the heart rate and stroke volume (CO = HR × SV).
- *Stroke volume*: this is the volume of blood ejected from either ventricle per heartbeat. At rest for an adult man, this is approximately 70 ml.

Each heartbeat involves a combination of muscle contraction, pressure changes within the heart chambers and changes to blood volume within the heart. These are coordinated via an organized intrinsic system of modified muscle cells that conduct electrical impulses through the heart muscle, leading to contraction of the myocardium. The mechanical events, pressure changes and associated blood flow that occur during each heartbeat are collectively known as the **cardiac cycle**.

The cardiac cycle involves periods when the heart muscle relaxes (**diastole**), enabling the ventricles to fill with blood, and periods when the heart muscle contracts (**systole**), when blood is pushed through and ejected from the heart. The cardiac cycle normally lasts 0.8 seconds, achieved by coordinated muscle contractions leading to pressure and blood volume changes. The coordination of atrial and ventricular contraction (systole) is achieved by a specialized system of non-contractile cardiac cells that conduct action potentials in a systematic way throughout the heart muscle. This intrinsic system is called the cardiac conducting system.

The cardiac conducting system

The major conducting pathways involved in cardiac conduction are illustrated in *Figure 9.11*. The electrical impulse that initiates heart muscle contraction commences in the **sinoatrial node** (SAN) located in the right atrium, inferior to the entrance of the superior vena cava. The cells of the SAN, as with other areas of the heart, have the ability to self-generate action potentials (electrical activity)

– described as intrinsic automaticity and rhythmicity. The SAN generates action potentials at a faster rate than other areas of the heart such as the atrioventricular node and Purkinje fibres. The SAN is therefore often called the 'pacemaker' of the heart. The action potential causing depolarization of the cardiac cells spreads to adjacent atrial myocytes, and a wave of depolarization spreads across the right and then the left atrium (position ① on *Figure 9.11*), stimulating atrial cells to contract (atrial systole). A band of parallel fibres, called Bachmann's bundle (also known as the interatrial bundle), conducts an excitation impulse from the SAN to the left atrium. Intrinsic SAN activity is modified by the autonomic nervous system. Stimulation by fibres of the sympathetic nervous system increases the frequency of activity of the SAN and thus increases the heart rate, whereas stimulation of the SAN by the parasympathetic nervous system slows down the heart rate and increases the time it takes for electrical impulses to pass from the atria to the ventricles via the atrioventricular node.

The wave of depolarization initiated from the SAN reaches another collection of specialized conducting cells called the **atrioventricular node** (AVN), which is located towards the posterior region of the right atrium on the right side of the septum, which separates the left and right atrium. The electrical impulse is conducted at a slower rate through the AVN (position ② on *Figure 9.11*), due to the organization of the conducting fibres in the node. It passes to a thick bundle of conducting fibres called the **atrioventricular bundle** (also called the **bundle of His**). The delay in conduction of the electrical impulse through the AVN ensures that the atria contract, adding blood to the ventricles before the ventricles contract; thus, the ventricles are filled optimally with blood before they contract. The combination of the AVN and the atrioventricular bundle forms a bridge that crosses the fibrous tissue supporting the heart valves, which separates the atrial muscle from the ventricular muscle. Effective conduction through the AVN and the atrioventricular bundle (position ③ on *Figure 9.11*) is crucial for the coordination

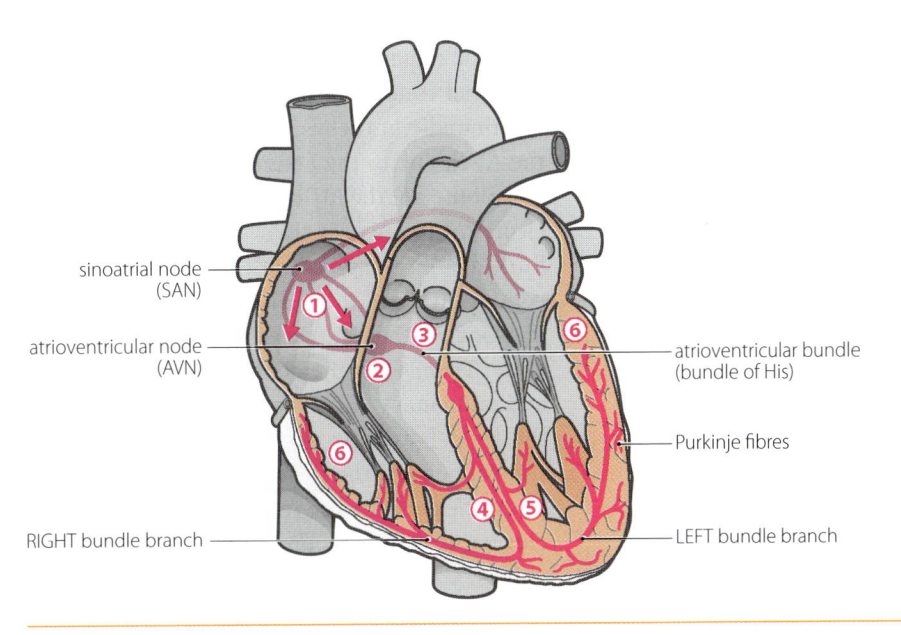

Figure 9.11 – **The cardiac conducting system.**

of atrial and ventricular contraction. Stimulation by the parasympathetic nervous system both slows the rate of SAN activation and increases the conduction time through the AVN, thus slowing down the heart rate.

From the atrioventricular bundle, the electrical impulse is conducted along the right and left bundle branches (positions ④ and ⑤ on *Figure 9.11*), which divide into a complex network of small conducting fibres called the **Purkinje fibres**. Activation of the ventricles occurs as electrical impulses are distributed through the ventricular myocardium via the Purkinje fibres (position ⑥ on *Figure 9.11*). An orderly and sequential spread of depolarization starts in the ventricular septum and then spreads through the ventricles, causing muscle contraction to be initiated at the apex and then work upwards towards the upper portions of the ventricles. There are minor differences between contraction of the right and left ventricles, but the coordinated contraction of each ventricle ensures that blood is pumped out via the pulmonary artery and aorta, respectively. The conduction of action potentials and associated wave of depolarization through the heart can be recorded using an electrocardiogram (ECG) (explained in *Box 9.4*).

The cardiac cycle: integration of mechanical and electrical events

The main phases of the cardiac cycle are shown in *Figure 9.13*, starting when the myocardium is completely relaxed. At the end of ventricular contraction, the ventricular muscle relaxes and the blood pressure in the ventricles decreases. This phase is called complete cardiac diastole. During this phase, as the atria fill with blood, returning from around the body, there reaches a point where the pressure of blood in the atria is greater than that in the ventricles and so the mitral and tricuspid valves open and the ventricles fill passively with blood. This is the early phase of diastole and approximately 80% of filling of the ventricles occurs during this phase. Towards the end of diastole, the SAN generates an action potential that spreads across the atria, causing the atria to contract (atrial systole). The contraction of the atria ensures maximal filling of the ventricles with the remaining 20% of blood. The wave of depolarization is captured by the AVN and conducted through the AVN and atrioventricular bundle to the left and right bundle branches. The delay in conduction of the electrical impulse through the AVN, due to the arrangement of the conducting fibres, ensures that the atria contribute to the filling of the ventricles before the ventricles contract. The electrical impulse is then conducted down both bundle branches and along the Purkinje fibres, spreading through the myocardium, stimulating the ventricles to contract (this is the period called ventricular systole). As a result, the pressure of blood in the ventricles increases, causing the mitral and tricuspid valves to close. Then, with the continued increase in intraventricular pressure, the aortic and pulmonary valves open, resulting in the ejection of blood from the heart into the aorta (systemic circulation) and pulmonary artery (pulmonary circulation), respectively. At the end of ventricular systole, the heart muscle relaxes completely (diastolic period). The resultant decrease in pressure within the ventricles leads to closure of the aortic and pulmonary valves, opening of the tricuspid and mitral valves, and filling of the ventricles. The ability of the myocardium to relax and for intraventricular pressure to decrease is a significant factor enabling filling of the ventricles.

SECTION 9.2 | WHAT YOU NEED TO KNOW – ESSENTIAL ANATOMY AND PHYSIOLOGY 283

> **BOX 9.4**
>
> ### Electrocardiogram
>
> The electrical activity conducted through the heart can be detected with surface electrodes attached to the skin and recorded via an electrocardiogram (ECG) (see *Figure 9.12*).
>
> Recording and monitoring of an ECG provides important information about the nature of the heart rhythm and identifies abnormalities in the rhythm and rate of the heart and the conduction of electrical activity through the heart (arrhythmias). 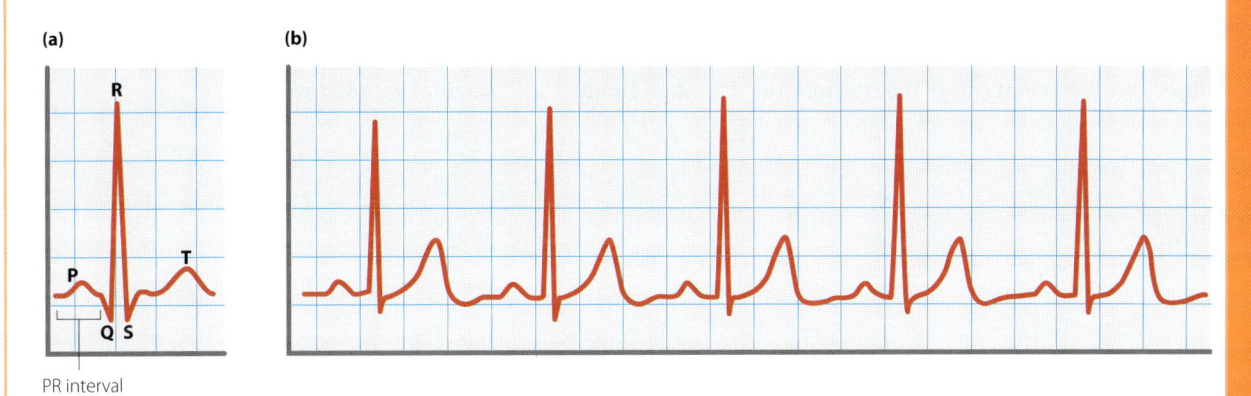
>
> **Figure 9.12** – (a) A normal ECG complex and (b) a rhythm strip showing normal sinus rhythm (five cardiac cycles are shown).
> The waves (also called deflections) that form the ECG complex are described using the letters P, Q, R, S and T. P = depolarization of atria; P–R interval = period corresponding to the time taken for the electrical activity from the SAN to spread across the atria, through the AVN and atrioventricular bundle and reach the bundle branches; QRS = depolarization of the septum and right and left ventricles; T = ventricular repolarization produced by the ventricular cells returning to their resting state. (Note that the deflection produced by atrial repolarization is usually too small to be seen.)

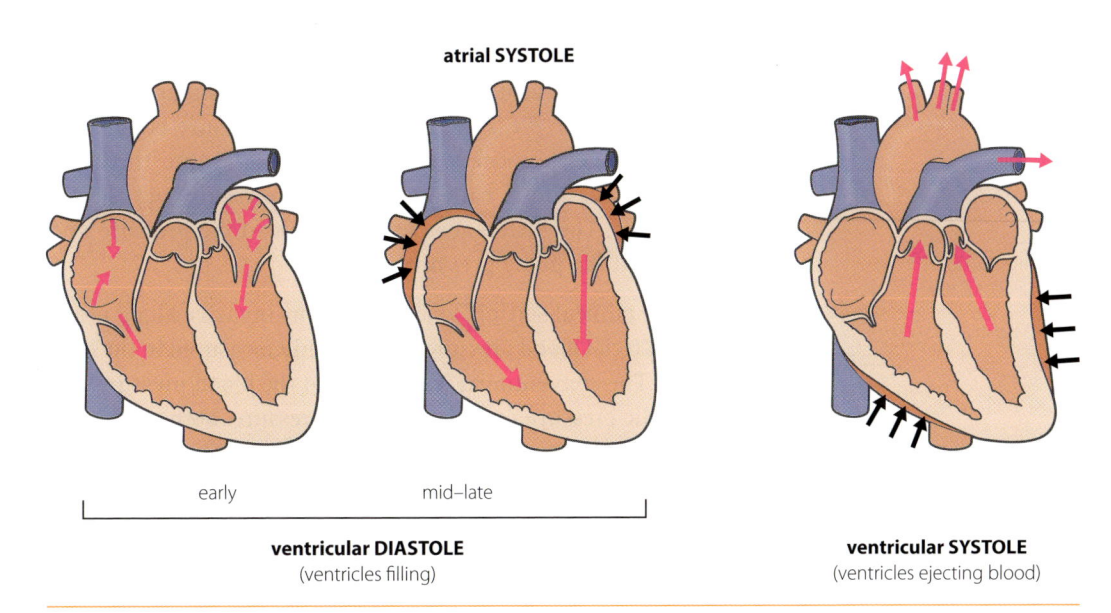

Figure 9.13 – The cardiac cycle.

The frequency of cardiac cycles is determined by the activity of the SAN, modified by the autonomic nervous system and by circulating hormones such as thyroxine and adrenaline (epinephrine). The normal heart rate and blood pressure for various age ranges and related terminology for abnormal values are shown in *Table 9.1*.

Table 9.1 – Normal heart rate (pulse) and blood pressure for various age ranges and related terminology for abnormal values

Heart rate		Blood pressure		
Age range	Normal range (beats/minute)	Age range	Normal values (mmHg)	
			Systolic	Diastolic
<1 years	100–160	Newborn	60–85	20–60
1–2 years	90–150	6 months	75–105	40–70
2–5 years	80–140	2 years	75–110	45–80
5–12 years	70–120	7 years	75–115	45–80
>12 years	60–100	Adolescent	100–145	60–95
Adult	60–100	Adult	Normally below 140/90	
Terminology	**Heart rate (beats/minute)**	**Terminology**	**Value (mmHg)**	
Tachycardia	Faster than normal: in adults >100	Hypertension	Higher than normal: in adults, ≥140/90	
Bradycardia	Slower than normal: in adults <60	Hypotension	Lower than normal: in adults, systolic <90	

Adapted from **Glasper, E. A., McEwing, G. and Richardson, J.** (eds) (2016) *Oxford Handbook of Children's and Young People's Nursing*, 2nd edn, tables on pp. 95 and 99, by permission of Oxford University Press; and the British Hypertensive Society guidelines IV (2004) (see *Further reading*).

9.2.4 Blood pressure

Blood pressure is commonly described as the pressure of blood exerted against the wall of a container. The container could be a blood vessel or the chambers within the heart and, as discussed previously in *Chapter 8*, blood pressure is an example of *hydrostatic pressure*. Arterial blood pressure is pulsatile (having a higher and lower value) because the heart ejects blood into the arteries intermittently. The higher pressure is called the systolic pressure and the lower value the diastolic pressure. The difference between the systolic pressure and the diastolic pressure is called the **pulse pressure**.

In the clinical setting, when using non-invasive blood pressure recording methods, the arterial blood pressure is commonly measured in the brachial artery of the upper arm. The conventional way to record the blood pressure is to write the value of the systolic pressure over the diastolic pressure, both expressed in units of millimetres of mercury (mmHg), for example 120 (systolic)/80 (diastolic). Contraction of the heart generates a pressure wave and blood flow, which are evident when feeling the arterial pulse. The normal ranges for blood pressure related to age are presented in *Table 9.1*. It is important to recognize that blood pressure is highly variable, depending on many factors including age, exercise, posture and emotions. Important clinical terms related to blood pressure are explained in *Box 9.5*.

SECTION 9.2 | WHAT YOU NEED TO KNOW – ESSENTIAL ANATOMY AND PHYSIOLOGY   285

> **BOX 9.5**
>
> **Blood pressure terminology**
>
> *Hypertension* refers to a higher than normal or expected resting blood pressure confirmed on at least two occasions. In adults, this is when the resting arterial blood pressure is greater than or equal to 140/90 mmHg. *Hypotension* is when the systolic arterial blood pressure is less than 90 mmHg (in adults). Both hypotension and hypertension can lead to serious health problems; for example, hypertension can lead to chronic kidney disease (see Marcus, Patient 8.1).

Determinants of blood pressure

As blood pressure fluctuates, it is usual to refer to the **mean arterial blood pressure** (MAP), which is the blood pressure averaged over time. However, this is not derived simply from the arithmetical mean between the systolic and diastolic blood pressure but is approximately equal to the diastolic pressure plus one-third of the difference between the systolic and diastolic pressure:

$$MAP = \text{diastolic pressure} + \frac{(\text{systolic pressure} - \text{diastolic pressure})}{3}$$

The MAP reflects two key physical factors: blood volume within the arterial system and the elastic qualities (compliance) of the arteries. These are affected by physiological factors, namely cardiac output (which is the product of heart rate and stroke volume) and peripheral resistance.

The interaction between these factors can be expressed by the equation:

$$MAP = \text{cardiac output} \times \text{peripheral resistance}$$

Cardiac output is determined by stroke volume and heart rate, and stroke volume is affected by blood volume; therefore, changes in any one of these can cause the blood pressure to change. For example, increasing the heart rate and the stroke volume through activation of the sympathetic nervous system will tend to increase blood pressure. A significant loss of blood volume (beyond the ability of regulatory mechanisms to compensate), for example by haemorrhage, may result in less blood returning to the right atrium, consequently reducing cardiac output and therefore blood pressure.

Peripheral resistance refers to those factors that impede or oppose blood flow through the circulatory system. Three principle factors influence peripheral resistance:

- Viscosity of blood: this is determined principally by the concentration of red blood cells and the volume of plasma (the greater the viscosity, the greater the resistance to the flow of blood).
- Length of blood vessels: the longer the vessel, the greater the resistance.
- Diameter of the lumen of blood vessels: as a tube becomes narrower (as in vasoconstriction), the surface area of the tube becomes greater in relation to the volume of fluid within the tube. This creates greater resistance to the flow of the fluid due to increased friction, in this case blood flow.

It is the diameter of the blood vessel lumen that has the predominant effect on peripheral resistance. Indeed, adjustment of the diameter of the arterioles is the most important response for the maintenance of blood pressure. For example, when the cardiac output decreases, the primary response is the vasoconstriction of arterioles to increase peripheral resistance and hence increase the blood pressure.

Regulation of blood pressure

Arterial blood pressure is regulated through a number of integrated responses, involving the autonomic nervous system, the central nervous system, the endocrine system and the renal system.

The short-term 'moment-to-moment' regulation of blood pressure is primarily via the autonomic nervous system mediated through a number of reflexes including the arterial baroreceptor and chemoreceptor reflexes. The more subtle longer-term regulation of blood pressure involves the endocrine and renal systems.

Short-term regulation of blood pressure involving the response of arterial baroreceptors to changes in blood pressure is illustrated in *Figure 9.14*. Arterial baroreceptors are stretch receptors located in the wall of the aorta and carotid arteries. These become more active when they are stretched, as blood pressure increases. When activated, sensory (afferent) impulses are delivered to the cardiovascular control centres within the medulla of the brainstem. Changes in sensory activity from the baroreceptors cause the cardiovascular control centres to modify sympathetic and parasympathetic nervous system responses. For example, when blood pressure increases, the arterial baroreceptors become more active and their rate of firing increases. The *increased rate of afferent* sensory impulses from the baroreceptors to the cardiovascular control centres in the medulla oblongata causes an *increase in efferent parasympathetic* activity, and *reduced efferent sympathetic* activity. As a result, the heart rate slows down and the force of ventricular contraction is decreased. Therefore, cardiac output decreases and at the same time arterioles dilate and peripheral resistance decreases. The overall effect is a reduction in blood pressure – this is an example of homeodynamics involving negative feedback (discussed in *Chapter 1*).

Long-term regulation of blood pressure occurs in response to a number of factors, from changes of blood pressure flowing through the kidneys to plasma volume and the composition of plasma. The renin–angiotensin–aldosterone system (RAAS), introduced in *Chapter 8*, regulates arterial blood pressure along with antidiuretic hormone released from the posterior pituitary gland and atrial and B-type natriuretic peptides produced by cardiac cells. The endocrine responses tend to either modify blood volume through effects on the kidney (see *Chapter 8*) or modify peripheral resistance within arterioles, or both. The response of the RAAS system to a fall in blood pressure or blood volume is illustrated in *Figure 9.15*. Renin is released from the juxtaglomerular apparatus in the nephron and cleaves angiotensinogen (a plasma protein produced by the liver) into angiotensin I. Angiotensin I is converted to angiotensin II by angiotensin-converting enzyme (ACE, a circulating enzyme that is secreted into the blood by renal and pulmonary endothelial cells). Two important physiological actions of angiotensin II are constriction of arterioles and stimulation of aldosterone secretion from

SECTION 9.2 | WHAT YOU NEED TO KNOW – ESSENTIAL ANATOMY AND PHYSIOLOGY 287

blood pressure (BP)

stimulus
↑ blood pressure

stimulus
↓ blood pressure

negative feedback
↓ blood pressure
• blood pressure returns to normal

negative feedback
↑ blood pressure
• blood pressure returns to normal

receptors
↑ stretch baroreceptors excited

receptors
↓ stretch baroreceptors less stretched (unloaded)

↑ afferent impulses

↓ afferent impulses

control centre
• medulla cardiovascular control centre

control centre
• medulla cardiovascular control centre

efferent impulses
↑ parasympathetic activity
↓ sympathetic activity

efferent impulses
↓ parasympathetic activity
↑ sympathetic activity

effectors: arterioles
• vasodilation
↓ peripheral resistance

effectors: heart
↓ heart rate
↓ stroke volume

effectors: arterioles
• vasoconstriction
↑ peripheral resistance

effectors: heart
↑ heart rate
↑ stroke volume

↓ cardiac output
↓ peripheral resistance

↑ cardiac output
↑ peripheral resistance

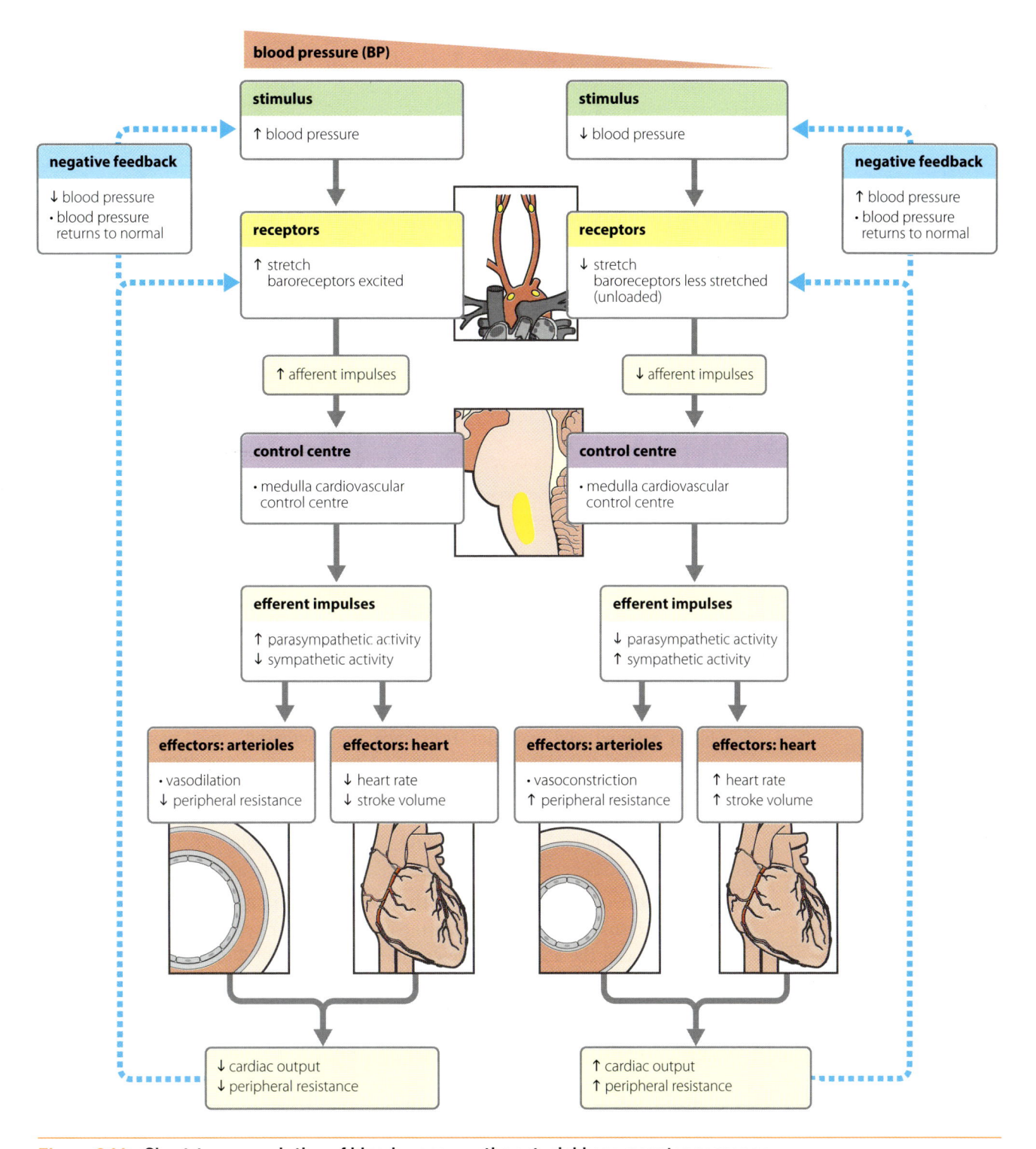

Figure 9.14 – Short-term regulation of blood pressure: the arterial baroreceptor response.

```
┌─────────────────────┐         ┌──────────────────────────┐
│ ↓ blood volume      │────────▶│ kidney                   │
│ ↓ blood pressure    │         │ (juxtaglomerular         │
└─────────────────────┘         │  apparatus)              │
                                └──────────────────────────┘
                                           │
                                           ▼
                                ┌──────────────────────────┐
                                │ renin                    │
                                └──────────────────────────┘
                                           │
┌─────────────────────┐                    ▼
│ angiotensinogen     │         ┌──────────────────────────┐        ┌──────────────────────────┐
│ (plasma protein made│────────▶│ angiotensin I            │        │ angiotensin-converting   │
│ in liver)           │         └──────────────────────────┘        │ enzyme (ACE)             │
└─────────────────────┘    renin converts angiotensinogen  ◀────────│ (from endothelium in     │
                           to angiotensin I                          │ lungs and kidneys)       │
                                           │                        └──────────────────────────┘
                                           ▼
┌─────────────────────┐         ┌──────────────────────────┐
│ adrenal cortex      │◀────────│ angiotensin II           │
│ stimulated to       │         │ (acts on ang II receptors)│
│ release aldosterone │         └──────────────────────────┘
└─────────────────────┘                    │
           │                               ▼
           ▼                    ┌──────────────────────────┐
┌─────────────────────┐         │ vasoconstriction of      │
│ aldosterone increases│        │ arterioles               │
│ renal reabsorption   │        │ (↑ peripheral vascular   │
│ of Na⁺ and H₂O       │        │ resistance and arterial  │
│ (↑ blood volume)     │        │ blood pressure)          │
└─────────────────────┘        └──────────────────────────┘
```

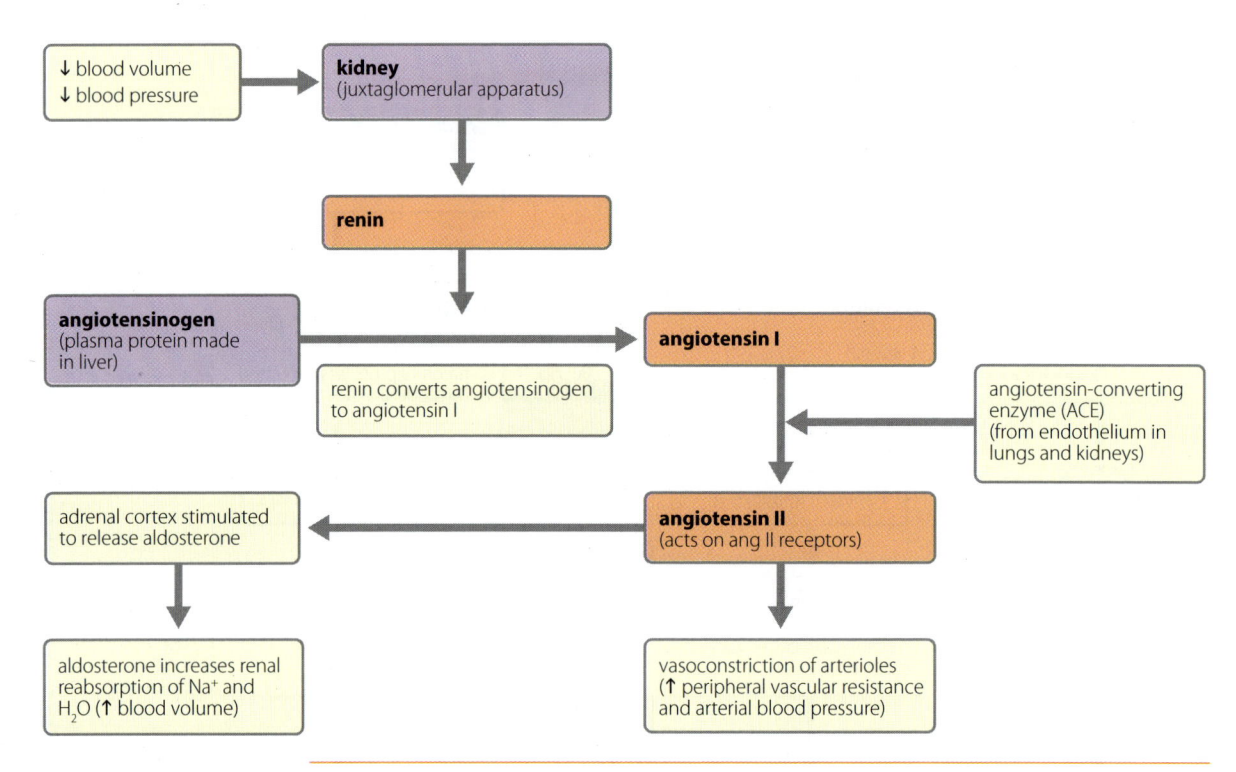

Figure 9.15 – The renin–angiotensin–aldosterone system (RAAS).

the adrenal cortex. Remember that aldosterone acts on receptors on the tubular cells in the distal convoluted tubule and collecting ducts of the nephrons in the kidneys to increase the reabsorption of sodium ions (Na^+). Through these actions, blood volume and vascular resistance are increased, thus increasing blood pressure. Drugs that interfere with the RAAS response include ACE inhibitors and angiotensin receptor blockers. These can be used to reduce blood pressure when a person is hypertensive (see *Marcus, Patient 8.1*) and to reduce the workload of the heart when a person has heart failure (see *Robert, Patient 9.1*).

Variation of blood pressure throughout the cardiovascular system

Blood pressure varies throughout the cardiovascular system. The blood pressure falls between the aorta and the capillaries (see *Figure 9.16*), creating a pressure gradient that enables blood to flow from the heart to the tissues. In addition, there is a change from a pulsatile to a steady-state flow as pressure continues to decline along the capillary. The pulsatile flow and blood pressure are dampened at the capillary level by the combination of the ability of large arteries to distend and the resistance produced by arterioles. As illustrated in *Figure 9.16*, the blood pressure in the left ventricle and arterial circulation is greater than that in the right ventricle and venous systemic circulation. Vascular resistance in the lungs is substantially lower than in the systemic circulation, and therefore the blood pressure is lower. Pulmonary arteries and arterioles are also shorter and have thinner muscular walls, which contribute to the reduced resistance. For this reason, the right ventricle is not required to generate systolic pressures to the same extent as the left ventricle, therefore the right ventricular wall is much

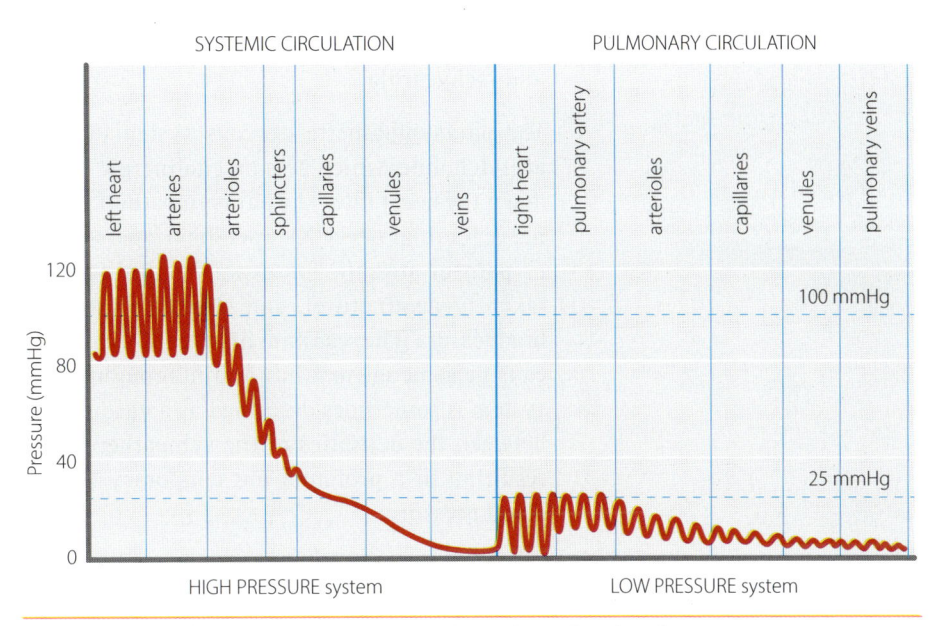

Figure 9.16 – Blood pressure variation throughout the circulatory system.

thinner. The left ventricle has a very thick wall that contracts in a very different way to the right ventricle, which works more like bellows contracting against the rigid septum. The thicker wall enables the left ventricle to generate a greater blood pressure to overcome the higher vascular resistance in the systemic circulation and the longer distances blood has to travel to reach the tissues of the body.

Autonomic nervous system effects on the cardiovascular system

Along with the endocrine system, the autonomic nervous system has an important role in the regulation of cardiovascular function. The sympathetic nervous system has an effect on both cardiac function and blood vessels, and this is mediated via the release of the neurotransmitter noradrenaline (norepinephrine) from nerve endings, which acts on specific adrenergic receptors. There are different types of adrenergic receptors: alpha (α) and beta (β). Within each type are subsets distinguished by numbers, such as α_1, α_2, β_1 and β_2 (see *Chapters 2 and 4*). Activation of the sympathetic nervous system increases the heart rate and force of contraction by acting on β_1-adrenoceptors, present on myocardial cells and the SAN. The effect of noradrenaline (norepinephrine) on the blood vessels is variable, depending on the type of adrenergic receptor stimulated; stimulation of α_1-adrenoceptors on skin arterioles causes vasoconstriction, whereas stimulation of β_2-adrenoceptors leads to vasodilation of the arterioles in muscles. Vasoconstriction of skin arterioles leads to a redistribution of blood flow into deeper and larger arteries and an increase in peripheral resistance. This is an important response to increase blood pressure when the arterial blood pressure decreases. As outlined in *Chapter 1*, peripheral vasoconstriction is also an important mechanism to conserve heat when the body temperature falls.

The activation of the sympathetic nervous system as a compensatory response to a sudden fall in blood pressure is illustrated in *Figure 9.14*. Some of the compensatory responses can present as cold and clammy skin, grey/pallid skin and tachycardia.

The parasympathetic nervous system, via the release of the neurotransmitter acetylcholine, which acts on cholinergic (muscarinic) receptors, principally slows down the heart rate. The parasympathetic nerve stimulating the heart is the vagus nerve (cranial nerve X). Specific triggers, such as emotional stress and unpleasant or painful stimuli, for example, the sight of blood or having a blood sample taken (venepuncture), can stimulate the vagus nerve, resulting in a profound bradycardia. The resultant bradycardia can lead to a dramatic fall in blood pressure, causing someone to faint. A faint brought on by activation of the parasympathetic system is sometimes described as a vasovagal episode; it represents an imbalance between the activities of the sympathetic and parasympathetic nervous system, resulting in a profound but temporary impairment in the normal regulation of blood pressure.

Venous return

Venous return is the flow of blood into the right side of the heart and occurs because of the pressure gradient between the capillaries and the central veins. Gravity, the diameter of the lumen of the vein (venomotor tone), the skeletal muscle 'pump' and respiration (respiratory 'pump') govern the distribution of venous blood between the peripheral veins and the thoracic veins, and this affects the volume of blood returning to the heart. The amount of blood that returns to the right side of the heart is important because this circulates through the lungs to the left side of the heart, filling the left ventricle and thus influencing the stroke volume.

Three functional adaptations influence venous return:

- the skeletal muscle 'pump'
- the presence of one-way valves in the major veins, which help overcome the effects of gravity
- the respiratory 'pump'.

The effects of the contraction of skeletal muscle and the valves in the veins on venous blood flow are illustrated in *Figure 9.17*. Contraction of skeletal muscles, for example calf muscles, compresses the veins that run through the muscles. As they do so, blood is squeezed along the veins towards the heart. Valves in the veins open due to the increased pressure, allowing blood to flow towards the heart. Once beyond the valve, the weight of the blood closes the valve and blood is prevented from flowing backwards. In this way, blood is shunted in segments towards the central veins and the heart.

The mechanics of breathing will be discussed and expanded on in *Chapter 10*, but it is important to recognize here that normal periodic breathing causes rhythmic variations in blood flow along the vena cava. Respiration provides an additional pump, promoting venous return. During respiration, the fall in the intrathoracic pressure expands the intrathoracic veins, reducing the central venous pressure and thus increasing the pressure gradient between the thoracic veins and veins outside the thorax. At the same time, contraction of the diaphragm increases the

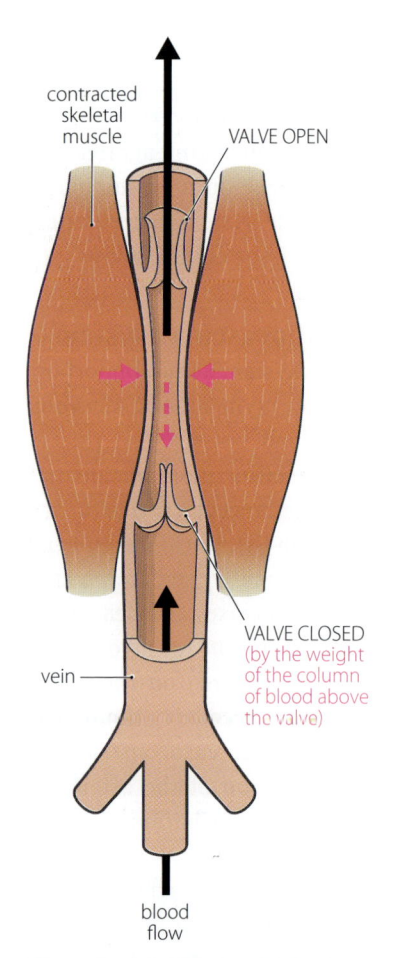

Figure 9.17 – Venous return: the skeletal muscle pump and the action of valves in the veins.

abdominal venous pressure, which also promotes venous blood flow from the abdomen into the thorax. Both mechanisms accelerate blood flow into the right atrium. During inspiration, while right ventricular stroke volume increases due to increased filling of the right side of the heart, left ventricular stroke volume falls. This is due to stretching of the pulmonary veins, causing more blood to remain in the pulmonary circulation and therefore reduced filling of the left side of the heart. Left ventricular stroke volume increases during expiration.

Effects of postural changes on venous return

When a person moves from a lying to a standing position and remains at rest, the blood pressure in the veins below the heart (such as the legs and feet) gradually rises over a period of 30–60 seconds. The slowness in the rise in venous pressure is due to the valves in the veins, which prevent any significant backflow of blood. The column of blood in the veins is supported at various points by the valves. Blood continues to flow into the veins from the arterial system, capillaries and venules and so the venous pressure continues to rise and the veins distend. This is often described as venous pooling. As the veins are highly distensible and as a result can hold a considerable volume of blood, the greatest effect of the change in posture is on the veins. Distension of the veins and redistribution of blood into the veins causes a reduction in the central blood volume and a reduction in ventricular filling, with a corresponding fall in stroke volume and cardiac output, which may lead to a fall in blood pressure. In response to the erect position, reflex compensatory adjustments are activated to correct the fall in blood pressure, leading to, for example, an increase in heart rate and vasoconstriction of arterioles (these are discussed previously in this chapter). Constriction of the veins also occurs, particularly in the veins from the spleen and intestines, helping to compensate for the venous pooling. When an individual with impaired reflex adaptations stands, the fall in blood pressure can be very severe, causing the person to feel dizzy or indeed faint on standing (this is called **orthostatic hypotension**). The risk of hypotension on standing is increased by vasodilation of the blood vessels of the skin (for example, when the ambient temperature is high), when the person is dehydrated or when the normal cardiovascular reflex response is impaired due to the effects of ageing or the action of drugs that slow the heart rate (such as β-adrenoceptor blockers). It is worth noting that the increase in venous pressure on standing does not occur when a person starts to walk. Contraction of skeletal muscle compresses the veins, forcing blood up the veins (aided by the valves) towards the heart.

Capillary fluid dynamics

Within capillaries, the movement of water and solutes between the blood and the interstitial fluid is a dynamic process and is carefully regulated. As stated in *Chapter 8*, the movement of water and solutes between the capillary and interstitial fluid is achieved through a balance of various forces, including the hydrostatic pressure exerted by the blood pressure and osmotic pressure within the capillaries, created by the presence of plasma proteins (more precisely called the oncotic pressure or colloid osmotic pressure). Hydrostatic pressure tends to push fluids across a membrane. Osmotic pressure counteracts hydrostatic pressure and is the force or pressure that stops water moving from a dilute solution into a concentrated solution when the two solutions are separated by a semi-permeable (or porous) membrane. *Figure 9.18* shows a simplified illustration of the balance of forces and the movement of water and solutes. Blood pressure decreases as blood flows along the length of the capillary, whereas osmotic pressure remains relatively constant. This means that at the arterial end of the capillary, hydrostatic pressure is greater than osmotic pressure (net pressure difference is +10 mmHg), leading to water and solutes moving en masse from the capillary into the interstitial fluid. In the middle of the capillary, the blood pressure equals osmotic pressure, allowing fluid to pass equally between the capillary and tissues. However, at the venous end of the capillary, due to the decrease in blood pressure, osmotic forces are greater (net pressure difference of −8 mmHg), leading to fluid moving back into the capillary. The change in these forces creates a bulk flow of water and solutes from the interstitial fluid back into the capillary, and creates a flow of fluid through the interstitial space. On balance, more fluid enters the interstitial fluid than moves back into the capillary, and this excess fluid is normally removed via lymphatic vessels that lie within the interstitial space between the blood vessels and cells. This fluid becomes part of the fluid in the lymphatic system and eventually is returned to the venous circulation via the right lymphatic duct, which drains lymph into the venous system at the junction of the right subclavian and internal jugular vein, and the thoracic duct, which drains into the junction of the left internal jugular and subclavian vein (see *Chapter 11*). Normal capillary fluid dynamics can become disrupted, leading to a collection of fluid in the tissues, for example when people develop swollen ankles (see Robert, Patient 9.1) or lymphoedema (see Sheila, Patient 2.3).

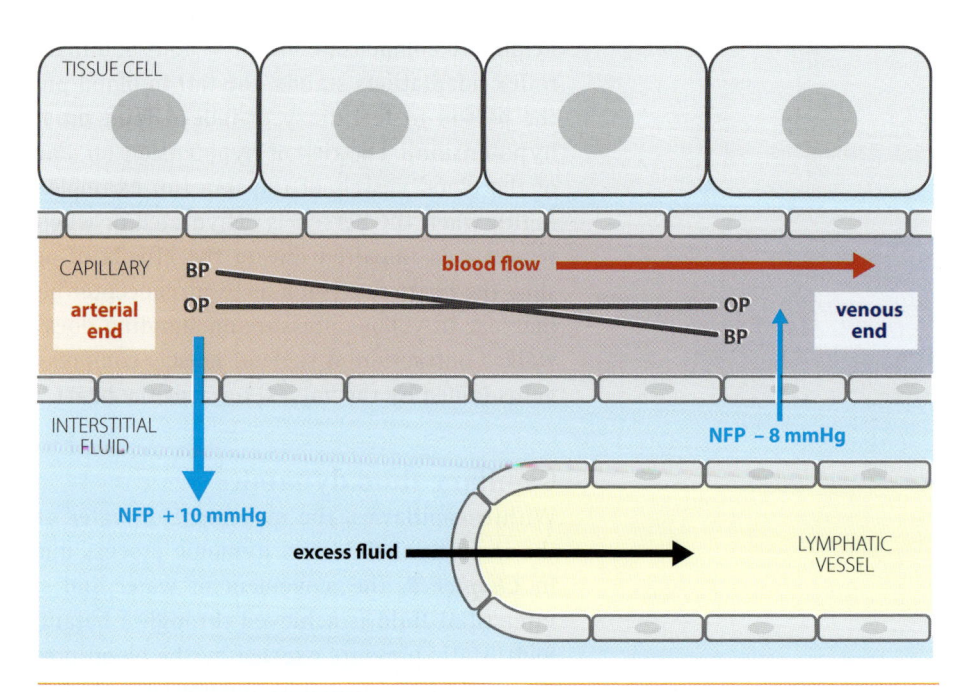

Figure 9.18 – Capillary fluid dynamics.
BP = blood pressure; OP = osmotic pressure; NFP = net filtration pressure; ➡ = direction of fluid flow.

9.2.5 Blood composition and function

Composition of blood

The importance of circulating blood should not be underestimated. The reduction of blood flow to any tissue can lead to cell injury and cell death within minutes. The average volume of blood in men and women is 5–6 and 4–5 L, approximating to 75 and 65 ml/kg of body weight, respectively. Blood accounts for approximately 8% of the total body weight and is composed of a mixture of cells suspended in a fluid called plasma. Plasma accounts for approximately 55% of the blood volume. Red blood cells account for 44% and the remaining 1% is composed of white blood cells and platelets (see *Figure 9.19*).

whole blood 8%	formed blood cells	red blood cells (erythrocytes) $4.5 – 6.5 \times 10^{12}/L$
	plasma 55%	platelets (thrombocytes) $150 – 400 \times 10^{9}/L$
		white blood cells (leukocytes) $4.0 – 11.0 \times 10^{9}/L$
BODY WEIGHT	VOLUME	NUMBER

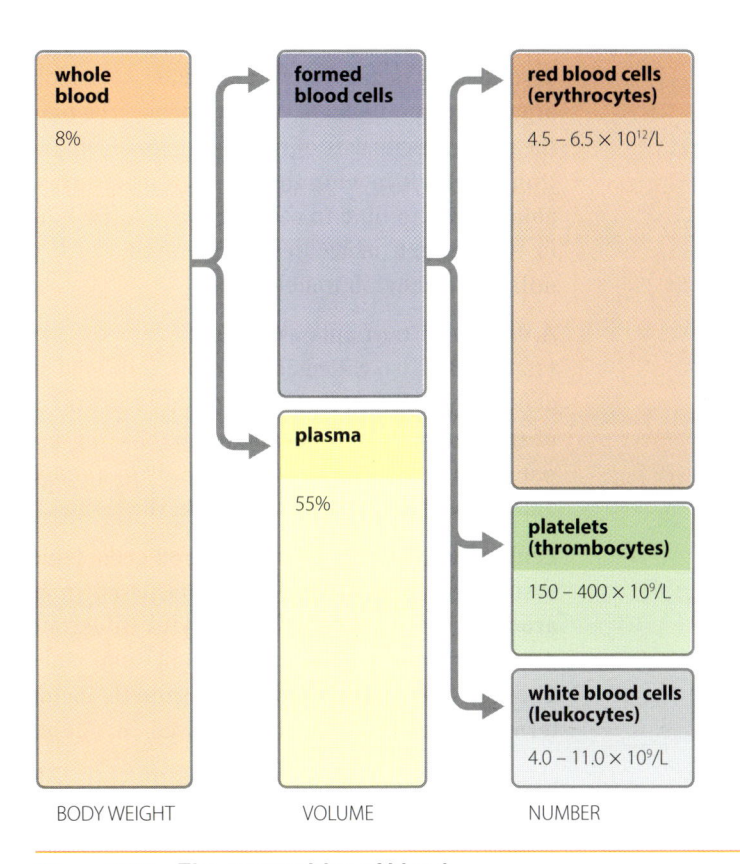

Figure 9.19 – **The composition of blood.**

Plasma is a pale, yellowish fluid of which 90% is water. The remaining constituents include:

- plasma proteins (such as albumin, antibodies, fibrinogen and prothrombin)
- hormones
- nutrients (glucose, amino acids, fatty acids, vitamins)
- electrolytes.

Figure 9.20 shows a smear of blood on a microscope slide. This smear reveals the main blood cells that comprise the formed elements of blood, which are:

- red blood cells (erythrocytes)
- white blood cells (leukocytes)
- thrombocytes (platelets).

Erythrocytes, also called red blood cells, are vitally important in carrying oxygen and carbon dioxide (discussed in *Chapter 10*). Erythrocytes have a biconcave shape, producing a lighter-coloured centre when viewed under the microscope. During the development of the erythrocyte, the nucleus is expelled to enable packaging of the cytoplasm with haemoglobin, and consequently erythrocytes cannot divide and have a limited lifespan of approximately 120 days. **Haemoglobin** is essential for the transportation of oxygen in the blood. Haemoglobin is described as a metalloprotein, made of a globular protein called *globin* and an organic compound called *haem*; hence, the name haemoglobin. The globin part of the molecule consists of four polypeptide chains; two α-chains and two β-chains. Iron (Fe^{2+}) is located in the haem group attached to each globin chain. One oxygen atom is able to bind to each Fe^{2+} and so each haemoglobin molecule can carry up to two oxygen molecules. Each single erythrocyte contains approximately 250 million haemoglobin molecules.

A variety of nutrients are essential for the synthesis of erythrocytes, including vitamin B_{12} (also called cobalamin), folic acid and iron (discussed in *Chapter 7*). A deficiency of any of these in the body can lead to abnormalities in the development of erythrocytes and haemoglobin, causing a variety of types of **anaemia**. The reduction in haemoglobin level leads to a reduction in oxygen-carrying capacity and reduced delivery of oxygen to the tissues.

Leukocytes, also called white blood cells, have an important role in the immune system for fighting infection (discussed in more detail in *Chapter 11*). There are a variety of types of leukocytes (illustrated in *Figure 9.21*). All blood cells develop from the same multipotent stem cells located in the red bone marrow. Through the action of specific growth factors, blood cells mature, becoming terminally differentiated (discussed in *Chapter 2*) into specific types of white

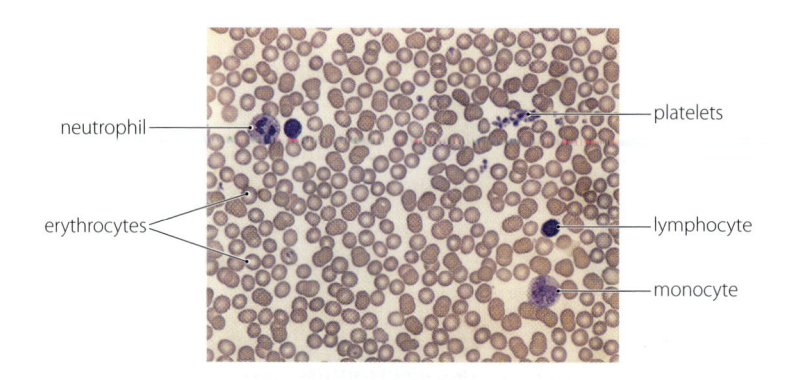

Figure 9.20 – **Photomicrograph of a human blood smear.**
Reproduced with permission from Science Photo Library.

SECTION 9.2 | WHAT YOU NEED TO KNOW – ESSENTIAL ANATOMY AND PHYSIOLOGY 295

blood cells. Leukocytes are classed as granulocytes and agranulocytes. When examined by microscopy, granulocytes are observed to contain a large number of cytoplasmic granules, which is not the case for agranulocytes. Granulocytes include neutrophils, basophils, eosinophils and mast cells; those classed as

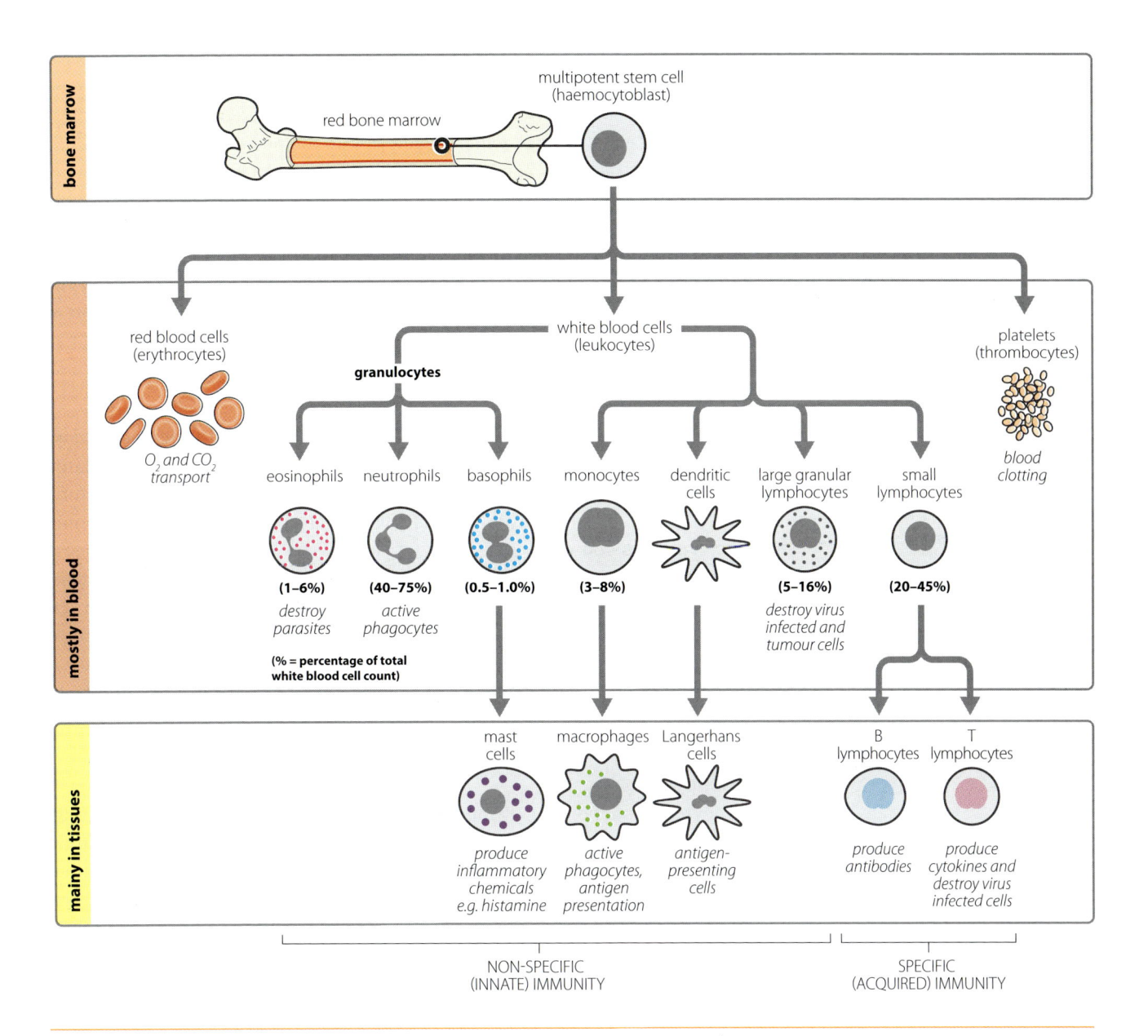

Figure 9.21 – Haematopoiesis (the formation of blood's cellular components).
Haematopoiesis starts with multipotential stem cells within the bone marrow. These cells provide a variety of progenitor cells which gradually differentiate to form a variety of mature cells. Differentiation is regulated by a complex network of cytokines, growth factors and hormones. *Note:* the lineage of mast cells and Langerhans cells is absent from the figure. The origin and maintenance of these cells is complex. Mast cells have a haematopoietic origin and can be renewed from multiple progenitor cells within tissues, while Langerhans cells (a type of dendritic cell) also have a haematopoietic origin, but in the early stages of embryonic and fetal development can be found within the developing skin, where they can be renewed throughout life.

agranulocytes include lymphocytes and monocytes. Monocytes migrate into the tissues and differentiate into macrophages. Neutrophils account for 50–70% of the total white blood cell count, while lymphocytes account for approximately 25–45% and monocytes 3–8%. Normal reference values for leukocytes present within the blood are presented in *Chapter 11, Table 11.1*.

Thrombocytes, also called **platelets**, are not really cells, but are anucleated cellular fragments, about a quarter of the size of a leukocyte, derived from much larger cells. They have an important role in the process of blood clotting and in wound healing. When a blood vessel wall is damaged, thrombocytes stick together and form an initial 'platelet plug', which develops into a blood clot (**thrombus**). They also release a variety of chemicals which act as growth factors and stimulate the immune system. Thrombus formation is a normal response to protect the circulatory system and stop blood loss. However, sometimes a thrombus can form that blocks the flow of blood through a blood vessel; as experienced by Robert (Patient 9.1), a thrombus can form at the site of atherosclerotic narrowing of the coronary artery, leading to obstruction of blood flow and possible development of a myocardial infarction.

Haemopoiesis

All blood cells develop from a common pluripotent stem cell called a **haemocytoblast** found within red bone marrow and the process is called haemopoiesis. Stimulated by specific chemical mediators such as hormones, cytokines and growth factors, stem cells divide by mitosis and become cells that are committed to form one specific type of blood cell – erythrocytes, leukocytes or thrombocytes. Once a cell is committed to a particular blood cell pathway, its development will remain on this pathway. This is governed by the presence of specific receptors on the cell membrane, which are stimulated by specific growth factors. The production of blood cells varies according to demand, for example when replacing destroyed blood cells, and physiological requirements, such as increasing the number of white blood cells when an infection is present.

Erythropoiesis

Erythrocyte production (erythropoiesis) occurs when a stem cell transforms into a committed cell called a pro-erythroblast. Through a series of mitotic divisions, the pro-erythroblast develops into an immature red blood cell called a reticulocyte (see *Figure 9.22*). A series of cell divisions results in the cell becoming smaller, and then towards the late stage of erythropoiesis, haemoglobin accumulates within the cytoplasm and eventually the cell nucleus collapses. The nucleus is ejected from the cell along with most of the organelles. The red blood cell adopts a biconcave shape. The process from the pro-erythroblast stage to the development of the reticulocyte takes about 15 days. Reticulocytes migrate from the red bone marrow into the blood, where they mature. The number of circulating erythrocytes is relatively constant, reflecting the extremely metabolically active red bone marrow as a balance is maintained between red blood cells removed from the circulation and the formation of new cells. Factors such as hypoxia (reduced oxygen levels in the tissues), due to impaired breathing or possibly due to the loss of red blood cells through bleeding, cause the release of **erythropoietin** from

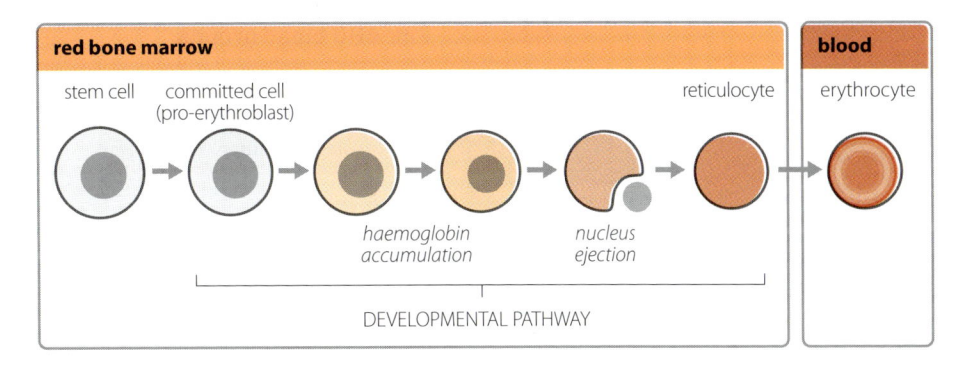

Figure 9.22 – **Erythropoiesis.**

the kidney, which stimulates erythrocyte production. Thus, a mechanism exists between the circulatory system, the kidneys and the bone marrow to regulate homeodynamic demands for oxygen capacity.

Blood groups

A person's blood group depends on genetically determined antigens (discussed in *Chapter 11*), which, when present on the cell membrane of erythrocytes, are called **agglutinogens**. These agglutinogens are able to bind to **agglutinins** to form a 'clump' or mass of cells. These agglutinins are specific antibodies (see *Chapter 11*) present in the plasma.

There are many blood grouping systems but the most commonly used are the ABO system and the rhesus system. The antigens of these two systems are responsible for most of the clinical effects encountered when incompatible blood is transfused, leading to transfusion reactions, which may be severe and can even cause death.

ABO system

The ABO system is based on the presence or absence of two antigens, A and B, on the membrane of the red blood cell and two antibodies in the plasma called anti-A and anti-B. The four groups identified under the ABO system are groups A, B, AB and O (see *Table 9.2*). For example, people with blood group A possess the A antigen on their red blood cell membrane and those with blood group AB possess both A and B antigens, while those with blood group O have neither type of antigen. The presence or absence of A or B antigens on erythrocytes is determined by genes inherited from each parent. For example, individuals with blood group A have the genotype AA or AO. You might recall from *Chapter 3* that the genotype influences the phenotype. In this case, AA represents the genotype and the expression of the antigen on the erythrocyte represents the phenotype, that is, the blood group of the person.

Antibodies are present in the plasma and these react to antigens on the membrane of the erythrocyte. For example, a person with blood group A has antibodies (agglutinins) in the plasma to blood group B or AB (see *Table 9.2*). The antibodies, known as anti-B, in the plasma react to erythrocytes that have the antigen B (an agglutinogen) on the plasma membrane. For this reason, it would not make any

Table 9.2 – The ABO blood groups

RBC antigens (agglutinogens)	plasma antibodies (agglutinins)	blood group
AB	none	AB
B	anti-A (a)	B
A	anti-B (b)	A
none	anti-A (a) anti-B (b)	O

DONOR (red blood cells) / RECIPIENT

	AB†	B	A	O
AB	✓	✗	✗	✗
B	✓	✓	✗	✗
A	✓	✗	✓	✗
O*	✓	✓	✓	✓

* universal donor = type O
† universal recipient = type AB

sense for a person to have antibodies in the plasma that would react to the antigens on their own red blood cells. Similarly, a person with blood group B has anti-A antibodies in their plasma. The reaction between antigens and antibodies forms the basis of transfusion reactions. An understanding of the blood group system is therefore imperative to ensure the safe transfusion of blood and blood products. Compatible blood groups are presented in *Table 9.2*. This table should help you understand why group O rhesus-negative blood (the rhesus system is discussed below) is used in an emergency before blood that has been typed (grouped) and cross-matched is available (see *Box 9.6*).

Rhesus system

Individuals are classified as having rhesus D-positive (Rh-positive) or rhesus D-negative (Rh-negative) blood, depending on whether or not the rhesus antigen

---

BOX 9.6

Blood typing (grouping) and crossmatching

Blood typing and crossmatching are done to ensure that a person who needs a blood transfusion receives blood that is compatible with their own. Blood typing is performed in a haematology or blood bank laboratory. The person's blood is mixed with commercially prepared serum containing specific antibodies. **Serum** is the plasma-like fluid component of blood left when the blood cells coagulate. When antigens on the person's red blood cells react with the antibodies in the serum, clumping of the cells occurs. Clumping indicates which antigens or antibodies are present – in other words, the blood group. Crossmatching is the second stage, where serum from the person who is to receive blood is mixed with serum from a potential donor (with the same ABO group and rhesus type). Lack of clumping indicates compatibility because the antibodies do not react to the antigens, and therefore the donated blood can be used for the transfusion. If clumping occurs, the blood is not compatible.

(called the rhesus or D factor) is present on their erythrocytes. An understanding of the implications of the rhesus system is particularly important in pregnancy. Normally, fetal blood and maternal blood circulate separately, with the transfer of nutrients and waste products occurring across the placenta (see *Chapter 14*). However, there are occasions when some fetal cells enter the maternal circulation, for example at the separation of the placenta following birth, or following damage to the placenta during pregnancy; both of these provide a 'sensitizing event'. If the mother is Rh negative and the fetus is Rh positive, the Rh-positive antigens in the fetal blood can provoke an immune response in the mother. She produces *maternal antibodies* against the *fetal D antigen* (anti-D antibodies), as illustrated in *Figure 9.23*. The mother is described as 'sensitized' and the anti-D antibodies can be identified in her blood using an *indirect Coombs test* (see *Box 9.7*). Maternal anti-D antibodies are small enough to pass across the placenta and to *enter the fetal blood*. If the fetus is Rh positive, the maternal anti-D antibodies react with the fetal D antigen on the fetal erythrocytes, causing **haemolysis**. This leads to the development of anaemia and jaundice, evident at birth as 'haemolytic disease of the newborn'. Severe forms of the disease can lead to death of the fetus. Usually, it is a baby from a subsequent pregnancy that is at risk of haemolytic disease of the newborn, because the process follows the primary and secondary responses to antigen (described in *Chapter 11*). When a sensitizing event occurs during pregnancy, maternal anti-D antibodies pass through the placenta into the fetal circulation and destroy the Rh-positive red blood cells. To prevent the development of anti-D antibodies, a woman who is confirmed to have Rh-negative

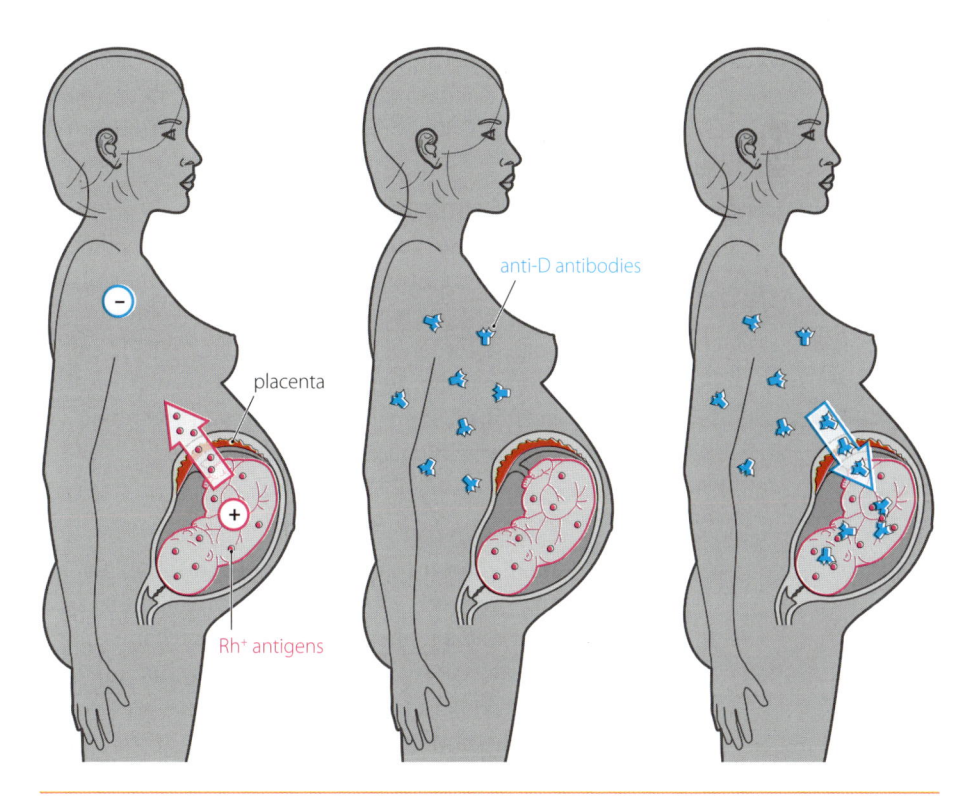

Figure 9.23 – **Rhesus factor: an illustration of the potential effects on baby and mother.**

> **BOX 9.7**
>
> **Indirect Coombs test**
>
> This test is named after Robin Coombs who first developed the technique for testing the effect of antibodies against other antibodies. It is also called an indirect antiglobulin test and is used to detect antibodies in the blood of the mother that may cross the placenta and cause haemolytic disease of the newborn. The indirect Coombs test allows anti-D antibodies to be identified before the maternal blood reacts with the fetal blood. In the past, the reaction between the antigens and anti-D antibodies was visualized as blood cells clotting in a test tube, but now more advanced technology to analyse proteins and detect the antibodies is used.

blood is offered an injection of anti-D antibodies during the pregnancy and after delivery or a sensitizing event, to 'mop up' or neutralize any Rh-positive antigens that might have entered the mother's blood during pregnancy.

Haemostasis and blood clotting

Haemostasis is essential to maintain an intact circulatory system and prevent the loss of blood, which can lead to acute and chronic health problems. Normally, haemostasis is rapid, controlled and localized. Haemostasis starts with damage to the wall of blood vessels, initiating three rapidly occurring events – vascular spasm, activation of platelets to form a platelet plug and coagulation.

Vascular spasm

Damaged blood vessels respond by constricting, thus minimizing blood loss from the damaged vessel. This effect can last 20–30 minutes, during which time platelets are activated and start to stick together (aggregate).

Activation of platelets

Exposure of collagen within the blood vessel wall due to damage to the endothelium activates a number of receptors on the wall of platelets, making platelets 'sticky'. Platelets stretch out as well as becoming sticky and release various chemicals such as adenosine diphosphate (ADP), serotonin and thromboxane A_2, which enhance the aggregation of platelets, forming a platelet plug. Platelet plugs are sufficient to seal small breaks in the blood vessel wall; however, to repair larger ruptures, blood clotting is required.

Coagulation

Coagulation (blood clotting) reinforces the soft platelet plug by forming a web-like network of fibrin threads that bind platelets. In the presence of calcium ions and factors released from activated platelets, coagulation occurs involving the activation of specific clotting factors in a controlled and ordered sequence. Most clotting factors are proteins produced in the liver and are identified by Roman numerals, for example factor VIII, factor X (Stuart–Prower factor), factor I (**fibrinogen**) and factor II (**prothrombin**). Vitamin K (see *Chapter 7*) is an essential vitamin for the production of prothrombin and factors VII, IX and X. Typically, clotting factors circulate in the blood in an inactive form. Once one clotting factor is activated, it activates the next clotting factor and a cascade of reactions results in the final blood clot. Calcium is vital in the coagulation process.

Activation of the clotting factors is initially by two pathways, called the intrinsic and extrinsic pathways, which come together at the formation of a prothrombin activator complex. From this point, a common pathway is followed. The intrinsic pathway is activated when the blood vessel wall is damaged, revealing underlying tissues such as collagen, and all of the factors needed for clotting are present in (intrinsic to) the blood. The extrinsic pathway is triggered when blood is exposed to a factor called **tissue factor** (factor III) found in tissue underneath the damaged endothelium. This pathway is called extrinsic because tissue factor is located outside of the blood. In the body, both pathways are usually triggered by damage to blood vessels and both pathways involve multiple steps to reach the common final pathway.

The common final pathway is shown in *Figure 9.24*. Prothrombin activator transforms prothrombin, a plasma protein formed by the liver in the presence of vitamin K, into the enzyme **thrombin**, which then transforms the soluble clotting factor fibrinogen into insoluble **fibrin**. Fibrin molecules form long fibrin threads that bind together to make a mesh-like framework, which glues platelets together and traps cells, thus forming the final clot. Within 30–60 minutes, the clot is stabilized further, and as the platelets within the clot contract, the clot becomes compacted and the edges of the damaged blood vessels are brought closer together to aid healing. Once the clotting cascade is activated, the clotting process continues until a clot is formed.

Following their useful purpose, clots are normally removed by a process called **fibrinolysis**. A fibrin-digesting enzyme called **plasmin** is activated by **plasminogen**, a plasma protein present within the blood clot. Typically,

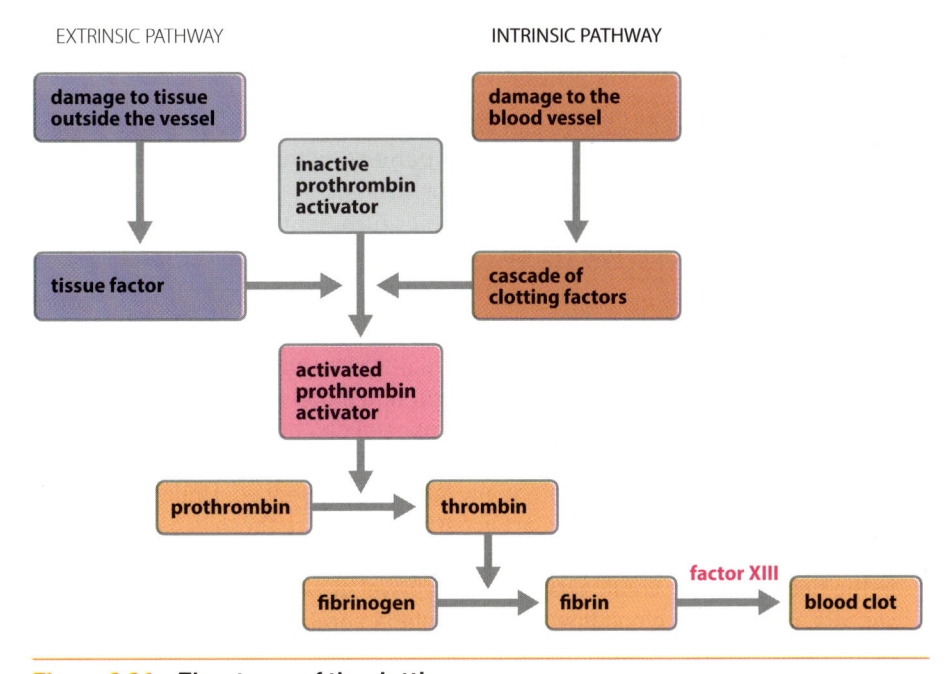

Figure 9.24 – **The stages of the clotting process.**

fibrinolysis starts within 2 days of the clot forming and continues for several days. Understanding the process of fibrinolysis has enabled the development of thrombolytic drugs as therapeutic agents. Thrombolytic drugs, which activate plasminogen to form plasmin, are used in specialist centres to dissolve blood clots in the acute phase of thrombo-embolic stroke (see Bessie, Patient 4.1), in major life-threatening pulmonary embolism and occasionally in acute myocardial infarction.

While clot formation is important for health, inappropriate clot formation must be prevented, and two mechanisms exist to control clot formation. First, clotting factors are quickly removed from the area, and secondly, activated clotting factors are inhibited. For example, the protein **antithrombin III** inhibits the action of thrombin that is not attached to fibrinogen to limit clot formation, while **heparin**, an endogenous anticoagulant found on the surface of endothelial cells and released from basophils and mast cells, inhibits the action of thrombin as well as the intrinsic pathway.

Problems can occur with the normal clotting process, leading to an increase in clot formation and an increased risk of stroke (see Bessie, Patient 4.1) and myocardial infarction (see Robert, Patient 9.1), or an increased tendency to bleed, for example the absence of specific clotting factors such as factor VIII, which leads to type A **haemophilia**. Indeed, through the use of specific anticoagulant drugs, such as heparin and warfarin, modification of the clotting process can occur to prevent the inappropriate formation of blood clots (see Katherine, Patient 3.3), for example following surgery for heart valve replacement or to prevent the development of deep vein thrombosis. A summary of selected blood clotting disorders and related terminology is presented in *Box 9.8*.

Summary of selected blood clotting disorders and related information

Thrombus

This is the formation of a blood clot within an intact vessel or on heart valves. The formation of a thrombus is enhanced in the presence of damage to the surface of a blood vessel wall, such as in atherosclerosis, damage to heart valves or damage to the valves in veins. Thrombi are also more likely to occur when blood flow is sluggish or turbulent. Some people have an inherent increased tendency for blood clots to form, as they have a deficiency in the production of antithrombin III.

Embolism

This is when a fragment of a thrombus breaks away and travels around the circulation until it becomes lodged in smaller vessels, obstructing blood flow. For example, a thrombus forming in the deep veins of the calf (deep vein thrombosis) can break away, travel to and through the right side of the heart and become lodged in one of the smaller branches of the pulmonary artery (pulmonary embolism), with potentially fatal consequences. Under particular circumstances when the endocardium of the heart is damaged, where there is damage to the heart valves or when there are heart rhythm abnormalities such as atrial fibrillation, thrombi can also form in the heart. If these break away, they can travel downstream and become lodged in smaller vessels, obstructing blood flow. For example, an embolus can travel from the left side of the heart up to the brain, causing a stroke.

BOX 9.8

Antiplatelet therapy

The binding together (aggregation) of platelets to form a platelet plug in arteries is dangerous because this can obstruct blood flow, causing ischaemia or infarction. The risk of this happening can be reduced by the use of antiplatelet drugs. Various antiplatelet drugs exist and work in a variety of ways, including blocking receptors on platelets to stop them binding together or inhibiting the production of chemical substances that enhance the stickiness of platelets. Antiplatelet drugs are particularly effective where blood flow is rapid, such as in the arterial circulation where thrombi are largely made up of platelets with little fibrin mesh.

Anticoagulant therapy

The main use of anticoagulants is to prevent thrombus formation or the extension of a thrombus in areas where blood flow is slow and where the thrombus contains a fibrin mesh. Heparin is a naturally occurring anticoagulant as well as a therapeutic agent, and inhibits the conversion of prothrombin to thrombin. As a therapeutic agent, heparin is commonly used and, in particular, low-molecular-weight heparin is preferred for routine use; for example, to prevent deep vein thrombosis. Oral anticoagulant drugs include warfarin, which inhibits the activity of vitamin K in the formation of clotting factors (see Katherine, Patient 3.3).

International normalized ratio

The international normalized ratio (INR) is the ratio of the time it takes a patient's blood to clot compared with a normal (control) sample. It is a standardized measure of the extrinsic and final common pathway of coagulation. The INR is typically used to monitor patients on anticoagulant therapy. The normal INR range for a healthy person not taking anticoagulants is 0.8–1.2. For those on anticoagulant therapy to prevent the formation of blood clots, a range of 2.0–3.0 may be the target.

D-dimer blood test

D-dimer is a fibrin degradation product that is present after a blood clot has been degraded by fibrinolysis. The presence of D-dimers can be detected, and this is used to confirm the presence of a blood clot. D-dimer blood tests are used to confirm or exclude the presence of thrombi, for example when there is a suspicion of deep vein thrombosis and pulmonary embolism.

Thrombocytopenia

This is a deficiency in the number of platelets, due to either a decrease in platelet production or an increased rate of destruction. Thrombocytopenia may occur as a result of radiotherapy, cancer chemotherapy and some leukaemias.

BOX 9.8 (continued)

9.3 Clinical application

Effective regulation of the cardiovascular system is of the utmost importance for health and homeodynamic processes. The flow of blood and perfusion of tissues for optimal cell function is affected by many factors. The regulation of the composition of blood, blood flow and blood pressure is necessary for health and can be altered due to various disease processes. The patients described in this chapter highlight how physiology explains a range of different clinical problems.

- **Sheila (Patient 2.3)** has breast cancer and has been offered surgery to remove the cancer, which could lead to the development of lymphoedema.
- **Katherine (Patient 3.3)** receives anticoagulant drugs to prevent the development of blood clots in the chambers of her heart. If these develop and are dislodged, they can travel to the lungs or brain, causing significant health problems.
- **Robert (Patient 9.1)** has developed heart failure following previous infarction of the myocardium. Impaired contraction of the heart muscle affects the maintenance of blood pressure, the flow of blood to the tissues of the body and effective oxygenation of the tissues.
- **Jane (Patient 9.2)** is concerned, along with her midwife, about the welfare of her baby, because her baby's rhesus status is different from her own. There is the risk that Jane could develop antibodies that would affect the baby's blood and therefore the baby's health.
- **Yasmeen (Patient 3.4)** has sickle cell disease and experiences episodes when erythrocytes in her blood adopt a sickle shape. This impairs blood flow, as the altered erythrocytes are unable to squeeze through small blood vessels. This causes obstruction to blood flow and tissue ischaemia, manifesting as acute pain.

| Patient 2.3 | Sheila | 30 | 54 | 59 | 93 | 267 | **304** | 448 | 473 |

- 47-year-old woman
- Recent diagnosis of breast cancer – biopsy shows cancer cells over-express HER2 protein
- Biological therapy with trastuzumab (Herceptin) to block HER2 action an option
- Is still offered surgery, chemotherapy and radiotherapy
- Agrees to add trastuzumab to chemotherapy plan
- Advised about surgery: lymphoedema a possibility

Sheila has been diagnosed with breast cancer. She had a fine needle aspiration of her right axillary lymph nodes and cancer cells were discovered in the aspirate (see *Chapter 14*). *HER2*-positive breast cancers tend to be more aggressive and are more likely to spread. She was therefore advised to have surgery to remove the cancer in her breast, with a 'wide local excision' of the breast. The surgeon also planned to remove all of her lymph nodes and perform a right axillary lymph node dissection (see *Chapter 14*). She was told that she could develop lymphoedema in her right arm following the surgery. Lymphatic vessels and nodes drain excess fluid away from tissues. When lymph nodes and vessels are removed or damaged during surgery, the draining of excess fluid can be compromised, with fluid accumulating within the tissues, which manifests as oedema. This is an example of a disturbance in normal capillary fluid dynamics (the key features of normal capillary fluid dynamics were presented earlier in this chapter).

Lymphoedema produces a tight or numb feeling with tingling in the arm or fingers. The arm can also feel heavy and ache, particularly when used to lift or carry objects. Lymphoedema cannot be cured, but a number of interventions are possible, including massage of the affected side, exercise and the wearing of compression sleeves. In addition, symptoms of lymphoedema can be reduced by avoiding heavy lifting or exercise in the affected arm and avoiding extreme changes in temperature, such as getting into a hot bath.

| Patient 3.3 | Katherine | 61 | 95 | 268 | **305** |

- 41-year-old woman
- Recent diagnosis of hypertrophic cardiomyopathy
- ECG shows arrhythmia and USS shows thickened left ventricle
- Given warfarin to reduce stroke risk and anti-arrhythmic drugs
- Genetic tests on one daughter

As Katherine has been prescribed warfarin, she attends her local anticoagulant clinic regularly to have her blood clotting (INR) status checked. Warfarin alters the action of vitamin K, inhibiting the synthesis of vitamin K-dependent clotting factors, which includes the formation of prothrombin in the liver. The consequence is a decrease in prothrombin and the amount of thrombin generated. The role of prothrombin and thrombin in the final common pathway of clot formation is illustrated in *Figure 9.4*.

Katherine was commenced on warfarin because one of her main problems with the genetic disorder of hypertrophic cardiomyopathy (HCM) is atrial fibrillation, an abnormal heart rhythm (arrhythmia), which increases the risk of stroke. Due to the rapid and altered heart rhythm that occurs with atrial fibrillation, blood flow through the heart becomes turbulent and there is a high risk that blood clots could form in her atria and ventricles. These might be pumped out of the heart and travel to the brain, causing a thrombo-embolic stroke, or to the lungs, causing a pulmonary embolism. To prevent this, Katherine's warfarin dose was adjusted to meet an INR target of 2.5. In view of her chronic arrhythmia and her HCM, Katherine is monitored by a cardiologist with expertise in HCM and she attends hospital for regular ECG and echocardiograph evaluation and review of her medications. Katherine and her family are supported by a genetic nurse counsellor and through a patient support group, as this heart condition might affect her extended family.

| Patient 9.1 | Robert | 268 | **305** | 448 | 474 |

- 56-year-old man with family history of CVD
- First MI at 38, stent at 45, and coronary artery bypass graft at 49
- ECG shows changes consistent with another MI; confirmed by biochemical marker tests
- Has hypotension and oedema
- Prescribed aspirin, atorvastatin, bisoprolol and perindopril
- Diet altered to reduce salt and fat and exercise levels increased

Robert has chronic heart failure due to his previous myocardial infarction and severe coronary heart disease. An echocardiogram confirmed that his heart was not contracting effectively, particularly the left ventricle. Damage to the left ventricle from the infarction has reduced the ability of the ventricular muscle to contract and therefore the force of contraction during systole. This has led to a reduction in stroke volume and cardiac output. As a consequence, Robert has a lower-than-normal blood pressure (hypotension). A number of responses to chronic heart failure arise in the cardiovascular system, including an increase in the activity of the sympathetic nervous system and the renin–angiotensin–aldosterone system (RAAS).

Additionally, because of failure of the right side of his heart, Robert has experienced swollen feet and ankles. The build-up of fluid in the interstitial space is called oedema, and in this context it is often called pitting oedema (see *Figure 9.25*) because when the swollen area is pressed, fluid is pushed away and an indentation is left in the skin. This then resolves after a few seconds as fluid returning to the tissues pushes the skin out. Peripheral oedema is an important indicator of a compromised circulatory system. Right-sided heart failure causes venous congestion and an increase in the venous blood pressure, and therefore the blood pressure at the venous end of the capillary is greater than normal. The balance between the osmotic pressure and hydrostatic pressure (capillary blood

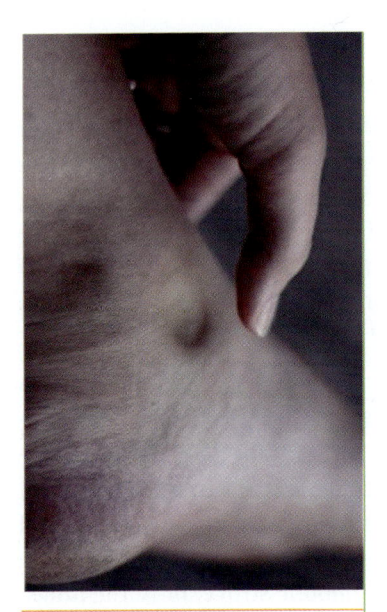

Figure 9.25 – **Peripheral (pitting) oedema.**
Reproduced from www.footiq.com.

pressure) is altered and consequently more fluid remains in the interstitial space. In this case, normal capillary fluid dynamics has been compromised by the heart failure.

Robert was prescribed a variety of medications to help reduce his risk from further acute coronary events and to improve the functioning of his heart. The medicines included aspirin because it has an antiplatelet action that reduces the risk of blood clot formation and therefore minimizes the possibility of a further acute coronary event. He was also prescribed atorvastatin to lower his blood cholesterol and to improve his lipid profile. Atorvastatin is an example of a group of drugs called statins, which inhibit the enzyme 3-hydroxy-3-methylglutaryl-CoA reductase (HMG-CoA reductase), an enzyme active mostly in the liver that controls the synthesis of cholesterol. Statins are particularly effective at reducing low-density-lipoprotein (LDL) cholesterol. The treatment of his heart failure included bisoprolol, a β-adrenoceptor blocker, which blocks the effects of the sympathetic nervous system on the heart with the effect of improving ventricular function, increasing stroke volume and preventing dilation of the ventricles. He was also taking perindopril, an angiotensin-converting enzyme (ACE) inhibitor that modifies the RAAS to reduce blood volume and vascular resistance, thus reducing blood pressure and improving the circulation of blood through the vasculature. Both drugs reduce the workload on the heart. Following advice from healthcare professionals, Robert modified his diet, reducing the amount of saturated fat and salt and increasing his consumption of fish, to increase his intake of omega-3 fatty acids (see *Chapter 7*). He also went out for a walk most mornings, lasting over 30 minutes. Regular exercise is very beneficial for people with chronic heart failure.

Patient 9.2 | Jane | 268 | **306**

- 28-year-old woman pregnant with second child
- Blood group O Rh −ve
- Given anti-D Ig at 28 weeks

Jane is rhesus negative. She was asked at the antenatal clinic whether she had a history of previous blood transfusions. Jane had not received any blood transfusions nor had she been 'sensitized', as her blood test was negative for anti-D antibodies. To prevent sensitization during the pregnancy, Jane was given anti-D antibodies in an attempt to prevent her body from making antibodies against her baby, which was rhesus positive. Anti-D antibodies (1500 international units) were administered intravenously. It is expected that this treatment will reduce the risk of Jane's baby developing haemolytic disease of the newborn.

Patient 3.4 | Yasmeen | 61 | 95 | 268 | **306**

- 17-year-old girl
- Has sickle cell disease but no long-term organ damage
- Discussed bone marrow transplant as treatment option
- Referred to clinical geneticist to find out more

Sickle cell disease may lead to various acute and chronic complications. The term *sickle cell crisis* is used to describe several acute conditions. Sickle cell disease causes anaemia and several forms of acute clinical conditions such as vaso-occlusive crisis. In vaso-occlusive crisis, sickle-shaped erythrocytes obstruct capillary blood flow to organs, resulting in pain, ischaemia, necrosis and possibly

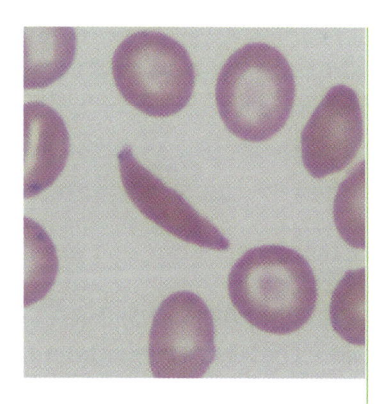

Figure 9.26 – **Blood film showing sickle shape of red blood cells in sickle cell anaemia.**
Reproduced under a CC BY-SA 4.0 International licence. Attribution: Gregory Kato.

organ damage (such as a stroke and kidney injury). The frequency and duration of the crisis varies in patients and with each crisis, but over time organ damage gradually accumulates.

Loss of elasticity of the erythrocyte cell membrane is central to the problems arising from sickle cell disease. Normally, erythrocytes are very flexible, allowing them to change shape as they squeeze through capillaries. When the concentration of oxygen in the blood is low, the abnormal erythrocytes adopt a sickle shape (illustrated in *Figure 9.26*). The alteration in shape arises from a single amino acid change in the β-chain of haemoglobin, producing an altered form of haemoglobin (discussed in *Chapter 3*). After repeated episodes of sickle cell crisis, the red blood cells might not resume their normal shape, remaining rigid as they pass through the capillary; this leads to blood vessel occlusion. In Yasmeen's case, sickle cell crisis presented as abdominal and chest pain. Fortunately, through effective self-care and regular review, Yasmeen did not have any end-organ damage.

Effective perfusion of the organs and tissues is essential for integrated function and for enabling homeodynamic adjustment with changing demands and over a lifespan. Understanding the nature and regulation of the cardiovascular system and the diverse factors that affect the perfusion of organs and tissues is essential for healthcare practice in order to provide effective care.

9.4 Summary

- Effective pumping of the heart and blood flow through the vasculature is essential to ensure that organs and tissues receive adequate blood flow and to deliver oxygen and glucose to meet the metabolic demands of the cells.
- Three main layers of tissue provide the structure of all blood vessels with the exception of capillaries (see *Figure 9.1*).
- Effective contraction of the myocardium and functioning of the cardiac valves are essential for the productive flow of blood through the heart to the lungs and around the systemic circulation.
- The emptying and filling of the heart during a cardiac cycle is coordinated by the conducting system of the heart (see *Figure 9.11*).
- The moment-to-moment regulation of blood pressure involves arterial baroreceptors (see *Figure 9.14*), while the long-term regulation of blood pressure involves the kidneys and the endocrine system (for example, the renin–angiotensin–aldosterone system).
- Blood cells are vitally important for health. They undertake a number of specific roles such as the transport of oxygen and carbon dioxide (erythrocytes), the response to infection and injury (leukocytes) and haemostasis (thrombocytes).
- The main blood groups are the ABO system (see *Table 9.2*) and the rhesus system.

9.5 Further reading

The following websites provide useful information about heart disease and the measurement and significance of arterial blood pressure:
British Heart Foundation: www.bhf.org.uk/
British Hypertension Society: www.bhsoc.org/

The following textbook provides the reference for the normal heart and blood values provided in this chapter:
Glasper, E. A., McEwing, G. and Richardson, J. (eds) (2016) *Oxford Handbook of Children's and Young People's Nursing*, 2nd edn. Oxford University Press, Oxford, UK.

The following web page provides some helpful information for professionals, families and carers about sickle cell disease:
www.nhlbi.nih.gov/health/prof/blood/sickle/sc_mngt.pdf

9.6 Self-assessment questions

Answers can be found at www.scionpublishing.com/AandP

(9.1) With reference to factors that aid venous return, identify which one option is correct.
 (a) Contraction of skeletal muscles
 (b) Decrease in intra-abdominal pressure
 (c) The presence of valves in the arteries
 (d) The creation of a positive intra-thoracic pressure
 (e) A thick smooth muscle layer present in the wall of veins

(9.2) With reference to the structure of the heart, identify which one statement is correct.
 (a) The myocardial septum separates deoxygenated blood in the left ventricle from oxygenated blood in the right ventricle
 (b) The tricuspid valve prevents the backflow of blood from the left ventricle into the left atrium
 (c) The pulmonary artery conducts deoxygenated blood to the lungs
 (d) Chordae tendineae are attached to the pulmonary artery valve
 (e) The tricuspid valve prevents the backflow of blood from the right ventricle into the pulmonary artery

(9.3) Identify the one correct statement.
 (a) Hypertension is when the systolic blood pressure is less than 90 mmHg
 (b) Bradycardia is when the heart rate is greater than 100 beats/minute
 (c) Cardiac output is the volume of blood ejected by each ventricle per minute
 (d) Tachycardia is when the heart rate is below 80 beats/minute
 (e) Venous return is the volume of blood returning to the left atria from the lungs

(9.4) With reference to the structure of the heart, identify which one statement describes correctly the function of chordae tendineae. Chordae tendineae:

(a) separate deoxygenated blood in the left ventricle from oxygenated blood in the right ventricle
(b) prevent the closure of the aortic valve
(c) conduct deoxygenated blood to the lungs
(d) ensure the tricuspid valve closes effectively to prevent the backflow of blood from the right ventricle into the right atria
(e) ensure the mitral valve closes effectively to prevent the backflow of blood from the right ventricle into the pulmonary artery

(9.5) Explain why blood that is group O and rhesus negative can be given in an emergency before blood that has been grouped or cross-matched is available.

(9.6) Explain why some people may experience dizziness and even pass out when they stand up suddenly.

(9.7) Why do children with the condition haemophilia tend to bruise easily and bleed into their knee joint if they bump their knee?

CHAPTER 10 | The body needs oxygen

Learning points for this chapter

After working through this chapter, you should be able to:

- Describe why regulation of oxygen and carbon dioxide in arterial blood is important for health
- Identify the structures that form the respiratory system
- Discuss the process and importance of pulmonary ventilation
- Describe how oxygen and carbon dioxide are exchanged within the lungs and tissue cells
- Describe how oxygen and carbon dioxide are transported in the blood
- Discuss how breathing is regulated

10.1 Introduction and clinical relevance

Each of the patients in this chapter highlights how effective oxygenation of the blood, perfusion of tissues and removal of carbon dioxide are necessary for health. The normal structure and function of the respiratory system are discussed, as this is essential knowledge for those involved in the care of patients such as Mary (Patient 2.1) and Sarah (Patient 3.1).

| Patient 2.1 | Mary | 29 | 53 | **311** | 330 |

- 57-year-old woman
- Chronic asthmatic on beclometasone dipropionate, salmeterol and salbutamol

Mary, aged 57 years, was diagnosed with chronic asthma. She is currently managed with beclometasone dipropionate (200 mcg taken as two puffs twice a day (BD)), salmeterol (50 mcg taken as one puff BD) and salbutamol (100 mcg taken as two puffs as required (PRN)). Her peak expiratory flow rate using a peak flow meter is normally around 480 L/minute.

| Patient 3.1 | Sarah | 60 | 94 | 195 | 237 | **311** | 333 |

- 17-year-old girl
- CF diagnosis at age of 1 year via a sweat test
- Frequent admissions for chest infections affecting breathing
- PERT added to meals to help digest her food

Sarah, aged 17 years, has cystic fibrosis and is assisted by her mother to complete a daily series of physiotherapy exercises to clear viscous mucus secretions from her lungs. Sarah has experienced very frequent admissions to hospital for exacerbation of her breathing problems due to the development of recurrent chest infections.

You are likely to meet individuals with a range of problems associated with breathing, such as asthma, chronic obstructive pulmonary disease (COPD), lung cancer and pneumonia. Mary and Sarah have very different stories, yet both have to cope with long-term respiratory disorders that affect their health and well-being. As a healthcare professional, you may be directly involved in assessing the pulmonary function of patients like Mary or Sarah. In order to provide the highest standard of practice, you need to have a clear understanding about the respiratory system and the regulation of breathing.

10.2 What you need to know – essential anatomy and physiology

As described in *Chapter 2*, oxygen (O_2) is vital for life and oxygen is utilized by the trillions of cells that make up the body to create chemical energy (ATP) that drives cellular activities. When cells use oxygen, carbon dioxide (CO_2) is produced. Carbon dioxide combines with water to form carbonic acid (H_2CO_3), which rapidly dissociates into a hydrogen ion (H^+) and a bicarbonate ion (HCO_3^-). The first reversible chemical reaction is catalysed by carbonic anhydrase, and can be presented as follows:

$$CO_2 + H_2O \rightleftharpoons H_2CO_3 \rightleftharpoons H^+ + HCO_3^-$$

carbon dioxide + water ⇌ (action of carbonic anhydrase) carbonic acid ⇌ hydrogen ion + bicarbonate ion

Accumulation of carbon dioxide in body fluids increases the H^+ concentration, which reduces the pH (making the pH of body fluids move towards the acid region of the scale), and this disrupts both the normal acid–base balance in extracellular fluid and normal cell functioning. For this reason, carbon dioxide has to be eliminated from the cells and extracellular fluid in order to regulate the concentration of carbon dioxide in arterial blood. The cardiovascular (see *Chapter 9*) and respiratory systems are fundamental to this regulatory process, which is essential in homeodynamics and for health:

- The respiratory system functions to ensure that oxygen is transferred from the atmosphere into the blood and that carbon dioxide is removed from the blood and exhaled into the atmosphere.
- The cardiovascular system is responsible for the delivery of oxygen to and the removal of carbon dioxide from the tissues.

Adaptation in the respiratory and cardiovascular systems can occur over time and this is exemplified in *Chapter 1*, where the response to poor availability of oxygen is discussed.

Both the respiratory and cardiovascular systems are responsible for maintaining the concentrations of oxygen and carbon dioxide in arterial blood within normal ranges. In a clinical setting, oxygen and carbon dioxide within arterial blood are referred to as arterial blood gases. Key points about arterial blood gases and the results obtained when analysing them are highlighted in *Box 10.1*.

> **BOX 10.1**
>
> ### Arterial blood gases
>
> A sample of arterial blood for analysis is often obtained from the radial or femoral artery. Analysis of the sample, using a blood gas analyser, provides important information on the quality of arterial blood, such as the concentration of oxygen and carbon dioxide and the pH. Typical results are illustrated as follows:
>
> - pH: normal range 7.35–7.45
> - PaO_2:   normal range 10.5–13.5 kPa
> - $PaCO_2$: normal range 4.5–6.0 kPa.
>
> PaO_2 and $PaCO_2$ are the partial pressure (P) of arterial (a) oxygen or carbon dioxide, respectively (i.e. the amount in arterial blood).
>
> ### Terminology
>
> - Hypoxaemia: an arterial content of oxygen lower than normal.
> - Hypercapnia: an arterial content of carbon dioxide greater than normal.
> - Acidosis: pH <7.35.
> - Alkalosis: pH >7.45.

10.2.1 Upper respiratory tract

The respiratory system (see *Figure 10.1*) comprises the nose (nasal cavities), pharynx, larynx, trachea, bronchi and lungs. The respiratory system can be described regionally as the upper and lower respiratory tracts. The **upper respiratory tract** refers to the airway above the vocal cords (the **glottis**), including the nasal cavities, **pharynx** and **larynx**. The **lower respiratory tract** includes the conducting airways in the thorax (the **trachea**, **bronchi** and **bronchioles**) and the **alveoli** (air sacs where the exchange of oxygen and carbon dioxide between the lungs and the blood occurs).

When inhaling, air flows into the nasal cavities. The nasal cavities are covered by the respiratory mucosa, which warms and moistens the air, and contains the olfactory receptors for sensing smell (see *Chapter 6*). From the nasal cavities, air flows into the pharynx that serves as a common passageway for air and food (see *Figure 10.2*). The pharynx has three regions: the nasopharynx, oropharynx and laryngopharynx. Air flows from the nasal cavities into the nasopharynx and oropharynx, after which it enters the laryngopharynx (also called the hypopharynx) and enters the larynx. The larynx directs air through the glottis (vocal cords) into the conducting airways. Air flowing over the vocal cords causes them to vibrate and as a result, sound is produced. Spasm of the laryngeal cords (known as laryngospasm) causes a sudden restriction of the airway when the vocal cords or area below the vocal cords are irritated by water, blood or mucus. Laryngospasm occurs suddenly and leads to difficulty in breathing and talking. During swallowing, to ensure that food or foreign objects do not enter the conducting airways causing laryngospasm or obstruction, the glottis opening of the larynx is covered by the **epiglottis** (a leaf-shaped piece of elastic cartilage attached to the larynx).

314 CHAPTER 10 | THE BODY NEEDS OXYGEN

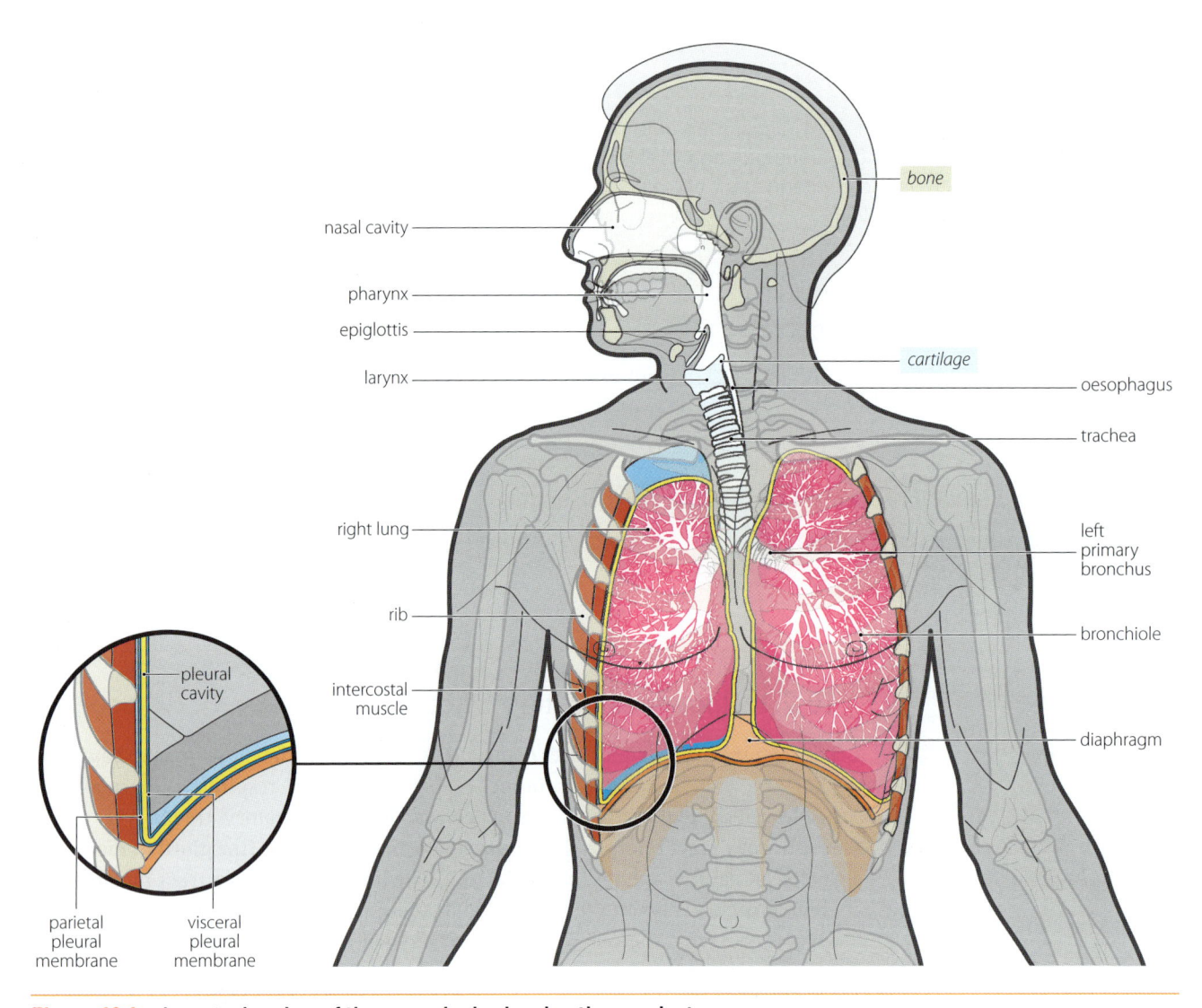

Figure 10.1 – **An anterior view of the upper body showing the respiratory organs.**

10.2.2 Lower respiratory tract

During inhalation, air from the upper respiratory tract flows into the trachea through the bronchi and bronchioles and finally arrives in the alveoli. The trachea is fairly rigid due to the presence of cartilage rings, which provide support to the wall of the trachea, thus keeping the airway open (see *Figure 10.3*). If you place your fingers on the larynx and gently run your fingers down the top part of the trachea, you can feel the firm cartilage rings. The cartilage rings in the trachea are described as incomplete rings as they are C-shaped; the break in the cartilage ring is orientated to the posterior region of the trachea where the oesophagus is located. This anatomical arrangement enables the oesophagus to distend as the bolus of food moves down the oesophagus into the stomach. The C-shaped cartilage ring structure continues into the bronchi. The right and left main bronchi, which are divisions of the trachea, continue to divide into smaller and smaller segmental branches as they spread out through the lungs. The right

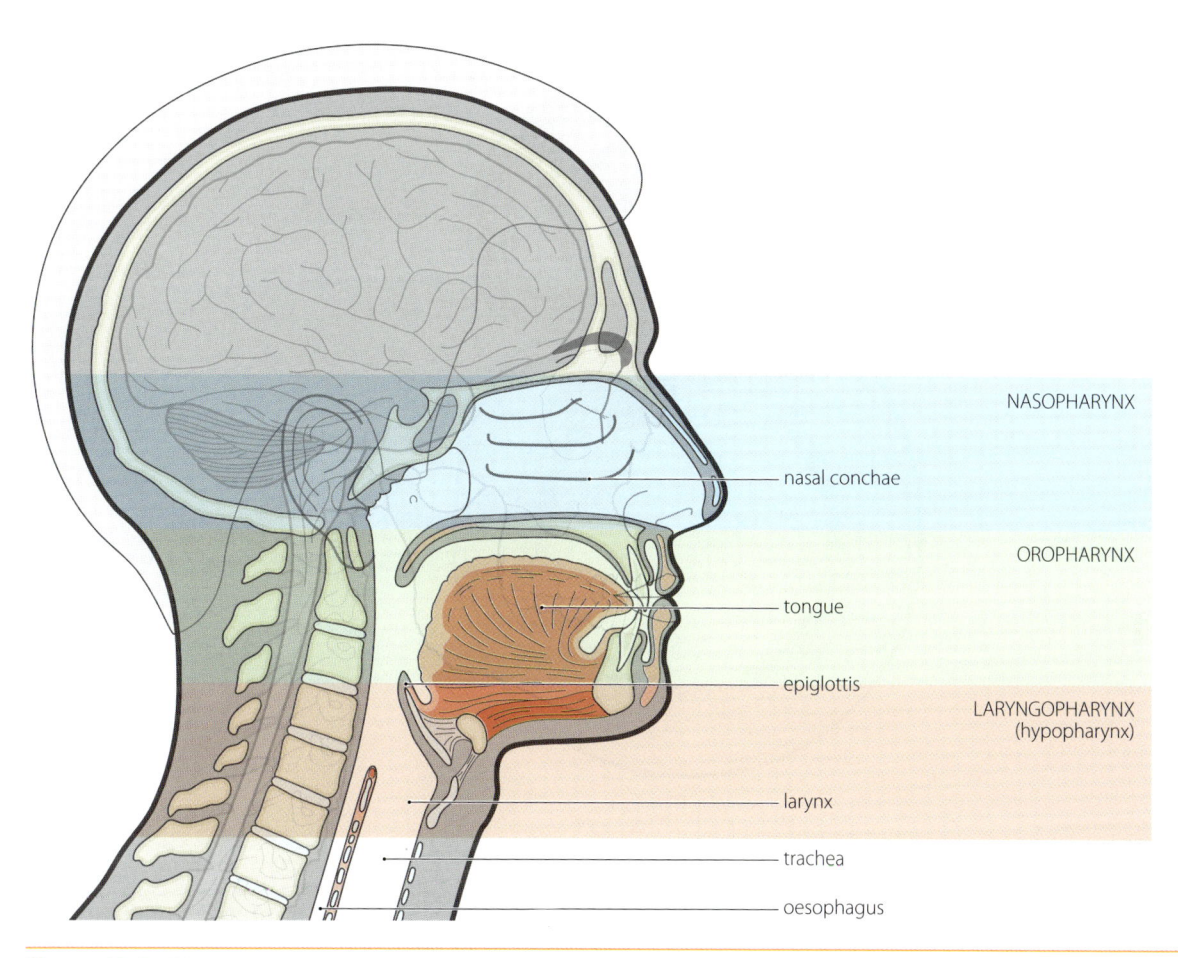

Figure 10.2 – **The structure of the pharynx.**

main **bronchus** is wider, shorter and more vertical compared with the left, which is more horizontal due to the position of the heart. Inhaled objects (as sometimes occurs in young children) are more likely to become lodged in the right bronchus.

The trachea and bronchi are lined by pseudostratified columnar epithelium comprising **ciliated columnar epithelial cells** and mucus-producing **goblet cells**. Mucus is a viscous fluid containing proteins called mucins, and the enzyme lysozyme, which has anti-bacterial properties (see *Chapter 11*). The presence of mucus helps to trap dust particles, microorganisms and other debris. Hair-like structures called cilia located on the columnar epithelial cells beat continuously (not dissimilar to a rowing motion) in a direction from inside the lungs towards the larynx. Together, the mucus-producing cells and cilia form the mucociliary escalator, which helps to trap and remove bacteria and harmful substances from the lung. The action of the cilia propels the mucus towards the upper airway where it can be coughed up and expectorated or swallowed, passing into the stomach to be destroyed by gastric enzymes and hydrochloric acid.

Ensuring the correct viscosity of mucus is complex and involves the movement of water and chloride (Cl^-) and sodium (Na) ions across the epithelial cell membrane. Specific protein channels within the epithelial cells that line the conducting airways

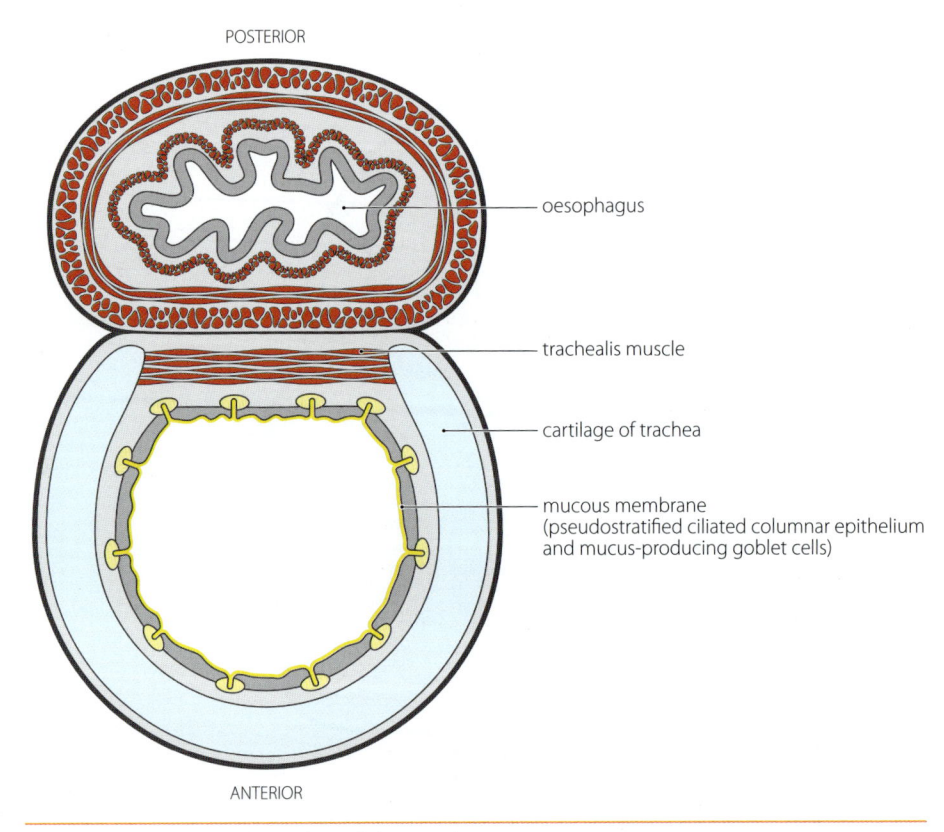

Figure 10.3 – A cross-section of the trachea.

facilitate the transport of the ions. The normal development and functioning of these channels are genetically determined; the importance of genetics on normal physiology and health is discussed in *Chapter 3*. Understanding the formation and the purpose of mucus is important underpinning knowledge when considering lung disorders such as cystic fibrosis (see *Chapter 3* and Sarah, Patient 3.1).

10.2.3 Lung tissue and the bronchial tree

The lungs fill the entire thoracic cavity, apart from the area in which the heart, major blood vessels and bronchi are located (an area known as the mediastinum). Each lung is divided into lobes; the right lung has three lobes, while the left lung has only two lobes due to the presence of the heart in the left side of the thoracic cavity. Each lobe is complete with discrete conducting airways and blood supply. The lung is composed of connective tissue, smaller conducting airways and alveoli. Surrounding each lung is a double-layered serous membrane called the **pleural membrane** (see *Figure 10.1*). The inner membrane (the visceral pleural membrane) covers the lung tissue, while the outer membrane (the parietal pleural membrane) is attached to the inner surface of the ribs and chest wall. Between the two pleural membranes is a space (the pleural cavity) containing a lubricating fluid (pleural fluid) that allows the two layers of pleura to glide over each other as the lungs expand and recoil, thus allowing the lungs to move relative to the chest wall. The membranes strongly resist being pulled apart and this physical effect is vitally important for normal breathing.

Within the lungs, the bronchi progressively divide into smaller branches until they become the bronchioles, which are the smallest conducting airways. The branching of the airways within the lungs leads to the commonly used description of a *bronchial tree*. As the airways divide and become smaller, the cartilage support becomes less organized within the smallest terminal bronchioles, and by the terminal bronchioles, cartilage support is lost; the terminal bronchioles are essentially muscular tubes. The muscle wall is composed of smooth muscle, which is under the control of the autonomic nervous system, and local factors, such as sensory receptors that respond to cold air or irritants. As the smooth muscle contracts, the lumen of the bronchioles becomes smaller in diameter – a process called *bronchoconstriction*. When the smooth muscle relaxes, *bronchodilation* occurs. In this way, airflow through the bronchioles to the alveoli is regulated.

As illustrated in *Figures 10.4* and *10.5*, the terminal bronchioles lead into alveolar ducts that connect to alveoli. The combination of terminal bronchioles, alveolar ducts and alveoli form respiratory zones in which the exchange of oxygen and carbon dioxide occurs. Alveoli are ideally suited for the exchange of gases by diffusion because the wall of the alveolus is very thin; in fact, the alveolus is composed of a single layer of squamous epithelium cells called **type 1 pneumocytes** supported by a very thin basement membrane.

A human lung has about 300 million alveoli and each is only 200–300 μm in diameter. Collectively, alveoli form a huge surface area estimated to be 50–70 m² and the outer surfaces of the alveoli are surrounded by a dense network of capillaries lying in close proximity to the alveolar wall. This intimate blood supply is vitally important to enable the effective exchange of oxygen and carbon dioxide by diffusion. The exchange of gases is further enhanced because the distance across the respiratory membrane (the alveolar wall, the interstitial space, the wall of the capillary and associated basement membranes) is extremely small – on average just 0.5 μm.

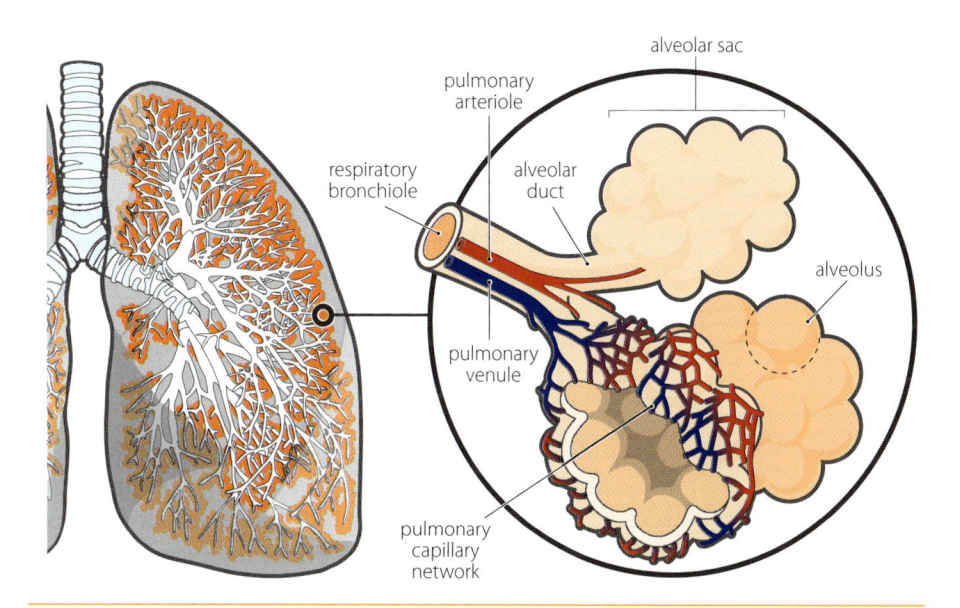

Figure 10.4 – **The structure of the bronchioles and alveolar sacs.**

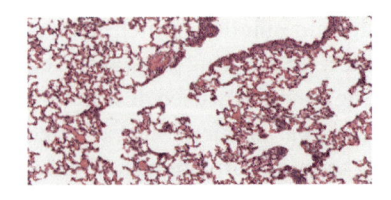

Figure 10.5 – Histology slide showing alveoli and alveolar ducts.
Reproduced under a CC BY-SA3.0 Unported licence. Author: OpenStax College.

10.2.4 Ventilation and the mechanics of breathing

Breathing involves the movement of air from the atmosphere into the lungs (inspiration) and out of the lungs (expiration); this is known as pulmonary ventilation. Pulmonary ventilation involves changes in lung volume and gas pressure within the lungs brought about through a sequence of mechanical events initiated by the nervous system. During restful breathing, expiration usually takes slightly longer than inspiration; for example, an inspiratory time of 2 seconds and an expiratory time of 3 seconds.

To understand fully the mechanics of inspiration and expiration, it is important to appreciate one aspect of the behaviour of gases: gas molecules will always fill the space in which they are contained. For example, the lungs form a chamber for the gas molecules of oxygen and carbon dioxide as well as nitrogen and water molecules. Where the chamber has a large volume, the gas molecules are further apart and therefore the pressure produced by the molecules in the chamber is lower. The converse is true when the chamber is smaller: the molecules are more tightly packed within the container and the pressure produced by the molecules is increased. This inverse relationship between lung volume and gas pressure is described by **Boyle's law**, which states:

> The volume of a given mass of gas is inversely proportional to the pressure to which it is subjected provided that the temperature remains constant

Provided the temperature remains constant, a fall in the volume of the gas will lead to an increase in its pressure and vice versa. Boyle's law helps to explain the mechanism that enables inspiration and expiration.

Two overlapping patterns are involved with breathing. There is a basic rhythm of inspiration and expiration, which is under the influence of the autonomic nervous system; however, this can be modified by behavioural (voluntary) influences and reflex responses such as sneezing. The basic intrinsic pattern of breathing is controlled by groups of neurones that form nuclei, collectively called the medullary respiratory centres. These neurones extend along the length of the medulla oblongata. Two additional groups of neurones in the pons of the brainstem modify the activity of the medullary respiratory centres (see *Figure 10.6*). The medulla contains two distinct groups of neurones called the **dorsal respiratory group** (DRG) and the **ventral respiratory group** (VRG). These two groups are involved in the generation of the respiratory pattern. The basic rhythm of breathing arises from cyclical bursts of nerve impulses produced by the VRG (which appears to be a rhythm generating and integration centre), stimulating inspiration. The VRG contains neurones involved with both inspiration and expiration; expiratory neurones are particularly active when forceful breathing is required. The VRG appears to be involved in triggering inspiration and the coordination of the rate, depth and rhythm of breathing, as specific cells located in the VRG may be involved in acting as a central pattern generator, setting the basic pattern of breathing. The DRG contains inspiratory neurones operating in an integrated way with the VRG. The DRG also integrates sensory impulses and in doing so, modifies the activity of the VRG. At the end of inspiration an 'off switch' event occurs where there is a decrease in firing of the inspiratory neurones. This pause in bursts of nerve impulses allows the muscles of respiration to relax, resulting in expiration.

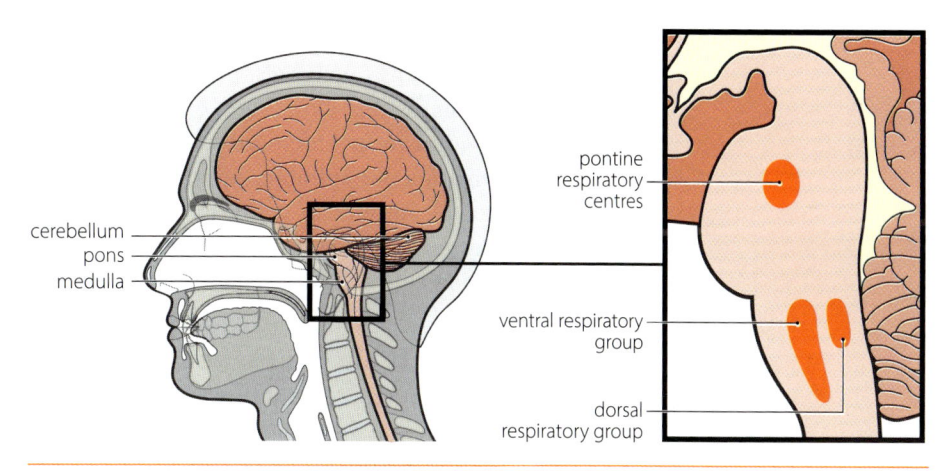

Figure 10.6 – **The brainstem and respiratory centres.**

Neurones in the pons that regulate breathing are classified as the **pontine respiratory group (PRG)** (formerly called the **pneumotaxic centre**) and the other more diffuse collections of neurones. The PRG inhibits the duration of inspiration by modifying the activity of the medullary inspiratory neurones. The switch between inspiration and expiration is not completely understood; however, rhythmic breathing seems to depend on activity from central pattern generator neurones and reciprocal inhibition of interconnected neural networks by impulses from pontine neurones and various areas of the cerebrum and afferent fibres. These include sensory impulses from stretch receptors, which are excited as the lung inflates, to prevent overinflation of the lungs. The breathing pattern is also modified to enable speech and eating, during exercise and when sneezing, as well as preventing harm to the lung tissue from overexpansion.

Motor nerve impulses generated by the inspiratory neurones in the medullary respiratory centres are conducted along the phrenic nerves to stimulate contraction and flattening of the diaphragm and at the same time along the external intercostal nerves to stimulate the contraction of the external intercostal muscles (between the ribs). During inspiration, contraction of the external intercostal muscles causes the ribcage and sternum to move upwards and outwards. These mechanical changes increase the size of the thoracic cavity, and importantly pull the pleural membranes (see *Figure 10.1*) outwards, thus increasing the volume of the lungs. In keeping with Boyle's law, as the lung volume increases, the gas pressure within the lungs (the intrapulmonary or alveolar pressure) decreases, eventually reaching a pressure *lower* than the atmospheric pressure, allowing air to flow into the lungs through the open conducting airways along the pressure gradient from the higher atmospheric pressure to the lower pressure in the alveoli.

Expiration is the reverse of the above process. During normal quiet breathing, expiration is passive, involving the relaxation of the muscles and elastic recoil of the lung tissue due to switching off of the nerve impulses from the inspiratory neural cells in the medulla. As a consequence, the diaphragm relaxes, becoming dome-shaped; the external intercostal muscles relax resulting in the ribs and sternum moving inwards and downwards, thus assuming the normal pre-inspiration position. This, coupled with the elastic recoil of the alveoli, results in a decrease in lung volume. In keeping with Boyle's law, the gas pressure within the lungs increases, this time to a level *higher* than atmospheric pressure. Consequently, air flows out of the lungs into the surrounding atmosphere. Expiration can be enhanced during times of exercise or difficulty in breathing by activation of expiratory neurones in the medulla, which stimulate the internal intercostal muscles to contract, thus enhancing expiration. A summary of the changes in gas pressure and lung volume that occur during inspiration and expiration is provided in *Figure 10.7*.

Factors that aid ventilation

The rigid structure of the trachea and bronchi and the extensive branching out of the bronchial tree also reduce the resistance to airflow and ensure that air is distributed to all parts of the lungs.

The integrity of the pleural membranes must be maintained to ensure normal inspiration and expansion of the lungs. The pressure between the two pleural membranes (the **intrapleural pressure**) is lower than the pressure inside the alveoli (the **intrapulmonary pressure**). This is due to opposing forces acting to collapse the lung (a combination of the elasticity of lung tissue and the surface tension of alveolar fluid) and to expand the thorax and lungs (the natural elasticity of the chest wall). The difference between the intrapleural and intrapulmonary

INSPIRATION ← **EXPIRATION**

intrapleural pressure **754** mmHg
alveolar (intrapulmonary) pressure **758** mmHg

intrapleural pressure **756** mmHg
alveolar (intrapulmonary) pressure **762** mmHg

atmospheric pressure **760** mmHg

- diaphragm and external intercostal muscles **contract**
- ribs move **up** and **out**
- diaphragm **flattens**
- lung volume **increases**
- alveolar (intrapulmonary) pressure **falls**
- air flows **into** lungs

- diaphragm and external intercostal muscles **relax**
- ribs move **in** and **down**
- diaphragm becomes **domed**
- lung volume **decreases**
- alveolar (intrapulmonary) pressure **increases**
- air flows **out** of lungs

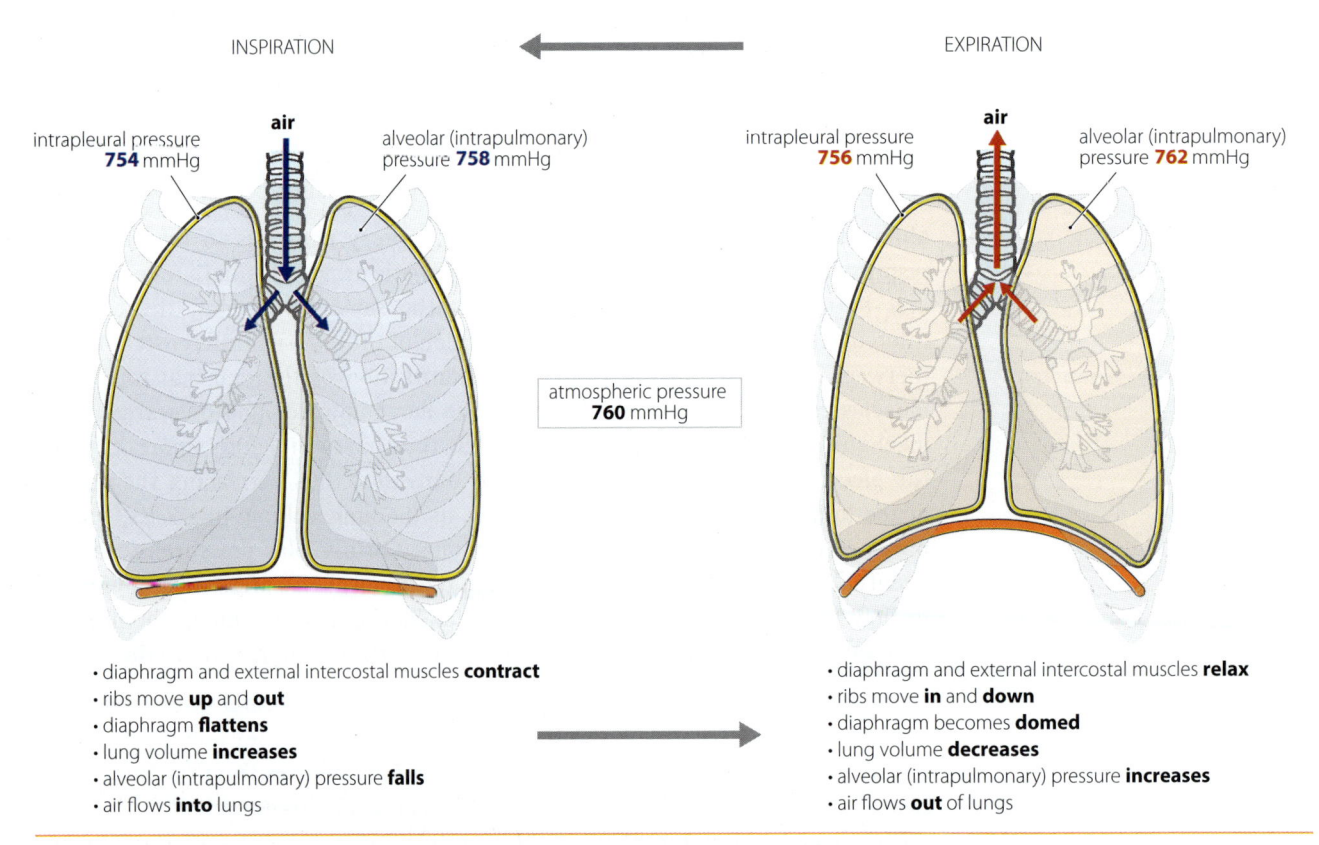

Figure 10.7 – **A summary of the events taking place during inspiration and expiration.**
During inspiration intrapulmonary pressure may fall by 1–2 mmHg (expressed as −1 to −2 mmHg) and during expiration it may rise by 1 to 2 mmHg above atmospheric pressure.

pressure helps to prevent the alveoli collapsing and reduces the work involved in breathing. Damage to the structure of the pleural membranes may result in air entering the pleural space, causing an increase in the intrapleural pressure. This is called a **pneumothorax**. The loss of the pressure gradient between the pleural cavity and the lungs prevents the lung from expanding during inspiration and, as a consequence, breathing can be seriously compromised. A pneumothorax can be corrected by insertion of a tube into the pleural space. The chest tube is connected to a drainage system that is designed to allow air to leave the pleural space, and so the pressure in the pleural space falls and it becomes possible to expand the affected lung.

Another factor that aids ventilation is the presence of **surfactant**, a phospholipoprotein fluid produced by special cells (**type 2 pneumocytes**) within the alveoli. A thin layer of water molecules, which aids the diffusion of gases, lines each alveolus, but, as outlined in *Chapter 2*, water molecules are attracted to the hydrogen atoms of other water molecules. This mutual attraction can be called a cohesive force. Cohesive forces exist between the water molecules on the surface of the layer of water, at the water–air interface. The pulling of the water molecules creates a **surface tension**, a force that tends to bring the walls of the alveoli together. Surface tension increases during exhalation as the alveoli decrease in size and the water molecules become closer together. Surfactant reduces surface tension and therefore *reduces* the tendency for alveoli to collapse, and in doing so reduces the work involved in inflating the lungs. The concept of surface tension is outlined in *Box 10.2*.

As surfactant is not normally produced in the alveoli of the fetus until week 30 of pregnancy, premature babies born before 30 weeks of pregnancy are at greatest risk of having alveoli that are unable to expand. Clinically, alongside other intensive support measures, synthetic surfactant can be administered down the **endotracheal tube** used for ventilating the premature baby. This helps to prevent the alveoli collapsing between each breath, assists inflation of the lung and reduces the work of breathing.

10.2.5 Respiratory volumes and capacities

Many factors affect lung capacity, such as a person's size, age, gender and physical condition. During normal restful breathing, approximately 500 ml of air is exchanged during inspiration and expiration, and this is termed the **tidal volume**. However, not all of the tidal volume that is inspired reaches and refreshes the air in the alveoli, because the conducting airways including the nose, larynx, trachea and bronchi contain air that mixes with the tidal volume. The volume of air in these conducting passageways is termed the **anatomical dead space** and is approximately 150 ml in volume. Thus, of all the air that is inspired during normal restful breathing (tidal volume), only approximately 350 ml reaches the alveoli and contributes to the exchange of oxygen and carbon dioxide between the alveoli and the pulmonary blood. Alveolar air contains less oxygen and more carbon dioxide when compared with atmospheric air.

Tidal volume can vary considerably; with forceful breathing, greater volumes of air can be inhaled or exhaled. Various lung volumes and capacities for an adult

322 CHAPTER 10 | THE BODY NEEDS OXYGEN

> **BOX 10.2**
>
> ### Surface tension
>
> Consider a drop of water sitting on a clean surface. Inside the main body of the drop, each water molecule is attracted to the hydrogen atoms in all of the other water molecules surrounding it (see *Figure 10.8*). Because each water molecule is surrounded by other water molecules, the forces are equally distributed. However, this is not true at the surface of the drop. A water molecule at the surface is subject to intermolecular cohesive forces, involving hydrogen atoms, from other water molecules inside the drop and from water molecules alongside it at the surface. Water molecules at the surface of the drop tend to be pulled inwards by molecules beneath. This mutual attraction between water molecules causes the water to adopt the smallest possible surface area. Surface tension is the term used to describe the behaviour of water molecules at the surface of the drop and how they cling to each other and resist being separated. 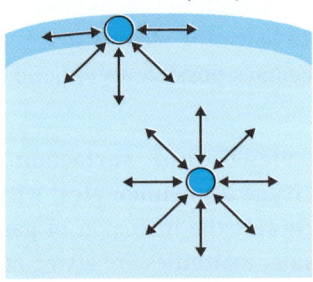
>
> **Figure 10.8 – Surface tension.**
> A water molecule in the body of the water drop is subject to cohesive forces from water molecules that surround it on all sides. In contrast, a water molecule at the surface is attracted to water molecules beside it on the surface of the drop and below it. 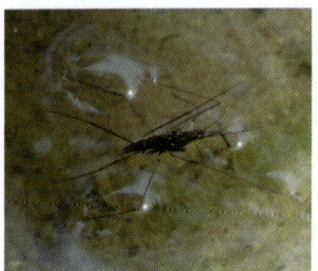
>
> An insect commonly called a pond skater can stand on water by making use of surface tension. Its legs have evolved so that it can spread its weight on the surface of the water without breaking the cohesive forces between the water molecules, so it literally walks on water (see *Figure 10.9*).
>
> **Figure 10.9 – A pond skater using surface tension to walk on water without sinking.**
> Reproduced under a CC BY-SA 3.0 Unported licence © Nevit Dilmen

male are illustrated in *Figure 10.10*. The volume of air above the tidal volume that can be taken in forcibly is called the **inspiratory reserve volume** (IRV) and is normally between 2100 and 3200 ml. The volume of air that can be forcibly exhaled is approximately 1200 ml and is called the **expiratory reserve volume** (ERV). Even after the most forceful expiration, about 1200 ml remains in the lung. This **residual volume**, which is determined by the elasticity of the lung tissue, the rigidity of the thoracic cavity and the presence of surfactant ensuring the alveoli do not fully collapse, helps to ease the work of breathing and allows the exchange of respiratory gases to continue between breaths. The sum of the IRV, ERV and tidal volume is known as the **vital capacity**, and this is the total volume of exchangeable air. This is normally approximately 4800 ml in healthy young men.

In a clinical setting, it is relatively easy to measure air flow out of the lung using devices such as a peak flow meter or spirometer (see *Figure 10.11*). The measurement of lung volumes and capacities (**spirometry**) is useful in the diagnosis of pulmonary disorders and evaluation of lung function (see Mary, Patient 2.1).

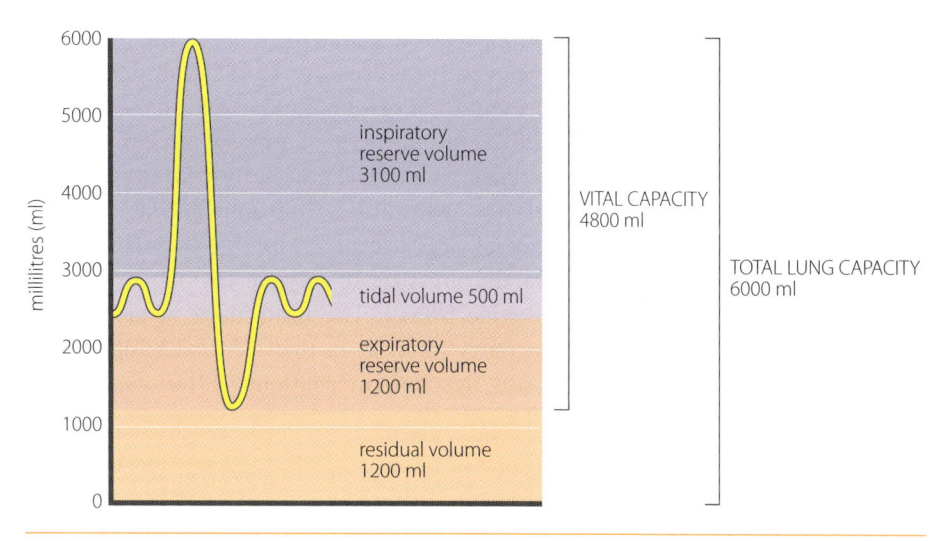

Figure 10.10 – **Lung volumes and capacities.**

10.2.6 Exchange and transportation of gases

The exchange of oxygen and carbon dioxide between the atmosphere and tissues can be described by the terms external and internal respiration. External respiration is the exchange of gases between the alveoli and pulmonary capillary blood, whereas internal respiration is the exchange of gases between tissue capillary blood and the cells. The transport of gases between the lungs and the tissues requires the cardiovascular system, with blood as the transport medium.

Gaseous exchange occurs by diffusion (see *Chapter 2*), with gas molecules moving from a place of high concentration to a place of lower concentration. Before considering this in detail, it is important to understand the way that gas concentration is described in physiology and measured in clinical practice.

Air in the atmosphere and in the lungs is a mixture of gases. Gases will try to fill the container in which they are held and in so doing exert a pressure on the walls of the container. Each gas in the mixture contributes to the total pressure. This is described by **Dalton's law**, which states that:

> The total pressure exerted by a gaseous mixture is equal to the sum of the partial pressures of each individual component in a gas mixture

The pressure exerted by each gas, the **partial pressure**, depends on the proportion of an individual gas within the mixture. Atmospheric air contains significant amounts of oxygen and nitrogen. Carbon dioxide, water vapour and insignificant amounts of inert gases such as helium make up the rest. Atmospheric air contains approximately 21% oxygen and 0.04% carbon dioxide. This means that oxygen exerts approximately 21% of the atmospheric pressure while carbon dioxide exerts 0.04% of the pressure. The air that is exhaled has a different composition (approximately 16% oxygen and 4.5% carbon dioxide). The different percentages reflect different amounts of gas molecules within the mixture. According to Dalton's law, the greater the proportion of a gas within the mixture, the greater will be the pressure it exerts within the container.

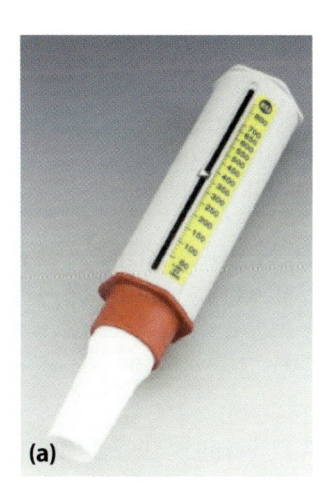

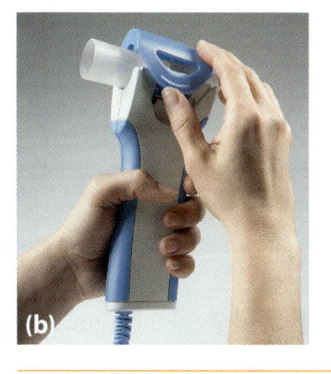

Figure 10.11 – **(a) A peak flow meter and (b) a digital spirometer.**
(a) Reproduced with permission from Clement Clarke International; (b) reproduced from www.midmark.com.

Dalton's law is a statement about the relative contribution that each gas makes to the overall gas pressure. Using atmospheric air as an example, there is more oxygen present than carbon dioxide and so oxygen makes a much greater contribution to the overall pressure of atmospheric air. At an atmospheric pressure of 760 mmHg, oxygen would exert an individual pressure of 160 mmHg (the partial pressure is 21/100 × 760 mmHg = 160 mmHg) and carbon dioxide would exert an individual partial pressure of 0.3 mmHg (0.04/100 × 760 mmHg). In atmospheric air, the partial pressure of oxygen (PO_2) is greater than the partial pressure of carbon dioxide (PCO_2). The units used to describe partial pressure are millimetres of mercury (mmHg) in the USA and kilopascal (kPa) in Europe and other countries using Système International (SI) units. (1 kPa is equivalent to 7.5 mmHg).

In a mixture of gases, each gas diffuses from a region of higher partial pressure to one of lower partial pressure; that is, gases diffuse down the partial pressure gradient. Differences in gas partial pressure exist throughout the respiratory system and the blood, and the partial pressure gradient determines the direction of movement of individual gases.

When considering the movement of oxygen and carbon dioxide across the respiratory membrane, a number of factors influence the gas exchange, particularly:

- the partial pressure gradients of oxygen and carbon dioxide
- the solubility of the individual gases within water and lipid (solubility is increased by temperature, hence the need to maintain a stable body temperature)
- the effectiveness of blood flow (perfusion) through the dense capillary beds surrounding the alveoli ventilated with air (i.e. matching ventilation and perfusion)
- the thinness of the respiratory membrane (the capillary cell wall, the interstitial space and the alveolar cell wall).

The alveoli are ideally suited for the exchange of gases because they form a large surface area, with each lung of an adult male containing approximately 500–700 million alveoli. Despite being composed of a number of tissue layers, the respiratory membrane is extremely thin (approximately 0.5–1.0 μm), thus helping to reduce the diffusion distance for gas transfer and, in so doing, maximize gaseous exchange.

The movement of oxygen and carbon dioxide at both the lung and tissue interfaces is illustrated in *Figure 10.12*, and can be summarized as follows:

- At the lungs, deoxygenated blood (which is low in oxygen (PO_2 = 40 mmHg/5.3 kPa) but high in carbon dioxide (PCO_2 = 45 mmHg/6 kPa)) becomes oxygenated blood that leaves the lungs rich in oxygen (PO_2 = 100 mmHg/13.3 kPa) and low in carbon dioxide (PCO_2 = 40 mmHg/5.3 kPa).
- On inspiration, due to the mechanics of breathing and the ventilation of the alveoli, the alveoli have a higher partial pressure of oxygen (PO_2 = 105 mmHg/14 kPa) compared with the blood entering the lungs (PO_2 = 40 mmHg/5.3 kPa) and so oxygen moves by diffusion from the alveoli into the pulmonary capillary blood.

- At the same time, carbon dioxide, which has a higher partial pressure in the blood entering the lungs (PCO_2 = 45 mmHg/6 kPa), moves from the pulmonary capillary blood into the alveoli where the partial pressure of CO_2 is lower (PCO_2 = 40 mmHg/5.3 kPa). Carbon dioxide is then exhaled during expiration.

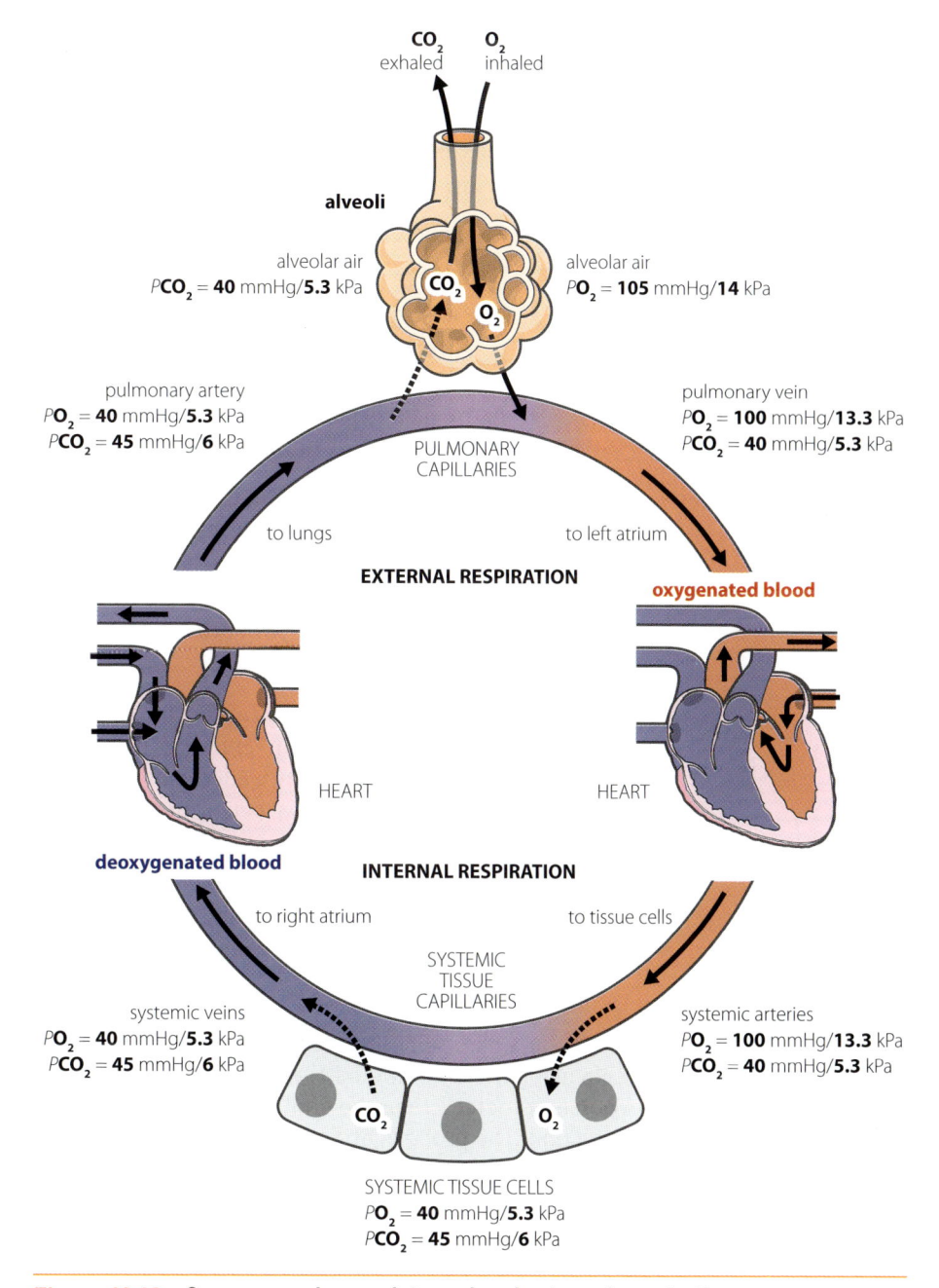

Figure 10.12 – Gaseous exchange: internal and external respiration.
Note that the partial pressure gradient for oxygen, and therefore the driving force, at both tissue level and at the alveolar interface is much greater than the partial pressure gradient for carbon dioxide. Carbon dioxide is considerably more soluble in water compared with oxygen and diffuses across the respiratory membrane much more readily.

- At the tissue level, arterial blood rich in oxygen enters the capillaries. Oxygen (PO_2 = 100 mmHg/13.3 kPa) moves from the capillaries into the tissue cells where there is a lower partial pressure of oxygen (PO_2 = 40 mmHg/5.3 kPa).
- At the same time, at the tissue level, carbon dioxide, produced by cellular processes as an end product during the production of chemical energy (ATP), moves from the higher concentration in the cell (PCO_2 = 45 mmHg/6 kPa) to the lower concentration in the capillary (PCO_2 = 40 mmHg/5.3 kPa).
- At the tissue level, oxygen is extracted from the blood and carbon dioxide is added so the blood that leaves the tissues via the venous system is low in oxygen and rich in carbon dioxide (deoxygenated blood).

Oxygen and carbon dioxide are carried between the lungs and tissues by blood. Oxygen is carried in two ways:

- The majority of oxygen (97–99%) binds to haemoglobin within the erythrocyte (red blood cell) to form **oxyhaemoglobin**, which is essential for carrying oxygen to the tissues.
- As oxygen is poorly soluble in water, only a small amount of oxygen (1–3%) dissolves in the plasma.

The amount of haemoglobin saturated with oxygen (oxygen saturation) can be measured non-invasively using an oxygen saturation probe attached to the ear lobe or finger. The process is known as pulse oximetry and is an important clinical procedure (see *Box 10.3*). As will be seen, the oxygen saturation levels of Mary (Patient 2.1) were lower than normal, reflecting the reduced oxygen content within her arterial blood.

Only a small amount of carbon dioxide, approximately 7%, dissolves directly in plasma. However, on entering the blood, the majority of carbon dioxide (approximately 70%) is converted rapidly into carbonic acid (H_2CO_3), which dissociates into bicarbonate ions (HCO_3^-) and hydrogen ions (H^+) (see *Figure 10.13*). Hydrogen binds to haemoglobin. Approximately 23% of carbon dioxide binds to haemoglobin to form **carbaminohaemoglobin**. As illustrated in *Figure 10.13*:

BOX 10.3

Pulse oximetry and oxygen saturation measurement

Pulse oximetry is used widely in a clinical setting to measure, non-invasively, arterial oxygenation in peripheral blood vessels using the different light-absorbing characteristics of haemoglobin and oxyhaemoglobin. A pulse oximeter is a probe emitting red and infrared light with a sensor attached to a computerized unit. The probe is attached to an area of the body that is relatively translucent such as the fingertip or ear lobe. The sensor, which is part of the probe, detects the amount of red and infrared light that passes through the body. Oxyhaemoglobin absorbs more infrared light, allowing red light to pass through. The oxygen saturation (SpO_2) can be calculated by measuring the relative amount of red and infrared light transmitted through the body area.

There are limitations to pulse oximetry because it does not measure the actual oxygen content of arterial blood. In patients with anaemia or severe circulatory impairment, pulse oximetry may not provide an accurate reflection of the actual amount of oxygen being delivered to the tissues. Normal oxygen saturation is above 94%.

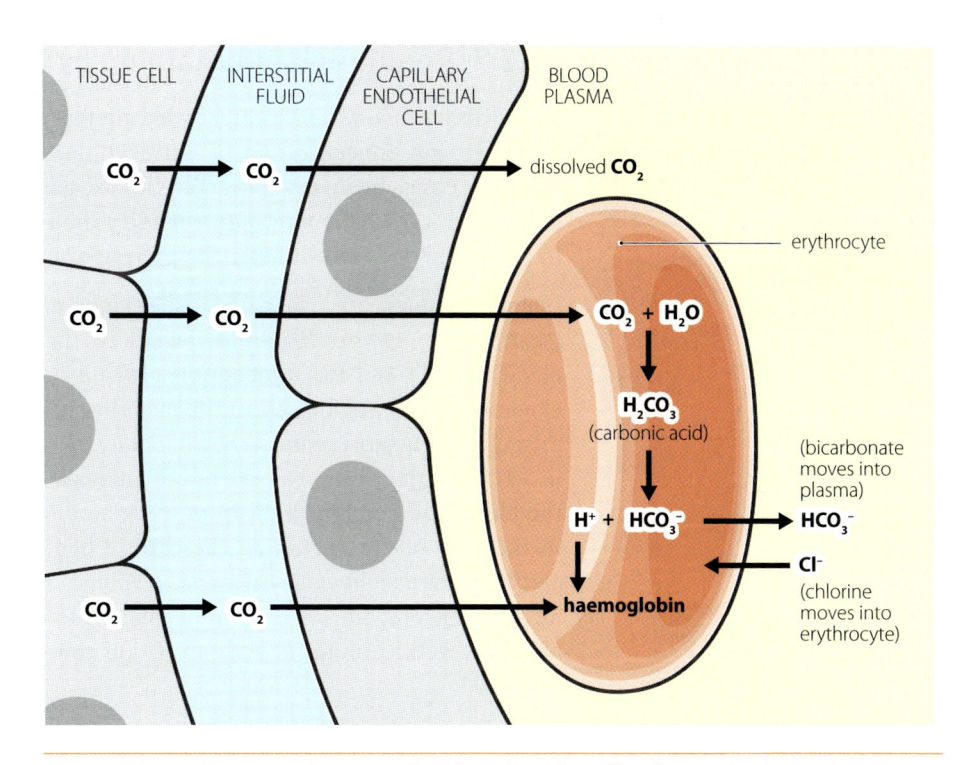

SECTION 10.2 | WHAT YOU NEED TO KNOW – ESSENTIAL ANATOMY AND PHYSIOLOGY

Figure 10.13 – Oxygen release and carbon dioxide collection at the tissue level.
Note: some CO_2 binds to haemoglobin to form carbaminohaemoglobin. Bicarbonate (HCO_3^-) moves into plasma and in return chlorine moves into the erythrocyte.

- When carbon dioxide diffuses into the watery environment of the erythrocyte, it encounters the enzyme carbonic anhydrase, which rapidly catalyses the combination of carbon dioxide and water to form carbonic acid.
- Once formed, carbonic acid instantly dissociates into H^+ and HCO_3^- ions.
- H^+ ions, which lower the pH of the blood, are removed by combining with haemoglobin within the erythrocyte, which acts as a buffer. Due to the buffering effect of haemoglobin, under resting conditions the pH of blood changes very little.
- HCO_3^- ions diffuse out of the erythrocyte into the plasma. To counterbalance the movement of negatively charged HCO_3^- ions into the plasma, negatively charged chloride ions (Cl^-) move from the plasma into the erythrocyte via a protein counter-transporter, exchanging one HCO_3^- ion for one Cl^- ion (this is called the **chloride shift**).
- The binding of carbon dioxide and H^+ ions to haemoglobin displaces oxygen, facilitating the unloading of oxygen at the tissues (the **Bohr effect**) and at the same time the affinity of haemoglobin for carbon dioxide is increased.
- The binding of H^+ ions and the release of HCO_3^- ions help to maintain the acid–base balance of blood.
- This chemical reaction is reversed at the lungs so that carbon dioxide is formed, which can then diffuse from the pulmonary capillaries into the alveoli for exhalation.

(a) central chemoreceptors

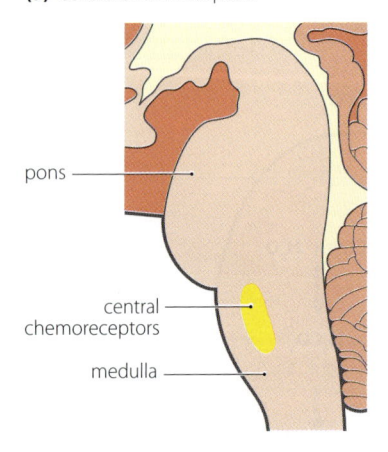

pons

central chemoreceptors

medulla

(b) peripheral chemoreceptors

sensory nerve fibres

carotid bodies chemoreceptor

left common carotid artery

aortic body chemoreceptor

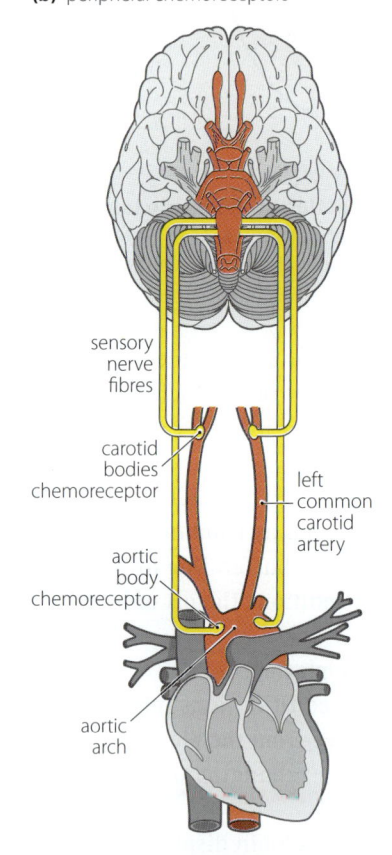

aortic arch

Figure 10.14 – **(a) Central and (b) peripheral chemoreceptors.**

10.2.7 Regulation of breathing by chemoreceptors

Specialized sensory nerve cells called **chemoreceptors** are stimulated by changes in the H⁺ ion concentration of extracellular fluid (blood and tissue fluid) and in some cases by a dramatic fall in oxygen content of arterial blood. Once stimulated, these chemoreceptors modify the activity of neurones in the medulla, in particular the DRG, to alter the pattern of breathing.

Chemoreceptors are classified as *peripheral* or *central*, depending on their location (see *Figure 10.14*). Increases in the concentration of CO_2 in arterial blood ($PaCO_2$) and CO_2 production provide the major respiratory drive. Central chemoreceptors are located in the medulla, in a region called the chemosensitive area. These chemoreceptors are excited by an increase in the H⁺ ion concentration in extracellular fluid, caused by an increase in the level of carbon dioxide in the blood and cerebrospinal fluid. Peripheral chemoreceptors, which are located in the arch of the aorta and the carotid bodies found at the bifurcation of the carotid arteries, have a different response and are often called the primary oxygen sensors; they are highly sensitive to a dramatic fall in PaO_2 in arterial blood, as well as to an increase in H⁺ ion concentration arising from an increase in $PaCO_2$.

Changes in ventilation in response to an increase in $PaCO_2$ are illustrated in *Figure 10.15*. When $PaCO_2$ rises, the H⁺ ion concentration of extracellular fluid increases, resulting in excitation of central (primarily) and peripheral chemoreceptors. This in turn leads to increased sensory (afferent) impulses to the DRG and VRG resulting in increased motor impulses down the phrenic and external intercostal muscle nerves, which increase the depth and rate of breathing and, as a consequence, increase alveolar ventilation. The increased alveolar ventilation maintains the effective partial pressure gradient to facilitate the rapid diffusion of carbon dioxide across the respiratory membrane into the alveoli and exhalation of carbon dioxide. Thus, the level of carbon dioxide in arterial blood decreases in keeping with the principle of homeodynamics.

Ventilation is normally closely matched to the production of carbon dioxide in the body, so that the level of carbon dioxide is kept within the normal parameters. For example, during exercise, ventilation increases. One reason for this is an immediate response to muscle contraction and the movement of joints. Sensory impulses from receptors in muscles and joints stimulate inspiratory neurones in the brainstem to send motor impulses to the diaphragm and external intercostal muscles. Secondly, there is an increase in ventilation in response to the increased production of carbon dioxide by exercising muscles. Both mechanisms ensure that the normal level of arterial blood gases is tightly maintained. Alteration in the normal regulation of breathing, due to disease or injury, may result in significant changes in the arterial blood gases. Dysfunction of the respiratory centres in the medulla and pons, for example due to drugs such as opiates or following a brainstem stroke, will depress breathing and indeed may cause breathing to stop, which is a medical emergency.

stimulus
- increase in arterial PCO_2

↓ pH
↑ H⁺
in extracellular fluid and cerebrospinal fluid

receptors
- central chemoreceptors excited

receptors
- carotid bodies, aortic bodies excited

↑ afferent impulses

control centre
- activation of medullary respiratory centres

negative feedback
- arterial PCO_2 and H⁺ return to normal
- reduced activity of receptors
- breathing pattern returns to normal

↑ efferent impulses down phrenic nerves and intercostal nerves

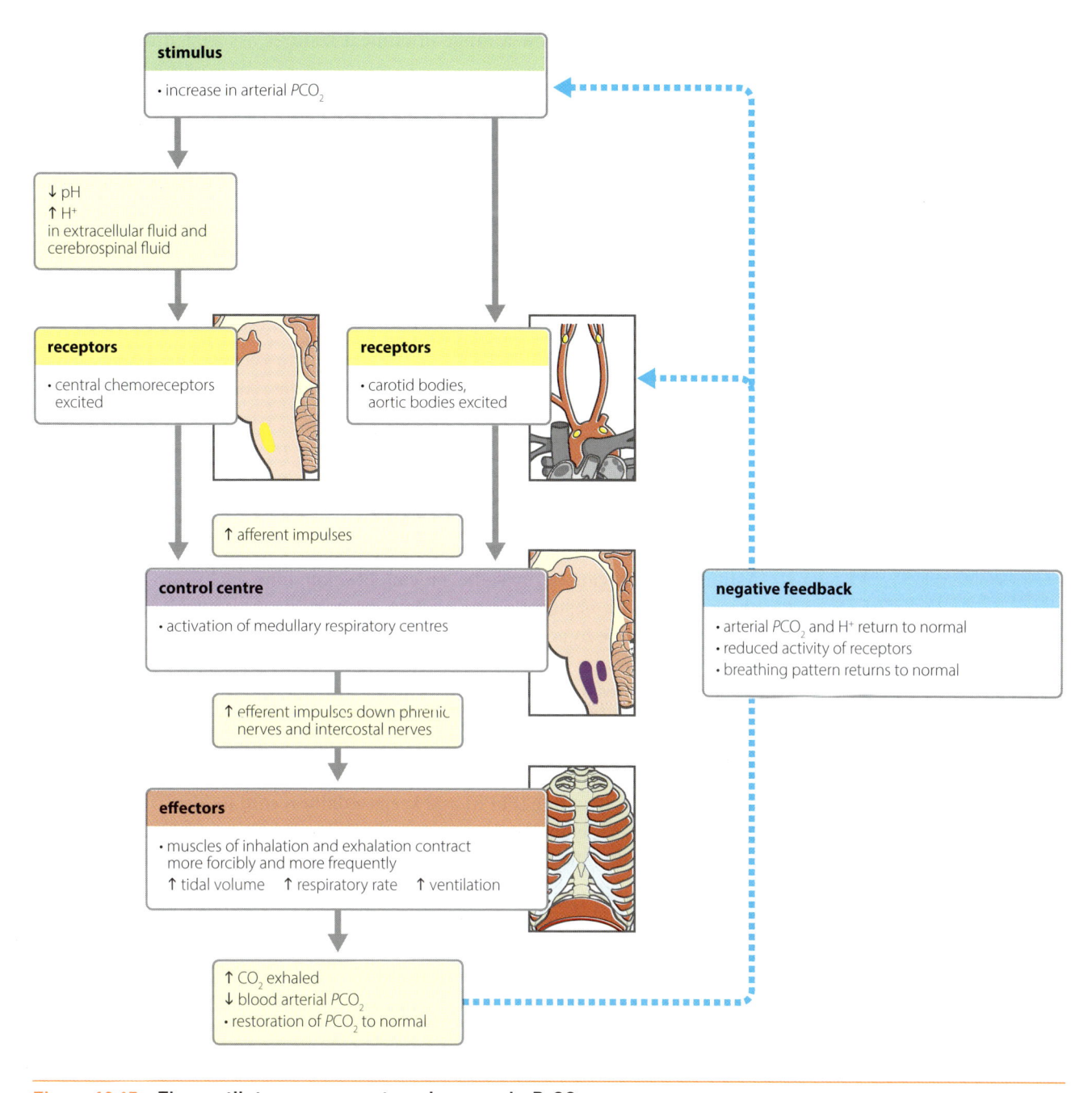

effectors
- muscles of inhalation and exhalation contract more forcibly and more frequently
  ↑ tidal volume   ↑ respiratory rate   ↑ ventilation

↑ CO_2 exhaled
↓ blood arterial PCO_2
- restoration of PCO_2 to normal

Figure 10.15 – The ventilatory response to an increase in $PaCO_2$.

10.3 Clinical application

Understanding the normal structure of the respiratory system, the regulation of breathing, and the normal exchange of oxygen and carbon dioxide between the lungs and the tissues is important in order that healthcare professionals can explain clearly the nature of the respiratory problem to patients. This can help them better manage their own breathing. An understanding also ensures that the most effective treatment to alleviate the difficulties can be provided. The patient cases in this chapter show a range of clinical features associated with impaired respiratory function:

- **Mary (Patient 2.1)** has chronic asthma, and with the help of healthcare professionals over a number of years has become an expert in understanding and managing her respiratory problem by adjusting the use of her inhaler medication to keep her feeling well. Understanding what triggers her asthma and the signs of worsening control, which require her to increase her medication and contact her family doctor, are an important part of her treatment plan and education. From time to time, her asthma worsens despite taking appropriate action. This leads to significant difficulties in her breathing.
- **Sarah (Patient 3.1)** requires daily physiotherapy to keep her lungs clear of viscous mucus to aid her breathing and reduce the risk of her developing a chest infection.

Patient 2.1 | Mary | 29 | 53 | 311 | **330**

- 57-year-old woman
- Chronic asthmatic on beclometasone dipropionate, salmeterol and salbutamol
- Has a cold and now presents with wheeze, tachycardia and green sputum
- Taking double usual amounts of salbutamol to keep asthma in check
- PEFR down to 180 L/min compared to usual 480 L/min

Mary has her respiratory function assessed regularly due to her chronic asthma. Asthma, which can be episodic or can develop into a chronic condition, is characterized by obstruction to airflow, especially on expiration. Individuals with asthma have hypersensitive airways (bronchioles) that are prone to go into spasm and constrict. This can be due to a variety of specific triggers; for example, a non-specific response to cold air or a specific allergic response to house dust mites. Any one of a range of triggers can lead to a reduction in airflow. The periodic measurement of Mary's expiratory airflow volume is important because it allows the assessment of airflow obstruction. Mary regularly measures her peak expiratory flow rate (PEFR) and keeps a daily record to identify any serious fluctuations. PEFR is the maximum rate of air flow measured in litres per minute generated during a forceful exhalation and is measured using a peak flow meter (see *Figure 10.11a*). Nomograms (graphical calculators) have been produced to reflect the normal expected variation in PEFR based on age, sex and height. These provide a guide for comparing actual patient recordings with expected recordings. PEFR tends to vary during the day and between days. During 1 week, Mary's PEFR diary indicated the following fluctuations, which is typical for her PEFR:

> Monday: 460 L/minute
> Tuesday: 480 L/minute
> Wednesday: 480 L/minute
> Thursday: 490 L/minute
> Friday: 470 L/minute

A serious reduction, for example by more than 20% from the average value of 480 L/minute, would indicate worsening airflow and deterioration in her asthma.

This would be an important indicator for Mary to seek professional advice or to adjust her inhaler medication, as indicated in her agreed treatment plan. In the past, Mary had episodes where her asthma control deteriorated and the reduction in airflow was evident in a significantly reduced PEFR.

Mary arrived at the health centre distressed, **tachypnoeic** (28 breaths/minute), wheezing, coughing up green sputum and **tachycardic** (115 beats/minute). She showed **central cyanosis** and was having difficulty speaking. For the past week, she had been suffering with a cold but had not sought treatment as she did not want to trouble the health centre. At one of her regular clinical reviews, Mary's treatment plan had been discussed and, in accordance with the plan, she increased her beclometasone (anti-inflammatory steroid inhaler) to four puffs BD. However, for the past two nights her asthma had disturbed her sleep and she now requires 8–10 puffs per day of her salbutamol (bronchodilator inhaler). Mary felt much worse today and her home PEFR was much lower than usual at 175 L/minute so she came to the health centre. Her PEFR was checked again using a peak flow meter and was found to be 180 L/minute; this reflected a significant reduction in the flow of air through her conducting airways. In the health centre, Mary was given salbutamol (5 mg) via a nebulizer and an ambulance was summoned.

In Mary's case, her asthma was exacerbated by the presence of a bacterial infection in her lungs, symptoms of which include coughing up green, purulent sputum and raised temperature. This was confirmed by sending off a sputum specimen to the microbiology laboratory so that the specific causative microorganism could be cultured and an appropriate antibiotic identified. Some of the important clinical features of impaired respiratory function are highlighted in *Box 10.4*. In Mary's case, not only did she expectorate green, purulent sputum, but she also had a faster than normal respiratory rate (tachypnoea), an expiratory wheeze and signs of central cyanosis. She also had difficulty completing a sentence when speaking. The term cyanosis refers to the blueish colour of the skin and mucous membranes in areas such as the lips and tongue, ear lobes, nose and nail beds. In people with heavily pigmented skin, cyanosis can be observed most easily in the tissues under the nail and in the inside of the mouth and tongue. Cyanosis reflects reduced oxygenation of arterial blood due to pulmonary disorders and/or poor circulation to the periphery (e.g. heart failure). Central cyanosis refers to cyanosis that is observed around the lips, the inside of the mouth and tongue, and reflects respiratory problems and/or circulatory problems.

Mary attempted to manage her worsening condition by altering her medications in accordance with the treatment plan negotiated with the healthcare professionals involved in her long-term care; the treatment plan was designed to prevent and relieve the obstruction in her airways. However, despite this, her condition deteriorated and she sought appropriate help. In hospital, Mary responded well to treatment and returned home with a revised treatment plan.

> **BOX 10.4**
>
> ### Indicators of respiratory impairment
>
> #### Abnormal respiratory rate of the patient
>
> Normal respiratory rates at rest are:
>
> - adult: 12–20 breaths/minute
> - 2–5 years old: 25–30 breaths/minute
> - under 1 year old: 30–40 breaths/minute.
>
> #### Abnormal breathing sounds
>
> Examples of these are:
>
> - wheeze – a high-pitched sound that occurs on inspiration and expiration due to obstruction of the airflow in the conducting airways; wheezing may be particularly evident during expiration
> - stridor – the sound produced during inspiration due to obstruction of the airflow (e.g. upper airway obstruction due to foreign body or swelling of the epiglottis).
>
> #### Difficulty in breathing
>
> This may be evident as:
>
> - the use of accessory muscles, for instance use of the shoulder muscles to help breathing
> - signs of skin retraction around the clavicle in children during inspiration
> - attempts to sit in an upright position.
>
> #### Signs of cyanosis (especially involving the tongue – evidence of central cyanosis).
>
> #### Abnormal secretions from the respiratory tract
>
> These may appear as:
>
> - thick green purulent sputum, indicating a probable bacterial infection
> - blood-stained sputum (haemoptysis), indicating a possible infection (e.g. tuberculosis, pulmonary infarction or lung tumour)
> - watery and frothy sputum, indicating pulmonary oedema.
>
> #### Pain associated with breathing
>
> This may be evident as pain on inspiration (pleuritic pain), which can be due to a number of causes (e.g. inflammation of the pleura (pleurisy)).
>
> #### Low oxygen saturation level (less than 94%).
>
> Oxygen saturation levels require careful interpretation particularly in the presence of a chronic obstructive pulmonary disease, where the target oxygen saturation for most patients is between 88 and 92%.
>
> #### Confusion due to reduced levels of oxygen delivered to the brain (cerebral anoxia).

Patient 3.1 — Sarah | 60 | 94 | 195 | 237 | 311 | **333**

- 17-year-old girl
- CF diagnosis at age of 1 year via a sweat test
- Frequent admissions for chest infections affecting breathing
- PERT added to meals to help digest her food
- Vigorous chest physio to remove excess mucus and improve ventilation
- Takes antibiotic and inhaled bronchodilators

Sarah has cystic fibrosis (CF), an autosomal recessive genetic disorder caused by a mutation in a gene called the cystic fibrosis transmembrane conductance regulator (*CFTR*), located on chromosome 7. As outlined in *Chapter 3*, Sarah inherited the genetic mutation from both parents.

The *CFTR* gene encodes a protein that forms an ion channel to facilitate the movement of chloride ions. The defective gene results in a disturbance of the normal movement of chloride, sodium and water between the cell and secretions from the cell such as mucus. The result is that the secretions are more viscous than normal, leading to a number of respiratory problems for Sarah, including the following:

- It is more difficult for her to cough up respiratory secretions (mucus) than normal. Individuals with CF have regular physiotherapy to help remove mucus and improve ventilation.
- She has impaired immune defence mechanisms, including alterations to ciliated epithelial cells in the lungs. This increases the risk of bacterial colonization and infection.

Due to the build-up of highly viscous and stagnated mucus in the smaller airway passages, Sarah is prone to developing chest infections, which in the long term could lead to detrimental changes to the respiratory epithelium and alveoli. Sarah has had a long history of repeated chest infections and has received long-term antibiotic therapy to prevent infection, with the aim of preserving pulmonary function. Vigorous and repeated chest physiotherapy at home, with careful positioning of the upper body to facilitate the draining of the excess mucus by gravity (postural drainage) is required to remove excess mucus from the conducting airways and help improve ventilation.

Sarah takes many medications, including long-term antibiotics and inhaled bronchodilators, to help counteract the effects of CF and to prevent the development of chest infections, and, as outlined in *Chapter 7*, pancreatic digestive enzyme replacement therapy and nutritional supplements to ensure that she receives the required amount of nutrients.

It is important for healthcare professionals to understand about the regulation of the respiratory system to ensure maintenance of the normal levels of oxygen and carbon dioxide in the blood to enable optimal cell functioning and health. As with all aspects of physiology, this understanding is continually being refined. This chapter covers the essential elements, but, as with all aspects of anatomy and physiology and healthcare, there is always more to know, especially for healthcare professionals involved in caring for people such as Mary (Patient 2.1) and Sarah (Patient 3.1).

10.4 Summary

- The respiratory system is essential for maintaining the normal levels of oxygen and carbon dioxide in blood and also the acid–base balance of blood, both of which are essential for life and health.
- Effective ventilation increases the oxygen content of arterial blood to the cells.
- Carbon dioxide, produced in the cells as a waste product of ATP production via cellular respiration, is removed from the cells and transported in the blood to the lungs, where it diffuses from the lung and is exhaled.
- The transportation of oxygen occurs primarily within the erythrocyte, where it is bound to haemoglobin.
- Breathing is an autonomic function controlled by groups of neurones (respiratory centres) in the medulla and pons of the brainstem. Breathing can be modified via the higher centres of the brain and various sensory receptors.
- Ventilation of the lungs is a combination of neural and mechanical events that change the gas volume and hence the gas pressure in the lungs.

10.5 Further reading

The British Thoracic Society provides comprehensive material on its website about the management of various respiratory disorders. Its guidelines on the management of asthma can be found here:
www.brit-thoracic.org.uk/clinical-information/asthma/asthma-guidelines.aspx

The Cystic Fibrosis Foundation website is a very useful resource, providing helpful information for individuals with cystic fibrosis and for carers and healthcare professionals:
www.cff.org

10.6 Self-assessment questions

Answers can be found at www.scionpublishing.com/AandP

(10.1) Identify the one correct statement. Dead space volume is the volume of air:
(a) remaining in the lungs after forced expiration
(b) inhaled after normal inspiration
(c) forcibly expelled after normal expiration
(d) not involved in gaseous exchange
(e) located in the bronchioles and alveoli

(10.2) Which one cell type produces the substance called surfactant?
(a) Microglial cells
(b) Islets of Langerhans
(c) Type 2 pneumocytes
(d) Thyroid gland cells
(e) Collagen

(10.3) Rearrange the following structures into the order that best describes the route for the flow of air into the lungs.
1. alveoli
2. larynx
3. nasal passages
4. secondary and tertiary bronchi
5. terminal bronchioles
6. primary bronchi
7. trachea

(a) 1 3 4 2 5 7 6
(b) 3 2 4 6 5 1 7
(c) 2 3 4 6 7 1 5
(d) 3 2 7 6 4 5 1
(e) 1 5 4 6 7 2 3

(10.4) Select the statement that best explains the response to an increase in $PaCO_2$:
(a) Central chemoreceptors are stimulated due to a fall in H^+ ions
(b) Tidal volume is reduced and respiratory rate increased
(c) Peripheral chemoreceptors are activated in preference to central chemoreceptors
(d) The increase in HCO_3^- ions stimulates central chemoreceptors
(e) There is increased efferent discharge from the ventral respiratory group

(10.5) Write brief notes on the structure and function of the regions labelled A and B on the diagram below.

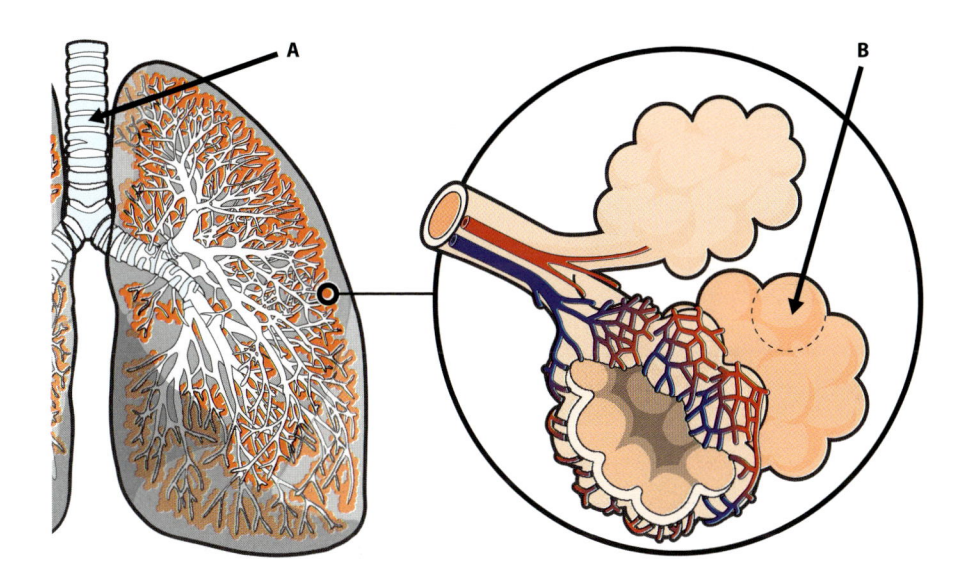

(10.6) Why is it important for Sarah (Patient 3.1) to receive regular physiotherapy to clear her bronchioles and bronchi of excess mucus secretions?

(10.7) Drawing on information in *Chapter 4*, outline how the drug salbutamol is an effective bronchodilator to improve the breathing of Mary (Patient 2.1).

CHAPTER 11 | Protection from harm

Learning points for this chapter

After working through this chapter, you should be able to:

- Describe the tissue, cellular and chemical elements of immunity
- Explain how physical defences provide an initial barrier to infection
- Discuss the contrasting features of innate and adaptive immunity
- Describe the acute inflammatory response
- Identify the role of lymphocyte populations in response to antigen
- Discuss the purpose of antibodies and explain how they are produced
- Apply knowledge of immunity to vaccination and changes to immunity over the lifespan

11.1 Introduction and clinical relevance

From the moment we are born, we encounter thousands of microbes as we go about our daily life. We also have living on and within our bodies trillions of these microbes, some causing disease, some protecting us from infection and others waiting for an opportunity to infect or cause disease. Damage to our body tissues from any cause requires repair and protection from infection. For this, we have an immune system comprising a complex network of cells and chemicals. This provides constant surveillance and response to tissue damage, and protects us from harm. Development of immunity occurs throughout the lifespan and an overactive or an underactive immune system can lead to poor health. Public health strategies such as vaccination stimulate protective immune responses that persist over many years and save millions of lives from potentially lethal infections. In this chapter, we aim to introduce core concepts to help you understand how crucial immunity is to health. Knowledge of this subject is developing quickly, and increasingly it is recognized that the immune system often has a role to play in both causing disease and protecting us from disease. The patient studies that follow illustrate some of the breadth of involvement of immunity in both health and disease, and highlight the knowledge required by healthcare professionals.

| Patient 1.3 | Francine | 2 | 21 | 194 | 235 | **338** | 371 |

- 40-year-old woman
- Crohn's disease – on steroids
- Presents with inflamed bowel and anaemia
- MRSA screen ahead of potential surgery
- TPN given IV to recovery during relapse
- Positive MRSA screen – decolonized over 5 days

Fluctuating periods of exacerbation and remission of Francine's Crohn's disease have been managed with potent anti-inflammatory medications, careful monitoring of her diet and occasionally with nutritional supplementation to counter the malabsorption of nutrients that sometimes occurs in patients with Crohn's disease. As a new admission to hospital and a potential candidate for surgery, Francine has been screened and found to be positive for colonization with meticillin-resistant *Staphylococcus aureus* (MRSA). Identifying any patient colonized with MRSA prior to admission to hospital is important for reducing rates of healthcare-associated infection and for protecting patients vulnerable to infection, such as the immunocompromised, very young, frail and elderly.

| Patient 11.1 | Albert | **338** | 372 |

- 81-year-old man
- Chest infection led to pneumonia
- Given IV antibiotics to rapidly improve symptoms
- In 6 days had severe foul-smelling diarrhoea – found to contain *C. difficile*

Albert is an 81-year-old gentleman, who was admitted to hospital with a severe chest infection that has developed into pneumonia. He lives with his wife, Ethel, in a bungalow, and describes himself as fit for his age. Intravenous antibiotic therapy was commenced, which improved his symptoms greatly. Four days after his admission, his temperature returned to normal for 24 hours and the administration of intravenous antibiotics was changed to oral antibiotics. Albert was beginning to feel much better; however, on the sixth day of his antibiotic treatment, he suddenly developed a severe offensive-smelling diarrhoea, which Albert found very debilitating and embarrassing. A stool specimen was sent to the laboratory because this is a typical presentation of an infection due to the bacterium *Clostridium difficile*. Albert was immediately isolated from other patients and moved into a side room.

| Patient 11.2 | Jerry | **338** | 374 |

- 30-year-old man
- Diagnosed with HIV at age 22
- Fall in CD4$^+$ count leads to discussion of treatment

Jerry is a 30-year-old man infected with human immunodeficiency virus type 1 (HIV-1). He was diagnosed 8 years ago after visiting his family doctor with symptoms of fatigue, fever and swollen glands. Initially, it was thought that Jerry might have glandular fever, but this was not the case and he was found to be HIV positive. Jerry's family doctor referred him to the centre for sexual health; since then, he has been attending the centre regularly for blood tests to monitor his condition. Although Jerry has lived with HIV for 8 years, he has not been prescribed any treatment, as his own immune system has been evaluated as sufficient to keep the levels of virus in his blood low, as indicated by high levels of a type of T-lymphocyte (also called CD4$^+$ cells, discussed later in this chapter). However, as his last two blood tests indicated a fall in the level of CD4$^+$ cells, the HIV specialist nurse at the centre now wants to discuss treatment options with him.

Immunity is the ability of the body to resist and eliminate infection and to recognize danger or stress to cells. The immune system is composed of a diverse array of physical, cellular and chemical defences that protect the body from infection caused by a wide variety of infectious disease-causing microorganisms, otherwise known as **pathogens**. Humans have evolved and adapted to survive with these microorganisms present in the environment. Our relationship with microorganisms is complex; on the one hand, we have developed protective mechanisms to limit the harm they can impose on our bodies, and on the other hand, we exploit the presence of microorganisms on our bodies to prime our immune cells and even metabolize substances within the gut. Immune responses are potentially harmful to the body, and so in eradicating infection, immune processes must be regulated so that damage to healthy tissue is avoided. If immunity is not carefully regulated, a variety of disease states can develop.

An immune system that is effective in protecting a person from infection is essential for health. Infectious diseases are a major cause of morbidity and mortality worldwide, and infection is the leading cause of death in children under 5 years. In addition, immune disorders acquired over the lifespan include many chronic disease states; for example, asthma is a disorder characterized by hypersensitivity reactions to various triggers, and rheumatoid arthritis is an example of an autoimmune disorder where the immune system damages the body's own tissues.

Healthcare professionals frequently encounter patients with a variety of chronic inflammatory diseases, such as Francine (Patient 1.3), or patients with infections, such as Albert (Patient 11.1). Healthcare-associated infection (HCAI; also referred to as hospital-acquired or nosocomial infection) is common, adding an extra burden on patients, clinical staff and the health service. Eradication of MRSA from the body is not easy to achieve reliably, and infection with *C. difficile* is not only unpleasant, but also dangerous to vulnerable patients such as the elderly or those with a compromised immune system. Each of the patients discussed within this chapter has a health problem that involves the immune system; knowledge of this system is important to better understand how we can optimize defences against infection.

The discovery and development of **antibiotic** compounds in the 20th century used as therapy to destroy pathogens quickly, despite a functional immune system, has saved a great many lives. However, the development of resistance by microorganisms to some of these agents has led to recognition in the early 21st century that resistance to antibiotics by pathogens has become a major threat to human health.

Compromised immunity can occur for a variety of reasons, and leaving the body unprotected against pathogens has a negative impact on physiological systems. All healthcare professionals have a responsibility to understand how best to prevent and limit infection in their practice.

11.2 What you need to know – essential anatomy and physiology

Immune mechanisms can be classified into two main groups. **Innate immunity** (also known as **non-specific immunity**) refers to immunity that is present from birth and is common to most animals including invertebrates. Innate immune mechanisms provide an immediate response to a wide variety of organisms by recognizing molecules present on potential pathogens, and they function to protect tissues from damage. **Adaptive immunity**, also referred to as **specific immunity**, is common to 'higher' vertebrates such as mammals, birds and fish. It also provides a response to potential pathogens, but unlike innate immunity it *develops* and *adapts* over the lifetime and is focused or restricted to *highly specific* molecules present on potential pathogens. The immune system is composed of mobile elements – cells and chemicals – supported by non-mobile structures that include lymphatic tissues and organs.

It is important always to bear the following points in mind as this chapter progresses:

- Innate and adaptive immune responses are fully integrated, working as a coordinated single immune system (see *Figure 11.1*).
- Protective mechanisms involve physical mechanisms – structural barriers to infection.
- Infectious agents that penetrate into the body will encounter:
  - immune cells
  - immune chemicals that exist in the body fluids – sometimes called humoral immunity (based on the ancient Greek theory that the body was filled with four fluids known as 'humours').
- Immunity must be carefully regulated to minimize damage to normal body tissue.

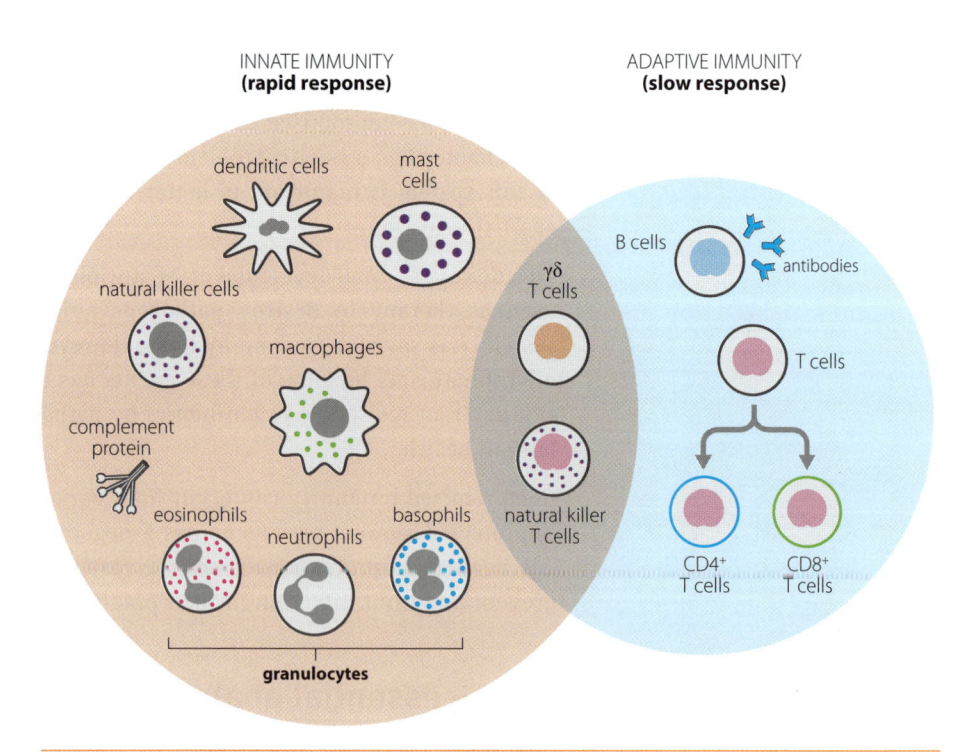

Figure 11.1 – Innate and adaptive immunity.
Innate and adaptive immunity mechanisms are fully integrated, providing cellular immunity supported by chemicals: complement in innate immunity and antibodies in adaptive immunity. Overall regulation is provided by cytokines, a diverse variety of soluble molecules.

11.2.1 Lymphatic structures support immunity

The lymphatic system is composed of a *low pressure* circulatory system together with organs operating in parallel with, but separate from, the blood circulatory system (see *Figure 11.2*).

Interstitial fluid collects within lymphatic vessels, forming a fluid known as lymph, which is distributed around the body. The vessels eventually merge to form two main lymphatic collecting ducts, the right lymphatic duct and the thoracic duct; lymph from the right side of the head, the right upper limb and the right thorax drains into the right lymphatic duct, while that from around the rest of the body drains into the much larger thoracic duct. These two ducts then empty into the venous circulation at the junction of the subclavian and jugular veins (on

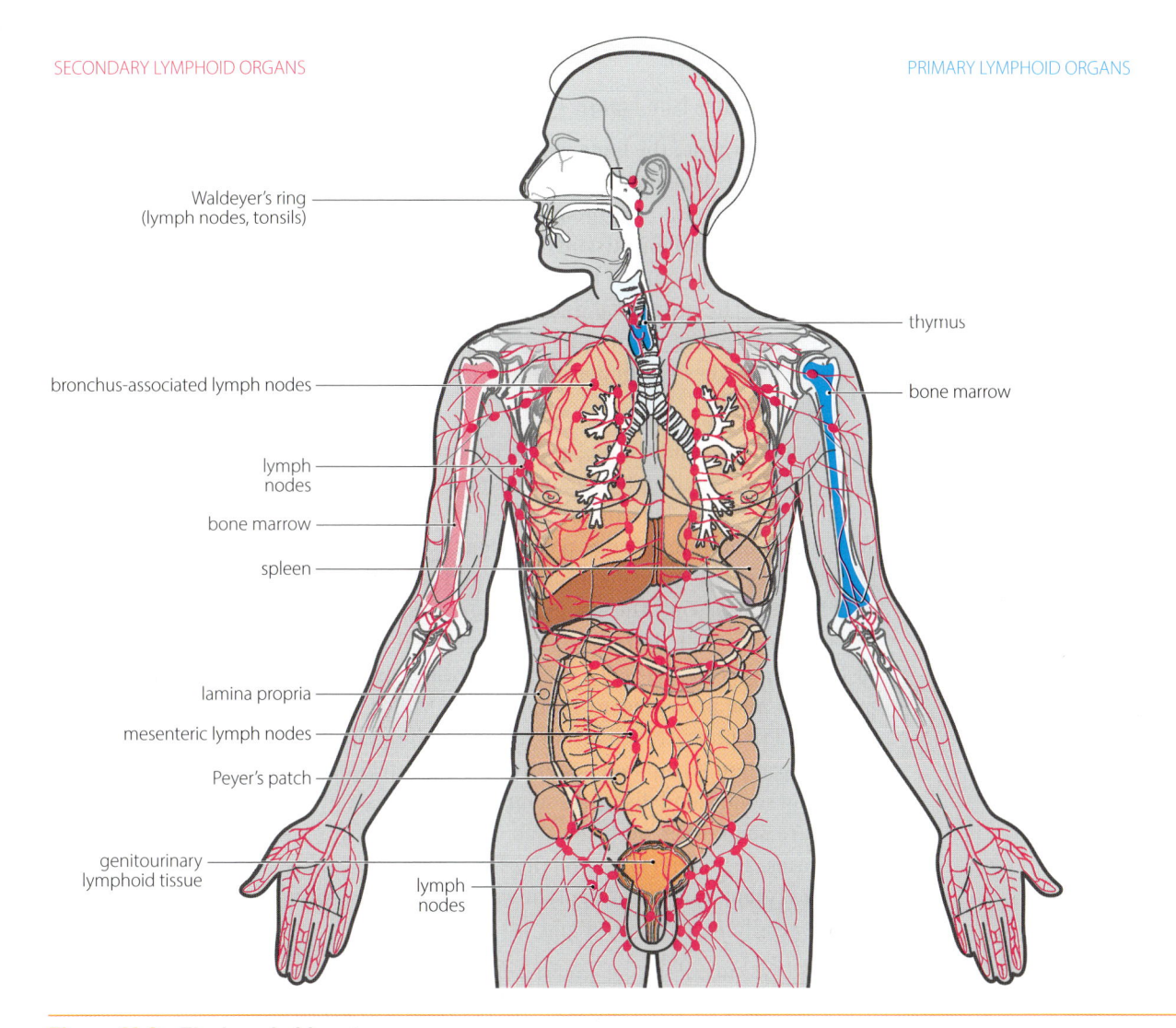

Figure 11.2 – The lymphoid system.
The lymphoid system consists of lymphatic organs and vessels that drain away low-pressure tissue fluid containing immune cells, which continually recirculates into the blood circulation.

the right and left sides of the body). This adds to the circulatory blood volume, returning excess lymph, proteins and cells back into the blood circulation. An effective lymphatic system is essential for the maintenance of normal blood volume and appropriate distribution of fluid between the circulating and tissue compartments. The composition of lymph is important for the regulation of the extracellular matrix (discussed in *Chapter 2*), and lymphatic vessels within the small intestine also absorb fat received from digestion in the gastrointestinal tract (see *Chapter 7*). The lymphatic system provides an integrating structure for immunity, providing a transport system for immune cells to move between blood, the tissues and lymph nodes. The circulation of lymph increases the interaction between elements of immunity and pathogens, and holds a reservoir of immune cells (approximately 90% of immune cells reside within lymphatic tissue). Immune cells within lymphatic fluid are not static, as in all other tissues; instead, they *recirculate*. Thus, they support immune cell development, differentiation and surveillance for pathogens and presentation of **antigens** (defined and discussed later in this chapter).

Lymphoid tissues (see *Figure 11.2*) include the following:

- Primary organs: the bone marrow and thymus gland. These form sites of lymphocyte development.
- Secondary organs: the lymph nodes, spleen, tonsils and **mucosa-associated lymphoid tissue** (MALT). These are sites of lymphoid tissue providing reservoirs of lymphocytes and a site of interaction with antigens. The urogenital and respiratory tracts contain MALT, and along the length of the small and large intestine, clusters of MALT termed **Peyer's patches** are important in protecting the body from food-borne pathogens.

Lymph nodes are found along all the major lymphatic vessels but are concentrated in the thoracic cavity and abdomen and also at the junctions of the extremities, including the arms, legs and neck (see *Figure 11.2*). Lymph nodes have a follicular structure, containing dense populations of immune cells. These are primarily lymphocytes but also macrophages and dendritic cells (these immune cells will be discussed as the chapter progresses). Mature lymphocytes constantly recirculate through lymph nodes, interstitial fluid and blood, averaging one to two circuits of the body each day. Antigens captured by immune cells are processed and presented to lymphocytes, which become activated in response to them. Lymphocyte activation becomes clinically evident when lymph nodes become swollen (**lymphadenopathy**) during infection and in other disease states including some blood disorders such as **lymphomas**. Biopsy and removal of lymph nodes are sometimes performed as clinically useful diagnostic and therapeutic procedures, respectively, especially for cancer. This is because cancer cells often travel to lymph nodes and remain within them (see discussion of Sheila, Patient 2.3, especially in *Chapters 9* and *14*).

11.2.2 Innate immunity – physical defences

There are four main **physical defences** that protect the body surfaces from infection (see *Figure 11.3*). These are:

- *barriers* to infection, e.g. external surfaces are protected by skin
- *chemical* defences, which destroy or limit infection
- *mechanical* defences, which remove potential infectious microorganisms or resist their entry into the body
- *normal flora*, microorganisms normally present on our body surfaces that help to exclude pathogens.

Anatomical barriers to infection are provided by the **epidermis**. The epidermis comprises a multilayered, keratinized epithelium, where dead **corneocytes** are constantly being shed from the surface while being renewed from lower proliferative layers. The epidermis provides a waterproof, abrasion-resistant layer (see *Chapter 12*); it is relatively dry, limiting the range of pathogens able to survive on it. Compounds released onto the surface of the skin also serve

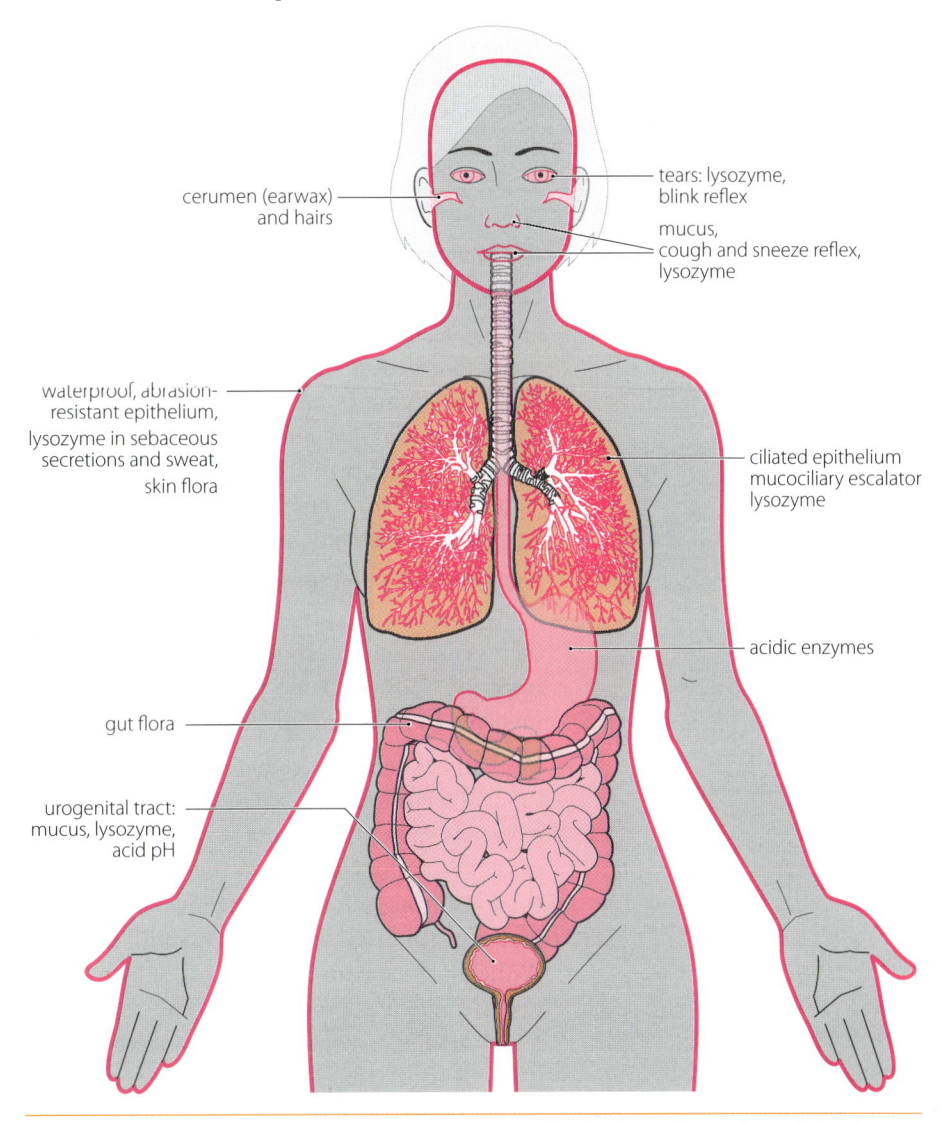

Figure 11.3 – The physical defences that protect the body surfaces from infection. These include physical, chemical, mechanical and microbial barriers. Penetration of these barriers by microorganisms results in activation of innate and adaptive immune cells and chemicals to limit infection and further tissue damage.

to limit microbial growth, for example by maintenance of an acidic pH in the range of 4–6. Sebum contains lactic acid and fatty acids, which support an acid skin pH. Skin is normally colonized by many species of microorganism, which collectively are called the normal flora (discussed later in this chapter). Evidence is accumulating to suggest that the normal flora of microorganisms on the skin's surface and within the gastrointestinal tract interact with immune cells and prime the immune system for defensive responses to pathogens. Thus, a symbiotic relationship exists between the normal flora and the body.

Mucosal surfaces within the body cavities of the respiratory, gastrointestinal and urogenital tracts are very thin and delicate and remain moist to allow the secretion and absorption of chemicals. The constant production and excretion of mucus limits the ability of microorganisms to colonize mucosal surfaces. In the respiratory tract, ciliated epithelium (see *Chapter 2*) assists in keeping the respiratory membrane free of microorganisms by moving particles trapped in mucus up into the upper airway where they can be coughed out or swallowed, to be destroyed by gastric juice in the stomach, thus limiting infection in the lung. Mucus contains a variety of compounds that limit the growth of organisms, including lysozyme, which is able to degrade bacterial cell walls, lactoferrin, which prevents bacteria utilizing the iron necessary for growth, and lactoperoxidase, which generates free radicals to destroy microorganisms.

Chemical defences against infection include hydrochloric acid in the stomach (gastric acid), which can have a pH as low as 1.5 (*see Chapter 7*). This destroys ingested microorganisms, which can be present in very high numbers in infected food. Lysozyme is an enzyme present in secreted fluid including breast milk, tears, saliva, sweat and mucus, and breaks down peptidoglycan, a component of bacterial cell walls, to cause osmotic lysis of bacterial cells. Lysozyme is also contained within some immune cells where it acts to protect against infection from within the body as well as at the surfaces.

Epithelial cells and immune cells produce a variety of host defence peptides such as defensins and cathelicidins, which interact with microorganisms to damage their cell wall or interfere with their metabolism, reducing their potential to cause infection. Host defence proteins can be found in secreted fluids and are also involved in modulating the responses of immune cells to infection.

Mechanical defences include any mechanism that removes microorganisms from the body. For example, coughing and sneezing expels mucus containing foreign materials (potentially microorganisms) that have irritated the mucosal surfaces of the respiratory tract into the environment. Vomiting forcefully expels gastric contents from the stomach, and can be stimulated as a response to bacterial toxins present in ingested food. Similarly, diarrhoea expels faeces out of the body. While diarrhoea might be provoked by an infection in the gut, and usefully helps to distribute a microorganism into the environment, it also reduces the load of microorganisms within the gut and can be regarded as a protective mechanism. It is important that the bladder is emptied or voided regularly. Urine is a warm, normally sterile fluid, with a composition suitable for microbial metabolism. Irregular and incomplete voiding of the bladder are associated with an increased risk of a urinary tract infection. Urinary catheterization to empty the bladder also increases the risk of infection (see *Box 11.1*).

> **BOX 11.1**
>
> **Minimizing healthcare-acquired infection (HAI)**
>
> Patients often undergo clinical interventions that require breaching the physical barriers, for example:
>
> - surgery may pierce the skin
> - artificial ventilation requires insertion of tubes into the respiratory tract, bypassing the normal protective respiratory epithelium
> - administration of intravenous fluids and drugs opens a pathway from the environment directly into the blood
> - urinary tract catheterization disturbs the fragile mucous membrane of the urethra, also providing a pathway into the urogenital tract that microorganisms can migrate into.
>
> Penetration of the physical defences can compromise immunity to increase HAIs. These HAIs can be dangerous for patients and exert a significant drain on health services; minimizing HAIs is an important target, closely monitored by regulatory agencies. *Figure 11.4* illustrates the common causes of HAIs; note the majority of HAIs are respiratory, urinary or surgical site infections and that approximately half of infections are sited at the mucosal surfaces of the respiratory, gastrointestinal and urogenital systems. These are very thin with easy access to body fluids and are easily damaged by clinical procedures or pathogens.
>
> Pie chart: primary bloodstream, 6.8%; skin and soft tissue, 10.5%; surgical site, 13.8%; urinary tract, 19.7%; other, 3%; respiratory, 20%; gastrointestinal system, 22%.
>
> **Figure 11.4 –** **The top sites for healthcare-acquired infection in England, surveyed by the Health Protection Agency (2012).**

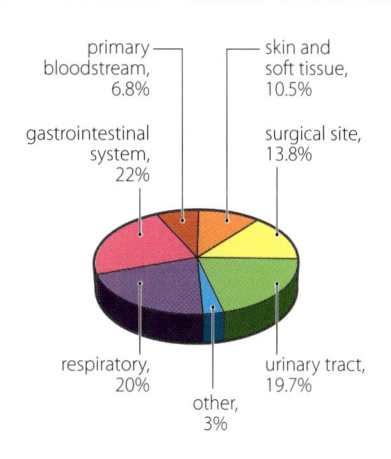

Normal flora is the term given to the organisms that normally reside on the body surfaces or within body cavities. Under normal conditions, these organisms are not pathogens. They occupy an ecological niche, in that their presence excludes pathogenic organisms. It is only when the population of normal flora is disturbed that pathogens are able to proliferate and cause disease. A good example of this is when the normal flora are killed by antibiotic therapy, allowing pathogenic organisms to proliferate (see Albert (Patient 11.1) and further discussion in *Box 11.4*).

The term normal flora is beginning to be replaced by the term **human microbiome** in recognition of the fact that these microorganisms are important beyond simply excluding pathogens. Within the gut, the normal flora assist with the digestion of non-starch polysaccharides and the provision of some vitamins such as vitamin K for blood clotting (see *Chapter 9*). They are also involved in the regulation of the enterohepatic circulation of bile acids (see *Chapter 7*). It is now recognized that microorganisms present on the skin, and on mucous membranes such as the gastrointestinal tract, also prime specific populations of immune cells in the body to proliferate and to secrete signalling proteins. The populations of microorganisms we are exposed to early in life are therefore involved in establishing the character of immune responses that individual people make when they encounter infectious organisms later in life. This has major implications for our susceptibility and resistance to infectious disease throughout our lives, and probably has an influence on other physiological systems, affecting the development of chronic diseases. The *potential* of microorganisms to influence health positively has reached public consciousness, and today the food industry provides a plethora of carefully marketed 'probiotic' foods in supermarkets for consumers. Following the initiative of the Human Genome Project (discussed in *Chapter 3*), the Human Microbiome Project is currently underway and aims to characterize the genomes of all communities of microorganisms that colonize sites of the body, so that we may understand more fully their role in health and disease.

Protection and maintenance of the physical defences is one of the most important factors to be considered within a healthcare environment, as disease and clinical interventions for diagnostic or therapeutic purposes often compromise these defences; some examples of this are provided in *Box 11.1*. The concept of the *chain of infection* (see *Box 11.2*) explains how to minimize the risk of infection.

> **BOX 11.2**
>
> **The chain of infection**
>
> Breaking the cycle or *chain of infection* is important for minimizing the risk of HAIs (see *Figure 11.5*).
>
> The six elements of the chain are:
>
> - **infectious agent**: any disease-causing pathogen
> - **reservoir**: the site where a pathogen resides and replicates; this could be water, food, a damp towel, animals, faeces, urine, pus, blood or vomit
> - **portal of exit**: the site where the transfer of the pathogen from the reservoir occurs, for example, the mouth, anus or a cut to the skin
> - **mode of transmission**: the mechanism of transfer the pathogen uses to leave the reservoir to the new host, such as:
>   - via a vector (parasite or sexual contact)
>   - direct contact with an infected person
>   - indirectly via contaminated surfaces, touch by an infected person or spread on unwashed hands
>   - aerosols (tiny fluid droplets from an infected person produced during coughing or sneezing; aerosols can be inhaled or can contaminate surfaces
>   - consumption of contaminated food/water or transferring pathogens from the hands into the mouth
>   - transfer of contaminated blood products from one person to another, accidentally or during therapy
> - **portal of entry**: the site where organisms enter the body; for example, the lungs when breathing, ingestion of food, breaks in the skin or mucous membranes caused by trauma or clinical procedures such as surgery, catheterization or cannulation
> - **susceptible host**: a patient may become exposed to pathogens when they are ill or their immune system is less effective; for example, poor nutritional status and therapy such as radiotherapy and chemotherapy (which destroys proliferating cells, including immune cells) can make the host susceptible; the very young and elderly are particularly vulnerable hosts.
>
> **Figure 11.5 – The chain of infection.**
> The chain of infection has six links. Each link represents an opportunity to break the link and interrupt the spread of infection.

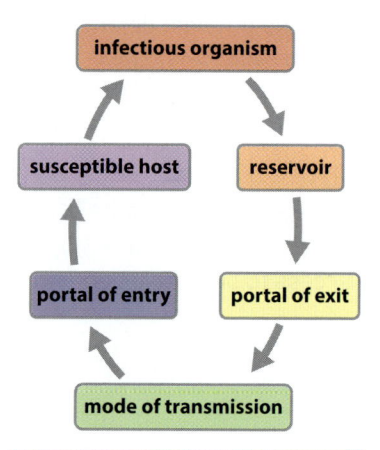

11.2.3 Recognition of microorganisms by innate immunity

Pathogens sometimes penetrate our physical barriers, gain entry to body fluids and proliferate to cause infection. Damage to physical barriers can occur in the following ways:

- physical damage – trauma such as accidental laceration to the skin or deliberate penetration during a medical procedure
- chemical damage – for example by acids or alkalis
- heat – burns (cold and thermal)
- radiation – via X-rays, ionizing radiation and ultraviolet light (sunlight)
- infection – some microorganisms secrete toxins and enzymes that lyse tissue.

In order to understand the cellular responses of innate immune cells to eliminate infectious microorganisms, it is necessary to consider how immune cells recognize them. A variety of molecules possessed by pathogens are recognized by elements of innate immunity when they enter the body; these are collectively called **pathogen-associated molecule patterns** (PAMPs). Innate immune cells possess **pathogen recognition receptors** (PRRs), which bind to a limited number of PAMPS that are common to a variety of microorganisms but *not present in humans*. An important variant of PRRs is the **toll-like receptor (TLR)**, which binds to PAMPs; binding of TLRs to one type of these PAMPS, such as **lipopolysaccharide**, a component of the cell wall of Gram-negative bacteria, acts as a signal to initiate a variety of *immediate* immune responses characterized by **acute inflammation** (discussed later in this chapter).

In this manner, the PRRs of innate immunity provide a non-specific mechanism to recognize 'non-self' molecules from the wide variety of microorganisms that could infect the body.

11.2.4 Innate immunity – cellular defences

Leukocytes (white blood cells) form all of the cells of both innate and adaptive immunity. They all originate from the haemopoietic stem cells within the bone marrow (see *Chapter 9*), which also provides erythrocytes and platelets. When bone marrow stem cells divide, they become committed to developing into cells that will eventually differentiate into cells of different lineages, descended from an original stem cell (see *Figure 11.6*). Two main lineages form leukocytes; the **myeloid** cell lineage provides innate immune cells, while adaptive immune cells are from the **lymphoid** cell lineage (discussed later in the chapter). A group of low-molecular-weight proteins called haematopoietic growth factors and haematopoietic cytokines regulate bone marrow stem cell differentiation to provide the correct balance of leukocytes required. Leukocyte production is very dynamic and can be rapidly increased by activated immune cells and other cells that release the cytokines in response to infection. Indeed, it has been estimated that 10^9 cells/kg of body weight of the type neutrophils (the most abundant leukocyte in blood) leave the bone marrow each day and enter the blood circulation. Alterations in the number and type of cells in blood can

348 CHAPTER 11 | PROTECTION FROM HARM

bone marrow

red bone marrow — multipotent stem cell (haemocytoblast)

mostly in blood

red blood cells (erythrocytes) — O_2 and CO_2 transport

white blood cells (leukocytes)

granulocytes

- eosinophils (1–6%) — destroy parasites
- neutrophils (40–75%) — active phagocytes
- basophils (0.5–1.0%)

(% = percentage of total white blood cell count)

- monocytes (3–8%)
- dendritic cells
- large granular lymphocytes (5–16%) — destroy virus infected and tumour cells
- small lymphocytes (20–45%)

platelets (thrombocytes) — blood clotting

mainly in tissues

- mast cells — produce inflammatory chemicals e.g. histamine
- macrophages — active phagocytes, antigen presentation
- Langerhans cells — antigen-presenting cells
- B lymphocytes — produce antibodies
- T lymphocytes — produce cytokines and destroy virus infected cells

NON-SPECIFIC (INNATE) IMMUNITY | SPECIFIC (ACQUIRED) IMMUNITY

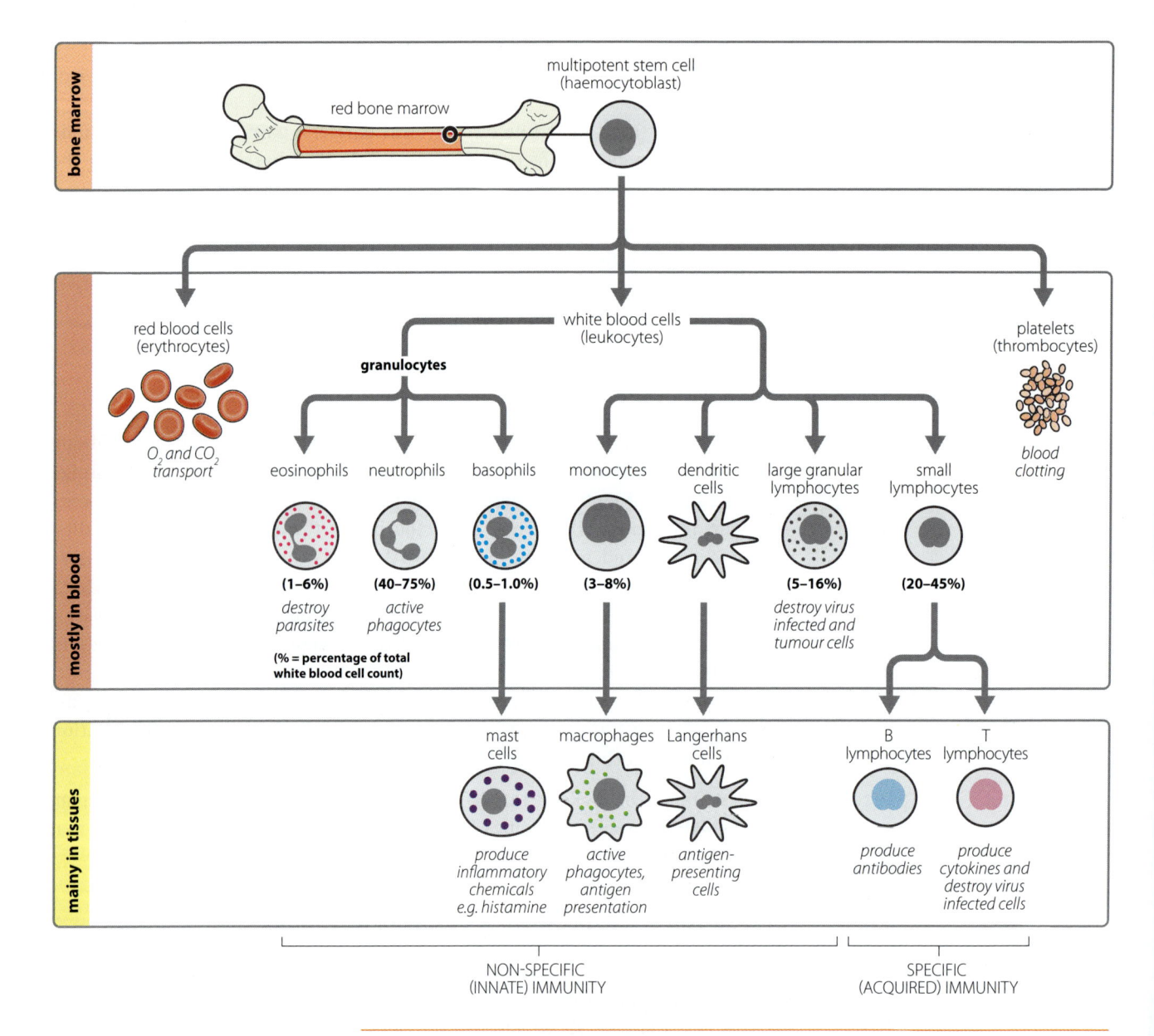

Figure 11.6 – Haematopoiesis (the formation of blood cellular components). Haematopoiesis starts with multipotential stem cells within the bone marrow. These cells provide a variety of progenitor cells which gradually differentiate to form a variety of mature cells. Differentiation is regulated by a complex network of cytokines, growth factors and hormones.

be very useful, and a blood test to determine the *full blood count* is one of the most common clinical investigations performed; typical values of leukocytes found in blood are listed in *Table 11.1*. However, blood values are affected by many factors such as age, gender, ethnicity and environmental factors including altitude and season. Reference ranges (usually in units of $\times 10^9$/L) differ between laboratories; therefore, the values quoted in *Table 11.1* should be considered as a guide only.

Table 11.1 – Normal values for leukocytes in blood (Caucasian adults)

Blood cell type	Normal range ($\times 10^9$/L)
Leukocytes	4.0–11.0
Neutrophils	2.5–7.5
Lymphocytes	1.5–3.5
Monocytes	0.2–0.8
Basophils	0.01–0.1
Eosinophils	0.04–0.4

Adapted from **Naushad, H., Marion, S. and Wheeler, T.M.** (2012) *Leukocyte count.* Medscape. Available at: http://emedicine.medscape.com/article/2054452-overview.

Myeloid cells

A fundamental function of innate immune cells is the destruction and removal, by the process of **phagocytosis** (discussed later in this chapter), of infectious organisms that have entered the body. The phagocytic cells are **neutrophils**, **macrophages** and **dendritic cells**.

Neutrophils are also called polymorphonuclear leukocytes (PMNLs) because, unusually, they possess a multi-lobed nucleus (see *Figure 11.7*). They are a type of **granulocyte** (a cell in which, when stained with a dye and viewed under a microscope, many granules can be seen filling the cytoplasm) and are the most numerous leukocyte found circulating in blood. They are also found in tissues and are able to leave the blood rapidly through tiny pores in blood vessel walls (facilitated by their multi-lobed nucleus) and migrate towards a site of infection to destroy microorganisms by phagocytosis. This involves releasing powerful antimicrobial compounds stored within preformed cytoplasmic granules onto microorganisms that have been transported into the neutrophil. The lifespan of neutrophils can be as short as a few hours during bouts of intense infection; as a result, the bone marrow can be expected to produce many billions of neutrophils per day when required.

Macrophages are also phagocytic cells that live much longer than neutrophils, and they are the largest leukocyte, with a characteristic horseshoe-shaped nucleus. Precursor cells in the bone marrow differentiate into **monocytes**, which circulate in the blood. These enter tissues, where they differentiate into macrophages. They provide a surveillance function, as they are able to respond quickly to tissue damage and infecting microorganisms. Macrophages kill other cells by phagocytosis and are also responsive to cells of the adaptive immune system, ensuring well-coordinated immune responses.

Dendritic cells develop from monocytes and are also found in tissues. When immature, they provide a phagocytic function, but when mature, they further differentiate and migrate into lymphatic tissue where their long branching cellular extensions, called dendrites, serve to trap and process non-self molecules. Dendritic cells also interact closely with multiple types of immune cells, providing a coordinating function to immunity, especially within the structures of the lymphatic system. Within the skin and mucosa, specialized dendritic cells called **Langerhans cells** interact with foreign molecules from microorganisms that are presented to them by other cells. It is likely that when microorganisms penetrate through body surfaces, the first immune cells they encounter will be Langerhans cells or macrophages resident in tissues; both macrophages and Langerhans cells also migrate to lymphatic tissue where they encounter cells of the adaptive immune system and activate a variety of responses to ensure quick and efficient clearance of microorganisms from the body.

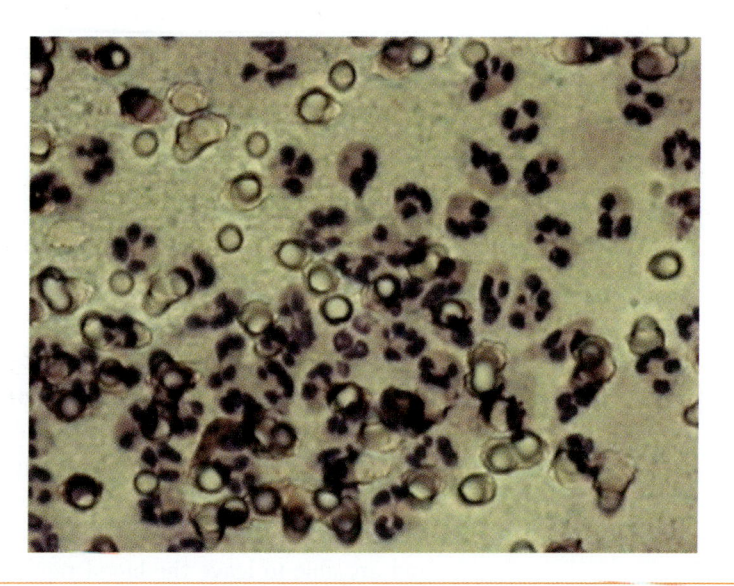

Figure 11.7 – **Neutrophils, also known as polymorphonuclear leukocytes.**
These short-lived cells have migrated through a porous membrane in response to a chemoattractant commonly found in bacteria. The multi-lobed nucleus is stained blue and the cytoplasm is stained pink. Original magnification ×400. Reproduced courtesy of Dr Jim Jolly, University of Leeds.

Basophils circulate in the blood and enter the tissues. They are stimulated by a variety of chemicals released during inflammatory processes when tissues become damaged. Like neutrophils, they are granulocytic cells, but only represent a small fraction of the total leukocytes found in blood. One important role of the basophil is to bind to a specific type of immune chemical called immunoglobulin E (IgE) (discussed later in this chapter). This immunoglobulin (a type of antibody, also described later in the chapter) causes basophils to *degranulate*, by releasing a variety of chemical mediators such as **cytokines**, and especially **histamine**, which stimulates tissue responses to infection and tissue damage.

Mast cells have a similar structure and function to basophils; however, they reside within tissues and are generally found close to blood vessels that are near to the surface of the skin and organs with a mucosal surface, such as the respiratory tract. Like basophils, they release a variety of chemical mediators including histamine and play a central part in inflammatory responses.

Eosinophils are found in relatively low numbers in the blood, but high numbers reside within tissues, especially the lymphatic system and along the gastrointestinal tract. Like basophils, they are granulocytic and degranulate when antibodies bind to them. However, eosinophils secrete a variety of powerful cytotoxic chemicals that are able to destroy organisms, especially those that are too large to be destroyed by phagocytosis, such as parasitic worms.

Together with basophils and mast cells, eosinophils are involved in generating inflammatory responses and have an important role in **allergy**. Excess histamine released from these cells is a common feature of allergies, and patients often benefit from taking *antihistamine* medications, which help to reduce inflammation, providing symptomatic relief.

Natural killer cells (NK cells) (also known as **large granular lymphocytes**) develop from lymphoid progenitor cells of the bone marrow. They are important for producing a rapid response to viral infection by eradicating cells infected with virus. When activated, NK cells release **perforins**, which are proteins that open pores within the plasma membrane, enabling other proteins such as **granzymes** to enter the cell and thus causing it to die by the process of **lysis**. NK cells provide a link between the innate and adaptive immune responses, ensuring an integrated response from both of the two main arms of the immune system. In addition, NK cells respond to a variety of cellular stresses as well as infection and are able to directly kill tumour cells; this has led to interest in their possible role against cancer.

11.2.5 Innate immunity – humoral defences

A diverse array of chemicals, known generically as chemical mediators, provide humoral immunity. They mediate between the activity of immune cells and tissues of the body in response to tissue damage or stress. They operate within a complex regulatory network within the fluid environment; many of them act as signalling compounds, while others assist with killing microorganisms. As there are too many to consider fully in this text, some important groups of chemical mediators will be selected for discussion in this chapter.

Eicosanoids are molecules synthesized from **arachidonic acid** released from phospholipids (see *Chapter 2*) by the action of phospholipase. The metabolism of arachidonic acid produces a wide variety of eicosanoids via three major metabolic pathways:

- cyclooxygenase – produces prostaglandins, thromboxanes and prostacyclin
- lipoxygenase – produces leukotrienes and lipoxins
- cytochrome P450 epoxygenase – producing epoxyeicosatrienoic acids.

Eicosanoids are very important in regulating cellular homeodynamics by autocrine and paracrine mechanisms (see *Chapter 5*). Synthesis of eicosanoids occurs very rapidly in most tissues as a response to specific stimuli such as cytokines or tissue damage, and their half-life is very short, in the order of minutes. Eicosanoids are important mediators in inflammation, influencing blood clotting, vasoconstriction and vasodilation, bronchoconstriction and the attraction of leukocytes to sites of tissue injury. They are also involved with the development of pain and fever. Non-steroidal anti-inflammatory drugs (NSAIDs) inhibit cyclooxygenase activity and the production of prostaglandins, reducing the inflammation, pain and fever.

Prostaglandins are produced by most tissues and their functions include vasodilation or vasoconstriction and control of platelet activation. They also stimulate inflammation and cell growth. **NSAIDs inhibit** cyclooxygenase enzymes, reducing **inflammation and pain.** Prostaglandins are converted to prostacyclins and thromboxanes. **Thromboxanes** are produced mostly by blood vessel smooth muscles, endothelium and platelets, promoting the formation of blood clotting. They are potent vasoconstrictors and bronchoconstrictors, whereas **prostacyclin** is a vasodilator and reduces aggregation of platelets.

Leukotrienes cause bronchoconstriction and vasoconstriction, and attract leukocytes. **Lipoxins** also attract leukocytes and stimulate free-radical production by neutrophils.

Epoxyeicosatrienoic acids stimulate proliferation of endothelial cells and have an anti-inflammatory effect.

Lysozyme is secreted principally by macrophages and is also found within excreted body fluids, supporting the physical defences described earlier in this chapter. It acts by splitting the peptidoglycan layer of the cell wall, mainly on Gram-positive bacteria, causing osmotic lysis of the bacterium. Many strains of bacteria have developed a resistant coating covering the peptidoglycan and so are resistant to the action of lysozyme; other immune mechanisms such as acute-phase proteins exist to deal with these.

Acute-phase proteins support innate immunity by limiting tissue damage caused by infection and inflammation. They are produced mainly by the liver in response to cytokines released from leukocytes and include: C-reactive protein (CRP), complement proteins, serum amyloid A (SAA), mannose-binding protein, metal-binding proteins, fibrinogen and protease inhibitors. Normally present in small amounts, the levels of acute-phase proteins in the blood increase rapidly by as much as 1000-fold during an infection. Detection of the level of CRP in blood is used clinically to monitor the progression or clearance of an infection and also to indicate the prognosis for a variety of disease states, such as cardiovascular disease, cancer and liver diseases. A group of acute-phase proteins, usefully illustrating the importance of humoral innate immunity, is the complement system.

Complement is a group of many plasma proteins, produced by liver cells, that are normally inactive until binding to the surface of a microorganism causes a cascade of enzyme-mediated events via one of three major pathways. These pathways are known as the *classical* (activated by antibodies), the *lectin* (activated by lectins – sugar-binding proteins on the cell wall of microorganisms) and the *alternative* (activated by a variety of factors including bacterial endotoxins, the cell walls of microorgansims and immune complexes) pathways (see *Figure 11.8*). These three pathways converge to form an enzyme complex called C3 convertase, which can activate a cascade of more C3 convertase to initiate and amplify a number of immune responses including:

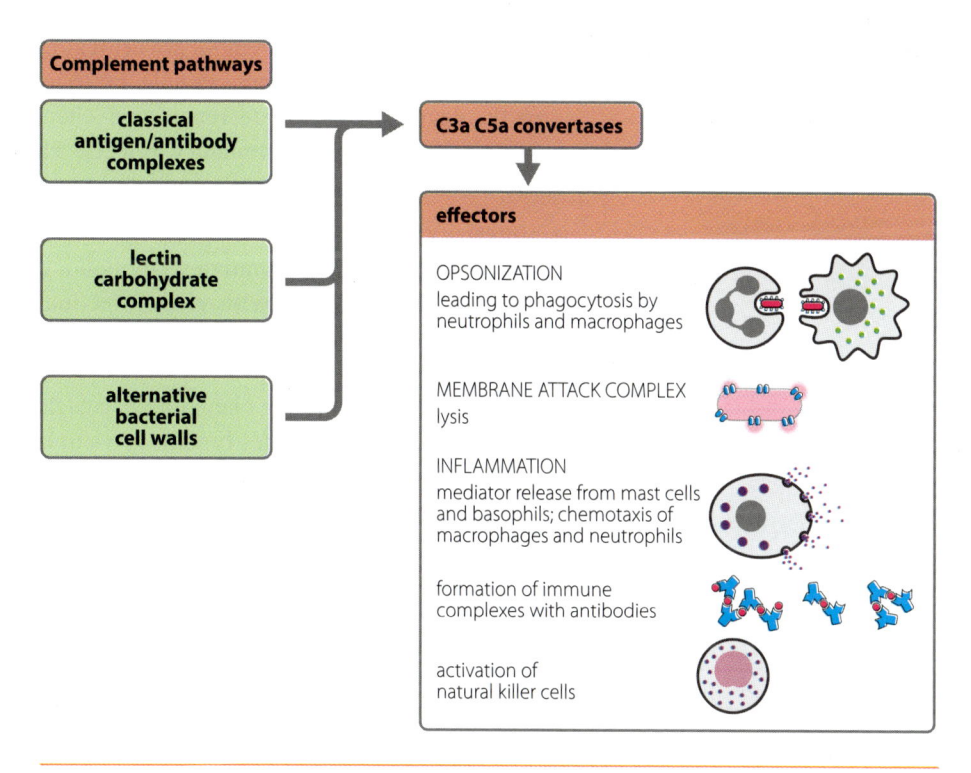

Figure 11.8 – The complement pathway (grossly simplified).
A series of proteins in plasma, when activated, converge on activated C3, via three main pathways, which together with activation of other components of the pathways provide a variety of effects to support immunity.

- initiation of acute inflammation
- attraction of neutrophils towards the microorganisms (**chemotaxis**)
- increased attachment of microorganisms to immune cells for stimulation of phagocytosis (opsonization)
- killing microorganisms by formation of a **membrane attack complex**, which causes cells to burst due to the effects of osmosis (known as lysis)
- activation and enhancement of adaptive immune cell activities.

Activation of complement is likely to be the first humoral element of innate immunity encountered by a microorganism as it enters through epithelial barriers and into body fluids. It is therefore an important initiating component of innate immunity; it also has significant potential for causing damage to normal body tissue. In addition, complement exerts effects on organ systems, and deregulation of the complement system is implicated in many diseases involving immunity, such as glomerulonephritis, systemic lupus erythematosus, multiple sclerosis and Alzheimer's disease.

Cytokines are small protein molecules secreted by cells in response to a stimulus. Their effect can be on the cell that produced them (**autocrine**) or on a cell fairly close to their site of production (**paracrine**) (see *Chapter 5*). They are only available for short periods of time (short half-life) and generally do not circulate in the plasma. Coordination of the activities of immune cells and cells of the tissues requires a complex network of cells that are able to respond to each other's signals.

Cytokines and cytokine receptors are critical to cell signalling, especially but not exclusively in immunity. For example, cytokines are involved in haematopoiesis, growth, development, tissue repair and chemotaxis, and are often classed as having *pro-* or *anti*-inflammatory effects. There are many cytokines, far too many to name here; they are organized into a variety of groups including:

- **interleukins** – signal leukocytes, e.g. interleukin-1 (IL-1) released from macrophages, which stimulates T-lymphocytes
- **interferons** – interfere with virus infection, e.g. interferons stimulate nearby uninfected cells to resist infection and activate immune cells such as macrophages
- **chemokines** – stimulate chemotaxis, e.g. the chemokine CCL19, expressed in lymph nodes, promotes lymphocytes to move towards lymph nodes
- **factors** – growth factors, colony-stimulating factors, tumour necrosis factor, and many others.

Cytokines can also be grouped by the type of cell that produces them; for example, lymphokines are produced by lymphocytes and monokines by monocytes.

Cytokines have multiple functions depending on which cell they influence. Generally, they alter gene expression of target cells, resulting in the desired effect. In terms of the immune system, this can include proliferation, adhesion, differentiation, apoptosis, modulation of inflammation or the production of cytotoxic chemicals.

Interferons are a class of pro-inflammatory cytokine produced by many types of cell in response to the presence of viruses and other microorganisms. They induce gene expression in cells, increasing resistance especially against virus infection. In virus-infected cells, they inhibit protein synthesis and so limit the formation of new virus particles, and increase the activity of NK cells, macrophages and T-lymphocytes (T-lymphocytes will be discussed later in this chapter), providing an early response to limit infection while other elements of immunity become activated. The ability of interferons to promote apoptosis in infected cells and to modulate immune responses has led to the therapeutic use of these compounds for the treatment of autoimmune diseases such as multiple sclerosis and as an adjuvant alongside chemotherapy and radiotherapy for cancer.

Cytotoxic factors in innate immunity

Phagocytosis is the main method employed by innate immunity to eradicate microorganisms when they succeed in penetrating epithelial barriers. The process, illustrated in *Figure 11.9a*, begins with binding of a phagocyte (primarily a macrophage or neutrophil) to a PAMP on the cell wall of a microorganism. The process is enhanced by a variety of molecules termed **opsonins** that serve to increase phagocyte binding and trigger phagocytosis, and include complement proteins and antibodies that also fix on to microorganisms.

Binding of a microorganism to a phagocyte triggers extensive cytoskeletal reorganization of the phagocyte, so that it is able to cause its plasma membrane to surround the organism and internalize it into the phagocyte (see *Figure 11.9a*). The organism, now enclosed within a membrane-bound compartment called a **phagosome**, is isolated from the rest of the body. The phagocyte then

(a)

1. microbe adheres to phagocyte
2. phagocyte forms pseudopods that engulf the microbe
3. phagocytic vesicle containing microbe (phagosome)
4. phagosome fuses with lysosome to form phagolysosome
5. microbe is killed and digested by lysosomal activity
6. residual material is expelled by exocytosis

(b)

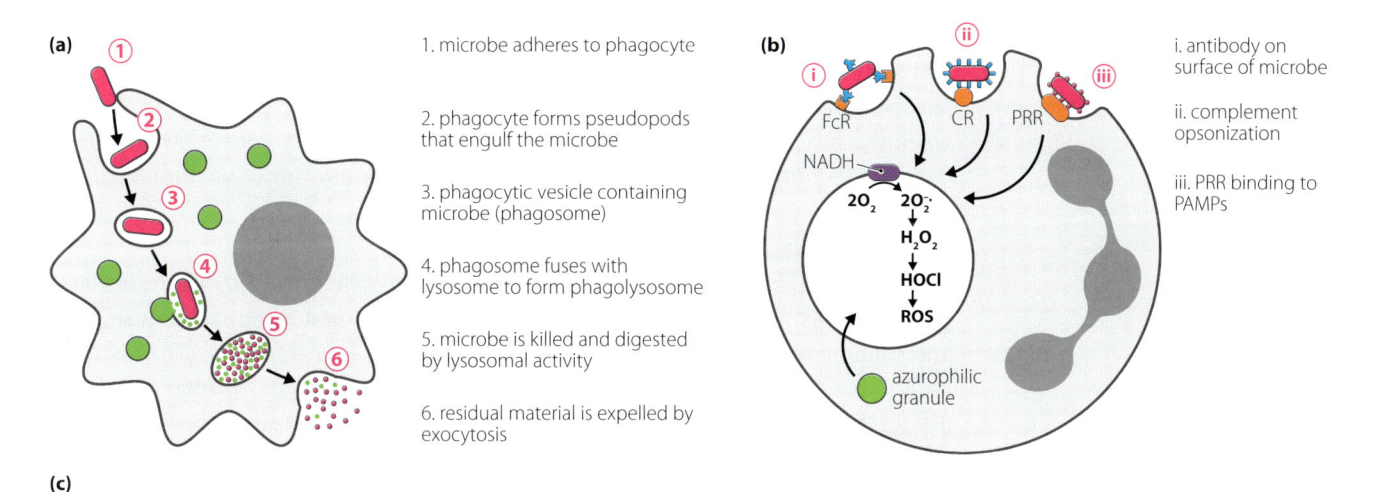

i. antibody on surface of microbe
ii. complement opsonization
iii. PRR binding to PAMPs

(c)

examples of some important reactive oxygen and nitrogen species (ROS/RNS)	
$O_2 + e^-$ ⟶	$O_2^-\bullet$ (superoxide)
$O_2^-\bullet + 2H^+ + e^-$ ⟶	H_2O_2 (hydrogen peroxide)
$H_2O_2 + e^-$ ⟶	$OH^- + OH\bullet$ (hydroxyl radical)
enzymatic conversion of L-arginine by nitric oxide synthase ⟶	$NO\bullet$ (nitric oxide)
$NO\bullet + O_2^-\bullet$ ⟶	$ONOO^-$ (peroxynitrite)

$\bullet$ = free radical e^- = electron

Figure 11.9 – Phagocytosis.
(a) Phagocytosis involves microbial attachment to a phagocyte, followed by internalization and destruction. (b) Antibody complexes and complement proteins opsonize microorganisms for phagocytosis and pathogen recognition receptors (PRRs) on phagocytes attach to microorganisms directly, causing the release of pre-stored granules into a phagolysosome, with the release of enzymes and generation of free radicals, which destroy internalized microorganisms. (c) Some important reactive oxygen and nitrogen species.

releases a number of granules or lysosomes into the phagosome (discussed in *Chapter 2*) to form a **phagolysosome**, where the killing of the microorganism occurs. Degranulation of proteases and hydrolytic enzymes along with other chemicals, such as **elastase** and **cathepsin**, into the phagolysosome begins destruction of the microorganism. Another group of important enzymes involved in killing microorganisms includes **myeloperoxidase** and **nicotinamide adenine dinucleotide phosphate (NADPH) oxidase**; these create large amounts of **free radicals**, such as superoxide, hydrogen peroxide and the hydroxyl radical, in what is termed the **oxidative or respiratory burst** (see *Figure 11.9b*). These free radicals (see *Figure 11.9c*) are highly toxic to microorganisms and also to phagocytes and even body tissue. Neutrophils are very short-lived cells that die soon after phagocytosis. A large proportion of pus, which is a sign of infection, is composed of dead leukocytes, especially neutrophils.

Cytotoxic factors exist in a wide variety of forms to support innate immunity. They include a broad group of host defence peptides and proteins, such as defensins and cathelidicins, polypeptides such as small alarm antiproteases, bacterial permeability factors, granzymes and perforin, lactoferrin, lysozyme and enzymes from granulocytes including elastase and cathepsin, and secretory phospholipase A2. It should be borne in mind that each of the cytotoxic factors not only acts to destroy microorganisms but also works in concert with innate and adaptive immunity, exerting an immune-modulatory role to varying degrees.

Free radicals

A free radical can be defined as '*any substance capable of independent existence that contains an unpaired electron*' (free radicals and their relationship to antioxidant chemistry is discussed in *Chapter 7*). Free radicals are unstable, highly reactive compounds involving oxides of oxygen or nitrogen and are often referred to as reactive oxygen or reactive nitrogen species (ROS/RNS). Free radicals are a *normal* product of cellular metabolism and at low levels have a beneficial role in physiology; for example, nitric oxide, a free radical, is also an important signalling molecule involved in regulating vascular tone, causing the smooth muscle surrounding blood vessels to relax. When free radicals are produced by immune cells at high concentrations, they can be sufficiently toxic to kill microorganisms and even body cells. A concentration of free radicals sufficient to harm tissue is described as **oxidative** or **nitrosative stress**. A variety of antioxidant defences exist to protect the body from oxidative stress and limit the damaging effects of high concentrations of ROS/RNS.

The enzyme NADPH-dependent oxidase is located on the plasma membrane of neutrophils. When stimulated by an opsonin or binding of a microorganism to a PRR to form a phagosome, NADPH is activated and transfers electrons onto oxygen to produce large amounts of the free radical superoxide into the phagosome (see *Figure 11.9b* and *c*). Another enzyme, myeloperoxidase, within cytoplasmic granules, which is also released into the phagosome, breaks down superoxide to form a mixture of free radicals including hydrogen peroxide, hypochlorous acid, the hydroxyl radical and singlet oxygen. Moreover, within neutrophilic granules are a variety of proteases, acid hydrolases and metalloproteinases that are released into the phagosome; it is this mixture of reactive compounds that provides the microbiocidal capacity of neutrophils.

11.2.6 Acute inflammation

Acute inflammation is a rapid coordinated response to tissue damage caused by trauma or infection, involving a stimulus such as recognition of PAMPs, activation of immune responses, resolution of inflammatory responses and healing of damaged tissue. These processes are overlapping and require careful regulation in order to avoid unnecessary effects on tissues; if these processes persist over a long time (months or even years), they create chronic inflammation, which is abnormal and causes chronic inflammatory disease states.

There are four recognized *cardinal* signs of inflammation; these are:

- heat
- erythema (redness)
- oedema (swelling)
- pain.

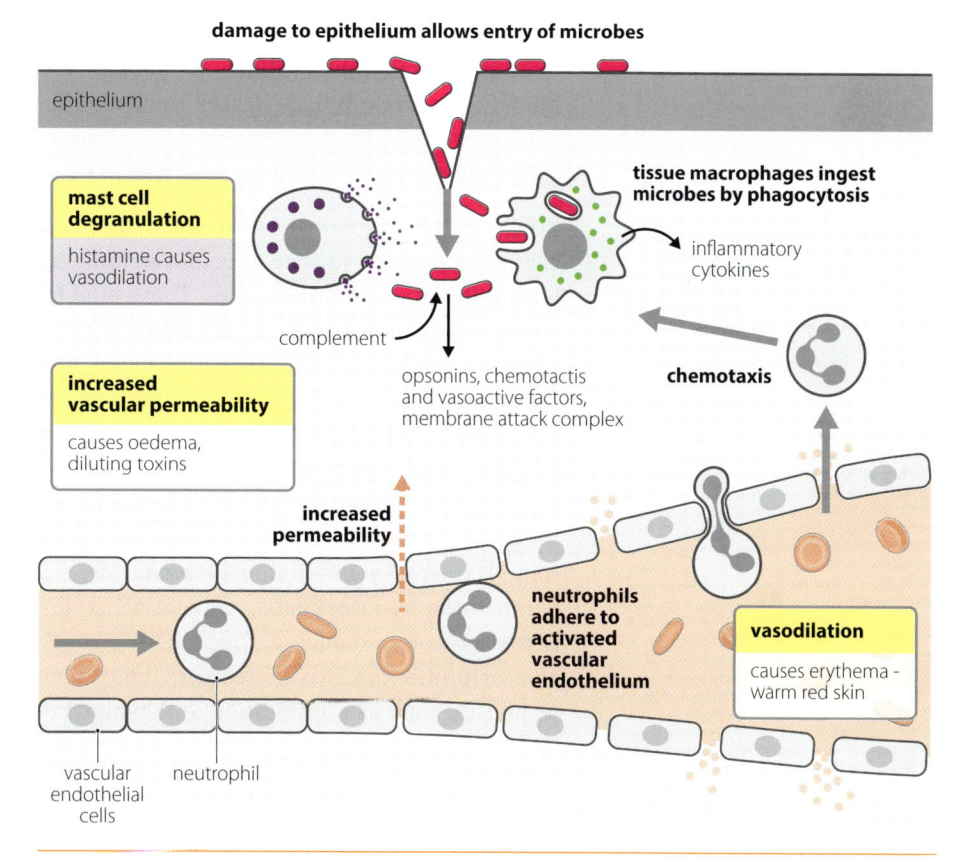

SECTION 11.2 | WHAT YOU NEED TO KNOW – ESSENTIAL ANATOMY AND PHYSIOLOGY

Figure 11.10 – **A breach in physical defences causing tissue damage stimulates a raft of primarily innate immune responses, resulting in acute inflammation.**

Sometimes a fifth sign is evident, that of loss of function.

How these symptoms arise is illustrated in *Figure 11.10*.

Physical damage to blood vessels causes bleeding, which often initiates two responses: a reflex contraction of blood vessels and clotting of blood, both of which are aimed at reducing fluid loss from the body. Damaged tissue releases **damage-associated molecular patterns** (DAMPs), which are detected by PRRs such as TLRs present on the surface of leukocytes and a variety of tissue cells. This triggers the secretion of a plethora of inflammatory mediators including cytokines and lipid mediators, which act as chemical messengers to trigger pro-inflammatory responses. These chemical mediators operate within complex signalling networks and exert effects on cells by autocrine, paracrine and/or endocrine mechanisms (see *Chapter 5*). For example, they might increase the rate of proliferation of cells, select cells to undergo differentiation and stimulate cells to migrate or produce additional cytokines.

Within tissues and in all vascular tissue are mast cells, which release a variety of pro-inflammatory chemical mediators, such as histamine. Histamine has a number of physiological roles; it acts as a receptor for regulating gastric acid secretion and airway muscle tone, and also functions as a neurotransmitter, but it is also very important in immunity and inflammatory processes. Within tissues, histamine, released primarily from mast cells, is a potent vasodilator, and it increases vascular permeability so that fluid can leak out of the circulation into the interstitial spaces. When released suddenly in large amounts, histamine can cause widespread vasodilation leading to a profound fall in blood pressure, a condition called **anaphylactic shock** (a type of hypersensitivity or allergic reaction).

When tissues are damaged, an important response is to activate phospholipase enzymes, which initiate the formation of lipid-based molecules such as prostaglandins and leukotrienes. These bind to vascular endothelial cells to cause vasodilation, increase the permeability of blood vessels and cause them to express adhesion molecules. The increased blood flow and the increased movement of fluid out of the blood vessels into the interstitial spaces cause the signs of *heat*, *erythema* and *oedema* (three of the cardinal signs of inflammation). Prostaglandins stimulate **nociceptors**, producing the sensation of pain (the fourth cardinal sign of inflammation). More fluid within the tissues and a greater blood flow also increase the pressure of fluid acting on nociceptors. Prostaglandins, some cytokines and some PAMPS, such as lipopolysaccharide, raise the temperature-regulating set point in the hypothalamus, causing a rise in core temperature and fever. Fever is useful, as by producing a high body temperature infecting organisms are less able to proliferate. An increase in body temperature also increases leukocyte responses, such as proliferation and phagocytosis.

These physiological effects are important aspects in acute inflammatory processes, allowing the rapid ingress of leukocytes into the site of tissue damage or infection, bringing nutrients to the area of damage and diluting toxins. Leukocytes flowing along the veins are interrupted by adhesion molecules secreted by endothelial cells in response to chemical mediators entering the circulation. Leukocytes, especially neutrophils, respond by secreting their own adhesion molecules and begin to attach to blood vessel walls. The attachment is initially weak, causing them to roll slowly along the blood vessel wall, until they are able to adhere sufficiently to stop and then migrate through spaces between endothelial cells lining the blood vessels and into the tissues. This process is known as leukocyte extravasation or **diapedesis**. The direction that leukocytes take as they migrate through tissues is determined by the chemicals (cytokines and PAMPs) produced at the site of tissue damage or infection. As the chemicals become dispersed through tissues, a concentration gradient is produced. Leukocytes detect this gradient and are able to orientate and travel towards the source of tissue damage or infection, following the concentration gradient, a process known as chemotaxis.

Acute inflammatory reactions are characterized by an influx of predominantly neutrophils followed by monocytes, this being determined by the pattern of inflammatory mediators released. Macrophages resident in tissues also converge on the site of tissue damage or infection to phagocytose particles of dead cells or microorganisms. The process is enhanced by antibodies, acute-phase proteins and complement proteins present within the fluid exudate, which enhance phagocytosis by opsonization.

When inflammatory responses have destroyed microorganisms and the levels of PAMPs and DAMPs fall, the stimulus for PRRs to drive leukocyte activity is reduced, and inflammation will begin to resolve. Excess neutrophils within the tissues undergo apoptosis and are phagocytosed by macrophages. Mechanisms to suppress inflammation also exist: cytokines bind to soluble receptors that limit cytokine and lipid mediator activity, and macrophages produce fewer pro-inflammatory cytokines and instead secrete transforming growth factor-beta (TGF-β), which inhibits TLR signalling in leukocytes.

Macrophages also stimulate wound healing processes by secreting *fibroblast growth factor* (FGF), *platelet-derived growth factor* (PDGF) and *insulin-like growth factor* (IGF). These growth factors help with the process of granulation and angiogenesis (see discussion of wound healing in *Chapter 12*). A variety of other cell types are involved in inflammatory processes, such as dendritic cells and lymphocytes, requiring coordinated activation and suppression via complex signalling networks. If microorganisms persist, the acute inflammatory response adapts by becoming dominated by an increased number of activated macrophages and recruitment of T-lymphocytes, leading to an abnormal state of chronic inflammation.

11.2.7 Adaptive immunity

The three key features that characterize adaptive immunity are *specificity*, *diversity* and *memory*. In contrast to innate immunity, which responds to a broad range of PAMPs, elements of adaptive immunity are able to respond to an incredibly diverse range of highly specific molecules called **antigens**. An *initial* encounter by cells of the adaptive immune system with a specific antigen prepares adaptive immunity to respond *more rapidly* to future encounters with the same antigen, even some years later. Thus, this arm of the immune system is *specific* and *adaptive*, developing and maturing over the lifespan in response to exposure to an antigen. The key features of adaptive immunity identified here are exploited in the practice of immunization, which makes an individual resistant to specific infections. Immunization is undoubtedly one of the most important public health interventions developed to improve human health and will be discussed later in this chapter.

Like innate immunity, adaptive immunity comprises cells and chemicals, but the cells are derived only from lymphoid precursor stem cells, which develop into **small lymphocytes**. The humoral component is represented by cytokines and a special group of glycoproteins unique to adaptive immunity, the **immunoglobulins**, which are also known as **antibodies**.

In order to understand adaptive immunity, the concept of **antigen** must be introduced. The term antigen was first used to refer to a substance that was able to generate the production of antibodies. Antigens are *usually* foreign to the host (the person exposed to the antigen) and are generally macromolecules (molecules comprising fats, carbohydrates, nucleic acids and proteins). The term antigen is now used to refer to *any substance* that is able to bind to antibody or to a **T-cell receptor**. Antigens are processed by all cells of the immune system, and some cells of the immune system such as dendritic cells, macrophages and B-lymphocytes are able to process antigens and present fragments of the antigen on their surface to T-lymphocytes in order to stimulate a coordinated response against the antigen. An immune cell that is able to process antigens so that fragments of the antigen are bound to its surface and are detectable by other immune cells is termed an **antigen-presenting cell** (APC).

Cells of adaptive immunity: small lymphocytes

There are two populations of small lymphocytes, **B-lymphocytes**, which mature in the bone marrow, and **T-lymphocytes** (see *Figure 11.6*), which travel from the bone marrow and mature in the thymus gland. These two populations of cells can be further grouped into subpopulations, depending on the molecules they express on their surface and their function. The major differences between B- and T-lymphocytes are that:

- B-lymphocytes produce antibodies and process *extracellular antigen* (extracellular infections); this is the *humoral* response
- T-lymphocytes process *intracellular antigen* (intracellular infections, especially viruses); this is the *cellular* response.

B-lymphocytes migrate from the bone marrow and reside within lymphoid tissue, such as the spleen, tonsils and Peyer's patches. B-lymphocytes bind antigen to a receptor on their plasma membrane called an immunoglobulin or antibody. Following binding, the B-lymphocyte processes the antigen and presents it on its surface together with an MHC II molecule (discussed later in this chapter). Some B-lymphocytes immediately respond by proliferating (T-lymphocyte independent), while others are influenced by a subset of T-lymphocytes called T-helper cells (T-lymphocyte dependent). T-helper cells recognize the processed antigen together with MHC II and stimulate the B-lymphocyte to proliferate (called clonal expansion – a clone is an *identical* copy) to form two populations of cells – plasma and memory cells (see *Figure 11.11*). **Plasma cells**, which produce and secrete large numbers of antibodies specific for the antigen, enter the body fluids, while **memory cells**, which produce antibodies on their surface that bind the specific antigen, do not secrete antibodies in large amounts and remain quiescent. Memory cells concentrate primarily within lymph nodes and when activated by antigen, they respond rapidly to produce antibodies. It is important to recognize that antibodies are produced in response to the binding of *only one specific antigen* and not any other antigen (illustrating the characteristic of *specificity*). The antibodies produced contain binding sites for the antigen and also a separate binding site for immune cells (see *Figure 11.12a* and *b*). There are approximately 10^{16} antibodies/ml in **serum**.

Plasma cells also *secrete* large numbers of antibodies into the body fluids, allowing free-floating antigens to be bound to free-floating antibodies to form clumps of antigen–antibody complexes.

The binding of antigens to antibodies has been likened to a neutralization reaction: by preventing microorganisms from adhering to body cells, they limit access to tissues and the potential for infection. Antibodies can also interfere with metabolic activity of the microorganism, and they can also bind viruses to prevent further infection of host tissue.

Multiple antigens and antibodies can be formed into *immune complexes* (see *Figure 11.8*), thus reducing the number of free antigens in the body. Furthermore, these immune complexes act as an opsonin to stimulate phagocytosis in particular, but also a variety of immune responses from the effector cells of the immune system.

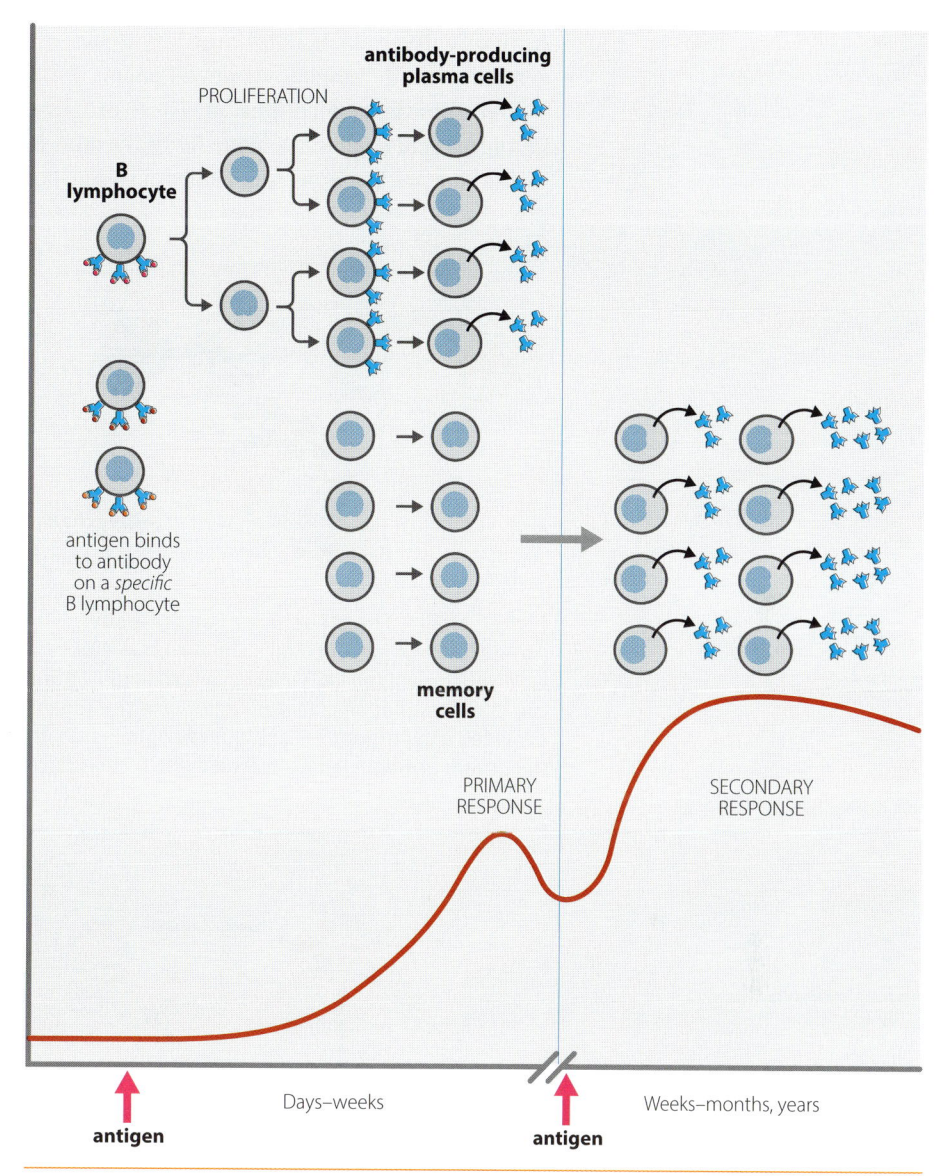

SECTION **11.2** | WHAT YOU NEED TO KNOW – ESSENTIAL ANATOMY AND PHYSIOLOGY 361

Figure 11.11 – **Clonal expansion of B-lymphocyte populations providing immunological memory.**
After the primary response, a later encounter with the same antigen elicits a rapid, sustained and greater secondary response.

The functions of antibodies can be summarized (see *Figure 11.13*) as:

- to clump antigens together to form an *immune complex* so that they can easily be phagocytosed
- to opsonize antigen to enhance phagocytosis
- to neutralize antigen, thus preventing infection or damage to host tissue
- to activate complement and inflammation
- to present antigen and stimulate cytotoxic cell responses against microorganisms containing the antigen.

Antibody diversity is determined by genetic mechanisms operating on antibody genes during B-lymphocyte development that include recombination (see *Chapter 3*) and **somatic hypermutation**. These processes generate many small differences in amino acid sequences made by individual B-lymphocytes. The consequence of this is that within a person, the pool of antibodies produced is diverse, estimated

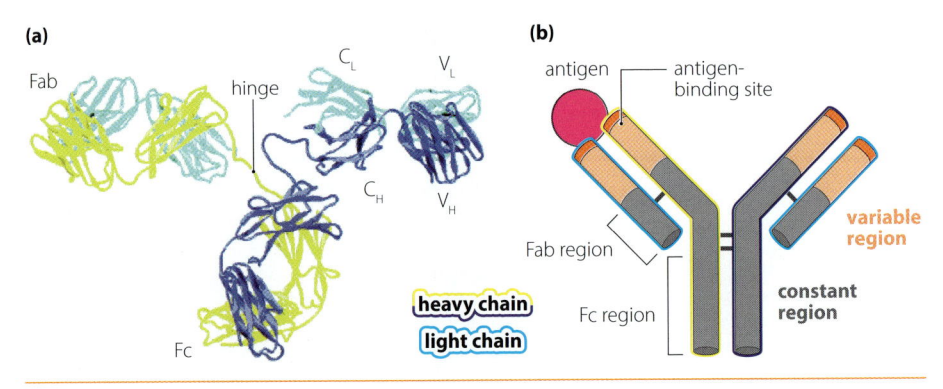

Figure 11.12 – **The structure of an antibody.**
Antibodies are glycoproteins. (a) A ribbon diagram of the first antibody (IgG) to be crystallized, based on X-ray crystallography, illustrating its Y-shape. (b) All antibodies are composed of an effector region (fragment crystallizable – Fc region), which provides attachment for cellular receptors and complement, and a recognition region (fragment antibody – Fab region), which recognizes specific antigen.

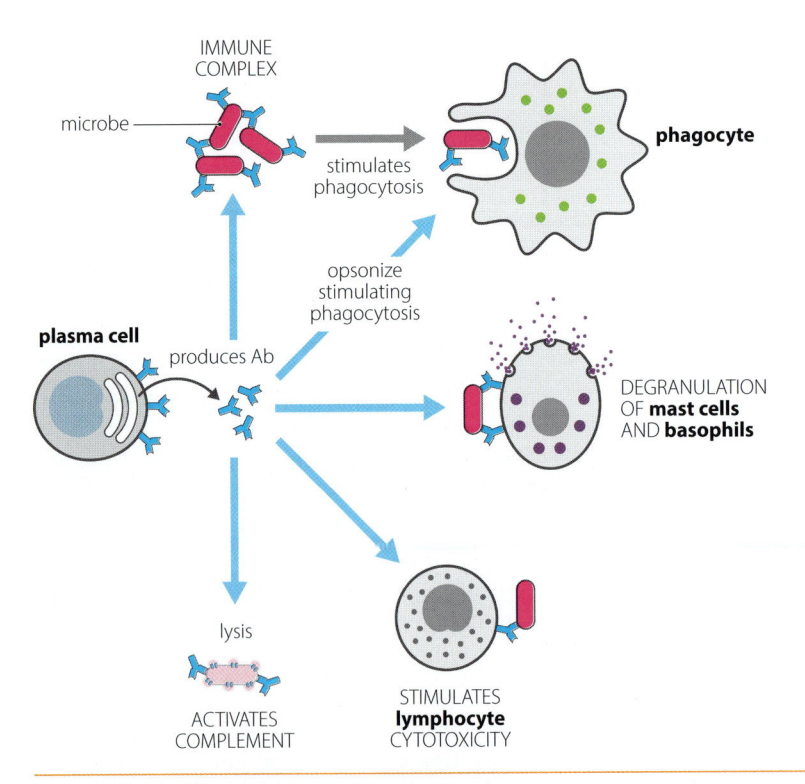

Figure 11.13 – **The functions of antibodies.**
Antibody directed against specific antigen functions to amplify immune responses and rapid clearance of antigens from the body; it also serves to integrate innate and adaptive immunity.

to be in the order of 10^8. As no two individuals will develop identical antibody repertoires, within the human population the capacity to bind to antigens is incredibly diverse. The diversity of antibodies a person is able to make defines to some extent their susceptibility or resistance to particular infections. Therefore, the maintenance of antibody diversity in the human population contributes to a survival advantage against pathogens.

Expansion of individual lymphocyte clones requires at least a few days from the initial stimulus to produce sufficient numbers of effector cells to elicit an evident effect. This is termed a **primary response** (see *Figure 11.11*). Subsequent exposure to the same antigen triggers a more rapid, greater and more persistent response than the initial encounter; this is known as the **secondary response**. The responses are entirely dependent on the specific antigen encountered by lymphocytes, so that exposure to an unrelated antigen from another microorganism will simply generate a new primary response.

The pattern of primary and secondary responses is a key feature of adaptive immunity, and the reasons for a delayed primary response are complex but include the following:

- Initial infection causes antigen to be processed by APCs such as dendritic cells, which migrate to lymph nodes to present the antigen to lymphocytes.
- Antigens often possess a variety of specific binding sites called **epitopes**; some epitopes are able to stimulate lymphocytes more or less strongly than others.
- Only a limited number of lymphocytes able to recognize a particular antigen are present initially; thus, a delay in response will be inevitable.
- An efficient response requires coordination with T-lymphocytes and a process of maturation of these within lymph nodes.

Antibody classes

The basic structure of antibodies (immunoglobulins) can be described as a Y-shape, consisting of four polypeptide chains. Two important receptor regions (see *Figure 11.12b*) within an antibody are the **fragment crystallizable** (Fc) and a variable region known as the **fragment antibody** (Fab). The Fc region has a conserved amino acid sequence in its structure, which varies only a little between antibodies and is attached to the B-lymphocyte at its surface, facing the Fab regions outward. When antibody is freely floating in body fluids, the Fc region acts as a point of interaction with leukocytes. The Fab regions have a *highly variable* amino acid sequence, which influences its structure and affinity for an antigen. There are two Fab regions within the basic antibody structure.

Five basic classes of antibody known as **isotypes** are observed in humans. These are IgG, IgM, IgA, IgD and IgE, and these differ by variations in the Fc portion, which has consequences for their overall structure and behaviour. Within these classes, antigen specificity remains unchanged, but the B-lymphocyte can change which isotype it produces. Initially, as a primary response to antigen, the first isotype produced is IgM, while in the secondary response the antibody produced is mostly IgG; isotype class structure and function are summarized in *Table 11.2*.

Table 11.2 – Immunoglobulin isotypes

Isotype		Function
	IgM	IgM is the first isotype produced in response to antigen and contains ten antigen-binding sites and has a serum half-life of 5 days. It is found predominantly in blood and tends to stay within the vascular space. It has a high avidity for antigens and is a very potent activator of complement. IgM can react with donated blood group antigens but cannot cross the placenta, so it also serves to protect the fetus from incompatibility between the mother and fetus.
	IgG	IgG is the main isotype produced in the secondary response and has two binding sites for antigen found in vascular and interstitial spaces. It is the most abundant isotype in blood and has a half-life of 23 days in serum. IgG can cross the placenta to protect the fetus and is also found in colostrum and breast milk. A very important opsonin, it activates phagocytes and complement proteins.
	IgA	IgA is the most abundant immunoglobulin and can be isolated within mucous membranes and secreted fluids such as breast milk, saliva, nasal secretions, tears and mucus of the genitourinary tract. IgA is able to block entry of bacteria across the gastrointestinal tract, binding antigens before they enter the internal environment. IgA has a serum half-life of 6 days and has four binding sites for antigen. IgA is a poor opsonin and only weakly stimulates complement.
	IgD	IgD is found on the B-lymphocyte membrane; production of IgD stops when IgM production commences. It has a half-life of 3 days, and two binding sites for antigen. Only very small amounts (<1%) of IgD are found in serum. The precise role of IgD remains unclear; however, it is known to enhance mucosal immunity and to enter the circulation and bind to basophils, stimulating pro-inflammatory responses.
	IgE	Only small amounts of IgE are found in serum because it binds (via the Fc region) to basophils and mast cells located within mucous membranes. It also binds to eosinophils and is found mostly in the interstitial spaces. It has a half-life of 2 days and two binding sites for antigen. IgE binding to antigen elicits cellular responses, resulting in inflammatory symptoms, including, in addition to the cardinal signs, pruritus, coughing, sneezing and mucus secretion. Allergies are commonly caused by overproduction of IgE in response to antigens from animal dander, pollen and venoms.

All antibodies (immunoglobulins) are based on a common Y-shaped structure in combinations that provide five main classes. These classes influence the location and biological activity of the antibody in addition to the antibody's ability to bind to specific antigens.

T-lymphocytes

T-lymphocytes (also called T-cells) form two major subpopulations of effector cells, each able to respond to specific non-self antigens.

Cytotoxic T-lymphocytes (CTLs) kill intracellular pathogens by destroying body cells that have become infected, usually with a virus but also with some forms of bacteria, such as the tubercle bacillus, which can also reside within body cells. CTLs are also able to kill cancer cells and cells from transplanted organs.

Virus-infected cells process viral antigen and present this on their surface. Recognition of antigen by T-lymphocytes requires antigen binding to the T-cell receptor and other receptors. CTLs then secrete perforins and granzymes, which destroy the infected cell. They also stimulate infected cells to undergo a form of programmed cell death called **apoptosis**. Debris from dead cells is then removed by phagocytes, and any free virus becomes bound to antibodies, thereby limiting the spread of virus and lowering the risk of further infection.

T-helper lymphocytes (T_H) are a heterogeneous population of cells that produce an individual profile of various cytokines in response to antigen presented to them by APCs and in doing so, generate specific immune responses tailored to eliminating pathogens or infected cells. T_H-lymphocytes are crucial in *helping* B-lymphocytes produce antibodies, activate macrophages and also initiate inflammatory responses. T_H-lymphocytes, therefore, through cytokine secretion and activation of APCs, perform a vital role in the orchestration of immune responses (see *Figure 11.14*).

A third population of **regulatory T-lymphocytes** (Treg) also exists; these regulate the development and activity of CTLs and T_H-lymphocytes and also reduce the potential of T-lymphocytes to react against **self antigens** and so avoid the development of **autoimmune** disease.

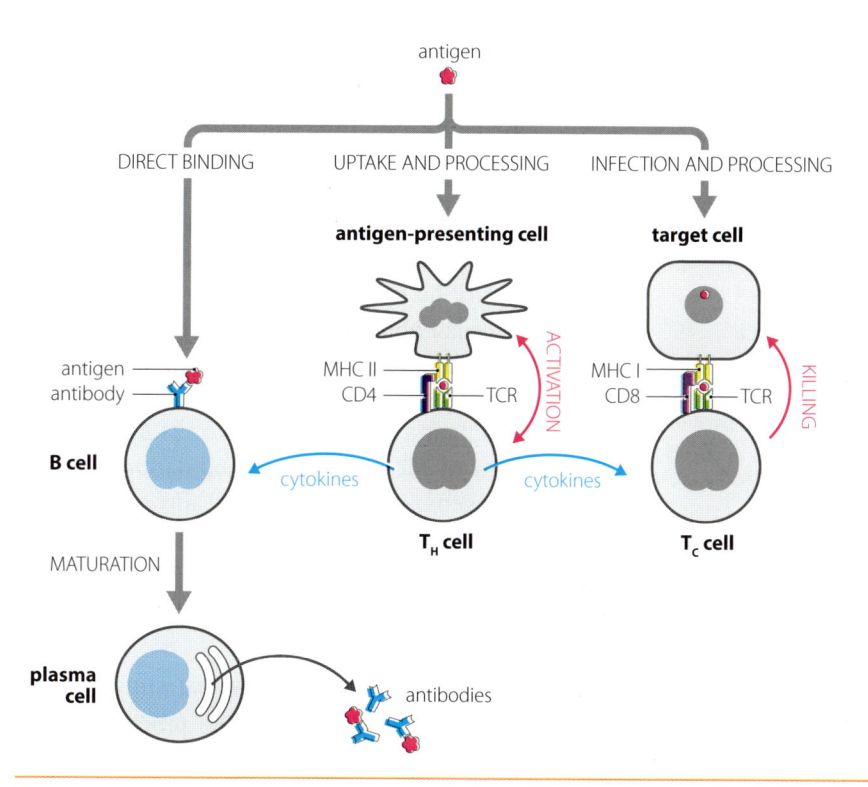

Figure 11.14 – Adaptive immunity processes specific antigens by directly binding to antibodies, activating T-helper (T_H) lymphocytes via antigen-presenting cells (APCs), or by destroying intracellular antigen by killing infected cells.
Note that the antigen requires processing and presentation with MHC proteins to the T-lymphocytes. TCR: T-cell receptor.

CTLs and T_H-lymphocytes express receptors on their surface called CD8 and CD4, respectively. CD stands for 'cluster of differentiation' and is a type of co-receptor involved with recognition of antigens. The level of CD8 and CD4 in the blood can be measured and used for monitoring and diagnosing immune disorders (see Jerry, Patient 11.2).

Concept of self and non-self: the major histocompatibility complex

Recognition of pathogens by T-lymphocytes requires the immune system to be able to discriminate between foreign (non-self) antigens and self antigens. Self antigens are antigens produced endogenously (by a person's own tissue) and are usually tolerated by the immune system, whereas non-self antigens are of exogenous origin (from foreign tissue) and are capable of inducing an immune response. Intracellular antigens are broken down and processed onto the surface of an infected cell by a cluster of proteins called the **major histocompatibility complex** (MHC). T-lymphocytes bind *simultaneously* to a complex of antigen and MHC proteins. MHC proteins are unusual in that they are structurally different between individuals in the population because the genetic code for MHC proteins is contained in highly polymorphic genes (see *Chapter 3*), such that it is exceedingly unlikely (except for identical twins) that any two people in the population will inherit the same form of alleles. There are two groups of MHC:

- MHC type I is present on the surface of nearly all body cells
- MHC type II is present on the surface of all leukocytes.

CTLs are *only* able to bind onto MHC type I proteins that *simultaneously* present antigen, while T_H-lymphocytes are *only* able to bind to *activated leukocytes* presenting antigen with an MHC type II molecule. This is termed MHC restriction, because T-lymphocytes are only able to react to fragments of antigen from intracellular infections, and it restricts and focuses T-lymphocyte activity to just a particular antigen. Importantly, it also reduces the risk of T-lymphocyte activity being directed against self antigens and the inappropriate destruction of normal body tissue. By regulating antigen presentation to T-lymphocytes, the MHC plays a fundamental part in adaptive immunity, influencing resistance and susceptibility to infection, the development of autoimmune disease and organ transplant rejection (see *Box 11.3*). The diversity of polymorphism in *MHC* genes enables the human population to be protected from a broad spectrum of pathogens; it is unlikely that any virulent lethal organism that evolves will be able to evade MHC processing in a cohort of the population and so MHC diversity is maintained by natural selection.

Acquiring immunity

Vaccination is the deliberate administration of a pathogen in order to stimulate an immune response. In the process, by activation of adaptive immunity, a person becomes immune. Vaccination is regarded as second only to clean water in terms of its impact on public health because it is able to reduce the rates of communicable diseases.

The administration of a microorganism, or a fragment of a microorganism, into the body so that adaptive immune cells can process the antigen generates the

BOX 11.3

The major histocompatibility complex (MHC) and tissue rejection

Humans did not evolve to accept organ transplants. Donor MHC molecules are strongly antigenic to a transplant recipient's host cells, causing immune-mediated rejection.

Organ rejection can be minimized by matching the donor and transplanted tissue as closely as possible for MHC compatibility. This is most likely to occur in closely related family members although exact matches are very unlikely. Transplanted organs can persist in an organ recipient by administering immune-suppressive drugs. These drugs can have significant adverse effects and leave a patient prone to opportunistic infections. However, donated organs such as kidneys and heart/lung transplants save lives. Currently, a successful kidney transplant typically lasts for 10 years for a deceased donor kidney and 12 years for a live related kidney.

Organ rejection occurs in a variety of ways; two important mechanisms are illustrated in *Figure 11.15*.

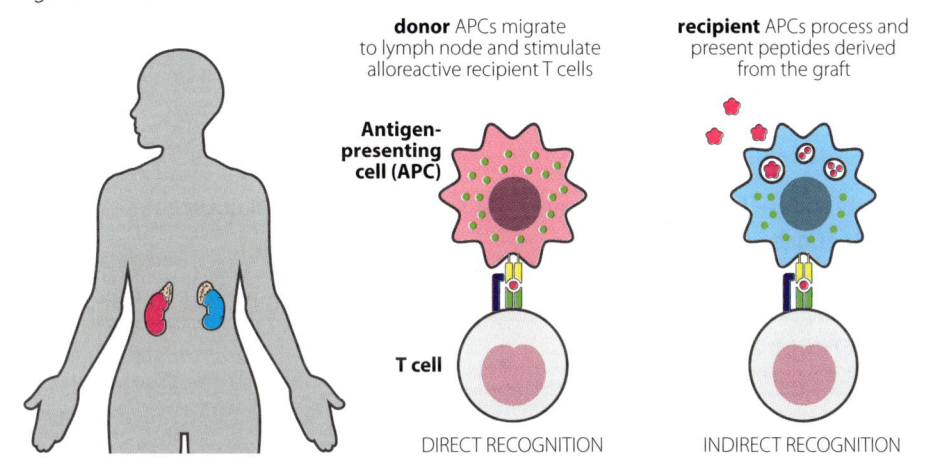

Figure 11.15 – Organ rejection.
(a) Passenger leukocytes in donated tissue travel to lymph nodes, stimulating host recipient T-lymphocytes. (b) Alternatively, recipient antigen-presenting cells (APCs) process donated antigens and present these to their own T-lymphocytes.

---

primary response discussed earlier. The microorganism in the vaccine is usually either killed, or live and attenuated (made less virulent) before administration to avoid the person getting the disease, but is still able to generate immune responses. Future exposure to the live pathogen causes a rapid secondary response, thus avoiding the disease or at least the worst effects of the disease. This is a form of **active immunity**, whereby inducing cellular responses provides long-term protection (months and years) against disease. Usually, the antigen is administered directly into muscle by injection, but the mucosal route, for example by nasal inhalation, is beginning to be used. This is more acceptable to many patients and parents of young children. Most vaccines are administered to young children, and several vaccines are usually combined in order to avoid multiple painful injections.

Vaccination provides an additional benefit by increasing the protection against infection of a population at risk (an example of a vaccine recently introduced to protect the population against the human papillomavirus is discussed in *Chapter*

14). The number of people immune to a particular infection will be defined by those who have previously been infected and those who have been immunized with a vaccine. This leads to a proportion of the population or *herd* that are immune. If this level of **herd immunity** is high enough, then the extent to which a microorganism can be transmitted to non-immune members of the herd will be lowered, decreasing the risk of uninfected and unprotected people becoming infected. High levels of herd protection are essential for the suppression of outbreaks of some infections and can even lead to total eradication of an infectious agent from the community, *without* actually vaccinating every individual. The level of protection within a population required to eliminate an infection can be calculated and for well-known infections is presented in *Table 11.3*. When vaccine uptake by the population falls, then herd immunity also falls and the incidence of reported cases increases. Vaccination rates against measles in the UK in 1995 reached 92% of the population, but this fell in subsequent years to 80%, due to speculation over the safety of the combined MMR (measles, mumps and rubella) vaccine. Since that time, rates of reported measles infections have increased, mainly in unvaccinated individuals.

Table 11.3 – Levels of herd immunity required to prevent outbreaks of particular infections

Infection	Herd immunity threshold
Diphtheria	85%
Measles	83–94%
Mumps	75–86%
Pertussis	92–94%
Polio	80–86%
Rubella	83–85%
Smallpox	80–85%

From **Fine, P. E. M.** (1993) Herd immunity: history, theory, practice. *Epidemiologic Reviews*, **15:** 265–302.

Immunity in neonates and infants

Infection is a leading cause of mortality in children under 5 years. Vaccination strategies are very useful in reducing child mortality, but because of the immaturity of infant immune systems, this is sometimes not entirely effective. While in the uterus, maternal and fetal immune systems are required to tolerate one another because they are genetically distinct. This tolerance is induced and mediated by mechanisms involving cytokine expression and T-lymphocytes. At birth, an infant moves from a sterile intrauterine environment to an antigen-rich *ex utero* environment where it needs to adapt rapidly to challenges from antigens from both benign microorganisms and pathogens.

Furthermore, at birth the skin is thinner and less resilient than adult skin, the normal flora are absent from the gastrointestinal tract and, although innate immune cells have developed, adaptive immunity remains largely naïve and unchallenged by antigen. However, some microorganisms can cross the placenta, especially viruses such as herpes simplex virus, rubella virus and human immunodeficiency virus (HIV). Maternal complement and IgG antibodies cross the placenta, and as these antibodies are largely formed during the secondary immune response, they represent responses to antigens from the environment that the mother has been exposed to and so will provide a degree of passive immunity, which persists at birth. Indeed, neonatal IgG levels exceed those of the mother by approximately 10% at birth, and vaccination of mothers against tetanus in endemic regions of the world has been shown to improve survival of their child by reducing neonatal sepsis.

The neonate obtains an additional boost in **passive immunity** via breast milk, especially from **colostrum**, the milk produced in the first few days of life. This is rich in secretory IgA, which is able to withstand gastric acid and is specifically sensitized (from the mother) to pathogens that typically infect the gastrointestinal and respiratory tracts. Breast milk also contains a wide variety of compounds with effects directly related to immunity; for example, vitamin B_{12}-binding protein in breast milk reduces the amount of vitamin B_{12} available for bacterial metabolism, and lactoferrin reduces the availability of iron, also required for microbial growth of some pathogenic microorganisms. Lysozyme, fatty acids, mucins and a variety of immune cells are also secreted into breast milk, serving to reduce pathogenic colonization of the respiratory and gastrointestinal tracts, while allowing colonization by the normal flora. The importance of breast milk in nutrition and immunity is underscored by the World Health Organization *strongly* recommending that all children should be exclusively breast-fed for the first 6 months of life.

Immunity in the older person

Immunosenescence is a decline in immunity with age, associated with greater susceptibility and severity from infection, together with reduced responses to vaccination. Generally, innate immunity is relatively well preserved, but adaptive immunity declines. The number of T-lymphocytes remains constant, and elderly people may have high levels of antibodies in their serum, reflecting a lifetime of exposure to antigen and immunological memory, but their responses to new antigens diminishes (summarized in *Table 11.4*). The causes for this are not entirely clear but include age-related mutations in genes within somatic cells, interference with gene expression over time caused by a history of virus infections (viruses disrupt host genes during infection) and age-related changes in a variety of organs. Other factors such as nutrition, particularly the availability of antioxidant vitamins, and age-related changes in hormones may also play a part. People over the age of 65 years are more likely to be affected by urinary tract, respiratory, abdominal and other infections, suffering mortality rates three times higher than the general population. Infection in elderly people is an important cause of reduced functional capacity, which also increases the risk of infection. In addition, febrile symptoms are sometimes not obvious in elderly patients. Despite a poorer response to vaccines, elderly people can benefit from them; currently, in the UK, people over the age of 65 years are recommended to receive a pneumococcal vaccine and a seasonal flu vaccine to protect against respiratory tract infection.

Table 11.4 – Age-related changes to immunity

Cell type	Age-related increase	Age-related decrease
Innate immunity		
Neutrophils		Oxidative burst, phagocytic capacity and bactericidal activity
Macrophages		Oxidative burst, phagocytic capacity
NK cells		Proliferative response to interleukin-2 (IL-2), cytotoxicity
Dendritic cells		Capacity to stimulate antigen-specific T-lymphocytes, migration to lymph nodes
Cytokines and chemokines	Serum levels of IL-6, IL-1β and TNF-α	
Adaptive immunity		
T-lymphocytes	Number of memory and effector cells, release of pro-inflammatory cytokines	Number of naïve T-lymphocytes, functional activities of naïve T-lymphocytes, diversity of the T-lymphocyte repertoire, expression of co-stimulatory molecules on APCs, proliferative capacity
B-lymphocytes	Autoreactive serum antibodies	Generation of B-lymphocyte precursors, number of naïve B-cells, diversity of the B-lymphocyte repertoire, expression of co-stimulatory molecules, B-lymphocyte switching of antibody isotype

Adapted from **Weiskopf, D., Weinberger, B. and Grubeck-Loebenstein, B.** (2009) The aging of the immune system. *Transplant International*, **22(11):** 1041–1050.

11.3 Clinical application

Coexistence with microorganisms places humans at perpetual risk of infection. This demands a robust immune system that is able to respond in diverse and complex ways to protect and repair the body from tissue damage. There is a fine balance to be achieved between tolerating colonization by microorganisms and infection. When this balance is disturbed, the implications for health can be profound. Paradoxically, inappropriate or excessive activation of the immune system can cause tissue damage, leading to autoimmune disease and chronic inflammation.

The dynamic interplay of the microbial world and immune responses has been brought into sharp relief by the emergence of HIV in the latter half of the 20th century. HIV infection can be successfully managed but not, as yet, eradicated. Having killed more than 25 million people in just three decades, HIV continues to pose a significant threat to global health; current estimates suggest that approximately 35 million people worldwide are infected with HIV.

Each of the patient cases discussed within this chapter illustrates how knowledge of immunity is essential to healthcare practice.

- Francine (Patient 1.3) is experiencing an acute exacerbation of her Crohn's disease, a type of inflammatory bowel disease. This disease involves inappropriate immune responses, which interfere with normal function of the gastrointestinal tract. It can often be managed, but not cured, with the administration of potent anti-inflammatory drugs that suppress activity of the immune system, allowing integrity and function of the bowel to be restored. This provides Francine with relief from the unpleasant symptoms of the disease.

- Albert (Patient 11.1) is infected with *C. difficile*; this could be fatal to him, unless the infection in his gastrointestinal tract is carefully managed. It is an opportunistic infection and an important healthcare-associated infection, requiring very high standards of infection control practice to limit its spread to other patients.

- Jerry (Patient 11.2) is infected with HIV and as a result has now become immunodeficient. He will be prescribed a combination of antiretroviral drugs to keep the levels of the virus in his blood low. This should allow Jerry's immune system to recover the capacity to protect him from infection. If Jerry is able to adhere to the treatment regime closely, he can look forward to a long life, as the development of new antiviral drugs has led to HIV no longer being regarded as a terminal disease but rather as a chronic disease.

Patient 1.3 | Francine | 2 | 21 | 194 | 235 | 338 | **371**

- 40-year-old woman
- Crohn's disease – on steroids
- Presents with inflamed bowel and anaemia
- MRSA screen ahead of potential surgery
- TPN given IV to recovery during relapse
- Positive MRSA screen – decolonized over 5 days
- Acute inflammatory episode – potent drugs given to reduce inflammation and try to avoid surgery
- Also given infliximab to reduce inflammation

On admission to hospital and for the following 5 days, in accordance with local guidelines, Francine followed a decolonization protocol using antibacterial compounds, in an attempt to eradicate MRSA from her body surfaces and nostrils – sites that MRSA most commonly colonizes. This is important because it will help to limit the risk of Francine developing a wound infection if she requires surgery and will limit the transmission of MRSA to other patients. Francine is anaemic, with a haemoglobin level of 8 g/dl (normal range: 11.5–16.0 g/dl) (anaemia is discussed in *Chapter 9*), and she is opening her bowels 8–10 times every day. She feels very weak and has been prescribed intravenous nutritional support (parenteral nutrition) where all required nutrients are infused directly into the blood, avoiding the gastrointestinal tract. This will help with alleviating Francine's symptoms and will reduce some of the inflammation of her bowel. The level of C-reactive protein (CRP, an acute-phase protein discussed earlier in this chapter) in Francine's blood was high at 16 mg/L (normally values are <5 mg/L), which suggests that Francine is experiencing an acute inflammatory episode. She has been prescribed potent anti-inflammatory drugs including intravenous steroids: hydrocortisone 100 mg every 6 hours, and an increase in her usual dose of azathioprine in an attempt to reduce the inflammation. In addition, Francine has been prescribed a monoclonal antibody (infliximab), administered intravenously. Infliximab is specific for the pro-inflammatory cytokine tumour necrosis factor-α (TNF-α), and so it blocks the action of TNF-α and also kills T-lymphocytes that express TNF-α, thus reducing inflammation.

The pathophysiological processes associated with Crohn's disease are not fully understood, although evidence suggests that it is associated with a defect in the epithelial barrier of the intestine and with abnormal signalling pathways that arise when PRRs on dendritic cells bind to PAMPs. This evidence is supported by the observation that patients with mutations in the genes that code for specific PRRs are more susceptible to Crohn's disease.

The epithelial lining of the intestine normally provides an important barrier function, keeping pathogenic microorganisms and the normal flora within the lumen, preventing them from causing an infection. To form a barrier, individual epithelial cells are held together tightly by proteins in the plasma membrane, forming tight junctions. Defective tight junctions allow microorganisms to penetrate the mucosa and initiate inflammation.

The epithelial barrier is not simply a static structure but is one in which immune cells interact with the intestinal environment and their activity is influenced by it. In Crohn's disease, abnormal signalling between immune cells and the intestinal environment leads to an overproduction of the pro-inflammatory cytokines TNF-α and interleukin-6 (IL-6).

Following her infliximab infusion and steroid therapy, Francine's symptoms improved greatly and the need for surgical removal of her affected bowel diminished. Her CRP level gradually reduced to normal levels, providing evidence of a resolution of inflammation, and her weight also increased due to the intravenous nutritional supplementation.

Francine was eventually discharged from hospital a few weeks later on a reducing dose of oral steroids. This is important, because long-term steroid therapy can exert many adverse effects. The anti-inflammatory effect of azathioprine takes a few months to become clinically evident but should maintain remission of her disease. Azathioprine inhibits DNA synthesis in T-lymphocytes by blocking the synthesis of the purine bases adenine and guanine (see *Chapter 3*), thus inhibiting adaptive immune responses.

| Patient 11.1 | Albert | 338 | **372** |

- 81-year-old man
- Chest infection led to pneumonia
- Given IV antibiotics to rapidly improve symptoms
- In 6 days had severe foul-smelling diarrhoea —found to contain *C. difficile*
- Developed colitis — result of antibiotic treatment

Albert is an 81-year-old gentleman with *C. difficile* infection of his colon, described as colitis. *C. difficile* is a Gram-positive, spore-forming **anaerobe**. The spores are able to survive harsh desiccating environmental conditions for long periods of time, which facilitates their survival and transfer between hosts (commonly hospitalized patients; see *Box 11.4*).

A stool specimen sent to the microbiology laboratory for testing confirmed *C. difficile* infection. *C. difficile* is notoriously difficult to grow in the laboratory – hence the name '*difficile*'. Current laboratory tests are based on detection of the toxins it is known to produce, rather than the organism itself. The toxins, called *C. difficile* toxin A (TcdA) and B (TcdB), damage the epithelial lining of the large bowel (colon) by stimulating the production of pro-inflammatory cytokines, including interleukin-8 (IL-8) and TNF-α. These activate mucosal mast cells, macrophages and neutrophils to trigger acute inflammation. An inflamed bowel has a reduced capacity to absorb nutrients and water, and prolonged exposure of the epithelial lining to *C. difficile* toxins results in cell death. In health, relatively few nutrients are absorbed via the colon, but up to 10% of water is normally reabsorbed (see *Chapter 7*), and Albert is at significant risk of becoming dehydrated.

Albert's colitis is likely to have developed as a result of the antibiotics he was prescribed. Although the antibiotics killed the pneumonia in his lungs caused by a streptococcal species of bacteria, the antibiotics also killed many of the normal flora living in his large bowel. In people colonized with *C. difficile*, the mixed population of organisms in the bowel maintains low numbers of *C. difficile* organisms through natural competition with the normal gut flora. When antibiotic therapy disturbs this flora, competition is reduced and the population of *C. difficile* increases. Once a critical level is achieved, colitis develops; hence, Albert's symptoms became apparent.

Clostridium difficile is an important source of healthcare-associated infection

BOX 11.4

The ability to produce spores is found in only a few species of bacteria, including *C. difficile*, *Clostridium tetani*, which causes tetanus, and *Clostridium botulinum*, from which we get the botulinum toxin 'Botox'.

Spore-producing bacteria exist in two states, the vegetative form and the spore form. Bacterial reproduction only occurs in the vegetative form, and for *C. difficile* this is the form present in the bowel. If the environment alters, such as a change in temperature, a lack of water or the presence of oxygen (*C. difficile* is an anaerobe), the vegetative form becomes spore-forming. This occurs when *C. difficile* leaves the body in the faeces and meets oxygen in the air. Spores exist in a dormant state; they are unable to metabolize or reproduce, but are able to resist harsh environmental conditions until the environment becomes more suited to growth, when they revert back to the vegetative form.

The only way to remove spores is by sterilization, which is achieved by exposing the spores to heat (134°C for at least 3 minutes), typically in an autoclave. As it is impossible to sterilize an occupied ward, the best that can be achieved is disinfection, which could leave some spores behind. These spores have the potential to be spread around the environment on the hands of patients or healthcare workers. Spores can also be ingested by patients or healthcare workers, reverting back to the vegetative state in the bowel and potentially causing infection. Hand washing, containment of the spores by putting the patient in a side room, and regular cleaning and disinfection of the side room are essential elements of infection control practice for this infection. Environmental disinfection is achieved by the use of a chlorine-based product.

Alcohol is ineffective for disinfection of *Clostridium* spores, and alcohol hand gel should not be used when caring for *C. difficile*-infected patients. Washing hands with a detergent physically removes spores, and all healthcare workers, patients and visitors should wash their hands with soap and water after contact with the patient or their environment.

Patient 11.2 — Jerry

- 30-year-old man
- Diagnosed with HIV at age 22
- Fall in CD4+ count leads to discussion of treatment
- Prescribed HAART

Jerry has been attending the sexual health clinic since the detection of HIV-1 antibodies in his blood some years ago. Infection by HIV can cause acquired immunodeficiency syndrome (AIDS). Discovered in 1983, the infection typically left people exposed to opportunistic infections by disrupting normal immune defences, and people frequently died within a couple of years of diagnosis. The current outlook for patients diagnosed as infected with HIV is much better, because antiretroviral therapy is able to extend life very effectively, so that infection with HIV has now been proposed to be a chronic and not necessarily a lethal disease.

Since receiving his diagnosis, Jerry has had regular blood tests at the clinic, measuring primarily CD4+ cells (T_H-lymphocytes) in his blood and the number of viral antigens detectable in his blood. These two measurements are related: as HIV replicates and destroys CD4+ cells, the number of these cells reduces and the viral load increases. Six months ago, Jerry's CD4+ cell count was reduced to 303 cells/ml and 4 weeks later it was still low at 312 cells/ml. It is usual to commence treatment when the CD4+ cell count is below 350 cells/ml, but a single measurement below this level is not sufficient to instigate treatment, as the CD4+ cell typically varies from week to week, depending on factors such as additional infections that are present. The normal CD4+ cell count in health is >500 cells/ml. Because Jerry's CD4+ cells had fallen below 350 cells/ml on more than one occasion, it was decided to prescribe antiretroviral medication.

Prior to treatment, blood was taken to provide a baseline for both CD4+ cell count and viral load, as a comparator for the success or failure of treatment over time. In addition, a genotypic resistance test was performed on his blood, to determine whether the particular strain of HIV that Jerry has is resistant to any of the antiretroviral drugs.

Approximately 2 weeks later, when the blood results were available, Jerry returned to the clinic and was prescribed a combination of antiretroviral drugs, described under the name of HAART (highly active antiretroviral therapy), because the biology of HIV makes it very difficult to eradicate from the body (see *Box 11.5*). It is vital that Jerry adheres to his drug regimen in order to reduce the chance of the virus developing resistance to the HAART. He also needs to take his tablets at the same time each day to maintain the optimum concentration of drug in his body. Jerry may find it difficult to stick to his medication pattern for the rest of his life, and it is vital that he establishes a routine where his tablet taking fits in with his lifestyle. He has found that using a daily pill box and keeping a supply of medication at his friend's flat helps him adhere to his medication.

Protection from harm is a core principle of healthcare, and yet interventions aimed at helping patients frequently place patients at risk of harm, particularly from healthcare-acquired infections. The immune system operates as a fully integrated

Table 12.1 – Functions of the skin: mechanisms and structure

Function	Mechanism	Structure/location
Barrier	Protection from physical damage, chemicals, microorganisms and ultraviolet radiation	Epidermis
Fluid balance	Evaporation of sweat	Epidermis
Metabolic	Group B vitamins and vitamin D synthesis	Epidermis
Temperature regulation	Multiple homeostatic mechanisms, including radiation, convection, conduction and evaporative water loss	Epidermis, dermis, blood vessels and sweat glands
Sensation	Pressure, pain, itch, heat	Nerve endings
Lubrication	Fluid, sweat and sebum	Sebaceous glands
Protection and grip	Nails, fingertips and hair	Epidermis
Insulation	Subcutaneous fat	Hypodermis
Shock absorption	Subcutaneous fat	Hypodermis
Calorie reserve	Subcutaneous fat	Hypodermis
Body odour	Secretions and microbial organisms	Apocrine sweat glands
Psychosocial	Structural variation affecting appearance; culturally defined	Skin, hair and nails
Drug absorption	Dependent on chemical properties	Epidermis and dermis

delay the appearance of ageing. Tattooing has been performed over centuries and continues to be practised by many cultures. Caucasian people often seek a darker skin tone through the use of 'tanning compounds' or exposure to ultraviolet light, even though they are aware of the dangers of sunburn to their skin. Conversely, some Asian cultures value and seek to protect a pale skin tone, while the use of skin bleaching compounds in some African communities has increased and is a concern for health. Emotional cues can lead to rapid changes in the skin such as facial 'blushing' during episodes of embarrassment. Thus, the skin has a more subtle and yet significant role in humans and their health than simply the maintenance of homeostasis.

12.2 What you need to know – essential anatomy and physiology

12.2.1 Structure of the skin

There are two principal parts to the skin: a very thin outer **epidermis** and below this the **dermis** (see *Figures 12.1a* and *b*). The dermis provides additional mechanical support to the skin, while the epidermis provides a barrier to water loss. The dermis lies on top of a layer of subcutaneous tissue known as the **hypodermis**,

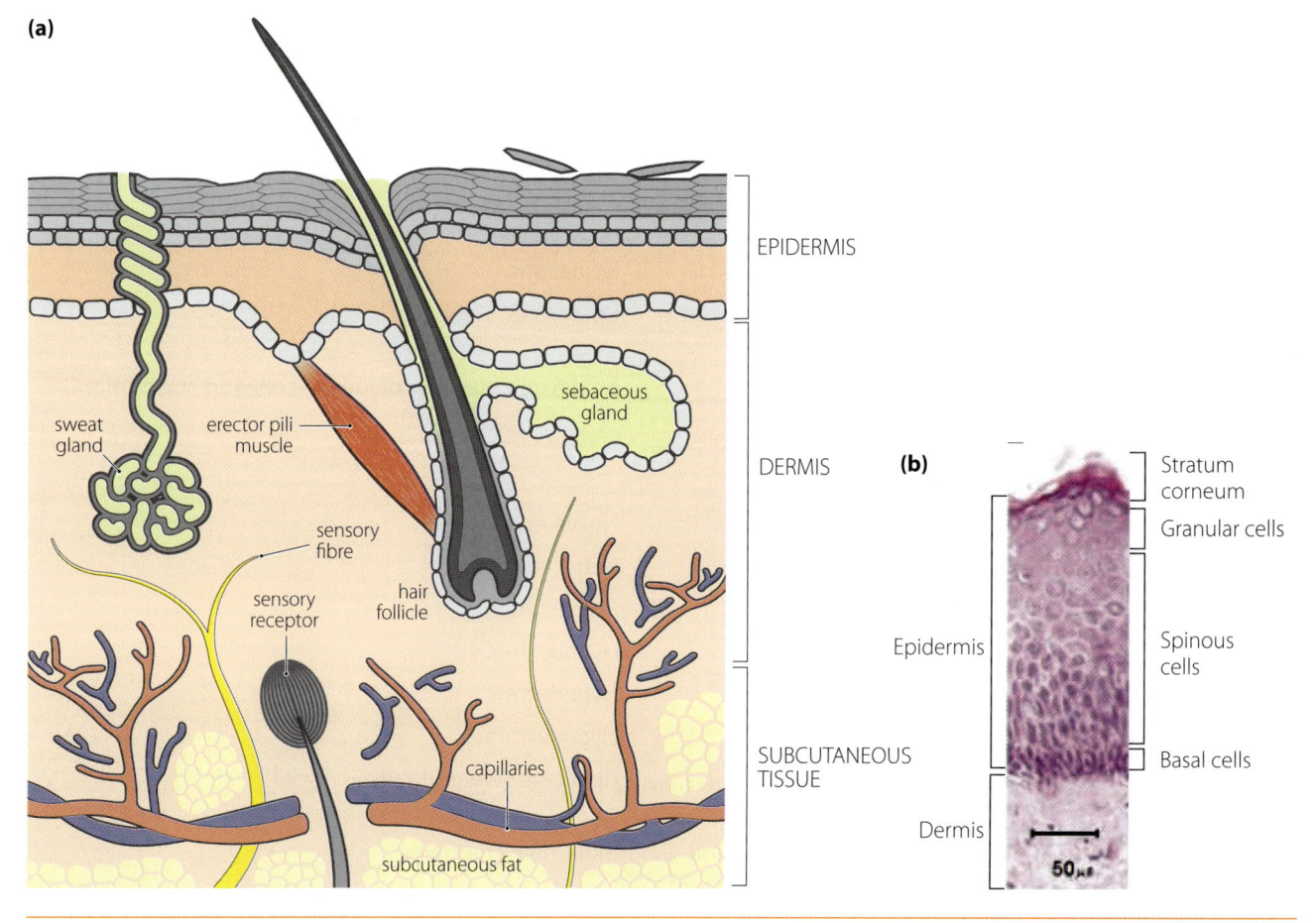

Figure 12.1 – (a) The structure of the skin, illustrating the structures found within it and (b) a photomicrograph illustrating the two main layers of skin.

The skin forms a protective barrier between the environment and the body. It has two main layers: the outer epidermis and the inner dermis, which lie on top of loose connective tissue. (b) reproduced from *Drug Discovery Today: Disease Mechanisms* 5(1), Lane, E.B., "Broken bricks and cracked mortar – epidermal diseases resulting from genetic abnormalities", pp. e93–101 (2008).

which is mostly connective tissue and is generally not regarded as forming part of the skin. The hypodermis provides a flexible basement for the skin, together with insulation and protection from mechanical shock to underlying organs, and as it is composed of adipose cells, it also provides a reserve of energy.

Structure of the epidermis

Despite being very thin, ranging from approximately 0.05 to 2.0 mm thick, the epidermis consists of a number of distinct, densely packed layers of cells (see *Figure 12.1b*). The epidermis is therefore a type of **stratified epithelium** (described in *Chapter 2*). The layers are formed mostly from **keratinocyte** cells, which produce and accumulate large amounts of an insoluble protein called keratin. It is this that provides the outer resilient surface of the epidermis known as the **stratum corneum**. Keratinocytes develop from mitotic cell division of epidermal stem cells from the lowest basal layer next to the dermis, called the **stratum basale** (see *Figure 12.1b*). As the newly divided cells mature, they become flattened, accumulate keratin and eventually die. These dead cells are called **corneocytes**. The corneocytes are gradually replaced by cells from below as cells are shed to the environment, a process called desquamation. Thus, there is a constant, gradual and upward movement of cells towards the outer epidermal surface, with the epidermal surface being progressively replaced approximately each month as corneocytes are rubbed and washed off.

The remaining cell types found within the epidermis are melanocytes, Langerhans cells and Merkel cells. Melanocytes are located within the stratum basale (innermost layer) and produce the pigment melanin, which is largely responsible for providing skin colour. The production of melanin is stimulated by exposure to ultraviolet light and functions to protect the DNA within skin cells from damage caused by the ultraviolet radiation contained in sunlight. Langerhans cells, located within the middle of the epidermal layer (the stratum spinosum), are responsive to the presence of microorganisms and interact with cells of the immune system to provide protection against infection. They are an example of an antigen-presenting cell (APC) (described in *Chapter 11*). Merkel cells are also located within the stratum basale and are involved with the processing of sensory information such as touch.

The densely packed cells that form the epidermis are held together by a complex matrix of proteins and lipids to form a highly organized watertight barrier that is also resistant to mildly irritant chemicals and infectious agents. This has been likened to a 'bricks and mortar' model, where keratinocytes of the stratum corneum form physically resistant bricks and a protein/lipid mixture forms the mortar that provides resistance to excessive water gain or loss (see *Figure 12.2*).

It is important to recognize that the epidermis is dynamic, flexible and able to renew cells and the surrounding matrix. It adapts to environmental changes such as ambient humidity, controlling the amount of water held within it or that which is lost to the environment. It contributes to the regulation of homeostasis by maintaining an effective barrier under a range of environmental conditions. The skin can become severely damaged by trauma or burning; when this happens, assessing the extent and depth of injury is very important and can be quite difficult (see *Box 12.1*).

Structure of the dermis

The dermis is thicker than the epidermis, approximately 3.0–5.0 mm. It lies on top of subcutaneous fat (see *Figure 12.1a*), also called the hypodermis, and is situated below the stratum basale of the epidermis. The dermis is largely made up of bundles of fibrous connective tissue (discussed in *Chapter 2*), such as the structural proteins elastin and collagen produced by fibroblast cells. These cells exist within a background 'gel-like' matrix of mucopolysaccharide ground substance. The fibrous connective tissue provides the skin with elasticity and strength, while the ground substance acts as a lubricant to allow the skin to move and to maintain water within the dermal layer. It also helps to provide resistance to physical stresses by absorbing shock and facilitating the movement of nutrients and chemicals required to maintain the dermis and epidermis.

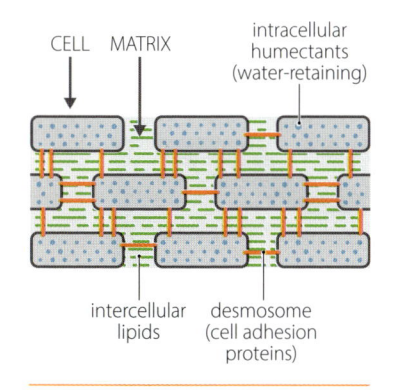

Figure 12.2 – The 'bricks and mortar' model of the epidermis.
Cells represent the bricks, which are held together by a matrix or 'mortar' of lipids and proteins, forming a water-resistant barrier.

> **BOX 12.1**
>
> ## Burns
>
> Estimating the extent of burns is difficult (see *Giuseppe, Patient 12.1*). The type of burn, extent and depth of a burn are important.
>
> There are three common methods of assessing the extent of a burn:
>
> - Wallace's 'rule of nines': the body is separated into nine regions; however, this is considered less reliable for children.
> - Palmar surface: the size of the patient's hand, with fingers extended but not splayed, represents approximately 0.8% of body surface area; this method is only useful for estimation of small burn areas.
> - The Lund and Browder chart (see *Figure 12.3*): this is commonly used instead of the methods above. This takes account of the age of the patient and the different proportions of the head and legs in children compared with adults.
>
> (a) 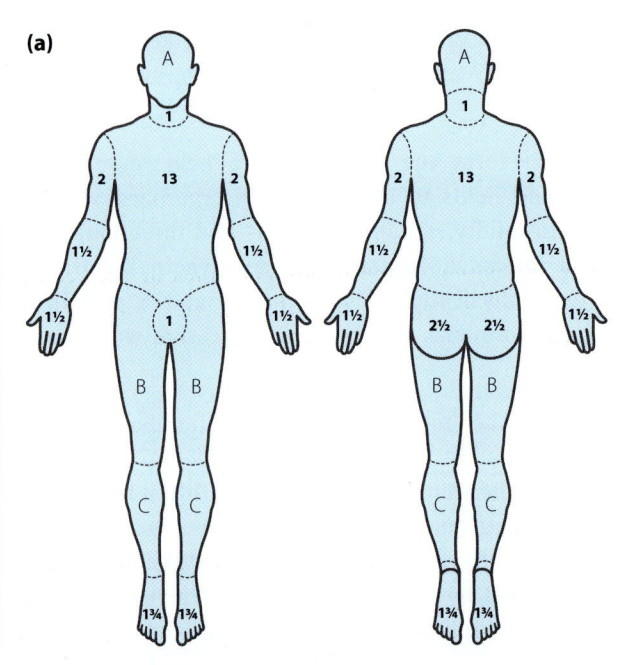
>
> | | % | |
> |---|---|---|
> | REGION | PTL | FTL |
> | head | | |
> | neck | | |
> | anterior trunk | | |
> | posterior trunk | | |
> | right arm | | |
> | left arm | | |
> | buttocks | | |
> | genitalia | | |
> | right leg | | |
> | left leg | | |
> | total burn | | |
>
> | AREA | age 0 | 1 | 5 | 10 | 15 | adult |
> |---|---|---|---|---|---|---|
> | A = ½ of head | 9½ | 8½ | 6½ | 5½ | 4½ | 3½ |
> | B = ½ of one thigh | 2¾ | 3¼ | 4 | 4½ | 4½ | 4¾ |
> | C = ½ of one lower leg | 2½ | 2½ | 2¾ | 3 | 3¼ | 3½ |
>
> **Figure 12.3 – Estimating the extent of burns.**
> (a) The Lund and Browder chart. (b) A superficial burn on the chest, plus a deep burn on a shoulder. The superficial burn will be very painful, but the area of the deep burn on the shoulder is not likely to be painful because the burn will have damaged pain receptors. Reproduced from "ABC of Burns: Introduction", Hettiaratchy, S. and Dziewulski, P. 328:1366–1368, 2004 with permission from BMJ Publishing Group Ltd.

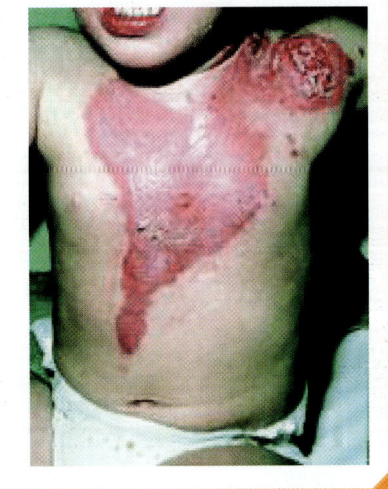

Between the fibrous connective tissue of the dermis is a network of structures, including blood vessels, lymphatic vessels, nerves and immune cells. Specialized structures unique to the skin are also embedded within the dermis. These include hair follicles, sebaceous glands and sweat glands (illustrated in *Figure 12.1a*).

Blood vessels supply the hair follicles, sebaceous glands and sweat glands. Under the control of the autonomic nervous system, these vessels have the capacity to dilate or constrict in order to assist with thermoregulation and wound healing. Loops of blood vessels reach up towards the upper papillary dermis, providing nutrients to epidermal cells by diffusion. Lymphatic vessels are also present; these assist with wound healing by facilitating the circulation of immune cells and the drainage of excess fluid (discussed in *Chapters 9* and *11*) that might otherwise accumulate in the skin. Various types of nerve fibres are present, providing sensory input for pain, touch, heat and **pruritus** (itching). In addition, chemicals and cytokines can affect nerve endings, causing the pruritus and pain associated with inflammation (discussed in *Chapter 11*).

Effective perfusion of blood to and from the skin is important in order to maintain skin integrity. Disruption of perfusion through sustained periods of pressure, chronic disease processes such as type 2 diabetes mellitus, peripheral vascular disease and trauma impairs blood flow to dermal tissue, resulting in the formation of ulcers, which, depending on their cause, can be hard to heal and may lead to surgical amputation of limbs.

Hair follicles are absent from the palms of the hands and soles of the feet, but otherwise they are found all over the body. Attached to each hair follicle is a muscle called the arrector pili and a sebaceous gland. Contraction of the muscle makes the hair stand up, allowing a layer of warm air to form very close to the body (discussed in *Chapter 1*). This mechanism helps to maintain body temperature in a cold climate; however, while humans retain this ability, they have much less body hair than most mammals. Therefore, it is a very poor warming mechanism in humans.

Sebaceous glands secrete a lipid-based compound known as sebum. A large amount of sebum is produced on the face and scalp and is responsible for the appearance of 'greasy' hair when not washed. Specialized glands in the ears and eyes produce sebum, forming a part of earwax (**cerumen**) and tears, respectively. The secretion of sebum contributes to the water-impermeable barrier of the epidermis and also ensures that the hair and epidermis remain flexible, so that the water barrier is not broken by movement or the cracking of dehydrated skin cells. Sebum contains antimicrobial compounds such as lysozyme and also contributes to maintenance of the acid epidermal surface (pH 5.4–5.9), which limits the growth of pathogens on the skin. Sweating, also known as diaphoresis, occurs via sudoriferous glands, commonly known as sweat glands. There are two types, **eccrine** and **apocrine** glands.

Eccrine glands are smaller and secrete sweat containing a hypotonic solution of water and electrolytes directly onto the skin. Sweating lowers the body temperature by the evaporation of water from the skin, taking heat away with it (discussed in *Chapter 1*). Eccrine glands are found all over the body except for parts of the genitalia, the ear canal and lips. The greatest density of eccrine glands is located on the palms of the hands, the soles of the feet and the forehead.

The activity of eccrine glands is regulated by the stimulation of sympathetic fibres via the autonomic nervous system. They are sensitive primarily to the neurotransmitter acetylcholine and to a lesser extent noradrenaline (norepinephrine), and also to adrenergic agonist drugs (introduced in *Chapter 2*). Drugs that affect the nervous system, hormonal changes associated with the menopause, some spicy foods and emotion can also cause episodes of sweating.

The volume of sweat produced is highly variable, depending on the ambient temperature, humidity and metabolic activity, and is increased during exercise. The amount and composition of sweat an individual produces changes as they adapt to environmental conditions. For example, the rate of sweating by manual workers has been estimated to reach up to 1.5 L/hour or 10–12 L/day under hot working conditions. Electrolyte losses, especially sodium, due to sweating can be large. The balance of sodium in the blood is regulated mostly by homeodynamic mechanisms involving the kidney (discussed in *Chapter 8*) and by replacement through dietary sources. If sweating causes excessive loss of water or electrolytes, this can affect the function of a variety of organ systems, including the regulation of blood pressure, activity of the nervous system and the kidneys.

Apocrine sweat glands are larger than eccrine glands and are located primarily around the areolae of the nipples, the genital areas and the axillae (armpits). They become active during puberty and secrete a viscous sweat that possesses a unique odour, via an opening through hair follicles. In mammals and perhaps also in humans, this may have a role in sexual attraction.

Unpleasant 'body odour' is produced from the interaction of microorganisms on the skin surface with sweat as they break it down. This is most pronounced in

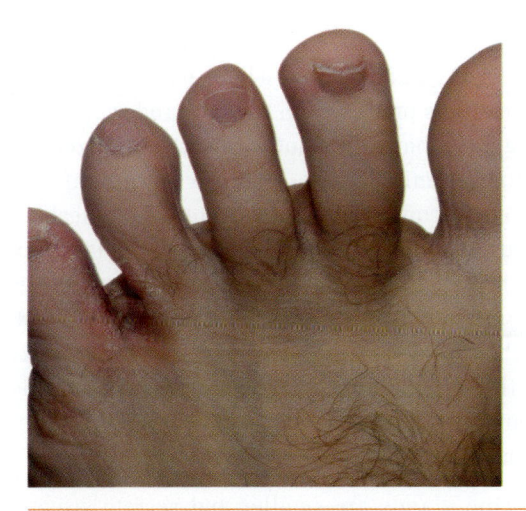

Figure 12.4 – **Athlete's foot, also known as tinea pedis.**
Note the flaking epidermis. This is due to a fungal infection and generally occurs in warm, moist skin folds of the feet and other parts of the body where evaporation of sweat is compromised, providing ideal conditions suited to the proliferation of microorganisms. Image © Roblan – stock.adobe.com.

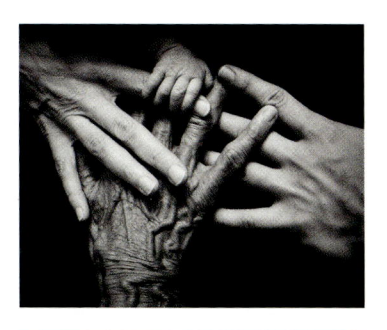

Figure 12.5 – **Four generations: the appearance of the skin changes with age.**
Reproduced from http://welearntoday.com.

the axillae and genital areas, because here the sweat produced contains more substances for microorganisms to feed on. A warm humid environment provides ideal conditions for a variety of microorganisms to proliferate, including bacteria, yeasts and fungi (an example of fungal overgrowth, tinea pedis, otherwise known as 'athlete's foot', is illustrated in *Figure 12.4*). Smelly feet tend to occur when feet are enclosed in socks and shoes, which limit the ability for sweat to evaporate, thus providing a greater source to support microbial metabolism.

12.2.2 Factors affecting the skin

Young skin

In comparison with older skin, in neonates the skin appears swollen and more transparent and has fewer wrinkles. This is because there are fewer elastic fibres, and increased water and sodium content in the skin helps to compensate for this. Neonates have a particularly high risk of sunburn if exposed to excessive sunlight as they produce less melanin. In infants, the immune system is not fully developed and the epidermal layers are thinner and less organized. As a consequence, the risk of physical damage and infection is therefore much greater than in older children or adults.

Preterm babies tend to possess **lanugo**, a fine downy hair, but this is often absent on full-term babies. The purpose of this hair is unclear, but other hairless mammals such as elephants and whales also produce offspring with lanugo; one hypothesis is that it is related to temperature regulation. The growth of lanugo-like hair is also a diagnostic feature of malnutrition, particularly when associated with some eating disorders such as anorexia nervosa (see Amy, Patient 1.1).

High levels of hormones circulating within the mother and the placenta may cause localized pigmentation in full-term babies, such that greater pigmentation on the breast and genitalia is sometimes apparent. Children possess the same number of sweat glands as adults, but the capacity to sweat is lower, possibly because the sweat glands of babies are smaller and are less sensitive to thermal stimuli than adults. Children also have a relatively high surface area : mass ratio in comparison with adults and so thermoregulation probably relies more heavily on convection and radiation than on the evaporation of sweat. Moreover, in addition to a higher surface area : mass ratio, physiological immaturity and other factors, such as the amount of body fat and levels of activity, play an important part in infant thermoregulation. Overall, infants are much more vulnerable to challenges of fluid and temperature imbalance than adults.

Ageing

The process causing skin to age is complex and is not well understood. Wrinkles, sagging loose skin, loss of elasticity, thin skin, blotches and grey hair are all signs of ageing skin (illustrated in *Figure 12.5*). Both the epidermis and dermis become thinner and more vulnerable to shearing forces with advancing age. Hereditary factors play a lesser role than environmental factors in ageing of the skin. There appear to be two main processes at work, involving intrinsic (from within) and extrinsic (from outside) factors.

Intrinsic factors

The junction between the epidermis and dermis contains a landscape of undulating ridges and furrows that provide a high surface area and a point of attachment for the epidermis. The ridges become flatter with age and contain reduced amounts of elastic tissue. Fibroblast cells become less efficient with age and collagen content falls. Collagen fibres also become densely packed and randomly organized. The ability of fibroblasts, keratinocytes and melanocytes to divide appears to reduce with age and gene expression for key proteins, such as elastin, is altered. In addition, the very efficient antioxidant systems present within the skin to protect it from the chemical damage associated with the activity of free radicals (discussed in *Chapters 7* and *11*) become less efficient. Over a lifetime, oxidized proteins, lipids and other chemicals associated with free-radical activity accumulate within the skin where they contribute to the ageing process. Thus, with age, both the cellular and matrix structure of the skin become progressively impaired, making it more vulnerable to the loss of cells and less able to repair itself.

Extrinsic factors

Exposure to sunlight. Sustained exposure to sunlight enhances changes in the skin associated with ageing. Indeed, it has been suggested that up to 80% of facial ageing might be due to exposure to direct sunlight. Photo-aged skin is characterized by deep wrinkles, dry rough skin with a loss of elasticity and the development of irregular areas of pigmentation (illustrated in *Figure 12.6*). The mechanism by which sunlight damages skin is not entirely clear and is subject to a great deal of research and interest, not least by the cosmetic industry. However, evidence is accumulating to suggest that the activity of a variety of enzymes and proteins within the skin involved with wound healing and dermal repair processes are all affected by ultraviolet light, especially the photosensitive pigment melanin.

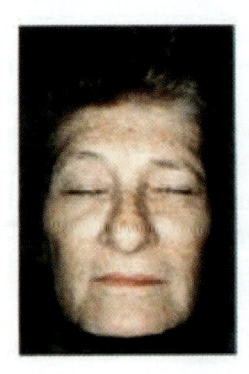

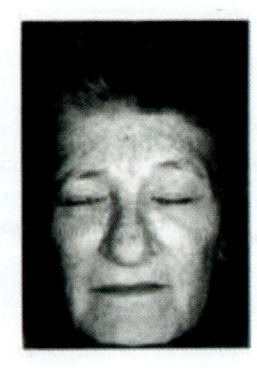

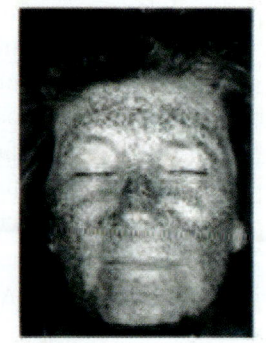

Figure 12.6 – Photo-aged skin revealed.
The two photographs on the left are taken with a normal camera. The image on the right is taken using UV photography. An ultraviolet flash can be used to capture irregularities in melanin to reveal the extent of damage about 3 mm under the surface of the skin. Photograph by David H. McDaniel, M.D., reproduced from www.insideoutsidespa.com.

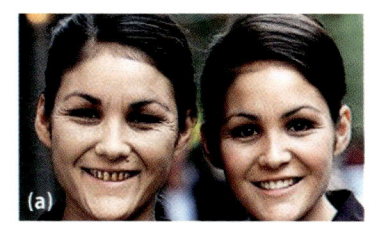

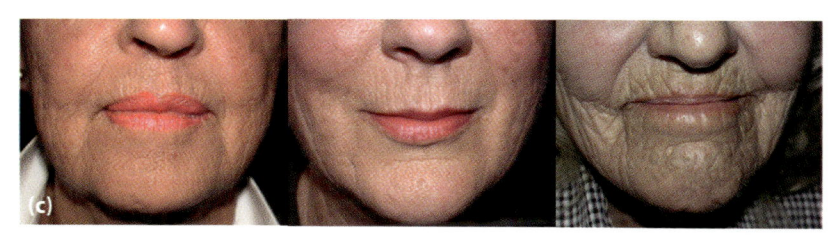

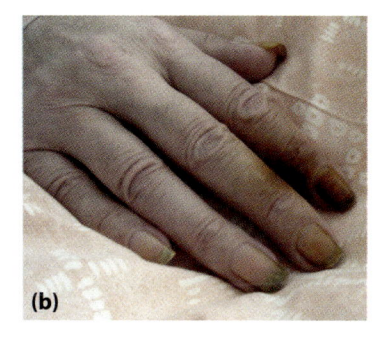

Figure 12.7 – The predicted change in an individual's appearance due to smoking. (a) In this image one 22-year-old twin has been made up to appear older and is compared with her sister, to show the expected effects of smoking. Reproduced from *Journal of Dermatological Science*, 48(3) Morita, A., "Tobacco smoke causes premature skin aging", pp. 169–175 (2007), with permission from Elsevier. (b) Yellow-brown pigmentation of the nails and fingers with hardening of the skin in a man with a long history of smoking. Reproduced from *BMJ Open*, John, G *et al.*, 3(11), 2013, with permission from BMJ Publishing Group Ltd (c) The gradual appearance of vertical wrinkles around the mouth associated with a history of smoking. Reproduced with permission from DermNet NZ.

Tobacco. Smoking tobacco has been observed to increase the depth and appearance of wrinkles (illustrated in *Figure 12.7*). Tobacco smoke contains many noxious substances that are absorbed into the body and can cause damage to tissues. In addition to lung cancer, emphysema and cardiovascular disease, these noxious substances are associated with a variety of dermatological effects, including:

- yellow-brown tobacco staining of the fingers and nails
- smoker's comedones – large open pores representing sebaceous gland ducts
- smoker's gingiva – discolouring of the gingival membranes of the mouth
- smoker's moustache – yellow-brown discolouring of facial hair
- smoker's face – characterized as deep wrinkles that radiate at right angles from the lips and corners of the eyes, together with numerous wrinkles over the face.

In long-term smokers, the facial bones eventually become more prominent, giving a gaunt appearance, and the skin becomes thin and discoloured (see *Figure 12.7*).

Hormones. The skin is sensitive to sex hormones, in particular oestrogen. Oestrogen replacement therapy has many effects on the skin, including the reversal of age-related epidermal thinning. Hormone replacement therapy has also been shown to improve the production of sebum, increase hydration and improve the elasticity of the skin in menopausal women. The most common effect of the menopause is skin flushes, known as 'hot flushes', caused by poor control of peripheral blood vessels due to reduced oestrogen production. A high level of oestrogen, as occurs during pregnancy, is associated with hair growth, while a low level of oestrogen, as occurs with the onset of the menopause, is associated with hair loss (alopecia).

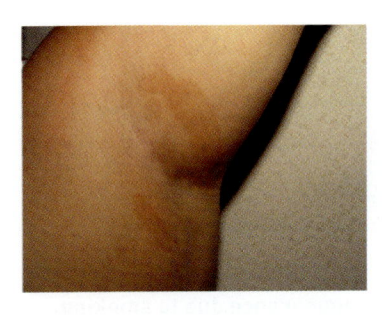

Figure 12.8 – **An example of axillary (armpit) intertrigo due to erythrasma.**
This rash occurs under skin folds and is associated with obesity. Reproduced with permission from DermNet NZ.

Food

Like any organ, the skin requires adequate nutrition to meet its metabolic needs and to maintain integrity and optimal function. Nutritional deficiency or excess can become evident in the skin; for example, the rapid weight gain of obesity can result in stretch marks and large skin folds on which a friction-induced rash commonly develops. This can become infected, giving rise to **erythrasma** or **intertrigo** (illustrated in *Figure 12.8*). Extreme forms of malnutrition are sometimes a cause of depigmentation or even hyperpigmentation of the skin and altered quality of hair, as in kwashiorkor, which is caused by inadequate dietary protein intake.

Vitamin deficiencies or excess can cause changes to the skin. Vitamin A is required for differentiation, proliferation and keratinization of the epidermis, while B-complex vitamins and vitamin C have a role in the maintenance of structural integrity. Vitamin C deficiency causes **scurvy** through impaired synthesis of collagen, affecting the skin, bones and blood vessels. Vitamin D is synthesized in the skin (discussed in greater detail later in this chapter). A micronutrient of importance for the skin is zinc; the skin normally accumulates approximately 20% of the total zinc in the body and most of this can be found in the epidermis. Within the skin, zinc acts to accelerate cell division and also functions as an antioxidant. Clinically, zinc supplementation is sometimes prescribed to patients in an attempt to accelerate wound healing, but strong evidence to demonstrate a clear benefit of this therapy has yet to be established.

Skin colour

Our understanding about the skin is mostly based on information gained from the study of pale Caucasian populations. This group tends to reflect a Western cultural obsession for attempting to delay the effects of ageing and has, to date, formed the largest consumer group for the marketing of cosmetic products. However, Asian

---

BOX 12.2

Factors affecting the care of skin in relation to colour and ethnicity

- Variation in colour – although darker skin possesses better defences against UV radiation, a good broad-spectrum sunscreen should be used with a protection factor of at least Sun Protection Factor (SPF) 15.
- Darkening of the skin called 'post-inflammatory hyperpigmentation' may occur after injury. Early treatment and regular sunscreen use can minimize this.
- Dry 'ashy skin' affects skin of all colours but can be a cause of distress with darker skin tones. Moisturizers can help. Pomades or hair oils can relieve a dry scalp and itching, but can also cause seborrhoea (oily skin) and acne.
- African hair is tightly curled on the head and beard. Excessive hair straightening and braiding can cause hair to become brittle and fall out.
- Shaving is associated with 'pseudofolliculitis barbae'. As hair grows, it can grow into the skin, causing irritation and inflammation. A careful shaving and washing regime can help to minimize this.

Table 12.2 – Ethnic differences in skin

Biological factor	Therapeutic implications
Epidermis	
Increased melanin content, melanosomal dispersion in people with skin of colour	Lower rates of skin cancer in people of colour Less pronounced photo-ageing Pigmentation disorders due to biological predisposition and cultural factors (for example, use of skin-lightening agents)
Dermis	
Multinucleated and larger fibroblasts in black compared with white persons	Greater incidence of keloid formation in black compared with white persons
Hair	
Curved hair follicle/spiral hair type in black compared with white persons, and fewer elastic fibres anchoring hair follicles to dermis in black compared with white persons	Pseudofolliculitis in black persons who shave Use of hair products that may lead to hair and scalp disorders in black persons Increased incidence of alopecia in black women

Adapted from **Taylor, S. C.** (2002). Skin of color: biology, structure, function, and implications for dermatologic disease. *Journal of the American Academy of Dermatology*, **46**: S41–S62.

populations and people with darker pigmented skin account for over half of the world's total population. Some biological differences and therapeutic implications for ethnic differences in skin are summarized in *Table 12.2*. *Box 12.2* also presents some factors relating to colour and ethnicity in the general care of skin.

Melanin, the principal pigment that determines skin colour, occurs in three main forms (see *Box 12.3*). Regardless of colour, all skin is susceptible to the effects of intrinsic and extrinsic processes, especially photo-damage due to exposure to sunlight. It is the distribution, type and amount of melanin produced by melanocytes that protects DNA against UV-induced photo-damage. The more melanin is produced, the darker the skin colour will be. This is genetically determined, but it is highly responsive to environmental stimulation by UV light, such that darker skin is more resistant to photo-ageing than lighter skin, and darker skin is probably less prone to the development of wrinkles. Melanin itself is composed of three distinct compounds that, in varying amounts, provide the main skin tones (see *Box 12.3*).

Skin can be classified according to the 'Fitzpatrick score', which predicts the resistance of skin to exposure to sunlight based on a subjective evaluation of skin colour (see *Table 12.3*); this classification system is commonly used by clinicians to predict responses to therapy and exposure to sunlight.

> **BOX 12.3**
>
> ### Skin colour
>
> Skin colour is varied, determined by a variety of compounds called chromophores. Melanin is the most important compound.
>
> | Chromophore | Responsible for: |
> |---|---|
> | Haemoglobin | Pinkish colour of Caucasians |
> | Oxyhaemoglobin | Pinkish colour of Caucasians |
> | Carotenoids | Yellow, orange and various shades in between in Asian and Mediterranean skin types |
> | Melanin | Black and suntanned skin |
> | Pheomelanin | – soluble, light yellow or red |
> | Eumelanin | – enriched, soluble, light brown |
> | Eumelanin | – enriched, insoluble dark brown or black |

Table 12.3 – The Fitzpatrick skin classification scale

Fitzpatrick classification	Skin type
Type I	Never tans, always burns (extremely fair skin, blonde hair, blue/green eyes)
Type II	Occasionally tans, usually burns (fair skin, sandy/brown hair, green/brown eyes)
Type III	Tans on average, sometimes burns (medium skin, brown hair, brown eyes)
Type IV	Usually tans, rarely burns (olive skin, brown/black hair, dark brown/black eyes)
Type V	Mostly tans, almost never burns (dark brown skin, black hair, black eyes)
Type VI	Never burns (black skin, black hair, black eyes)

Sunlight and vitamin D

Some wavelengths of ultraviolet sunlight are able to penetrate the skin sufficiently to even reach circulating blood cells, and these wavelengths possess sufficient energy to damage DNA within cells. Most of this damage can be repaired by endogenous DNA repair processes. If the damage is extensive, then cell death might occur by apoptosis and this will prevent the accumulation of mutations in DNA being passed to future generations of cells. However, excessive exposure to sunlight over time is associated with an accumulation of DNA 'photolesions' in skin cells and suppression of immune responses, increasing the risk of developing skin cancer (see *Box 12.4*). Diagnosis of malignant melanoma, a form of skin cancer, has increased rapidly since 1970, and statistics summarized by Cancer Research UK estimate that 37 people are diagnosed with malignant melanoma in the UK every day. Some of this is due to better surveillance and early detection, but most of this is considered to be linked to greater sun exposure, an increase in foreign holidays and greater use of sunbeds. Thus, sunlight can be thought of as a potent carcinogen. This increase is thought to be related primarily to an increased exposure of skin to sunlight, brought about by altered clothing habits and an increase in the length of time spent in direct sunlight.

> **BOX 12.4**
>
> ### The ABCDE of moles
>
> Moles (melanocytic naevi) are skin lesions composed of a collection of melanocytes. The ABCDE method can be used to check moles for the following signs, which may indicate a melanoma:
>
> - **A**symmetrical – the melanoma has two very different halves and is an irregular shape
> - Irregular **B**order – unlike a normal mole, a melanoma has a notched or ragged border
> - Two (or more) **C**olours – the melanoma will be a mix of two or more colours
> - Large **D**iameter – unlike most moles, melanomas are larger than 6 mm in diameter
> - Raised **E**levation – the melanoma will feel slightly raised above the surface of the skin
>
> Images of melanomas for comparison purposes can be found at:
> www.nhs.uk/Tools/Documents/mole_a_visual_guide.html

Exposure to sunlight is the most important source of vitamin D, but dietary sources (oily fish, such as salmon, is the richest dietary source of vitamin D) can be important, especially when factors such as seasonal changes, living at high latitudes, ageing and a dark pigmented skin limit vitamin D synthesis in the skin.

Approximately 90% of vitamin D is obtained from sunlight. Ultraviolet B radiation (wavelength 290–315 nm) converts 7-dehydrocholesterol into pre-vitamin D, which is quickly converted within the skin into vitamin D_3. This circulates in the blood until it reaches the liver and eventually the kidneys, where it is converted into the active form 1,25-dihydroxyvitamin D_3. The amount of vitamin D produced is dependent on the time of day that sun exposure occurs, latitude, season, use of sunscreen, age, how much skin is exposed and skin colour. People with black African skin (Fitzpatrick classification IV–VI; see *Table 12.3*) can produce up to 99% *less* vitamin D than Caucasian people exposed to the same amount of UV light.

In cells that express the vitamin D_3 receptor, vitamin D performs a variety of roles; for example, in intestinal cells, the vitamin D_3 receptor increases calcium absorption and interacts with osteoblasts in bone to regulate calcium homeostasis

> **BOX 12.5**
>
> ### Factors that can damage skin
>
> - Mechanical – pressure and friction, including stress and shear forces
> - Chemical – urine, faeces, soaps and cosmetics
> - Vascular – insufficient blood flow, diabetes, peripheral vessels and trauma
> - Infection – *Candida* (yeast), impetigo (bacterial), herpes simplex (virus)
> - Allergy – exposure to an irritant, inflammation, blistering and rashes
> - UV radiation – inflammation, blistering, DNA damage and cancer risk

(see *Chapter 13*). Vitamin D also interacts with immune cells and regulates production of the hormone renin. The levels and activity of vitamin D are important in the development of a wide range of disorders including bone diseases such as rickets and osteoporosis, susceptibility to infection, and autoimmune and cardiovascular diseases.

It is unclear how much sunlight a person should receive, as it is not known how much sun exposure is actually required to maintain healthy levels of vitamin D. Current advice is to follow the 'SunSmart' campaign guidelines (www.sunsmart.org.uk). This advice is aimed at avoiding UV-induced skin damage and therefore reducing the increased incidence of skin cancers observed in the UK population over recent decades. However, the majority of the UK population has been estimated to be deficient in vitamin D, and so a sensible balance of exposure to sunlight is required: sufficient to allow adequate vitamin D synthesis but without incurring damage to skin (this includes seeking a suntan). Nutritional supplementation with vitamin D is currently recommended in the UK for pregnant and breast-feeding mothers and for their children, from the age of 6 months to 5 years. The Department of Health also recommends that people over the age of 65 years not be exposed to the sun, and also take a daily vitamin D supplement.

Skin hygiene and vulnerability

The maintenance of skin integrity can be described by the bricks and mortar model described earlier, (see *Figure 12.2*) with the cells (bricks) and surrounding matrix (mortar) functioning to maintain an effective barrier to water loss and retain the correct amount of water in the skin; failing this, skin can become too dry or too moist.

Dry scaly skin is often due to the loss of water from the stratum corneum, resulting in skin that is less flexible and more easily damaged. This can be induced by frequent or aggressive washing; soaps often have a high pH (>pH 7.0), which, by leaving irritant residues on the skin, can dissolve lipids, denature proteins and reduce the thickness of the stratum corneum. In addition, vigorous towel drying further removes cells by mechanical forces. These factors each facilitate the loss of water from the epidermal matrix, contributing to dry skin conditions. A variety of factors that contribute to skin damage are listed in *Box 12.5*.

Employees exposed to excessive amounts of cleaning agents, such as hairdressers, workers in the food and engineering industries, and healthcare workers, are at increased risk of damage to the skin. Patients suffering with incontinence requiring frequent washing are especially at risk. Urine and faeces are highly irritating, acting to reduce the integrity of the stratum corneum, which becomes compromised further by frequent washing (see Bessie, Patient 4.1).

Excessive hydration of skin exposed to water for long periods reduces the barrier function of the epidermis because the normal balance of water content within the skin is disturbed. The penetration of irritants may increase, facilitating the development of contact dermatitis, and the growth of normal flora may also be altered, supporting the growth of pathogens. In extreme cases, the skin can become **excoriated**, that is, the epidermal surface can be removed, and this can be made worse by mechanical forces, especially over areas prone to pressure ulcers

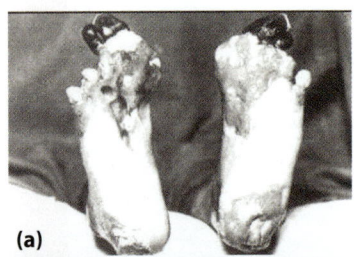

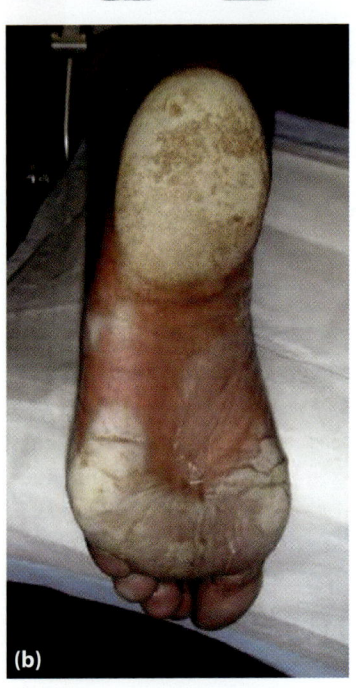

Figure 12.9 – Examples of immersion foot.
(a) A severe case of immersion foot, a type of non-freezing cold injury leading to excoriated and macerated skin. (b) Mild forms of immersion foot still occur today, for example in military personnel unable to change or dry their boots, or in homeless people, and have even been reported in people attending music festivals! Reproduced with permission of MSN, FNP-BC, Neighborhood Service Organization, Detroit, MI.

in immobile patients. A severe form of injury known as 'trench foot' or 'immersion foot' can occur when feet are kept wet for long periods of time (see *Figure 12.9a*). The skin becomes macerated (essentially, waterlogged), skin integrity is lost and layers of the skin easily shed from the body (illustrated in *Figure 12.9b*).

Moisturizing agents, often applied as creams and ointments, are available in a variety of forms. They are used to prevent further loss of moisture and also to attract water to the skin. These agents help to make the skin supple and aid repair of a damaged epidermal barrier. They are also commonly used to protect the skin from further irritant damage with patients who experience faecal and urinary incontinence. There are two main types of moisturizing agents:

- Occlusive moisturizers physically prevent water loss from the stratum corneum by limiting evaporative water loss and simultaneously may also help to restore the normal lipid barrier of the skin.
- Humectant moisturizers prevent water loss by attracting water molecules from the deeper dermal structures to the epidermis and also restore the lipid composition of the skin.

Moisturizing preparations may also have additional lubrication, soothing and softening properties, and some contain antimicrobial compounds. They provide a useful addition, along with other considerations (considered in *Box 12.6*), for the maintenance of skin hygiene and integrity, especially in people with sensitive skin or those vulnerable to a loss of skin integrity.

12.2.3 Wound healing

The skin is a dynamic organ responsive to physical damage. Any physical damage or loss of skin must be repaired to limit fluid loss from the body and reduce the risk of infection. Wound healing can be observed to involve a series of complex overlapping physiological phases, with the goal being to restore an effective barrier and normal function (see *Figure 12.10*):

BOX 12.6

General tips for looking after the skin

- Assess for risk such as sensitive skin, immobility and incontinence
- Assess for sensitivity
- Wash only when necessary
- Remove irritants such as urine and faeces as soon as possible
- Use just enough non-perfumed soap with a neutral pH – consider the use of oil or an emollient instead
- Avoid very hot water and change this frequently. Avoid long periods of soaking skin in water, such as a bath
- Dry with minimal friction – patting dry might be best
- Apply an emollient or barrier preparation *sparingly, without rubbing* as soon as practicable, to limit water loss and protect the epidermal barrier

- **Inflammation**: changes in local blood supply occur, together with inflammatory processes (described in *Chapter 11*). This prepares the wound for healing by the process of phagocytosis, which removes foreign material such as dirt and microorganisms from the wound. Inflammatory processes also stimulate and regulate the other phases of wound healing.
- **Proliferation**: following acute inflammation, wounds are filled with new cells to replace those lost to trauma and infection. New blood vessels begin to form (**angiogenesis**) and fibroblasts prepare new connective tissue by secreting the fibrous proteins elastin and collagen. This provides some structural strength to the wound and causes the edges of the wound to contract.
- **Epithelialization**: gradually, epithelial cells begin to migrate across the wound surface, and when completely covered, the epithelial cells begin to differentiate, forming a multi-layered epidermis.

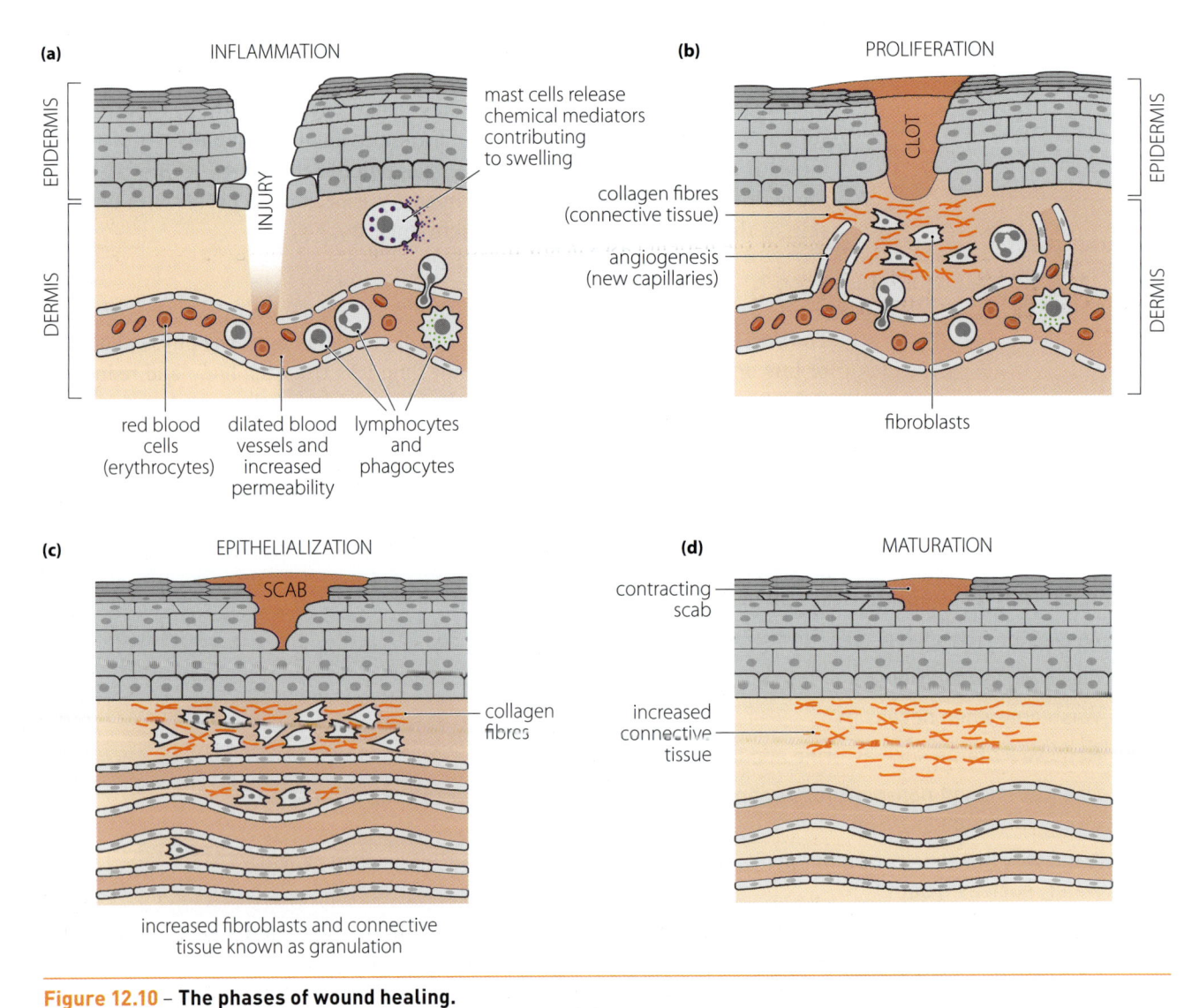

Figure 12.10 – **The phases of wound healing.**
(a) Inflammation; (b) proliferation; (c) epithelialization; and (d) maturation. Note that these phases can often overlap.

- **Maturation:** in this final stage, fibroblasts become less active, connective tissue becomes more organized and the wound gains greater strength. Larger amounts of connective tissue and a reduction in inflammatory responses often leave newly healed wounds with a pale, smooth and flat appearance (scar). Scars become visibly evident when a wound is large and extensive connective tissue forms a scar.

Some wounds can be very hard to heal, and the factors that influence this include ageing skin, effects of disease processes such as inflammatory disease, circulatory disorders and diabetes mellitus (see David, Patient 5.1). High glucose levels cause microvascular changes, which reduce blood flow in patients with diabetes. This causes complications including wounds that are slow to heal, typically in the legs or feet; diabetes is one of the leading risk factors for amputation of a lower limb. In addition, hormonal or nutritional status and the effects of medication such as oral steroids can influence wound healing. Social and psychological factors are also important, as some patients might not be able to recognize that their skin integrity has deteriorated, or they may have lost the motivation or ability to care for their own skin.

12.3 Clinical application

The skin is an interface between the external and internal environments and as such it must provide a competent epidermal barrier to protect the tissues beneath. Each of the patient cases below illustrates compromised integrity to the epithelial barrier in different ways.

- Bessie (Patient 4.1) has developed macerated skin from long-term exposure to irritant body fluids.
- Giuseppe (Patient 12.1) has thermal burns from misadventure while cooking.
- Daphne and Joe (Patients 12.2) are at risk of sunburn.
- Audrey (Patient 12.3) has cut her hand – her skin has become vulnerable due to the effects of ageing.

Each of these patients requires a detailed and specific response from healthcare professionals, not only to protect the skin but to limit further tissue damage and to aid repair of the epithelial barrier.

Patient 4.1 | **Bessie** | 99 | 130 | 379 | **397** | 403 | 441

- 71-year-old woman
- Lifelong smoker –20 cigarettes per day
- Found unconscious with stroke and hemiplegia
- Skin damage and incontinence suggests unconscious for >24h
- Macerated skin dressed
- Pressure ulcers will develop without extra care

After having her immediate clinical needs taken care of, Bessie was gently washed with a pH-neutral soap and water. The skin surfaces were thoroughly rinsed with fresh warm water and her skin carefully dried by gentle patting with a warm soft towel. A lipid-based barrier compound was sprayed onto the non-macerated areas of her skin without rubbing and dry non-adherent dressings were applied to cover and protect the macerated areas, prior to further detailed assessment by the tissue viability team. Ongoing care for Bessie is likely to be complex, requiring careful assessment, planning, implementation and evaluation of nursing and clinical care that will take account of how best to improve and maintain her physiological and holistic needs.

Bessie is a patient with a high risk of developing pressure ulcers due to her age and probable impaired mobility as a result of her stroke. Reference to up-to-date clinical guidelines for the management and prevention of pressure ulcers, such as those available from the National Institute for Health and Care Excellence (http://www.nice.org.uk/guidance/cg179), would be very a useful resource, to inform the management of this patient.

Patient 12.1 — Giuseppe — 380 | 398

- 41-year-old man
- Badly burnt on head, chest and arms
- Lund and Browder chart estimates burn area at 27%; increased risk of hypovolaemic shock
- Lost fluids replaced via IV cannula

Giuseppe suffered a mixture of deep and superficial burns to his head, both arms and chest. First aid was rapidly provided by irrigating Giuseppe's upper body with copious amounts of water. The aim of this was to help cool the skin tissue quickly and to minimize skin loss.

On arrival at the hospital, assessment of the burn area was estimated using the Lund and Browder chart to be 27% (see *Figure 12.3*). Giuseppe's skin appeared red, and was painful and very sensitive. Although extensively burnt, Giuseppe's burns were initially assessed as superficial burns affecting the epidermis only. Deep burns are generally not painful because of the destruction of nerve endings.

Due to the extent of the burns (in excess of 15% of body surface area), fluid loss increased the risk of **hypovolaemic shock**. Two major potential complications of extensive burns are fluid loss and an increased risk of infection, simply due to loss of the epidermal barrier. The larger the surface area of a burn, the greater the risk.

Clinical staff inserted an intravenous cannula and assessed Giuseppe for replacement of lost body fluids by the intravenous route. A variety of intravenous solutions are available and a number of formulae are used to help clinicians decide how much fluid to administer to a patient, taking into account the extent of burns, the size of the patient and other related factors.

Some serum-filled blisters, which occurred over a period of hours, were left intact where possible in order to minimize the risk of infection and of causing additional pain. Fluid collected in blisters assessed as likely to burst, or present in awkward areas such as skin folds, was selectively aspirated under aseptic conditions.

Patient 12.2 — Daphne and Joe — 380 | 398

- Newly-wed couple going to Australia for 3 months
- Found SunSmart advice to minimise sun damage while there

Joe found the 'SunSmart' sun behaviour recommendations so that he and Daphne could enjoy their holiday in Australia, while minimizing the risk of sun damage to them both. He also found a simple guide to help recognize the difference between a normal mole on the skin and an abnormal, possibly cancerous lesion such as a melanoma (see *Box 12.4*).

SunSmart recommendations:

- Spend time in the shade between 11:00 and 15:00
- Use clothing to cover up exposed skin and use shade wherever possible
- Obtain sunscreen that is classified as at least SPF 15 and use generously and regularly

CHAPTER 13 | Achieving movement

Learning points for this chapter

After working through this chapter, you should be able to:

- Describe the general structure and function of the skeleton
- Describe the classification of bones and explain the process of bone formation
- Describe the structure of the synovial joint
- Discuss the similarities and differences between different types of muscle
- Describe the microscopic structure of skeletal muscle and the events leading to muscle contraction
- Discuss how bones and muscles enable movement and how movement is coordinated

13.1 Introduction and clinical relevance

Each patient in this chapter highlights the importance of movement and the way this is achieved by the function of bones and muscles, together with associated structures such as ligaments and tendons. The role of the nervous system in coordinating any movement is illustrated by Bessie (Patient 4.1) who was unable to move because of muscle weakness, by Graham (Patient 4.3) who developed tremor in both of his hands with rigidity and by Sally (Patient 6.1) who needed to use a wheelchair because of her inability to move. The three patients in this chapter illustrate how the structure, organization and function of bones, joints and muscles enable movement to occur in a person and what can happen when some of these structures are damaged by disease processes, as in Sally (Patient 6.1).

| Patient 4.1 | Bessie | 99 | 130 | 379 | 397 | **403** | 441 |

- 71-year-old woman
- Lifelong smoker —20 cigarettes per day
- Found unconscious (>24h) with stroke and hemiplegia
- Macerated skin dressed
- Pressure ulcers will develop without extra care

Bessie was found unconscious on the floor of her kitchen. She regained consciousness while in the ambulance but her speech was slurred and she had saliva drooling from her mouth. On arrival at the hospital, Bessie was observed to have weakness to the limbs on the right side of her body (right hemiplegia) caused by a left-sided stroke.

| Patient 4.3 | Graham | 100 | 132 | **404** | 442 |

- 57-year-old man
- Gradual onset of trembling in left hand
- Family doctor referred him to neurologist
- Diagnosis of Parkinson disease led to depression
- MRI has excluded other causes
- Prescribed bromocriptine to help with Parkinson symptoms

Graham, a 57-year-old man who was working as a carpenter, noticed that his tremor was getting worse in both hands and he told his family doctor that he feels some rigidity in the joints, he is more tired and experiences some pain in his hands. His family doctor decided to start Graham on treatment for Parkinson's disease and discussed this with him and his wife. Graham now takes co-beneldopa capsules three times a day. Co-beneldopa capsules contain a mixture of benserazide hydrochloride 25 mg and levodopa 100 mg.

| Patient 6.1 | Sally | 167 | 188 | **404** | 443 |

- 50-year-old woman
- Has MS and is now a wheelchair user
- Burning sensation in her hands and double vision
- MRI confirms plaques in her brain consistent with MS

Sally was a school teacher who, at the age of 35, developed problems with her vision and had a burning sensation in her hands. Following a long period of investigations, which included a lumbar puncture, visual evoked potentials and magnetic resonance imaging (MRI), a diagnosis of multiple sclerosis was reached. Now at the age of 50, Sally is disabled. She uses a wheelchair and requires hoisting from bed to chair and into the bath. Sally has a long-term self-retaining (indwelling) catheter as she has lost the ability to control micturition.

An evolutionary process (see *Chapter 1*) resulted in *Homo sapiens* (humans or modern man) evolving from moving on all four limbs to an erect position. It has been suggested by paleobiologists that the adoption of the erect posture was necessary to enable humans to view objects much farther away and to use their upper limbs for other functions such as improved manual dexterity.

The intricate manoeuvres of a gymnast performing on a beam not only demonstrate spatial awareness but are also achieved by the coordinated functions of bones of the skeleton and their attachments, which include muscles, ligaments and tendons. Indeed, while talent and practice are important to achieve the delicate movements, coordination of the movements is necessary for completing daily tasks requiring spatial awareness and integration by the nervous system (see *Chapter 4*).

13.2 What you need to know – essential anatomy and physiology

13.2.1 Bones

General structure of the skeleton

The human skeleton (see *Figure 13.1*) is divided into two main divisions, namely the **axial skeleton** and the **appendicular skeleton**, and is made up of 206 bones. The axial skeleton forms the axis of the skeleton or the trunk from which other bones are anchored, and is made up of the skull, ribcage, sternum and spinal column, while the appendicular skeleton is made up of the bones of the limbs and girdles. Joints are formed where bones meet, and other tissues such as **cartilage**, **ligaments** and **tendons** complete the structure of the joints, ensuring that various forms of movement are possible.

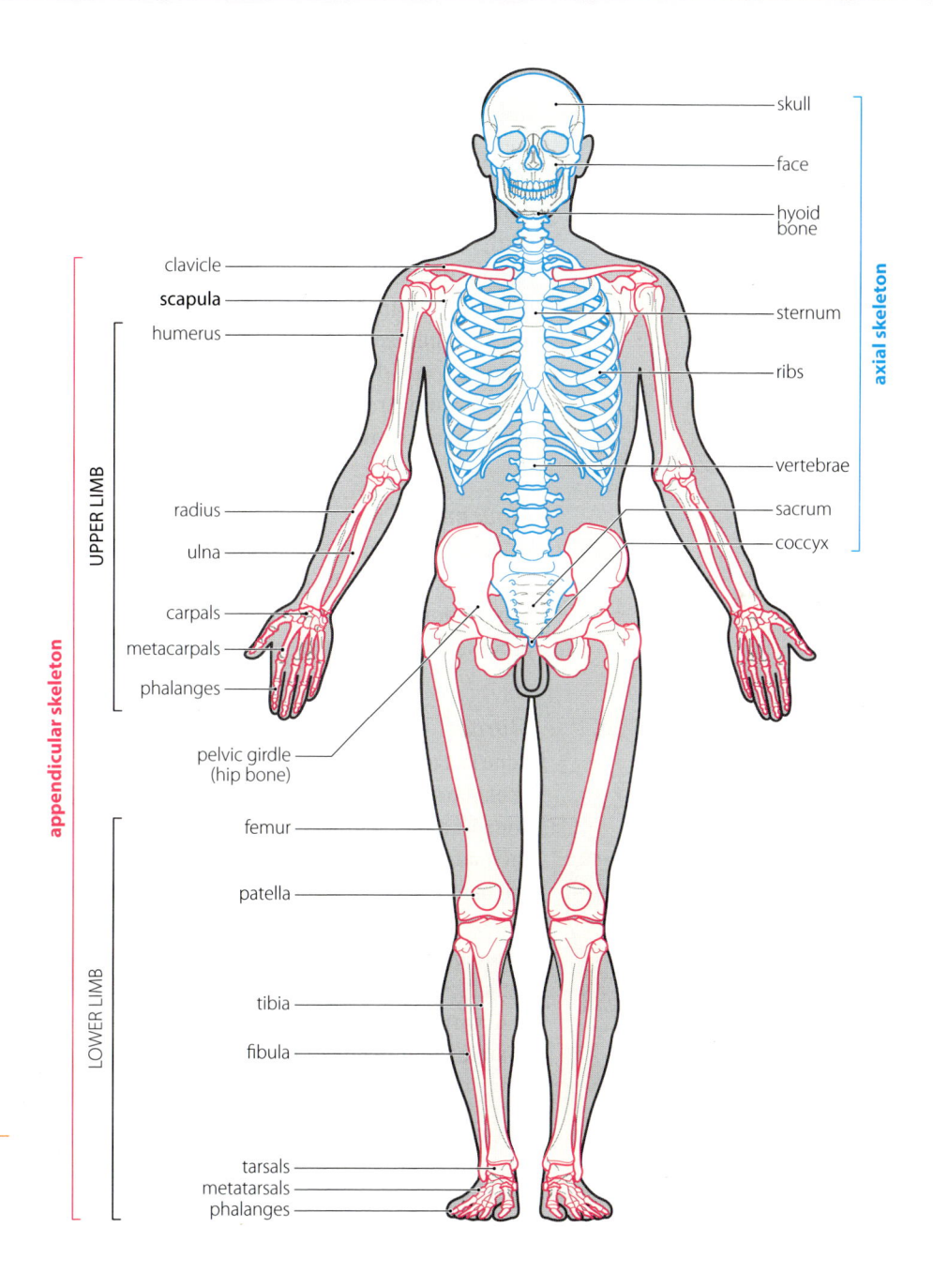

Figure 13.1 – The skeleton, showing the axial and appendicular skeletons.

Functions of the skeleton

Support
The skeleton is the framework of the body from which other soft tissues are supported and anchored.

Protection
Delicate tissues and organs such as the brain and spinal cord are protected by the skull and spinal column, respectively. The ribcage protects delicate organs within the thoracic cavity such as the lungs and the heart.

Formation of blood cells

Haematopoiesis, or the formation of blood cells, occurs from stem cells in the red bone marrow. In infants, all bone marrow is red and is found in all flat bones, in the medullary cavity of all long bones and in cancellous (spongy) bone. As the child grows, some of the red bone marrow is converted to yellow bone marrow. In adults, the red bone marrow in the medullary cavity of long bones is replaced by fat and hence the marrow is known as yellow bone marrow. As a result, red bone marrow is found only in the flat bones such as the cranium, ribs and scapula, at the epiphyseal end of long bones such as the femur and humerus, and in the spongy bone (**diploë**) of the sternum and the coxal (hip) bone. The coxal bone and the sternum are the major sites for haematopoiesis in adults, whereas the femur and humerus are major sites in children.

Movement

It is the attachment of ligaments and tendons to bones and muscles that forms lever systems, enabling varying degrees of movement to be achieved. However, it is important to remember that it is the brain that initiates and regulates the process of coordinated movement (discussed in *Chapter 4*).

Storage

Bone is a major reservoir for important minerals, the most abundant being calcium, phosphorus and magnesium (see *Chapter 7*). The movement of minerals from bone to blood and vice versa is a homeodynamic process influenced by hormones such as parathyroid hormone and calcitonin (see *Chapter 5*). For example, during the menopause, oestrogen levels decline, resulting in reduced bone density due to loss of calcium. This increases the risk of osteoporosis, a condition in which bones become weak and fragile. Adequate calcium intake in adolescence increases bone density, reducing the risks associated with osteoporosis in later life. Thus, calcium and hormone metabolism throughout the lifespan determine the homeodynamic changes that occur to bone.

Classification of bones by shape

The bones of the human skeleton can be classified according to their shape (see *Table 13.1* and *Figure 13.2*).

Structure of bones

The long bones, such as the humerus and femur, have a tubular shaft in the middle that is known as the **diaphysis**, and an expanded head at each end called the **epiphysis** (see *Figure 13.3*). The diaphysis is made of **compact (dense) bone** and has a cavity of bone marrow known as the **medullary cavity**. The outermost part of the compact bone in the diaphysis region is surrounded by a double-layered membrane called the **periosteum**, to which ligaments and tendons attach. Perforating collagen fibres, also known as **Sharpey's fibres**, attach and secure the periosteum to the underlying bone structures. An opening known as a **nutrient foramen** is found in the diaphysis, and through this opening, blood vessels, lymphatic vessels and nerves enter the periosteum.

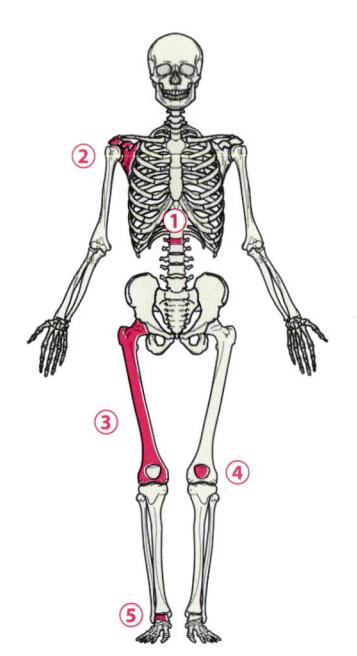

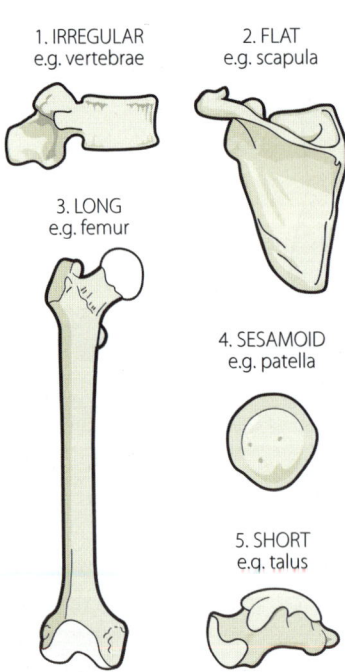

Figure 13.2 – Classification of bones by shape.
(1) Irregular bones (e.g. vertebra, coxae); (2) flat bones (e.g. skull, scapula); (3) long bones (e.g. femur, humerus); (4) sesamoid bone; and (5) short bones (e.g. tarsals, carpals).

Table 13.1 – Classification of bones by shape

Classification	Description
Long bones	The long bones consist of the bones of the upper limbs, namely the humerus, radius and ulna, and those of the lower limbs, namely the femur, tibia and fibula. These bones have a proximal part and a distal part (see *Chapter 1*). They have a head at both extremities and a shaft in the middle. Long bones are compact.
Short bones	The bones of the wrist and ankles are all short bones, are less compact and are made of spongy bone. Short bones usually have the shape of a cube.
Flat bones	As the name suggests, flat bones are flat and generally thin. They have spongy bone in between two thin layers of compact bone. Examples of flat bones include the skull, the sternum and the ribs.
Irregular bones	Other bones such as those of the vertebral column (spine) and the hip bones, which do not fit any of the classes described above, are known as irregular bones.
Sesamoid bones	Sesamoid bones are short, small, flat bones that are found near joints of the upper and lower limbs at the hands, knees and feet. They usually develop within tendons. The patella, commonly known as the kneecap, is an example of a sesamoid bone that develops within the quadriceps tendon.

The medullary cavity contains yellow bone marrow in adults. The part of the epiphysis that forms the joint is covered with articular hyaline cartilage. An **epiphyseal line** (see *Figure 13.3*) is found between the diaphysis and each epiphysis. The epiphyseal line represents the remains of an **epiphyseal plate** consisting of hyaline cartilage, which is responsible for lengthening the bone during childhood. The epiphysis is typically formed of cancellous or spongy bone. This has a honeycombed appearance formed by a lattice of **trabeculae**. The spaces within cancellous bone provide a highly vascular matrix facilitating haematopoiesis.

Bone formation, growth and development

Bone growth starts as hyaline cartilage, at a site known as the **primary ossification centre** (*Figure 13.4*). Chondrocytes secrete hyaline cartilage resulting in a cartilaginous matrix within the primary ossification centre of the shaft. As chondrocytes enlarge, more hyaline cartilage is produced causing the cartilaginous matrix to enlarge. The cartilaginous matrix surrounding the chondrocytes calcifies forming a cartilaginous calcified matrix. The enlarged chondrocytes stop producing cartilage and begin producing alkaline phosphatase, an enzyme needed to enable mineral deposition. As the cartilaginous matrix becomes increasingly calcified, diffusion of nutrients or waste products reduces and the chondrocytes eventually die. However, blood vessels grow into the area surrounding the shaft of the cartilage, and blood supply to the periosteum increases, facilitating the migration of fibroblasts into the cartilage. These fibroblasts differentiate into **osteoblasts**, which are bone-building cells. Osteoblasts also originate and differentiate from stem cells called **osteoprogenitor cells**. They synthesize proteins and other organic material such as osteocalcin and osteopontin that make up the bone matrix together with the minerals. This organic matter of bone matrix produced by osteoblasts is known as **osteoid**. The osteoblasts produce

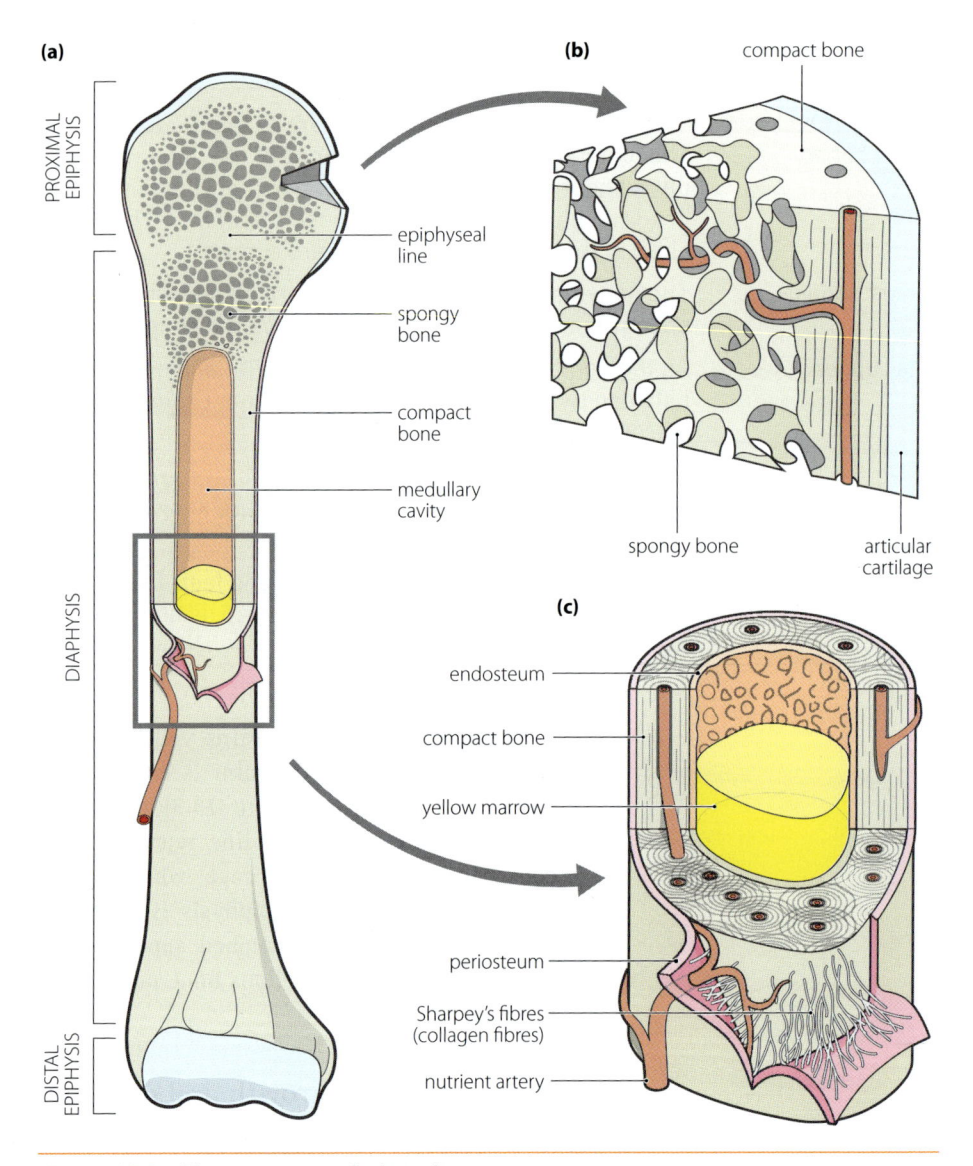

Figure 13.3 – The structure of a long bone.
(a) Anterior view with longitudinal section cut away; (b) three-dimensional view of spongy bone; and (c) cross-section of the diaphysis.

spongy bone, which replaces the calcified cartilaginous matrix as it disappears. Eventually, bone-remodelling cells called **osteoclasts** appear and create the marrow cavity by eroding the trabeculae. Osteoclasts secrete proteolytic enzymes and acids that dissolve bone matrix, thus remodelling the bone as well as releasing stored minerals. Primary ossification proceeds inwards from the external surface of the bone. This type of ossification in which hyaline cartilage is broken down as ossification proceeds and is replaced by bone occurs in the majority of bones with the exception of flat bones and is known as **endochondral ossification**.

During fetal growth and development, as the diaphysis elongates and a medullary cavity is formed, new centres of spongy bone growth known as secondary ossification centres form. From the diaphysis form the epiphyseal regions (see

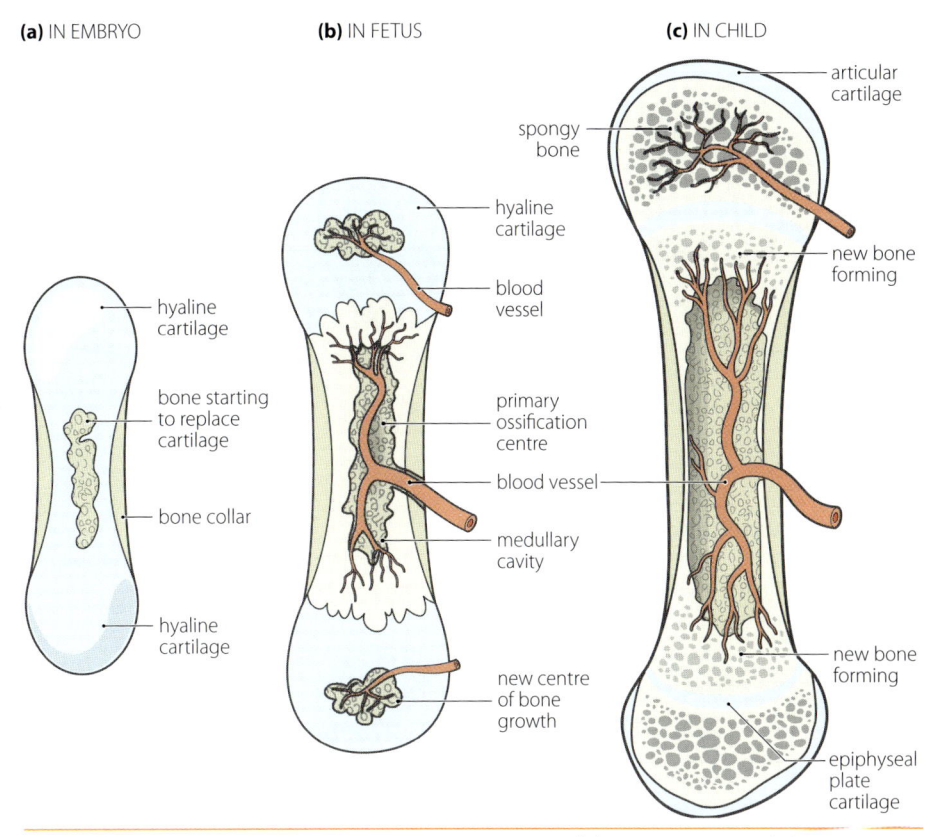

SECTION **13.2** | **WHAT YOU NEED TO KNOW – ESSENTIAL ANATOMY AND PHYSIOLOGY** 409

Figure 13.4 – **Stages in the formation of long bones (a) in the embryo, (b) in a fetus and (c) in a young child.**

Figure 13.4), which are separated from the diaphysis at either end by two narrow regions of epiphyseal cartilage called the epiphyseal plates. These form in a region called the metaphysis. The length of the bone will continue to increase as long as the epiphyseal cartilages continue to grow, which push the epiphyses further away. Osteoblasts invade the cartilage, continuously replacing it with bone, and secondary ossification occurs outwards from the centre of the epiphysis towards the outer part of the bone surface. During the growth spurt at puberty, bone growth is accelerated by the presence of growth hormone, thyroid hormones and the sex hormones.

In flat bones such as the skull, during fetal development a process less complex than endochondral ossification occurs, known as intramembranous ossification (see *Figure 13.5*). Cartilage is not present during intramembranous ossification. Instead, mesenchymal cells initiate intramembranous ossification by producing fibrous connective tissue, and they also differentiate into osteoblasts to form an ossification centre. The osteoblasts secrete osteoid (bone matrix), which quickly becomes mineralized. Some of the osteoblasts are trapped in the bone matrix, and these develop into osteocytes. As the bone matrix is laid between blood vessels, a network of trabeculae is formed. Cavities of cancellous bone containing red marrow are formed.

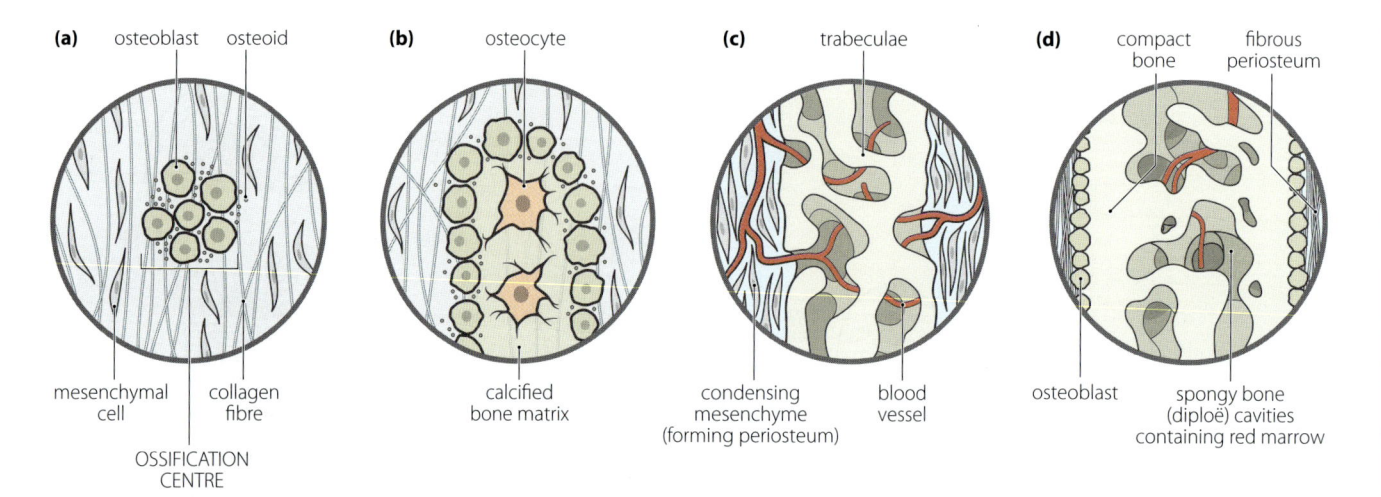

Figure 13.5 – Ossification of bone.
(a) Ossification in fibrous connective tissue; (b) bone matrix or osteoid in the fibrous membrane; (c) a network of trabeculae formed from accumulating osteoid (bone matrix); and (d) formation of compact bone and red bone marrow cavities.

Histology of bone

Compact bone

Bone is a type of connective tissue known as **osseous** tissue (see *Chapter 2*). When viewed under a microscope, the structure of compact bone appears as an arrangement of units known as **osteons**, which form the **Haversian system** consisting of a canal in the middle surrounded by concentric rings known as **lamellae** (singular = lamella) (see *Figure 13.6*). The **central canal**, also known as the **Haversian canal**, contains blood vessels and nerves. Collagen fibres and minerals are found in the lamellae; these are tough and flexible, allowing bone to bend a little without breaking. Mineral deposits, especially calcium phosphate, provide added density. The incorporation of magnesium, sodium and fluoride salts into the inorganic calcium salt hydroxyapatite forms approximately half the weight of the bone. Adequate consumption of calcium-rich foods during teenage years is required, especially in females, because bone density in females is promoted during this period with the help of hormones such as oestrogen. If the development of bone density is poor in adolescent years, particularly in girls, then osteoporosis may develop in later life around the onset of the menopause.

Within the periosteum are found other openings or canals that link up blood vessels and nerves of the periosteum with those of the central canal. Hollow spaces known as **lacunae** occur at the junctions of the lamellae, and the lacunae are connected to one another by a network of canals called **canaliculi**. The canaliculi also connect the lacunae to the central canal. Bone cells known as **osteocytes** are found in the lacunae. The homeodynamic function of osteocytes is to maintain the integrity of bone matrix by supplying it with nutrients such as proteins and minerals, and to respond to any stresses that could result in bone being damaged. Osteocytes ensure that information is relayed to osteoblasts and osteoclasts when bone damage has occurred, so that it can be repaired.

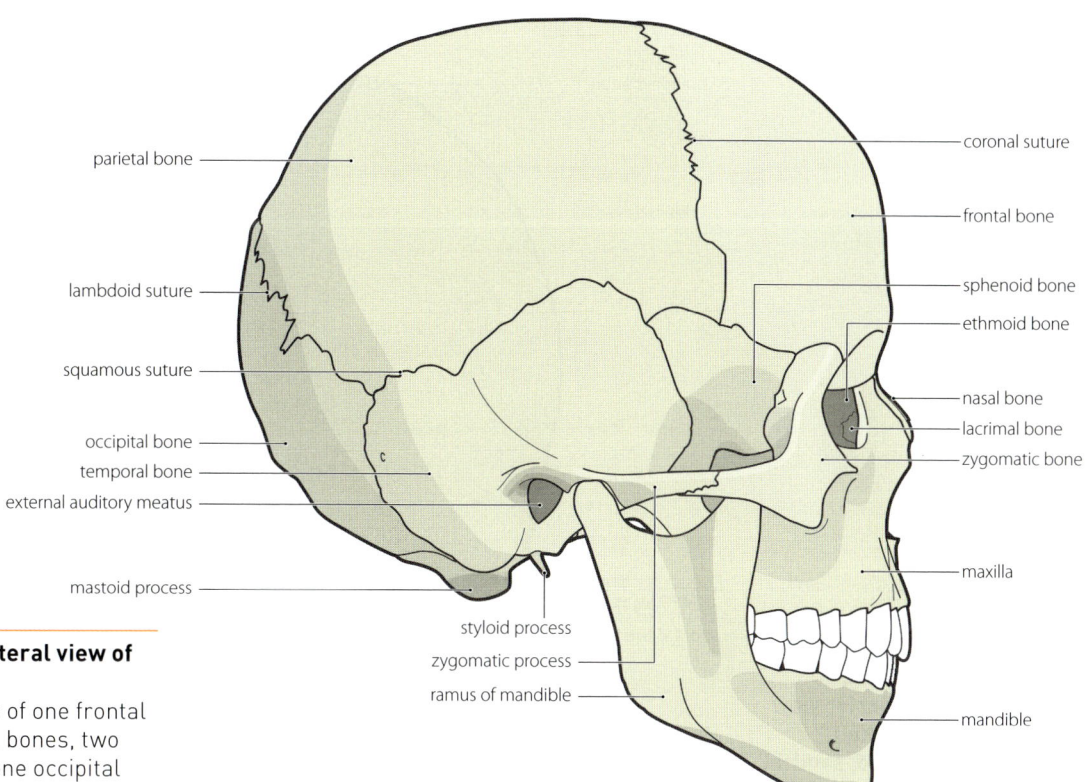

SECTION **13.2** | WHAT YOU NEED TO KNOW – ESSENTIAL ANATOMY AND PHYSIOLOGY 413

Figure 13.8 – **A lateral view of the human skull.**
The skull consists of one frontal bone, two parietal bones, two temporal bones, one occipital bone, one sphenoid bone and one ethmoid bone.

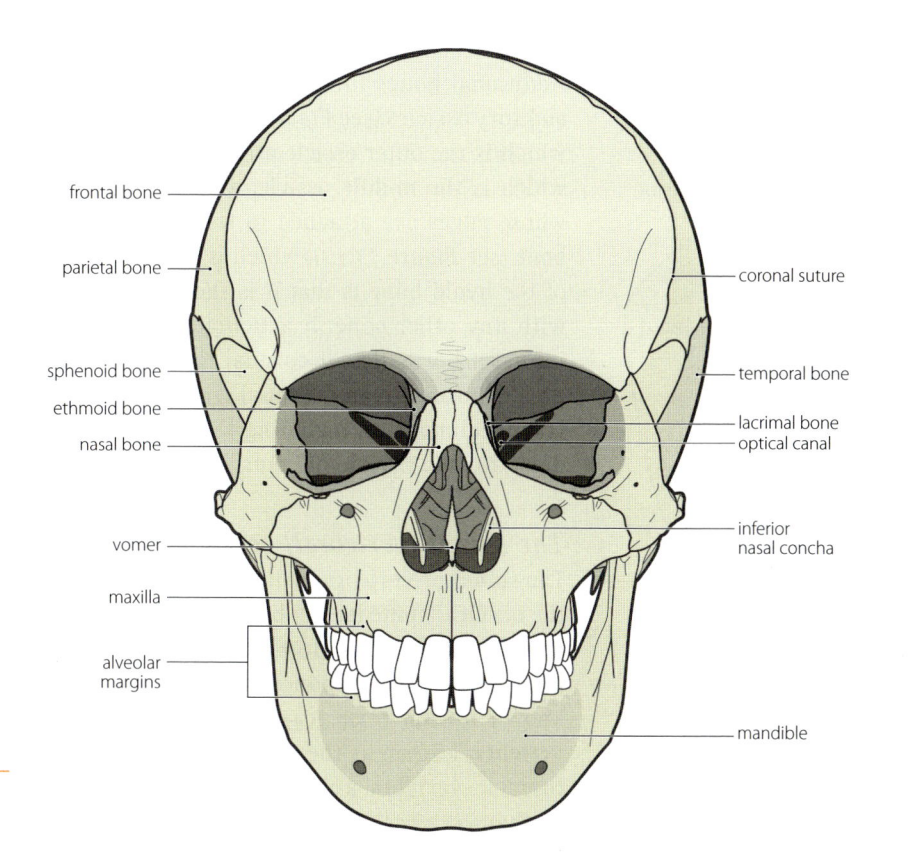

Figure 13.9 – **An anterior view of the human skull.**

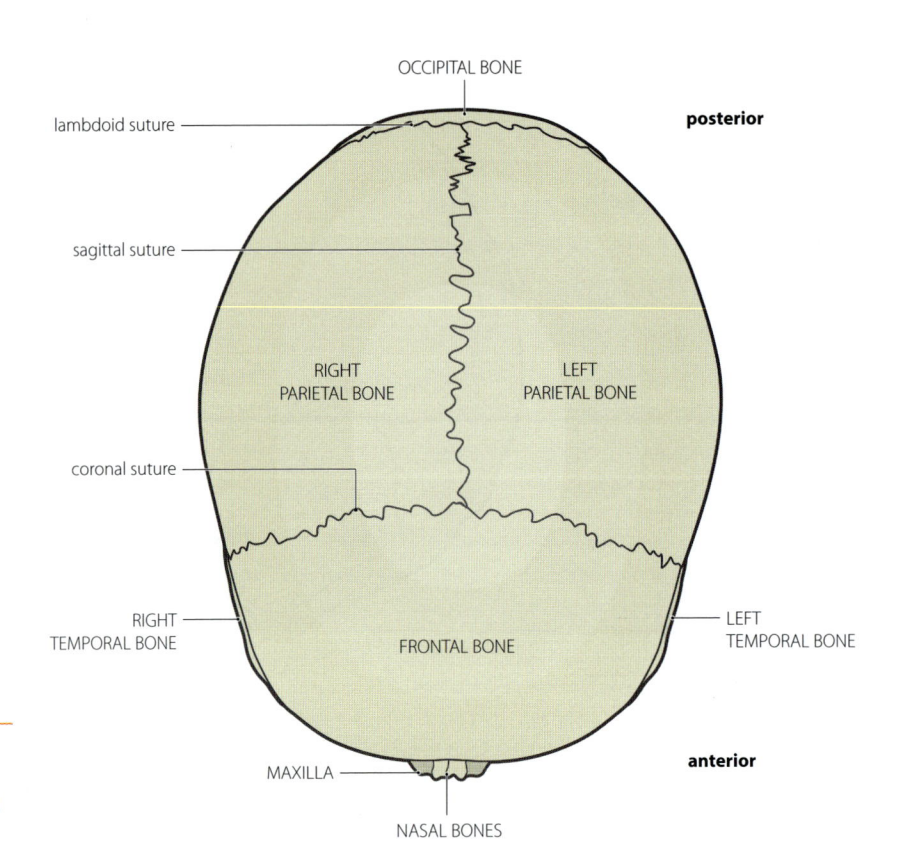

Figure 13.10 – A superior view of the adult human skull, showing the lambdoid, sagittal and coronal sutures.

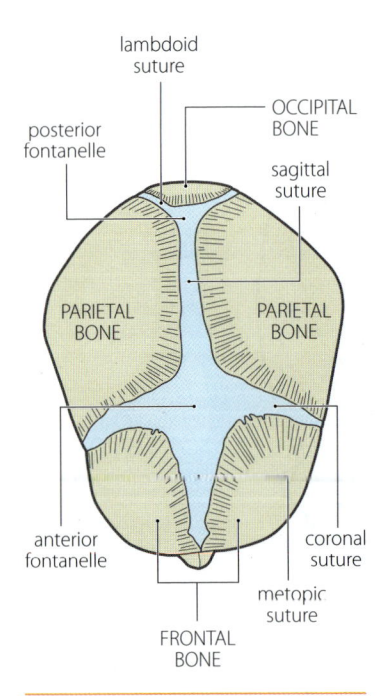

Figure 13.11 – A superior view of an infant skull, showing the anterior fontanelle and posterior (occipital) fontanelle.

Additional bones linked to the skull, also discussed in *Chapter 6*, are the three auditory ossicles (see *Figure 13.12*) of the middle ear, namely the malleus (hammer), which is the outer ossicle attached to the tympanic membrane, the incus (anvil), which is the middle ossicle, and the stapes (stirrup), which is the inner ossicle whose edges are attached to the oval window. An additional bone is the hyoid bone (see *Figure 13.13*), which is located in the neck. A very special characteristic of the hyoid bone is that it is the only bone in the body that does not articulate with any other bone. It articulates with the stylohyoid ligaments, which attach its lesser horns (lesser cornua) to the inferior aspect of the temporal bones. The greater horns (greater cornua) serve as attachment sites for several pharyngeal and laryngeal muscles, including the pharyngeal constrictor, hyoglossus, stylohyoid, digastric and mylohyoid muscles, as well as anchoring the tongue.

The spinal (vertebral) column

The spinal or vertebral column (see *Figure 13.14*) consists of 33 bones comprising the cervical spine (seven bones), thoracic spine (twelve bones), lumbar spine (five bones), sacral spine (five fused bones) and coccyx (four fused bones). All the individual vertebral bones articulate with each other. The first cervical vertebra, known as the atlas, carries the head, and it rotates on the second cervical vertebra, known as the axis. The seventh cervical bone articulates with the first thoracic vertebra and likewise the twelfth vertebra articulates with the first lumbar vertebra. The fifth lumbar vertebra articulates with the sacrum, which

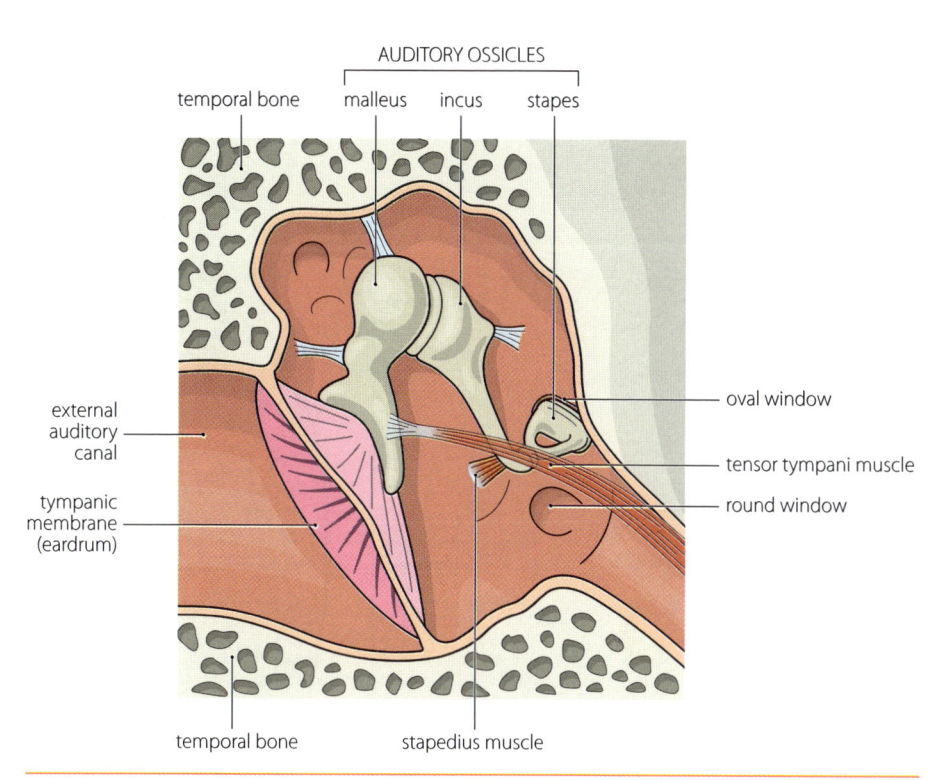

Figure 13.12 – **The ossicles of the middle ear.**
The positions of the malleus next to the tympanic membrane, the incus in the middle and the stapes near the oval window are shown.

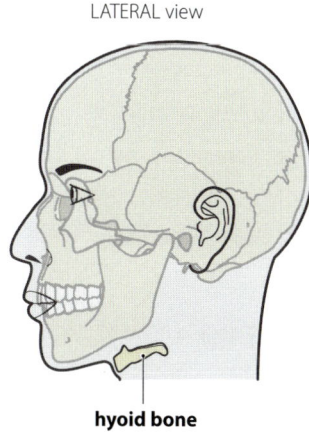

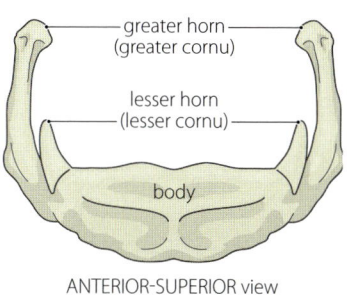

Figure 13.13 – **The hyoid bone.**
The hyoid bone is the only bone in the body that does not articulate with any other bone.

in turn articulates with the coccyx. The bones of the sacrum and coccyx remain unfused in childhood and adolescent years. Fusion occurs in early adulthood when individuals are in their 20s.

Each vertebra has a vertebral body, vertebral foramen, spinous process, transverse process, articular facets and transverse foramen (see *Figure 13.15a, b* and *c*). The vertebral body ensures that weight is transferred along the axis of the spinal column. Vertebral bodies are held together by ligaments, while the vertebral foramina of the vertebral bones form the vertebral canal in which the spinal cord is found. The spinous processes project outwards (posteriorly) and can be seen in very thin people as knobbly protrusions along the spine, especially when bending forwards. The transverse processes project laterally, and together with the spinous processes, serve as sites for the attachment of ligaments and muscles that stabilize and move the vertebral column, respectively.

The vertebrae are separated by intervertebral discs (see *Figures 13.16* and *13.17*). An intervertebral disc is made up of two parts. The inner layer is gelatinous and is called the **nucleus pulposus**; it makes the disc elastic and is easily compressible without being damaged. The outer layer that surrounds the nucleus pulposus is called the **annulus fibrosus** and is made up of fibrocartilage and collagen fibres. Its role is to minimize the extent to which the annulus pulposus can expand during compression of the spine. The role of the discs is to act as shock absorbers during everyday physical activity and vigorous activity, such as sport and manual work (see *Box 13.1*).

416 CHAPTER 13 | ACHIEVING MOVEMENT

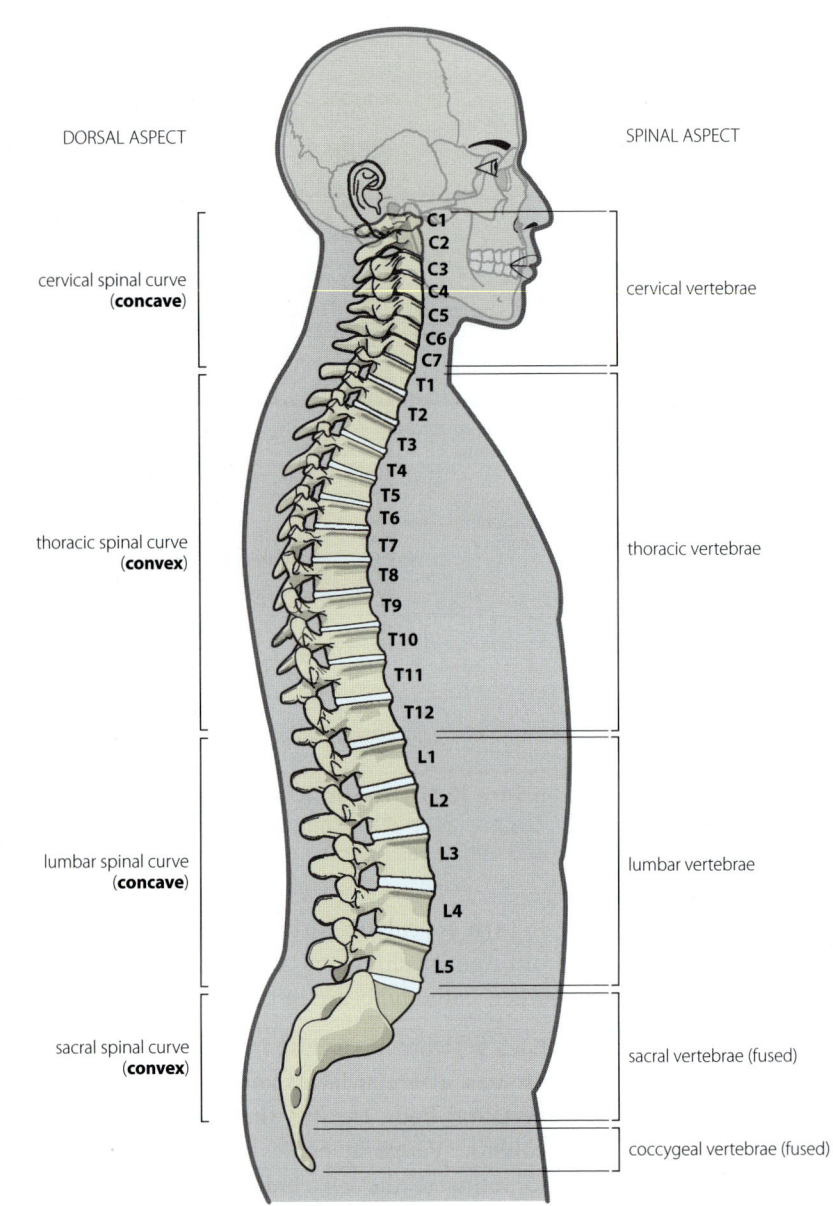

Figure 13.14 – The vertebral column regions showing the four spinal curves.
The four spinal curves comprise the cervical spinal curve, the thoracic spinal curve, the lumbar spinal curve and the sacral spinal curve. The cervical and lumbar are concave, while the thoracic and sacral are convex. Concave means curving in, while convex means curving out.

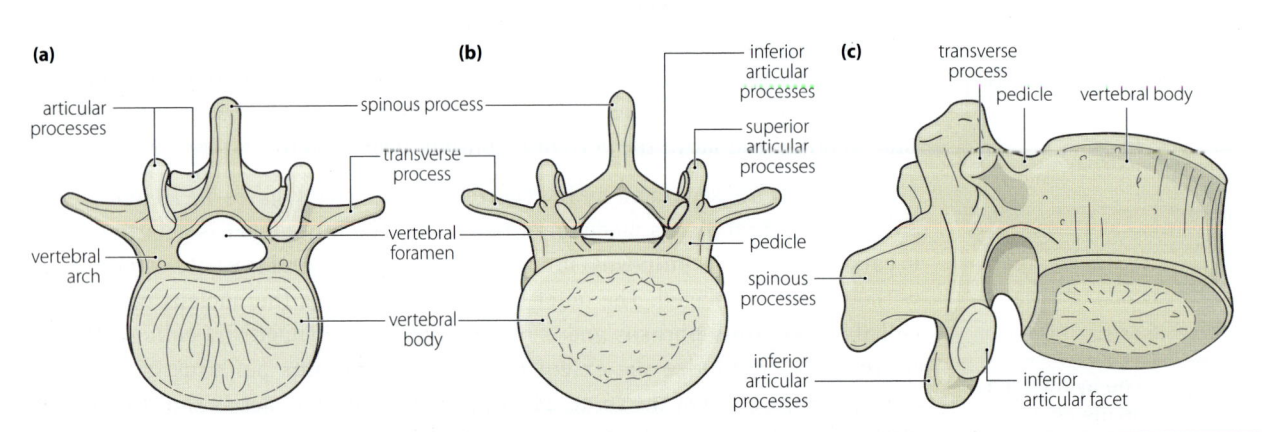

Figure 13.15 – The structure of the vertebrae showing (a) a superior view, (b) an inferior view and (c) lateral and inferior views.

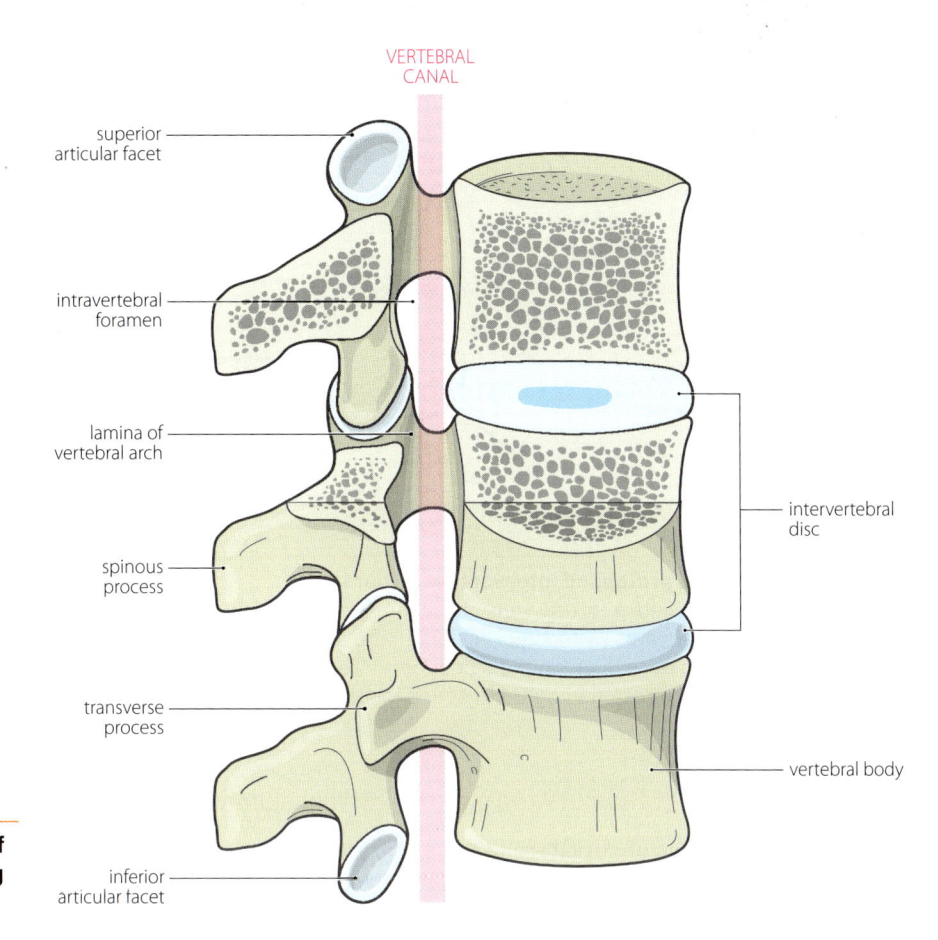

SECTION **13.2** | WHAT YOU NEED TO KNOW – ESSENTIAL ANATOMY AND PHYSIOLOGY **417**

Figure 13.16 – A lateral view of articulated vertebrae showing the intervertebral discs.

> **BOX 13.1**
>
> ### Moving and handling
>
> The principles of moving and handling emphasize the fact that appropriate posture and natural curves must be maintained at all times when handling and moving objects. This means avoiding any movement such as bending, twisting and over-reaching that will lead to damage to the spinal bones or discs of the vertebral column. A **prolapsed** (or **slipped**) **disc** (see *Figure 13.17*) usually results when excessive pressure is exerted on the discs when bending the spine while lifting a heavy object. Back injury, due to incorrect moving and handling, can lead to many hours of lost work and is a huge cost to employers. This is recognized to be so important that specific legislation exists to limit the risk of injury from manual handling. Many employers invest resources to train their employees in how to adopt the correct posture when sitting down and the appropriate procedures when moving and handling objects in the workplace. In a healthcare setting, moving patients in different situations should be a well-thought-out and planned manoeuvre to protect patients and staff. Appropriate equipment designed for specific purposes may be needed in healthcare settings to ensure that moving and handling is done without serious damage to the spine.

The spinal column is not straight but is curved in four regions: the cervical, thoracic, lumbar and sacral regions. This enables the body weight to be distributed and transmitted to the hips and lower limbs. The curves ensure that the spine is not rigid but is flexible and resilient, allowing the distribution of weight to be in line with the axis of the body (see *Box 13.2*).

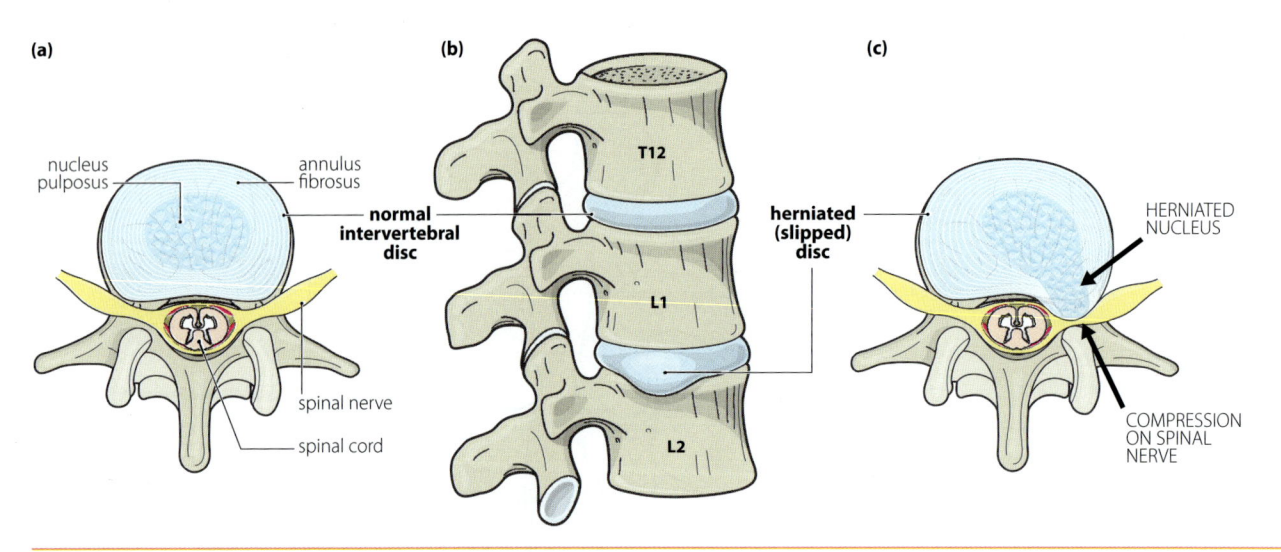

Figure 13.17 – Normal and prolapsed intervertebral discs.
(a) Intact intervertebral disc; (b) a lateral view of the lumbar region, showing herniated intervertebral disc; and (c) a sectional view of a herniated disc with compression on the spinal nerve. The prolapsed disc shows the herniated nucleus pulposus, which causes compression on the spinal nerve resulting in pain such as sciatica. A prolapsed disc can be detected by magnetic resonance imaging (MRI) scans including in adults who may be asymptomatic.

Conditions that affect the curvature of the vertebral column

Although small degrees of curvature of the spine are normal, some developmental and/or pathological conditions can lead to abnormal curvature of the spine. Normal curvature of the spine is illustrated in *Figure 13.14* and abnormal curvatures of the spine are illustrated in *Figures 13.18–13.20*.

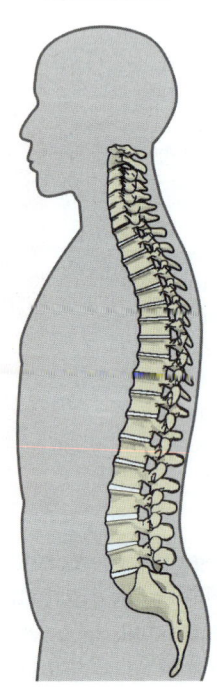

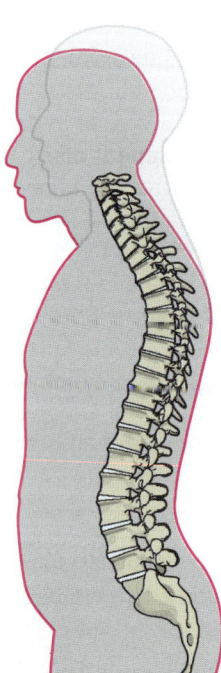

Kyphosis

Kyphosis ('hump back') refers to the posterior exaggeration of the normal convex curvature of the thoracic curve. Kyphosis can result from abnormal growth of the vertebral bones, either in the womb or during adolescence due to poor posture such as slouching. In later life, especially in women, kyphosis occurs due to osteoporosis, leading to bone compression fractures of the anterior portions of the vertebral bodies, and can be caused by chronic contraction of the muscles attached to the vertebrae.

Figure 13.18 – Kyphosis.

BOX 13.2

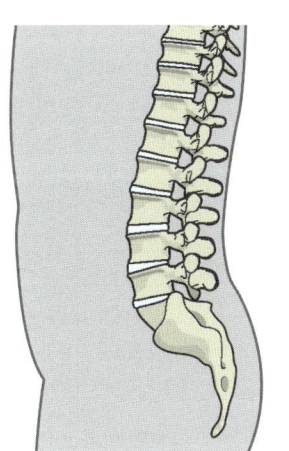

SECTION **13.2** | WHAT YOU NEED TO KNOW – ESSENTIAL ANATOMY AND PHYSIOLOGY   419

BOX 13.2 (*continued*)

NORMAL SPINE   LORDOSIS OF THE SPINE

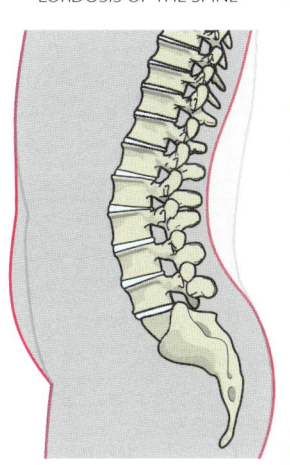

Lordosis

Lordosis ('swayback') occurs as a result of anterior exaggeration of the concave lumbar curvature, which makes the buttocks more prominent. Lordosis can result from weakness in the muscles of the abdominal wall or from abdominal (truncal) obesity.

Figure 13.19 – **Lordosis.**

NORMAL SPINE   SCOLIOTIC SPINE

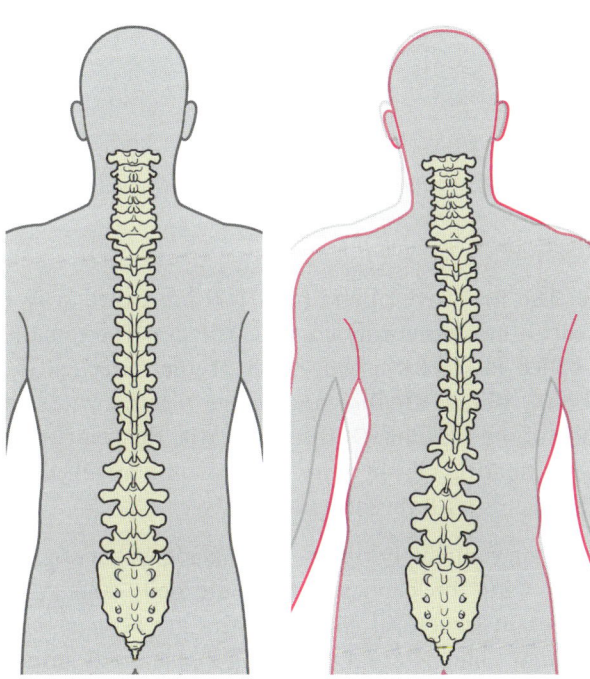

Scoliosis

In scoliosis ('hunchback'), there is abnormal lateral curvature of the spine of more than 10°. It can occur in more than one area of the spine, resulting in a curve. This results in one shoulder blade being higher than the other if the scoliosis is in the thoracic region, and likewise one hip appears higher than the other if the scoliosis is in the lumbar region. It can occur during developmental stages such as the growth spurt at puberty, due to incomplete formation of the vertebrae. Alternatively, it can occur in later life, due to muscle paralysis affecting one side of the back. Scoliosis can be idiopathic or due to neuromuscular causes and is the most common of the disorders described.

Figure 13.20 – **Scoliosis.**

The thoracic cage

The **thoracic cage** (see *Figure 13.21*) consists of the ribs, the sternum and the thoracic vertebrae. It protects the heart, lungs and other soft organs within the thoracic cavity. It stabilizes the vertebral column and also serves as an attachment for the muscles of respiration and those that allow movements of the upper limbs. The ribs and sternum form the **ribcage** whose function is discussed in respiration (see *Chapter 10*).

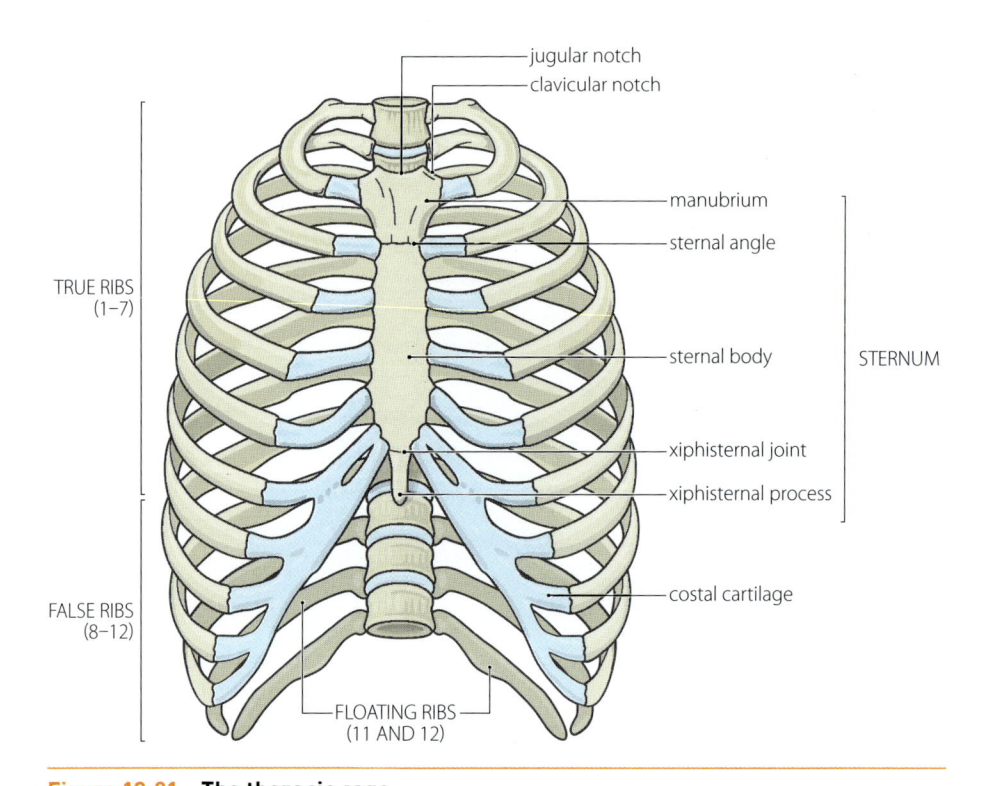

Figure 13.21 – The thoracic cage.
The false ribs (ribs 8–12) are shown, of which ribs 11 and 12 are known as floating ribs.

There are 12 pairs of ribs. The first seven pairs (ribs 1–7) are called **true ribs** because they are connected to the sternum by costal cartilages. The remaining five pairs (ribs 8–12) are called **false ribs** because they are not attached to the sternum directly but three (8, 9 and 10) fuse and merge together with rib 7 cartilages before they attach to the sternum. Of the false pairs, the last two pairs (ribs 11 and 12) are known as **floating ribs** because they are only attached to the vertebrae and have no attachments with the sternum.

The sternum is a flat bone approximately 15 cm long, made up of an upper **manubrium** that articulates with the clavicles, a middle body and a lower **xiphoid process**. Three important structural characteristics are associated with the sternum, namely the jugular notch, sternal angle and xiphisternal joint. The *jugular notch*, which is superior to the xiphisternal joint, is at the level of the intervertebral disc between the second and third thoracic vertebrae (T2 and T3), which is at the point where the left common carotid artery originates from the aorta. The *sternal angle* is where the manubrium joins the body of the sternum and is at a level approximate to the intervertebral disc between the fourth and fifth thoracic vertebrae (T4 and T5). This is at a level approximate to the second pair of costal cartilages that attach to the second ribs. The *xiphisternal joint* is where the body of the sternum and the xiphoid process meet and is in line with the ninth thoracic vertebra (T9).

The appendicular skeleton
The appendicular skeleton is made up of the bones of the pectoral girdle, the upper limbs, the pelvic girdle and the lower limbs.

The pectoral girdle
The pectoral (shoulder) girdle (see *Figure 13.22*) is made up of the **clavicles** and the **scapulae**. The clavicles (collar bones) are long bones that are felt easily on palpation and are located anteriorly with one end (the medial end) attached to the axial skeleton at the sternum while the other end called the **acromion** articulates with the scapula (distal end). The clavicles anchor many muscles and ligaments. They also channel forces from the arms to the axial skeleton when the arms are involved in physical work.

The scapulae (shoulder blades) are thin triangular flat bones located posteriorly. The scapula has a protruding or prominent part called the **spine** that terminates as an enlarged projection called the acromion, which forms the **acromioclavicular joint** with the clavicle. The scapulae are held on to the vertebral column and the thorax by muscles only. Each scapula forms a shallow joint known as the **glenoid joint** with the humerus, thus allowing free movement of the arms. It is this shallowness of the joint that gives poor stability to the joint and makes it relatively easy for a person to dislocate a shoulder. Shoulder dislocations are very common in rugby and football (soccer) players if they fall awkwardly.

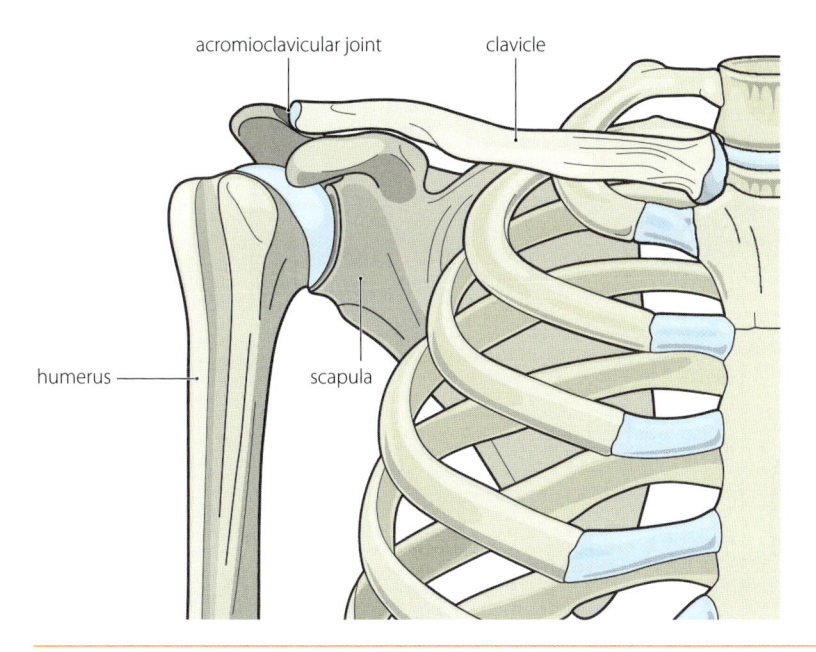

Figure 13.22 – The pectoral girdle.
The positions of the clavicle and the acromioclavicular joint are shown.

The upper limbs

Each upper limb (see *Figure 13.23*) is made up of the arm, the forearm and the hand. The arm is made up of the **humerus** (see *Figure 13.24*), which is the largest and longest bone of the upper limb. The humerus articulates with the scapula at the **proximal** end (the shoulder) and with the radius and ulna at the **distal** end. The humerus has a head at the proximal end that forms the glenoid joint with the scapula, an anatomical neck and a surgical neck. Almost halfway along its long shaft, the humerus has a roughened area known as the **deltoid tuberosity**, which is a point of attachment for the big deltoid muscle from the shoulder. There are two condyles (bone protrusions) known as the **capitulum** and the **trochlea**, as well as two depressions, the **coronoid fossa** and **olecranon fossa** (see *Figure 13.24*), at the distal end that articulate with the bones of the forearm.

The **forearm** is made up of the **radius** and **ulna** (see *Figure 13.25*). These two bones run parallel to each other. The radius is thin at the proximal end where it articulates with the humerus and widens as it reaches the distal end. It has a **head**, a **neck**, a **radial tuberosity** where biceps muscles attach and a **styloid process** at the distal end for the attachment of ligaments. The radius is in line with the bones of the thumb at its distal end, articulating with the ulna at the ulnar notch and with the bones of the wrist. The radial artery is easily felt here because it lies over the radial bone close to the surface and can easily be palpated. For this reason, the radial artery is often palpated in clinical practice to determine the pulse. The ulna, being slightly longer than the radius, forms the elbow. At the proximal end (see *Figure 13.25*), it has the **olecranon process** and the **styloid process**, which

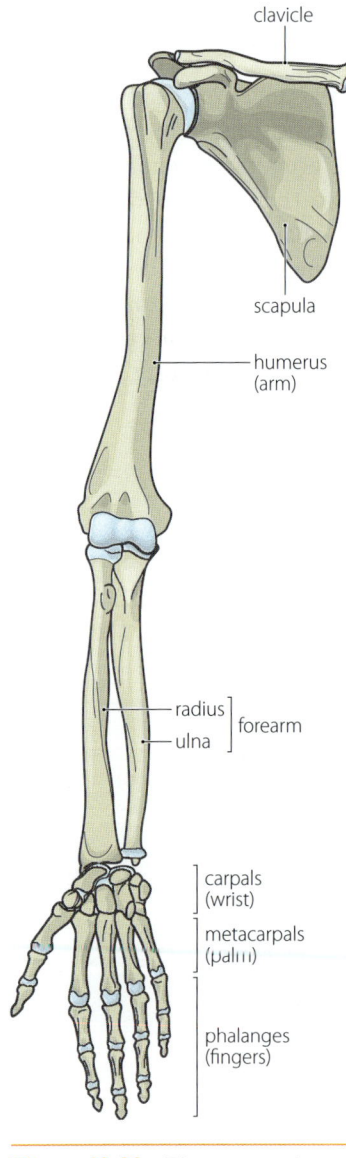

Figure 13.23 – The pectoral girdle and upper limb.
The bones of the upper arm, forearm, wrist and hand are indicated.

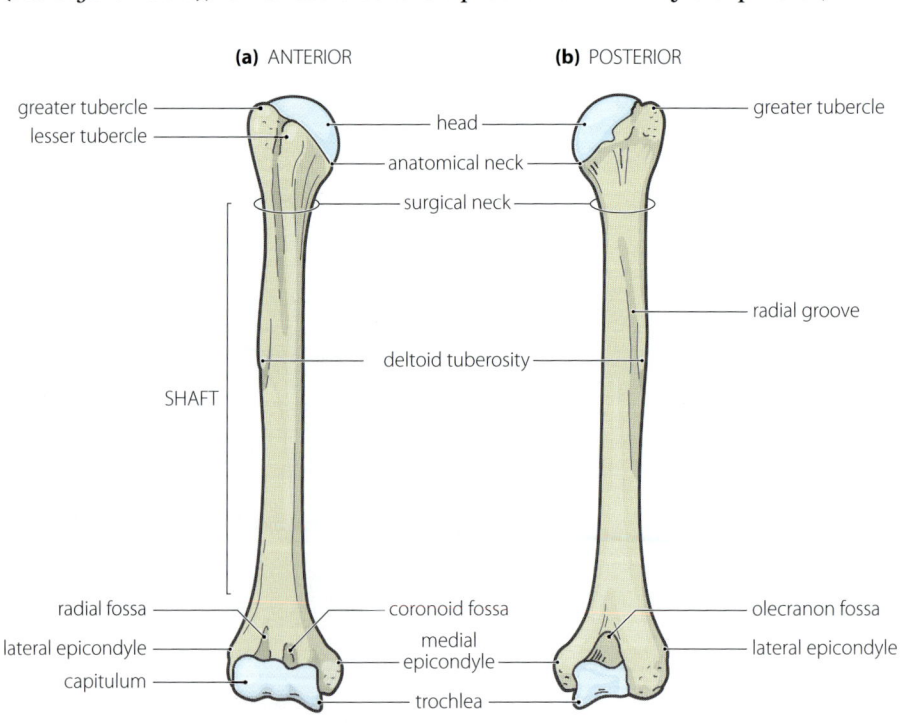

Figure 13.24 – (a) Anterior and (b) posterior surface views of the right humerus.
(a) The anterior surface view shows the relationship of the coronoid fossa to the medial and lateral epicondyles. (b) The posterior surface view shows the relationship of the olecranon fossa to the medial and lateral epicondyles.

form joints with the coronoid fossa and olecranon fossa of the humerus, as well as a deep **trochlear** notch that enables the elbow joint to be formed with the humerus (see *Figure 13.25*).

The bones of the **hand** (see *Figure 13.26*) include the **carpals** (wrist bones), the **metacarpals** (bones of the palm) and the **phalanges** (bones of the fingers). Each finger is made up of a distal phalanx, a middle phalanx and a proximal phalanx. There are eight short bones that make up the carpals of each hand. These bones articulate with each other, but the **scaphoid** articulates with the radius and the **lunate** articulates with the ulna. The **trapezium**, which lies in between, articulates with the scaphoid, **capitate** and first metacarpal. The **trapezoid** articulates with four bones, namely the scaphoid at the proximal end, the second metacarpal at the distal end, and the capitate and trapezium on either side. In addition to articulating with the trapezoid and scaphoid, the capitate also articulates with three other bones, namely the third metacarpal, the **hamate** and lunate. The **triquetral** (also known as **triquetrum**) is a triangular bone that articulates with the hamate, lunate and another small bone called the **pisiform**. Collectively, these bones provide a full range of movement in three dimensions, involving pronation–supination, flexion–extension and rotation (see *Table 13.3* later in the chapter).

The **palm** of each hand is made up of **five metacarpal bones** numbered I to V. Metacarpal I articulates with the thumb phalanges and metacarpal V articulates with the phalanges of the little finger. Metacarpal bones have a base that articulates with the carpals and a head that articulates with the phalanges and protrudes as a knuckle when a fist is made.

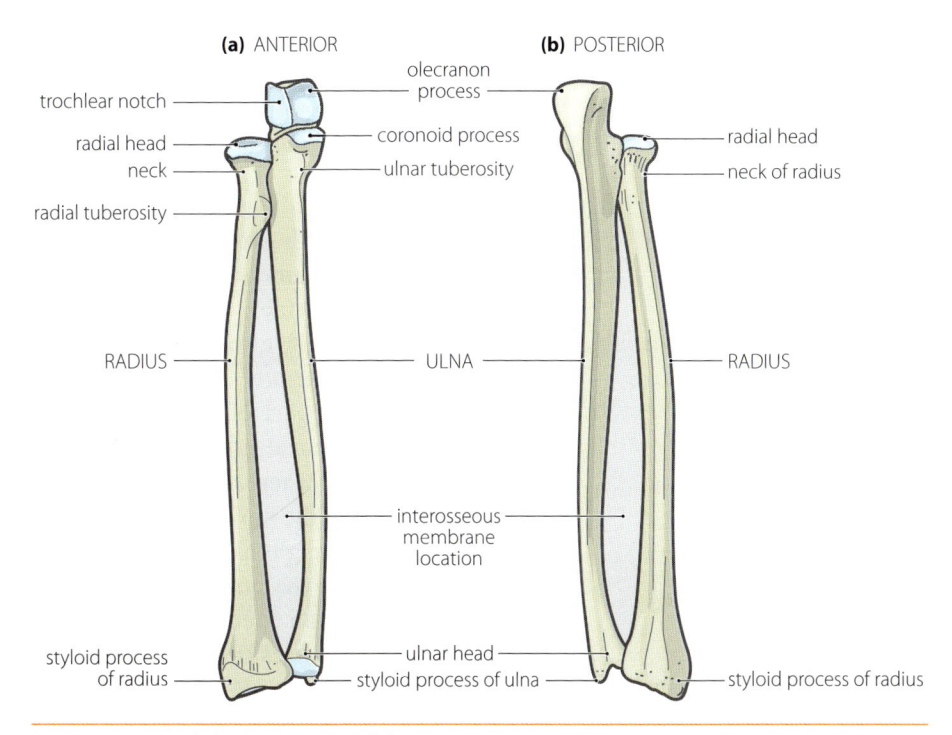

Figure 13.25 – (a) Anterior and (b) posterior surface views of the radius and ulna of the right forearm.

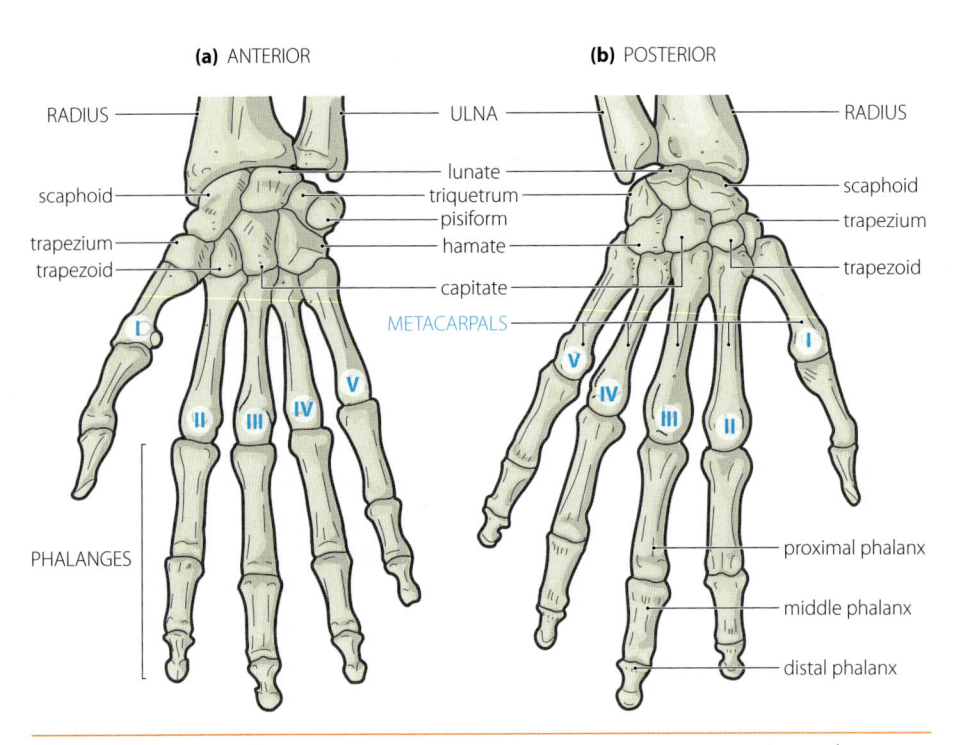

Figure 13.26 – (a) Anterior and (b) posterior views of the bones of the hand (wrist, palm and fingers).
By convention, the thumb is identified as I while the little finger is V.

Likewise, the fingers are numbered I to V starting with the thumb. In total, there are 14 bones of the fingers in each hand that make up the phalanges. This is because there are only two phalanges that make up the thumb – the proximal and distal phalanges, while each of the remaining four fingers has three phalanges.

The pelvic girdle

The role of the **pelvic (hip) girdle** (see *Figure 13.27*) is to attach the lower limbs to the axial skeleton. Both femurs are held firmly in the **deep sockets** of the pelvic girdle with **strong ligaments** that hold the bones together. These characteristics make the joint more stable and minimize the chances of dislocation. The **hip bones** (see *Figure 13.27*), also known as **coxal bones**, unite anteriorly and connect with the sacrum posteriorly. The coxal bones, sacrum and coccyx form the **bony pelvis**. The superior part of the coxal bone is the *ilium*, while the posterior-inferior part of the coxal bone forms the *ischium*. A deep socket known as the **acetabulum** is found where the *ilium*, *ischium* and *pubis* meet (see *Figure 13.28*). The strongest part of the hip bone is the **ischial tuberosity (ischium)**, which is the part that takes the weight of the body when in a sitting position. Anteriorly, just above the ischium is the **pubic bone (pubis)**. The shape of the ischial and pubic bones helps to create an opening called the **obturator foramen** that enables blood vessels and nerves to pass through.

The pelvis bones surround the pelvic cavity, which contains the urinary bladder, located anteriorly. The reproductive organs, pelvic colon and rectum are located posteriorly. The cavity has two lateral walls, an anterior inferior wall, a posterior wall and an inferior wall (the pelvic floor). The major blood vessels, muscles and nerves that serve the pelvic organs are found in the pelvic cavity. The pelvic girdle encloses a space known as the lesser pelvis (true pelvis), which is bounded in front and below by the pubic symphysis; it is in this cavity that the urinary bladder, pelvic colon and rectum are found.

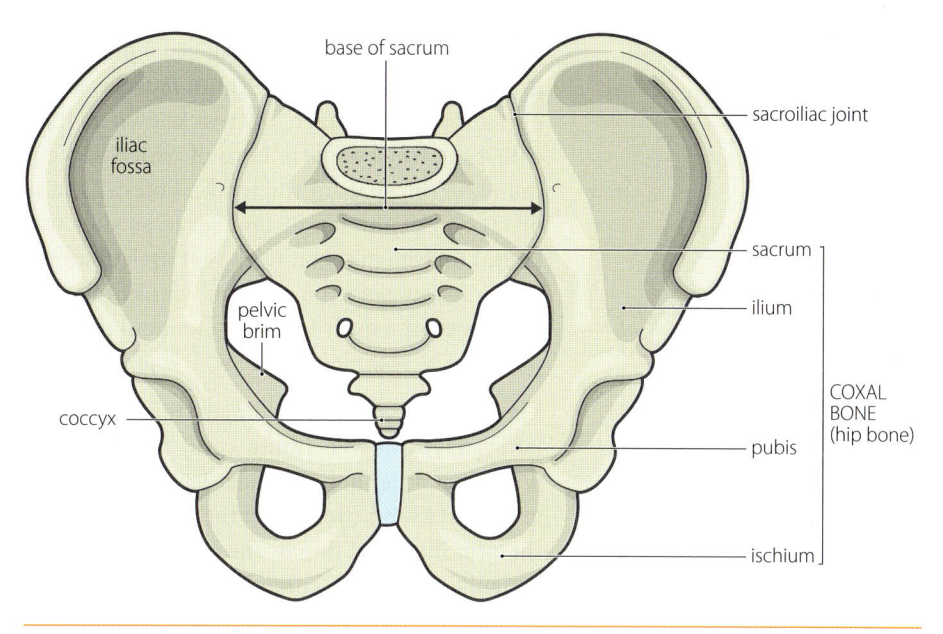

Figure 13.27 – **The pelvic girdle and sacrum.**

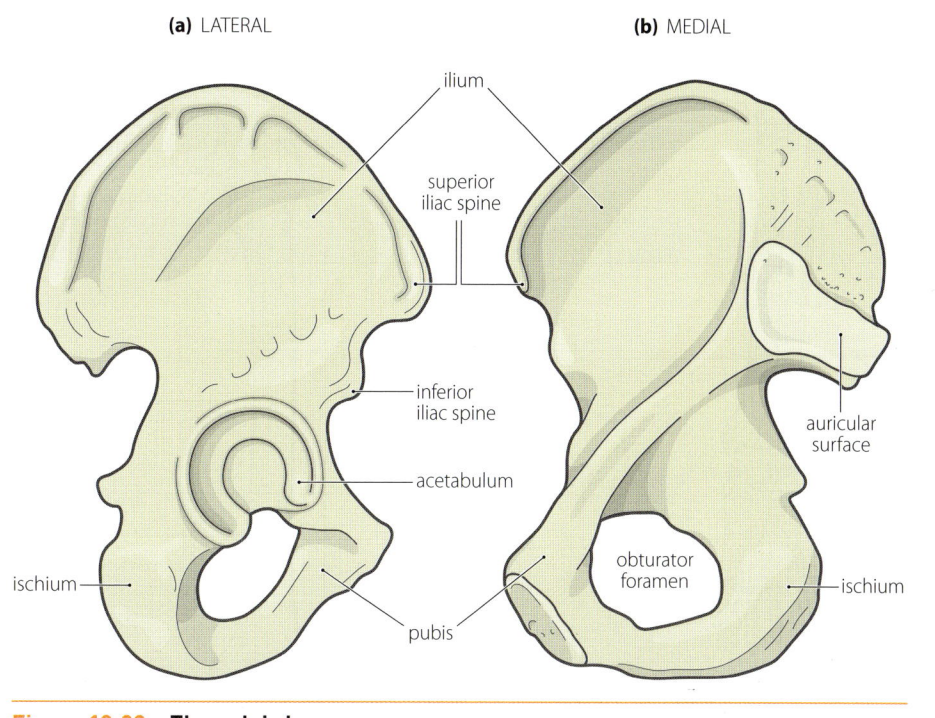

Figure 13.28 – **The pelvic bones.**
(a) Lateral view of right hip bone; and (b) medial view of right hip bone.

The lower limbs

The lower limbs are made up of the **thigh**, the **leg** and the **foot** (see *Figure 13.29*).

The **thigh** is made up of the **femur** (see *Figure 13.30*), which is the largest and longest bone in the body. The femur is surrounded by many muscles that enable the limb to perform its functions. It has a **head** at its proximal end that articulates with the hip bone. Attached to the head is the neck, which is the weakest and most frequently broken part of the femur. Two projections are present, namely the **greater trochanter**, where thigh muscles attach, and the **lesser trochanter**, where buttock muscles attach. A crest known as the **gluteal tuberosity** and a long ridge called the **linea aspera**, both of which serve as points of muscle attachment, are found on the shaft of the femur. **Lateral** and **medial epicondyles** are found at the distal end of the femur and serve as sites for muscle attachment, as well as the lateral and medial condyles that articulate with the tibia. On the anterior aspect of the femur between the condyles is found a smooth patellar surface, while on the posterior aspect is the intercondular fossa. As stated earlier in *Table 13.1*, the **patella** is a **sesamoid** bone, which protects the knee joint.

The **leg** consists of two bones that run parallel to each other called the **tibia** (shinbone) and the **fibula** (pin) (see *Figure 13.31*). These two bones articulate with each other at both ends. The tibia is the weight-bearing bone of the leg, as it articulates with the femur; the fibula does not bear weight. The tibia is broader at the proximal end due to the presence of the **medial** and **lateral condyles**, which articulate with the condyles of the femur. Between these two tibial condyles is found the **intercondylar eminence** and below the condyles is a roughened area known as the tibial tuberosity, which acts as an attachment point for the patellar

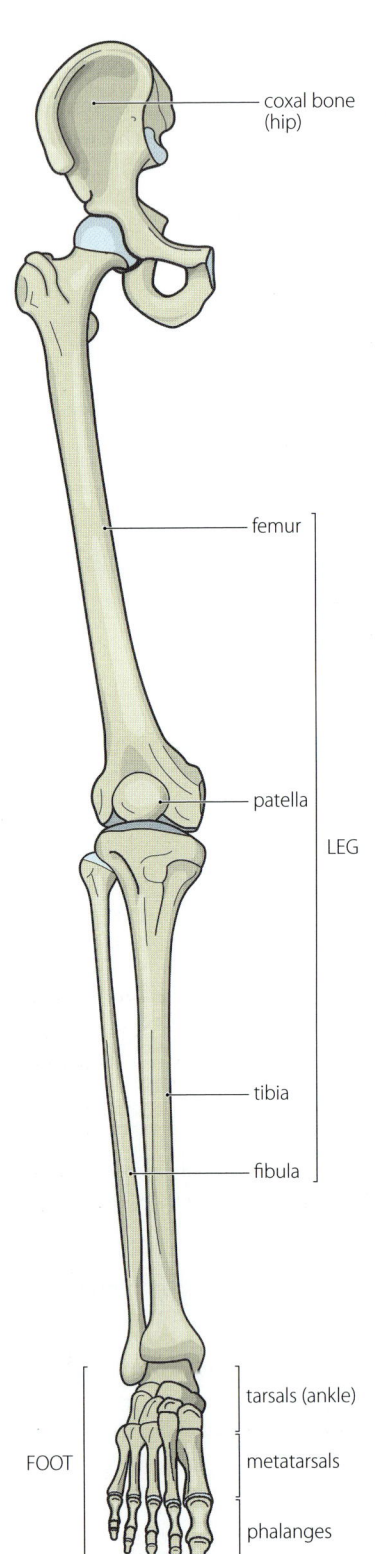

Figure 13.29 – An anterior view of the pelvic girdle and the right lower limb.

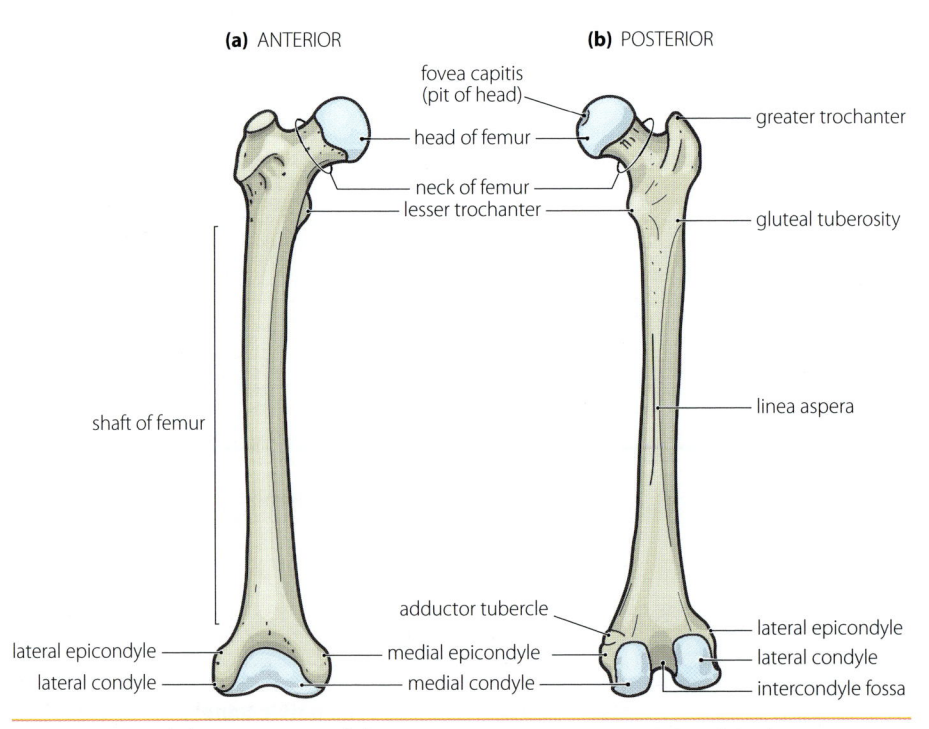

Figure 13.30 – (a) Anterior and (b) posterior surface views of the right femur.

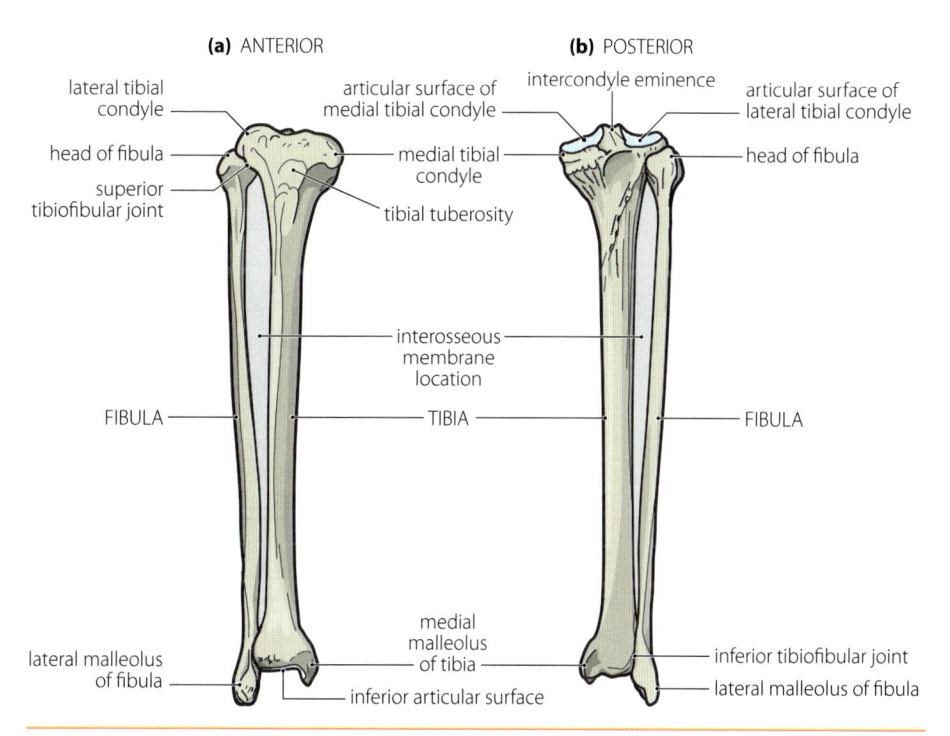

Figure 13.31 – (a) Anterior and (b) posterior surface views of the tibia and fibula of the right leg.

ligament. At the distal end of the tibia is the **medial malleolus**, which presents itself as a bulge in the middle of the ankle. The fibula is thinner than the tibia and is wider at both ends, with a **head** at the proximal end and a **lateral malleolus** at the distal end that articulates with the talus.

The **foot** (see *Figure 13.32*) is made up of 26 bones consisting of seven **tarsal bones**, five **metatarsal bones** and 14 **phalanges**. The seven tarsal bones make up the posterior part of the foot. One of the two largest of the tarsal bones is the **talus** (*ankle bone*), which articulates with both the tibia and the fibula. The other large tarsal bone is the **calcaneus** or *heel bone*, which is located below the talus. The Achilles tendon, which attaches the calf muscles to the calcaneus, is located here. The other five tarsal bones are the **cuboid**, **navicular** and the **medial**, **intermediate** and **lateral cuneiform** bones.

There are five **metatarsal bones** (see *Figure 13.32*) that run parallel to each other, usually identified by Roman numerals I–V, with I being the metatarsal in line with the great toe. The metatarsal bones articulate with the proximal phalanges of the toes. The phalanges make up the toes and each toe is made up of three digits, with the exception of the big toe (the **hallux**), which has two digits.

13.2.2 The joints

Bones articulate or meet with each other to form joints that enable movement. Joints can be classified by their structure into fibrous, cartilaginous and synovial joints, or by function into immovable joints (**synarthroses**), slightly movable joints (**amphiarthroses**) and freely movable joints (**diarthroses**) (see *Table 13.2*).

428 CHAPTER **13** | ACHIEVING MOVEMENT

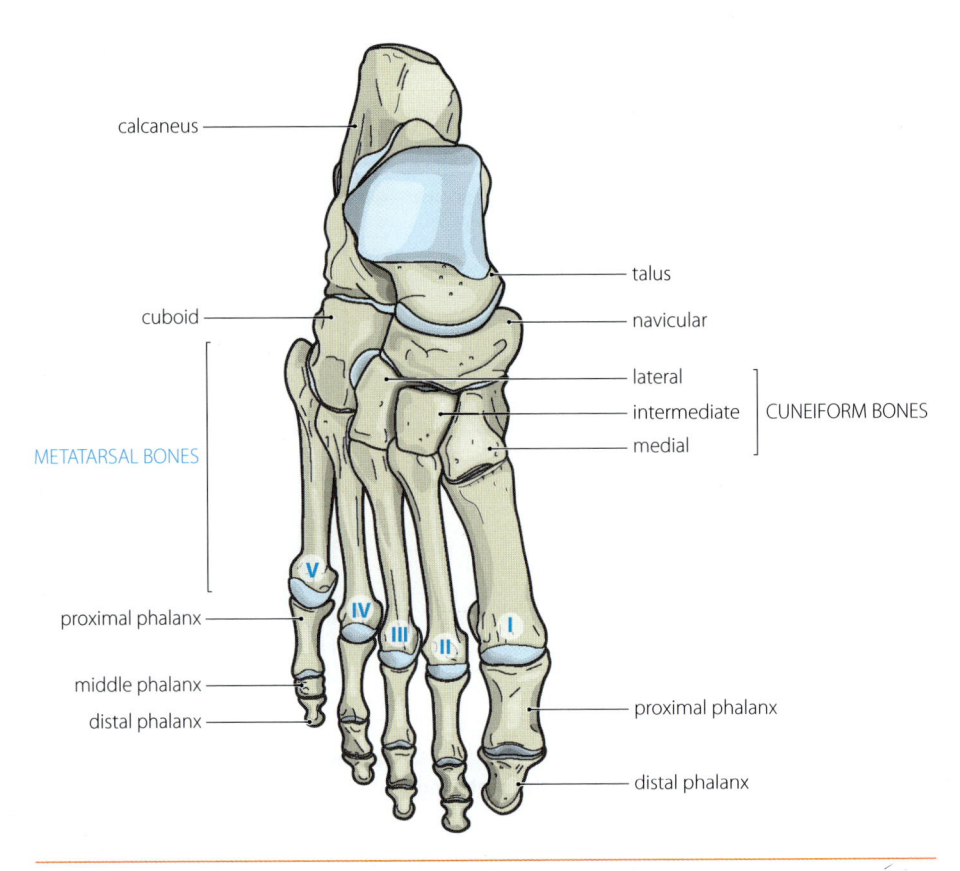

Figure 13.32 – **A superior view of the bones of the right foot.**
Note the position of the proximal, middle and distal phalanxes.

The immovable and slightly movable joints are found in the axial skeleton, while the freely movable joints are found in the appendicular skeleton.

The synovial joint

A synovial joint (see *Figure 13.33*) has a joint cavity containing synovial fluid, with the opposing surfaces of the joint bones covered by hyaline cartilage, which acts as a shock absorber. Synovial joints also have an outer fibrous capsule of dense irregular connective tissue and an inner synovial membrane made up of loose connective tissue. The outer fibrous capsule is attached to the periosteum of the bones making the joint, to ensure that the bones stay connected. Examples of synovial joints are all the joints of the limbs. The synovial membrane cells secrete synovial fluid, which lubricates the joint surfaces and reduces friction. Synovial fluid also provides nutrients to the cells in the cartilages and contains low numbers of phagocytic cells (see *Chapter 11*) that protect the joint cavity.

The stability of a synovial joint depends on three main features, namely the shape of the articular surfaces, the number of ligaments and muscle tone. Joints with shallow sockets are less stable than those with deep sockets. Generally speaking, the more ligaments there are to support a joint, the more stable the joint is. Muscles are connected to bones by tendons, while ligaments join bone to bone at joints. The small amount of contraction present in relaxed muscles at all times

Figure 13.33 – **The synovial joint.**

Table 13.2 – Classification of joints

Structural classification	Functional classification	Joint characteristics and examples
Fibrous joints	Immovable (synarthroses)	No joint cavity Connective tissue fibres unite bones, or ligaments connect bones *Sutures* – wavy junction of the skull bones *Syndesmoses* – joint between distal ends of tibia and fibula; ligament connects the ends *Gomphoses* – tooth articulating in bony socket
Cartilaginous joints	Slightly movable (amphiarthroses)	No joint cavity Cartilage unites articulating bones *Synchondroses* – a plate of hyaline cartilage unites the bones, such as the epiphyseal plate between diaphysis and the epiphysis of long bones *Symphyses* – hyaline cartilage, which is fused to fibrocartilage, covers articulating surfaces; limited movement is allowed by the fibrocartilage, which acts as a shock absorber
Synovial joints	Freely movable (diarthroses)	Hyaline cartilage covers opposing bone surfaces Cavity separates articulating bones Cavity contains fluid Joint capsule containing an outer fibrous capsule of dense irregular connective tissue and an inner synovial membrane made up of loose connective tissue Reinforcing ligaments present *Diarthroses* – joint cavity present (limb joints)

is known as muscle tone, ensuring that the tendons are kept taut by the muscles attached to these tendons.

Types of synovial joints

There are six different types of synovial joints. The joints formed between the atlas and the axis of the skull and between the head of the radius and the ulna are known as **pivot** joints. This joint allows rotational movement only. **Gliding** joints are found in the bones between the articular surfaces of the vertebrae and those found in the carpal and tarsal joints. **Condyloid** joints have oval surfaces and allow different angular movements, such as are found at the wrist joints and the knuckle joints.

The **saddle** joint is made by the meeting of bones that have a concave and convex shape, which snuggle together to form a saddle, thus allowing a high amount of free movement. An example of a saddle joint is that between the carpals and metacarpals of the thumb. A **hinge** joint allows movement in one plane such as the bending and straightening of the elbow and the knee (see *Figure 13.34*). Finally, a **ball-and-socket** joint is described as multiaxial (many axis), which means that it allows movement in all directions or planes. Examples are the shoulder joint and the hip joint (see *Figure 13.35*).

430 CHAPTER **13** | ACHIEVING MOVEMENT

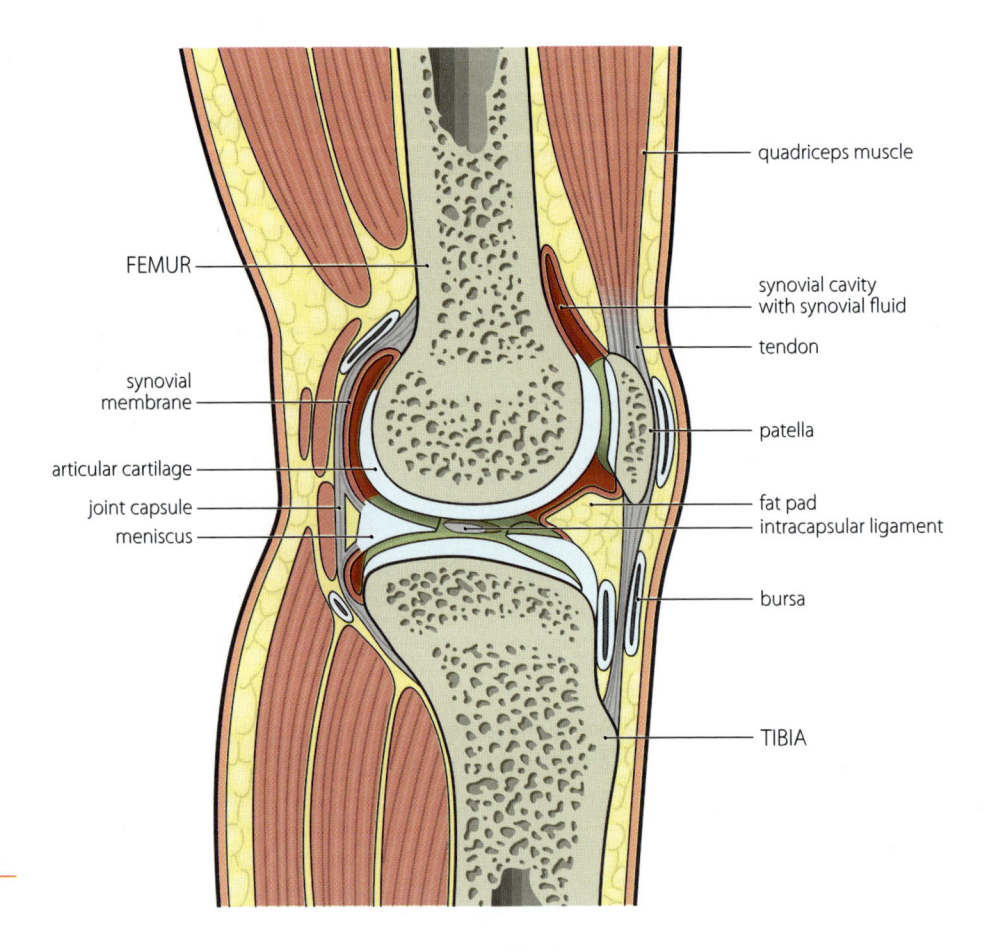

Figure 13.34 – **The knee joint.**

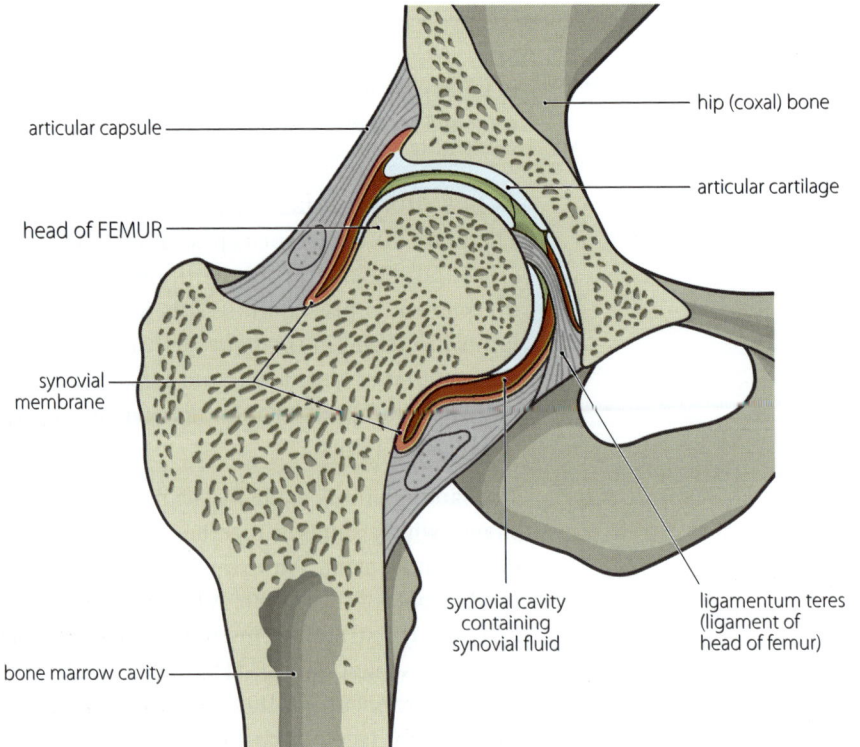

Figure 13.35 – **The hip joint.**

Table 13.3 – Joint movements

Movement	Description of movement	Examples
Angular movements		
Flexion	Bending along a sagittal plane; the angle is decreased	Moving head downwards towards chest; elbow; trunk; knee
Extension	Movement extending body part along a sagittal plane; the angle is increased	Lifting head upwards at the neck; straightening elbow; knee
Abduction	Movement of limb away from the midline	Raising arm; lateral movement of leg and thigh; spreading of fingers
Adduction	Movement of limb towards the midline	Dropping arm; inward movement of leg and thigh
Rotation	Turning a bone around its axis	Atlas movement on its axis; movement at the shoulder and hip joints
Circumduction	Movement of the end of a limb in a circle (cone-like movement); this incorporates the other four movement types described above	Circular movement of limb with shoulder or hip almost stationary
Special movements		
Pronation	Turning forwards – rotating the forearm medially such that the palm of the hand faces posteriorly	Movement of radius around the ulna
Supination	Turning backwards – rotating the forearm laterally such that the palm of hand faces anteriorly	Movement of radius around the ulna
Inversion	Movement of the foot	Sole of the foot is turned medially
Eversion	Movement of the foot	Sole of the foot is turned laterally
Protraction	Non-angular movement of mandible (lower jaw)	Mandible moved forwards
Retraction	Non-angular movement of mandible	Mandible moved to original position
Elevation	Moving a body part upwards	Moving arm superiorly
Depression	Moving a body part downwards	Moving arm inferiorly

Forms of movement at synovial joints

Joint movements are either angular or specialized. Angular movements reduce or increase the angle at the joint, while specialized movements occur at a number of joints (see *Table 13.3*).

13.2.3 Muscles

Muscle tissue constitutes nearly 50% of the body's mass. It has the capability of transforming chemical energy in the form of ATP (discussed in *Chapter 7*) into mechanical energy, facilitating mechanical coordination of physiology such as respiration, cardiovascular function and control of gastrointestinal activity, in addition to locomotion, thus contributing to homeodynamic regulation. The names and locations of many of the superficial muscles of the body are illustrated in *Figures 13.36a* and *b*.

Characteristics of muscles

Muscles enable movement to occur and are capable of exerting force through their contraction. Muscles have the ability to respond to stimulus (**excitability**); they can contract due to their ability to shorten (**contractility**), and they can extend, as they possess the ability to be stretched (**extensibility**) and are elastic, giving them the ability to recoil to their original resting state after being extended (**elasticity**).

Types, characteristics and functions of muscle

Skeletal muscle enables **voluntary movement** and is made up of cells (myocytes), which are multinucleated due to fusion of adjacent cells. Myocytes, sometimes referred to as muscle fibres, have a long, striated and cylindrical appearance when viewed under a microscope (*Figure 13.36a*). The striated appearance is due to the arrangement of the **sarcomeres**, units that form the basic functional unit of muscle cells. Each skeletal muscle is a discrete organ with its own blood vessels, nerves and tendons. Skeletal muscle provides stability to the skeleton and helps to maintain posture, enables movement, generates heat during contraction, protects internal organs and forms external sphincters that are found at the orifices, such as those of the digestive system and urinary tract. For example, muscles of the head and neck enable movement of the head and neck, facial expressions, chewing, swallowing, eye movement and speech. Some muscles enable gross motor movements, while others enable fine movement.

Smooth muscle enables **involuntary movement** and is made up of short, spindle-shaped cells that are distinct from skeletal muscle by the absence of striations when viewed under a microscope. Smooth muscle contains a single nucleus in the centre of the cell (*Figure 13.36b*). Smooth muscle is found in the walls of blood vessels and in many organs of the digestive, respiratory, reproductive and urinary systems. Contraction and relaxation of smooth muscle enables substances such as blood, food, urine and other secretions to be moved along blood vessels and through other hollow organs and openings. Messages to the smooth muscles in Sally's (Patient 6.1) bladder were affected by the multiple sclerosis, such that Sally felt the urge to urinate frequently, had a tendency to dribble urine involuntarily and was unable to empty her bladder completely before she was catheterized. Smooth muscle also regulates the diameter of the lumen of the respiratory passageways. The use of bronchodilator drugs relaxes smooth muscles, causing the diameter of the bronchioles to increase (see *Chapter 10*). Likewise, smooth muscle forms internal sphincters at urethral and anal orifices.

Cardiac muscle, found only in the heart, is involuntary and is made up of short, striated cells that are branched and usually contain a single nucleus (see *Figure 13.36c*). The cardiac muscle contains **intercalated discs**, which are special regions where the membranes of the cells are held together by adhesional complex proteins, known as **desmosomes**. These are complexes of membrane proteins that provide cell adhesion (see *Chapter 2*). Cardiac muscle cells have **innate rhythmicity**, which means that they have the ability to initiate and establish a regular rate of contraction independent of a stimulus by the nervous system.

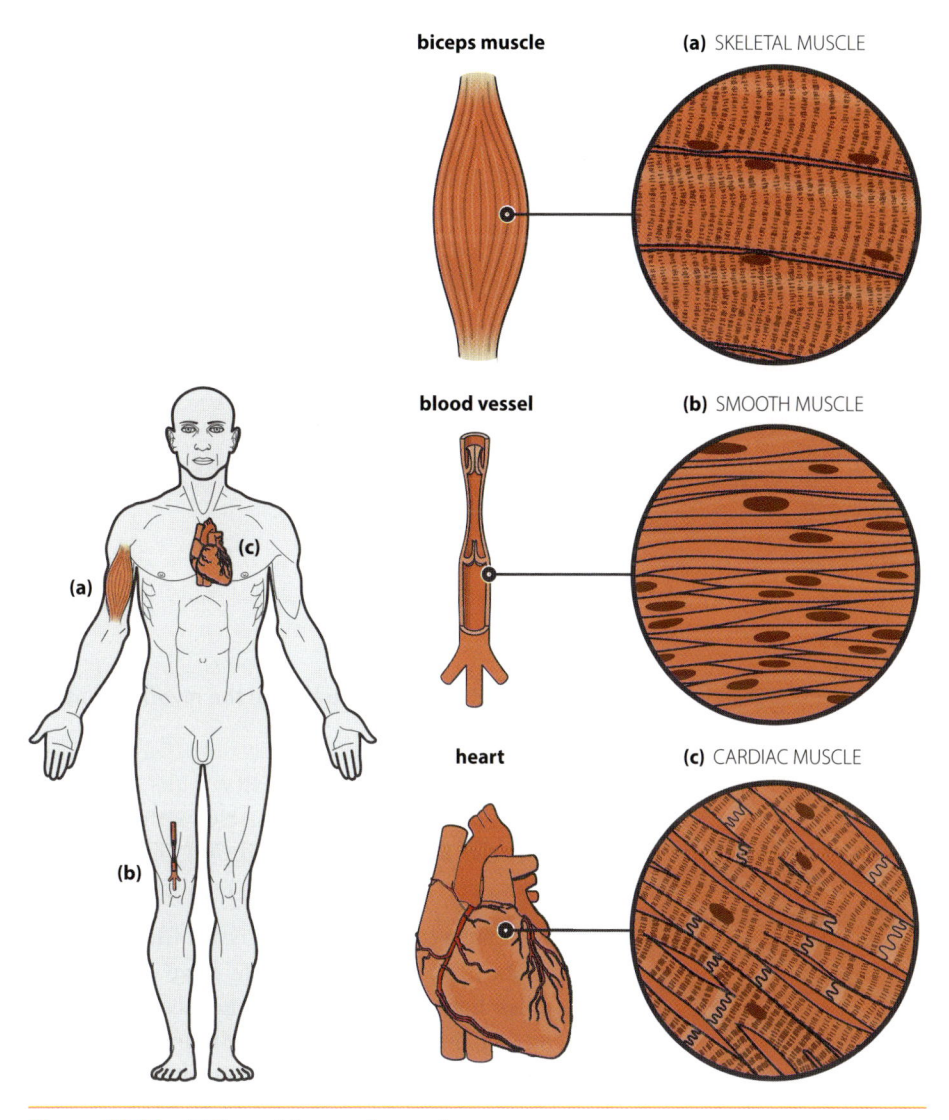

SECTION **13.2** | WHAT YOU NEED TO KNOW – ESSENTIAL ANATOMY AND PHYSIOLOGY 433

Figure 13.36 – Different types of muscle.
(a) Skeletal muscle, such as the biceps of the upper arm; (b) smooth muscle, such as the wall of a blood vessel; and (c) cardiac muscle, found in the walls of the heart.

Structure of skeletal muscle fibre, myofibrils and myofilaments

The cell membrane of a muscle fibre is called a **sarcolemma**, while the cytoplasm of a muscle fibre is known as the **sarcoplasm** (see *Figure 13.37a*). Inside each muscle fibre are found hundreds of cylindrical structures known as **myofibrils** that extend along the entire length of the muscle fibre. These myofibrils are made up of bundles of thin protein myofilaments called **actin** and thick protein myofilaments called **myosin** (see *Figure 13.37b*). Actin has subunits called globular actin (G actin), which possess the active sites where myosin heads attach during contraction. Myofilaments are organized into repeating units called sarcomeres. The contraction of muscle is due to the shortening of these myofibrils. Exercise and bodybuilding may involve hypertrophy of the sarcoplasm, which is characterized by either growth of sarcoplasm and non-contractile proteins or myofibril hypertrophy, which involves the enlargement of muscle fibres with an

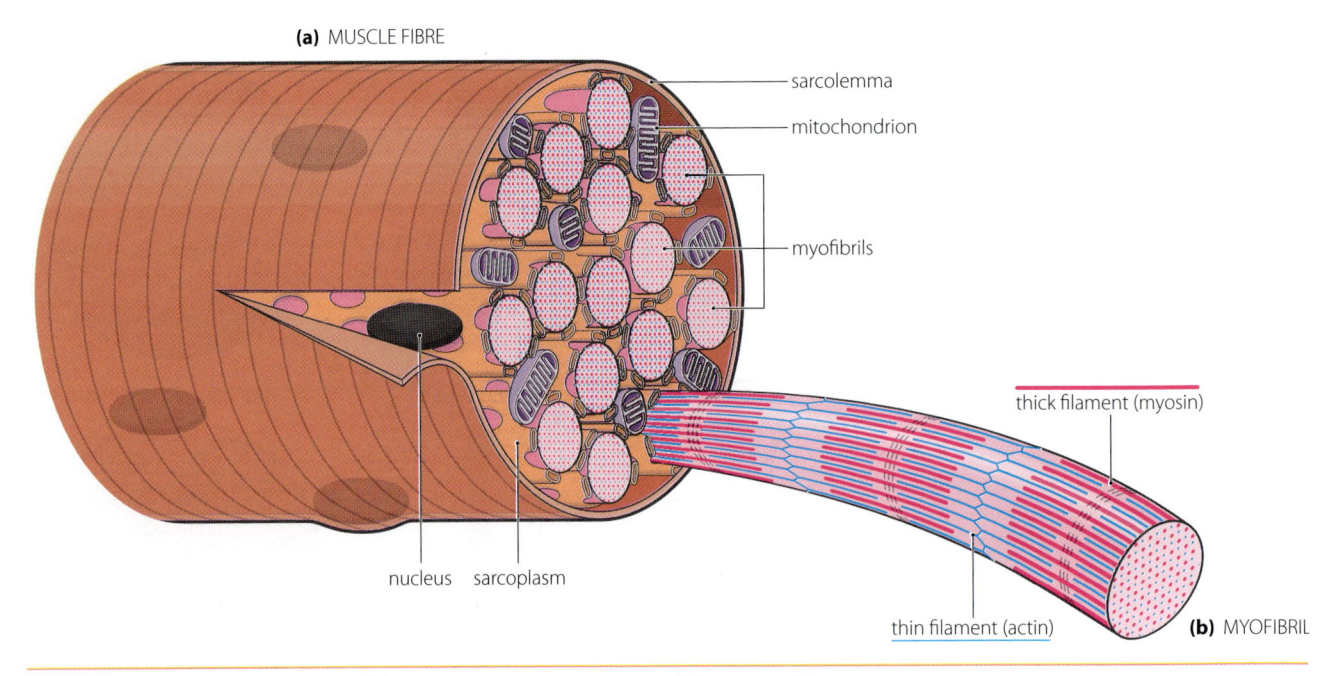

Figure 13.37 – **The structure of (a) skeletal muscle fibre and (b) the myofilaments.**

increase in filament density. Thus, endurance training increases the oxygen-carrying potential of muscle without significantly affecting the size of the muscle. Resistance training, on the other hand, increases the total size of the cross-section of myofibrils, resulting in an increase in muscle size and mass.

The structure of muscle tissue illustrated in *Figure 13.36* shows that skeletal muscle and cardiac muscle have a striated appearance, while smooth muscle does not. This is because the fibres in smooth muscle interlace to form sheets rather than bundles: the actin and myosin filaments are organized in a random arrangement instead of being organized into repeating units of myofilaments. This random arrangement in smooth muscle gives it more elasticity and allows it to dilate and shorten as well as to elongate and constrict during contraction of the longitudinal layer and circular layer of the smooth muscle, respectively (see *Chapter 7, Figure 7.13*).

The sliding filament theory of contraction

Contraction of a muscle represents shortening of the muscle because the two fibrous proteins, actin and myosin, are able to slide over each other – this is described as the sliding filament theory of muscle contraction. Although the thin filaments, usually 5–6 nanometres in diameter, are generally referred to as actin filaments, they are made up of several proteins that include **tropomyosin** and **troponin** as well as actin (see *Figure 13.38*). The binding of myosin to actin is regulated by tropomyosin, which covers the site on actin where myosin is able to bind. Tropomyosin is made up of two twisted polypeptide strands that look like two twisted ropes. The tropomyosin molecules are regulatory, as they prevent interaction between actin and myosin at the binding sites for myosin heads. When the muscle is at rest, the level of intracellular calcium is low and tropomyosin

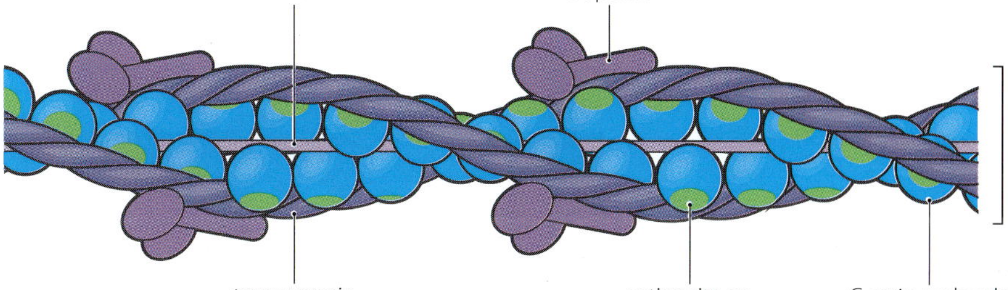

Figure 13.38 – The structure of a thin filament showing the positions of the F filament, nebulin, tropomyosin and troponin.

binds to one molecule of troponin, forming a *troponin–tropomyosin complex*. This prevents the binding of myosin heads to active sites on actin. One subunit of troponin binds to tropomyosin, while another binds to intracellular calcium ions. Muscle contraction only occurs when the position of the troponin–tropomyosin complex changes to reveal the binding site for myosin heads on actin, as occurs following calcium binding. When muscle tissue becomes damaged, troponin can enter the blood. A myocardial infarction, also known as a 'heart attack', results in damage to heart muscle; elevated levels of troponin in blood can be a clinical indicator of this (see *Box 13.4*).

The thick filaments are approximately 10–12 nanometres in diameter and are made up of myosin molecules. Each myosin molecule has two subunits twisted around each other and has a free head that projects towards a thin filament, and a long tail that binds it to other myosin molecules within the thick filament. The connection between the tail and the head is flexible; this enables hinge movement, with the tail acting as a pivot for the head (see *Figure 13.39*). ATP that is bound to myosin is hydrolysed by the enzyme ATPase to ADP and inorganic phosphate, with the release of energy, which activates the myosin head. The myosin head binds to the exposed active site on the actin filaments and pulls the actin filaments along. Shortening of the muscle occurs as the filaments are pulled across each other. The binding of ATP causes the actin–myosin bond to be destabilized and results in detachment of myosin from actin. The hydrolysis of ATP on the now-detached myosin activates the myosin, which binds to free active sites on actin, and the process is able to start all over again. During muscle contraction, the pivoting allows the myosin head to swing back and forth, with the head forming cross-bridges as it interacts with the thin filaments, thus allowing the thick and thin

---

Troponin

Troponin is made up of three different forms of regulatory proteins (isoforms). Troponin T (TnT) binds to tropomyosin, troponin I (TnI) is an inhibitory protein that binds to actin and troponin C (TnC) binds to calcium. Both cardiac troponin T (cTnT) and cardiac troponin I (cTnI) are released into blood when the myocardium is damaged. Therefore, they can be useful diagnostic markers of myocardial infarction.

BOX 13.4

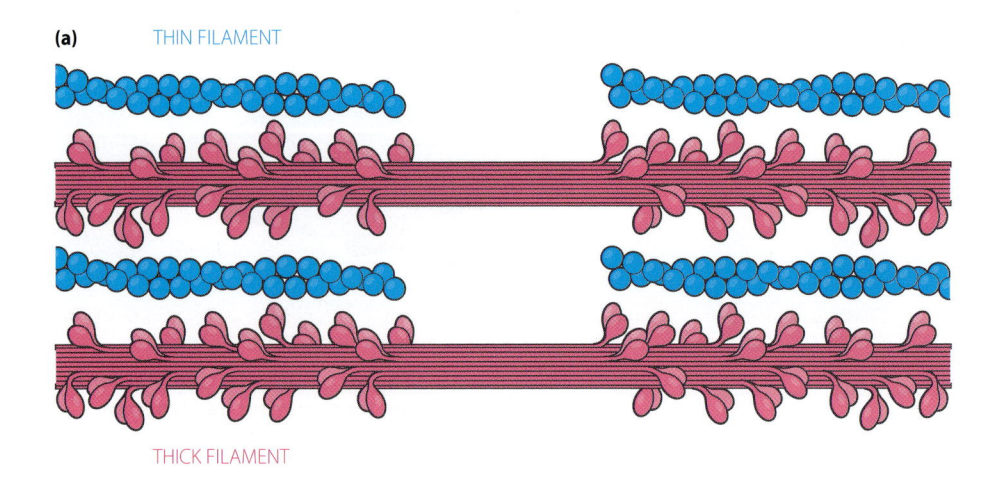

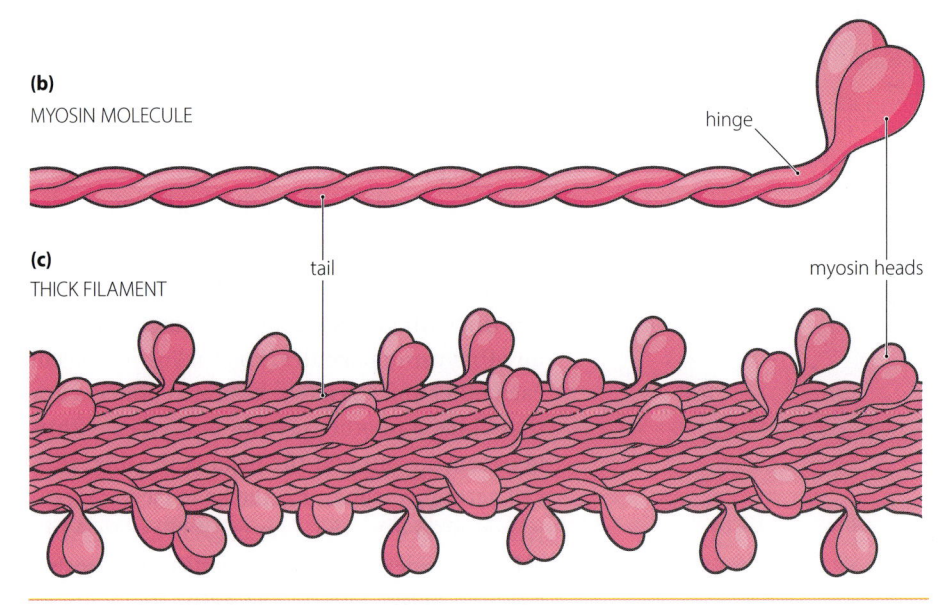

Figure 13.39 – Sections of myofilaments, myosin molecule and a thick filament. (a) Sections of a myosin filament in one sarcomere of a myofibril; (b) a myosin molecule; and (c) a portion of a thick filament.

filaments of the sarcomere to overlap to a great extent. This mechanism is known as the **sliding filament theory of contraction**.

Muscle biomechanics

Biomechanics is the study of movement of living animals using the science of mechanics, a branch of physics that describes motion and how forces create motion. Muscles and bones work in partnership to form lever systems, which operate by applying forces that enable movement to occur. A lever is a rigid structure such as a bone moved by a muscle acting as a force (also known as the **effort**) at a joint or fixed point called the **fulcrum**; the object being moved is the **load**. Joints such as the knee joint and the hip joint act as fulcrums and the effort that moves the load is provided by muscle contraction. The load is the bone (and the object, if any) to be moved.

In the human body, different lever systems are identified by how muscles are attached to a bone at a joint (see *Figure 13.40*). Generally, when a muscle is inserted further away from the fulcrum, more leverage is provided and less effort is needed to move the bone or load. In some lever systems, the fulcrum is found between the effort and the load, such as is seen in a seesaw in a playground. An example in the body is the skull, which acts as the lever, while the posterior neck muscles provide the effort to lift the head (the load). In other lever systems, the load is between the fulcrum and the effort, resulting in less effort being needed to move the load. A person standing on tiptoes is using the toe joints as a pivot and the foot as the lever. The effort is transmitted through the Achilles tendon from the contraction of the calf muscles, while the body weight is the load. In another type of lever system, the effort is nearer the fulcrum than the load or the load is further away from the fulcrum than the effort. Such a lever system is illustrated well by a bent arm, with the elbow representing the fulcrum, the forearm forming

(a) FIRST CLASS LEVER

when tilting the head upwards, the effort is provided by posterior neck muscles

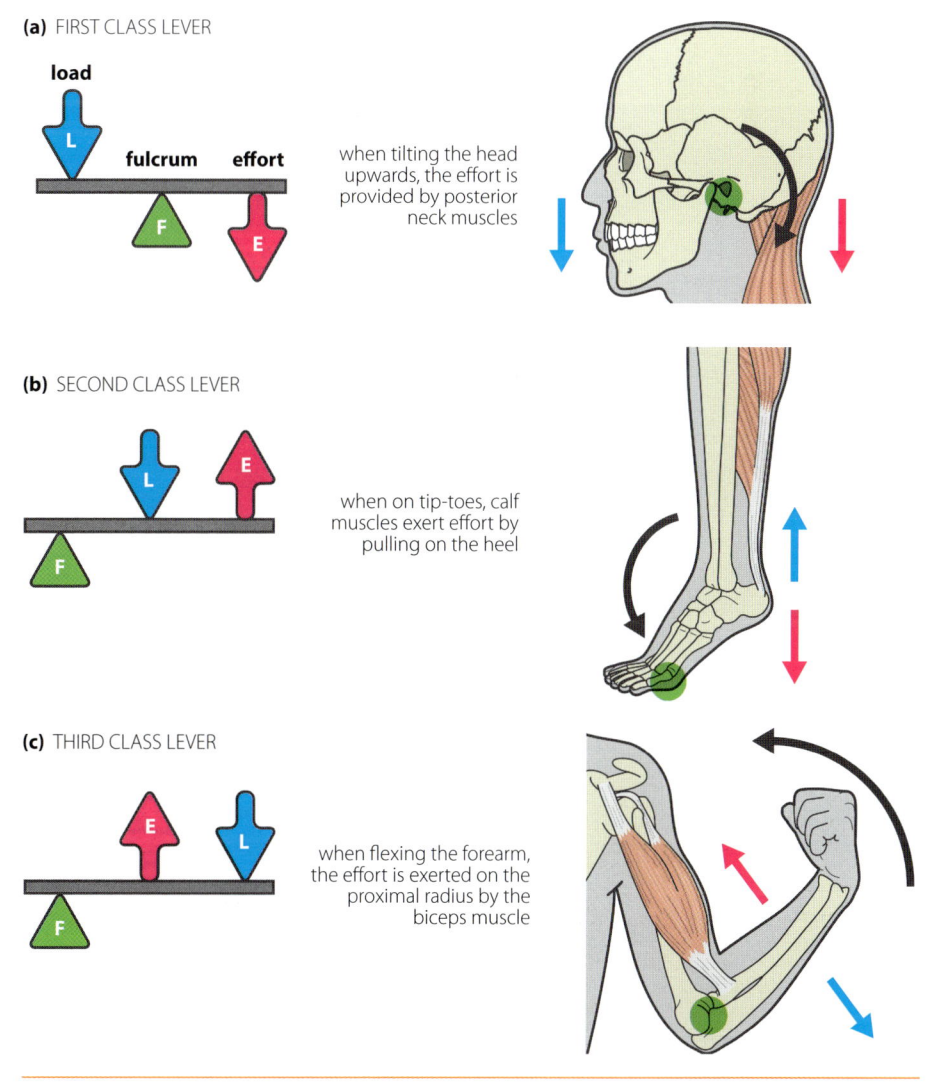

(b) SECOND CLASS LEVER

when on tip-toes, calf muscles exert effort by pulling on the heel

(c) THIRD CLASS LEVER

when flexing the forearm, the effort is exerted on the proximal radius by the biceps muscle

Figure 13.40 – **Skeletomuscular levers that differ in the arrangement of the fulcrum, load and effort.**

the lever and the biceps muscle providing the effort that bends the arm with any load that is being carried (see *Figure 13.40*). This type of lever system enables greater speed of movement than in other lever systems.

An understanding of muscle biomechanics helps to ensure that there is reduction of injury and improved performance in a workplace where moving and handling is performed routinely, as well as during sport and exercise. The different anatomical structures that have been described in this chapter – muscle, bone, cartilage, ligaments and tendons – all have biomechanical properties. In both moving and handling, as well as in sport and exercise, the outcome very much

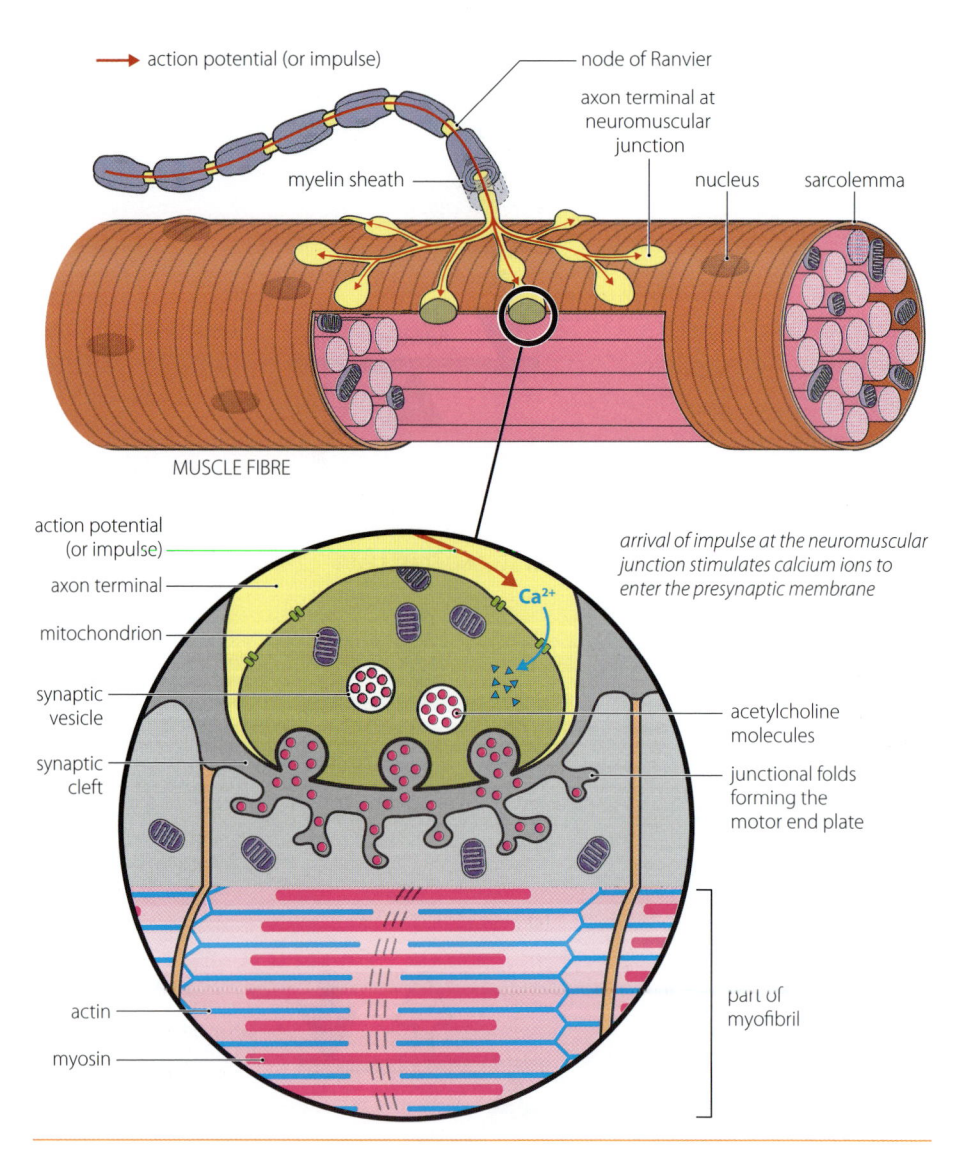

Figure 13.41 – **The neuromuscular junction, showing details of the process that occurs at the synapse.**
The arrival of an impulse at the neuromuscular junction stimulates calcium ions (Ca^{2+}) to enter the presynaptic membrane. This stimulates vesicles containing acetylcholine to be released by exocytosis. Acetylcholine diffuses across the synaptic cleft and binds to its receptors on the junctional folds of the postsynaptic membrane.

depends on the relationship between the applied force and the tissue tolerance to the applied force. An activated muscle generates a force by pulling on its attachments equally. It is the force produced in muscle that powers movement. Bessie (Patient 4.1) illustrates how muscle contraction is affected by lack of coordination and spasticity, while Sally (Patient 6.1), who is experiencing muscle stiffness, spasms, pain and spasticity, illustrates the consequences of lack of coordination.

The neuromuscular junction

Unlike cardiac muscle, skeletal muscle fibres lack the ion channels required for spontaneous membrane depolarization. Therefore, skeletal muscle requires a nerve impulse in order to contract. The synapse formed by motor nerves to muscles is called a neuromuscular junction (see *Figure 13.41*). The postsynaptic membrane, made of folds of the sarcolemma, forms the motor end plate.

The arrival of a nerve impulse at the neuromuscular junction also allows calcium ions (Ca^{2+}) to enter the presynaptic membrane and to stimulate the vesicle containing the neurotransmitter acetylcholine to be released by exocytosis from the vesicles. Acetylcholine diffuses across the synaptic cleft and binds to its receptors on the junctional folds of the postsynaptic membrane of the sarcolemma (see *Figure 13.41*), allowing the muscle to contract. ATP breakdown provides the energy that enables muscle contraction to occur. The process of muscle contraction is summarized in *Box 13.5*.

However, this is short lived because the acetylcholine is destroyed by an enzyme found at the neuromuscular junctions, called acetylcholinesterase (see *Chapter 4*). The destruction of acetylcholine stops continuous muscle contraction and ensures

---

The process of muscle contraction

1. The arrival of a nerve impulse at the neuromuscular junction stimulates the release of acetylcholine, which causes depolarization of the motor end plate and the release of calcium ions (Ca^{2+}) from the sarcoplasmic reticulum.

2. Ca^{2+} binds to one isoform of troponin, causing it to change its shape, resulting in the removal of tropomyosin from the active site of actin. This allows myosin filaments to attach to actin filaments and actin–myosin cross-bridges to form.

3. ATP hydrolysis provides the energy that enables the myosin filaments to pull the actin filaments inwards to shorten the muscle.

4. Myosin filaments detach from the actin filaments, breaking the cross-bridges, when the ATP binds to the myosin heads. Further ATP breakdown allows a myosin head to bind to another actin-binding site further along the actin filament, resulting in repeated pulling of an actin filament over a myosin filament. This repeated pulling is sometimes referred to as a ratchet mechanism.

5. Muscle contraction continues as long as Ca^{2+} and adequate ATP are present, but when the Ca^{2+} dissociates from troponin and returns to the sarcoplasmic reticulum, the muscle relaxes and lengthens.

BOX 13.5

> **BOX 13.6**
>
> **Multiple sclerosis**
>
> Multiple sclerosis is an autoimmune, neurodegenerative condition of the central nervous system characterized by poor conduction of nerve impulses as a result of hardened sclerotic lesions, also known as plaques, that develop in it. The condition usually affects young adults, with first symptoms being experienced between the ages of 20 and 40 years. It is more prevalent in colder climates than warmer climates and affects about 0.1% of the population. The myelin sheaths of nerve fibres, which form the white matter of the nervous system (see *Chapter 4*), become damaged in a process known as demyelination, but the axons remain intact. The exact cause of demyelination is still not clear. However, demyelination results in abnormal conduction of nerve impulses such as *reduced conduction velocity* or *blocked conduction*, affecting muscle function. The areas that may be implicated include the cerebral cortex, affecting muscles of speech and swallowing; the optic nerve, affecting vision; cerebellar tracts, affecting muscles involved in coordination and gait; and corticospinal tracts, whereby the strength of muscles is affected.
>
> *Pathological changes* in multiple sclerosis include: degeneration of myelin sheath and the formation of plaques of demyelination.
>
> *Presenting features* are: gradual loss of vision, a burning sensation, painful eye movements, spasms and stiffness, spastic paralysis (spasticity), poor coordination, ataxia, vertigo, vomiting, frequency and urgency of micturition.
>
> *Complications* include: fatigue, spasticity, tremor, constipation, speech disturbances, bladder dysfunction, erectile dysfunction, depression and memory loss.

that it only occurs when there is nerve stimulation (see *Figure 13.41*). Conditions such as multiple sclerosis (see *Box 13.6*) demonstrate that whenever nerve impulse propagation to muscles is compromised by disease, muscle contraction is affected, leading to lack of coordination and spasticity as some of the presenting features and complications.

13.3 Clinical application

The musculoskeletal system protects organs, generates heat and supports homeodynamic processes. The skeleton and the muscles form lever systems at joints that enable movement to occur in a coordinated manner with the help of the central nervous system (CNS). In addition, careful coordination of the muscles facilitates digestion and elimination. The homeodynamic relationship between the nervous system, cardiovascular system and muscular system is demonstrated by the cases presented in this chapter. A good blood supply to both muscles and the CNS ensures that muscle function is regulated effectively.

- A stroke caused Bessie (Patient 4.1) to have profound difficulty in speaking and walking because she lost control of her muscles. Clinical management included medication to thin her blood, physiotherapy to strengthen her muscles and improve her movement, and speech therapy to strengthen her swallowing muscles and improve her speech.

- **Graham (Patient 4.3)** has a tremor in both hands, rigidity (stiffness) and tiredness caused by Parkinson's disease. His movements have become slower, so that it takes him much longer to fulfil his activities of daily living. His family doctor prescribed co-beneldopa, medication that helps reduce the tremor in his hands and rigidity, together with his other medication for depression (see *Chapter 4*).
- **Sally (Patient 6.1)** has multiple sclerosis, an autoimmune and neurodegenerative condition that has affected the coordination of her muscles and her mobility. Sally experiences spasms and stiffness in some of her muscles and now uses a wheelchair because she has lost her mobility. The damage to some of her neurones is such that her bladder control has been affected and she now has a self-retaining catheter to maintain continence.

Patient 4.1 | **Bessie** | 99 | 130 | 379 | 397 | 403 | **441**

- 71-year-old woman
- Lifelong smoker –20 cigarettes per day
- Found unconscious with stroke and hemiplegia
- Skin damage and incontinence suggests unconscious for >24h
- Macerated skin dressed
- Pressure ulcers will develop without extra care

A stroke can be caused by narrowing and blockage of a cerebral blood vessel (cerebral thrombosis), by a blood clot formed in another part of the body arriving in the brain, or by cerebral haemorrhage (a ruptured artery in the brain). When this happens, the supply of oxygen to the brain is impaired and necrosis of CNS tissue can occur. The blockage to cerebral blood flow can be determined by angiography, a procedure in which a radio-opaque dye is injected into the cerebral arteries; this allows the lesion to be located by X-rays. Bessie highlights the symptoms that are experienced following a stroke. Bessie had right hemiplegia, slurred speech and was drooling saliva with a loss of voluntary movement, following her stroke. The hemiplegia in her right arm was due to impaired motor responses from the brain as a result of poor blood supply to part of the left side of her brain. The reason for the opposite side being affected is because motor neurones cross over from one side to the other in the medulla oblongata, known as decussation. Motor neurones travel from the cerebral cortex to limbs and other parts of the body such as the face to enable voluntary movement. When the nerve impulses are blocked, weakness (paresis) or paralysis develops on one side of the body (hemiplegia). Physiotherapy can usually help to improve mobility in the majority of cases, although residual weakness remains in many individuals, depending on the site and extent of the damage.

The drooling of saliva is due to motor impulses to the face being affected, resulting in weakness in the facial muscles. The centre for initiation of speech is located in the left side of the brain in most people. Loss of speech is called aphasia. Following a stroke, people will have difficulty understanding speech (receptive aphasia) or difficulty in expressing themselves (expressive aphasia). The slurred speech is a result of facial muscles being affected. In many people, loss of speech is temporary and significant recovery can be achieved with the help of speech therapy.

Patient 4.3 — Graham

- 57-year-old man
- Gradual onset of trembling in left hand
- Family doctor referred him to neurologist
- Diagnosis of Parkinson disease led to depression
- MRI has excluded other causes
- Prescribed bromocriptine to help with Parkinson symptoms

Parkinson's disease usually affects people over 50 years of age, although people under the age of 50 are also affected. Up to approximately 5% of Parkinson's disease is associated with certain genes with an inheritance pattern that is thought to be autosomal recessive, while 95% is thought to be multifactorial in origin, including environmental factors such as undetected viruses. It does appear that Graham has Parkinson's disease that is multifactorial in origin, as there is nobody else in his family who has the disease. People affected by Parkinson's disease do not produce enough of the neurotransmitter dopamine in their brain, especially in the substantia nigra, which is part of the basal ganglia (see *Chapter 4, Table 4.1*). Dopamine modulates the activity of muscarinic (cholinergic) neurones, which activate skeletal muscles, resulting in suppression of undesired movements of the skeletal muscles. Graham's tremor is more prominent when he is at rest, and it is observed to disappear with intentional movement. The tremor can interfere with coordination, causing him, for example, to spill a drink; this makes him embarrassed and frustrated. He has found that taking co-beneldopa (Madopar) capsules stops him from shaking and his movements have also improved, such that he does not take as long to perform his activities of daily living as he used to before he started taking this medication. Taking dopamine orally would not help Graham because dopamine cannot cross the blood–brain barrier. However, taking co-beneldopa helps because it is made up of two drugs: benserazide and levodopa, the amino acid precursor of dopamine, which can cross the blood–brain barrier. Benserazide is an extracerebral DOPA decarboxylase inhibitor – it stops levodopa from being converted to dopamine peripherally (outside the brain) by blocking the enzyme DOPA decarboxylase, ensuring more levodopa enters the brain where the brain neurones can use it to make more dopamine. Benserazide does not cross the blood–brain barrier, which is helpful. Levodopa is converted to dopamine in the brain, and this replaces the dopamine that has been lost due to Parkinson's disease. When Graham first started taking co-beneldopa, he noticed that he felt nauseous, which he discussed with his family doctor and Parkinson's nurse. The Parkinson's nurse suggested that Graham might want to try taking his capsule with a small amount of protein food but to eat most of the protein in the evening meal. Such a change in his routine has helped to reduce the feeling of nausea. Eating too much protein at the time of taking the co-beneldopa can reduce the amount of drug that is absorbed. Should the nausea get worse, Graham may have to be prescribed domperidone which reduces nausea and vomiting. Graham will benefit from care that focuses on helping him to maintain flexibility and reduce joint rigidity, such as exercise and other forms of physical therapy. Emotional support will be important to Graham in order to boost his mental wellbeing.

Patient 6.1 | Sally | 167 | 188 | 404 | **443**

- 50-year-old woman
- Has MS and is now a wheelchair user
- Burning sensation in her hands and double vision
- MRI confirms plaques in her brain consistent with MS

Sally's case demonstrates that in multiple sclerosis, which results in demyelination of the neurones, mobility is greatly affected and reduced due to muscle weakness. Multiple sclerosis affects more women than men, although the reasons for this are not clear. Sally, who is now disabled, has lived with multiple sclerosis for 15 years since she was diagnosed. She has muscle spasms, stiffness and joint pain, and has lost the ability to move her legs due to progression of the disease, such that she relies on a wheelchair to get about. A hoist has to be used to help transfer Sally from bed to chair and in and out of the bath. Muscle tightness and pain are experienced, causing spasms in Sally, while in other cases spasticity occurs where muscles become stiff and resistant to movement. Spasms and spasticity cause pressure on muscles and joints, resulting in pain. In severe cases of multiple sclerosis, all muscle coordination is lost and the affected person may require the support of a wheelchair, as has happened in Sally's situation. Bladder control is eventually lost due to the demyelination in the CNS and poor conduction of nerve impulses to the bladder. This has happened in Sally's case so a urinary catheter has been placed into her bladder. Sally has regular catheter care to minimize infection and her catheter is changed every 3 months. Sally benefits from taking baclofen 10 mg three times a day to limit the spasticity. Baclofen is a skeletal muscle relaxant that works on the CNS and helps to relieve spasms and spasticity. It inhibits transmission at the spinal level. The overall aim of Sally's care is to improve her quality of life.

The focus of this chapter has been to explain how movement is achieved by the coordinated function of bones and their attachments. These include muscles, ligaments and tendons. Bones and their attachments form lever systems that enable voluntary movement by skeletal muscles to occur. The importance of adequate nutrition and the role of hormones to maintain integrity of bones through calcium and phosphorus regulation should not be underestimated, in particular during adolescence in young females, when bone density is reinforced by hormonal action such as that of oestrogen. The patients discussed in this chapter illustrate how diseases that affect muscle functioning affect movement.

13.4 Summary

- Movement is a complex process achieved by the coordinated functions of the bones of the skeleton, their attachments and the nervous system.
- The skeleton provides the framework in which levers and joints enable movement to occur with the help of muscles, ligaments and tendons (*Figure 13.40*).
- Bones articulate with each other to form joints, some of which are immovable and others which are slightly movable or freely movable (*Table 13.3*).
- Bones store important minerals such as calcium, phosphorus and magnesium, and some hormones are involved in the homeodynamic storage and release of minerals by bones.

- Skeletal muscle is voluntary and has striations, while smooth muscle is involuntary and has no striations (*Figure 13.36*).
- The meeting of a nerve fibre and a muscle forms a neuromuscular junction where the neurotransmitter acetylcholine is released to enable muscle contraction (*Figure 13.41*).

13.5 Further reading

The following website has many interactive pictures on the human body and gives information on the skeletal system and its attachments and how movement is allowed at joints:
www.innerbody.com

The website of the UK National Osteoporosis Society highlights the factors influencing who is at risk of osteoporosis and fractures. It also suggests foods and nutrients that are important for bone health, as well as other measures that people can take, such as physical activity, to improve the health of their bones:
www.nos.org.uk/

The UK Multiple Sclerosis Society website has information on how individuals living with multiple sclerosis can access support and specialist healthcare. It also contains useful publications on the condition for both the public and health professionals, including evidence from recent research:
www.mssociety.org.uk/

Parkinson's UK is a charitable organization in the UK that gives advice to individuals newly diagnosed with Parkinson's disease, as well as to those living with the condition and their relatives. Furthermore, information is made available on the website regarding local peer support services that can be accessed. The contact details and location of Parkinson's nurses are also given:
www.parkinsons.org.uk

13.6 Self-assessment questions

Answers can be found at www.scionpublishing.com/AandP

(13.1) Select the one correct answer. What is the tubular shaft in between each end of a long bone, such as the femur and the humerus, called?
    (a) Medullary cavity
    (b) Epiphysis
    (c) Diaphysis
    (d) Periosteum
    (e) Compact bone

(13.2) Select the one correct answer. What is the name that is used when classifying joints to describe joints that are slightly movable, such as cartilaginous joints?
    (a) Diarthroses
    (b) Sutures
    (c) Syndesmoses
    (d) Gomposes
    (e) Synchondroses

(13.3) Which one of the following is not a function of muscle?
  (a) Heat generation
  (b) Maintenance of posture
  (c) Enabling movement
  (d) Holding bones together at joints
  (e) Formation of sphincters

(13.4) Select the one correct answer. Which muscle protein has specificity for cardiac muscle and is used to identify damage to myocardial muscle following myocardial infarction?
  (a) Actin
  (b) Acetylcholine
  (c) Troponin
  (d) Tropomysium
  (e) Myosin

(13.5) Mark each statement either true or false:
  (a) Fibrous joints have a joint cavity and are immovable.
  (b) The stability of synovial joints depends on the shape of articular surfaces, number of ligaments and muscle tone.
  (c) A hinge joint allows movement in one plane only.
  (d) Adduction is movement of limbs away from the midline.
  (e) Hyaline cartilage acts as a shock absorber.

(13.6) Mark each statement either true or false:
  (a) The bones of the foot are referred to as carpals and metacarpals.
  (b) The insertion of a muscle further away from the fulcrum provides more leverage, enabling less effort to move the load.
  (c) During muscle contraction, the binding of ATP to myosin heads enables filaments to detach from the actin filaments.
  (d) Smooth muscle has no striations and contains intercalated discs.
  (e) In multiple sclerosis, the axon is damaged while the myelin sheath remains intact.

(13.7) Select the one correct answer. Which of the following bones is not part of the hand?
  (a) Capitate
  (b) Hamate
  (c) Scaphoid
  (d) Talus
  (e) Trapezium

(13.8) Describe the process that results in bone development.

(13.9) Describe the characteristics of a synovial joint and how it is suited for its function.

CHAPTER 14 | From one generation to the next

Learning points for this chapter

After working through this chapter, you should be able to:

- Name and identify the structures of the male reproductive system
- Outline the role of accessory glands in the production of semen
- Describe the regulation of spermatogenesis
- Name and identify the structures of the female reproductive system
- Describe the ovarian and menstrual (uterine) cycles
- Describe the early hormonal changes associated with pregnancy
- Describe the interplay of hormones between the fetus and mother that are associated with labour and birth
- Describe the development of the breast during puberty and pregnancy

14.1 Introduction and clinical relevance

Each of the patients discussed in this chapter illustrates how normal reproductive physiology can be altered, leading to health problems that are commonly encountered. The cases help to identify the underpinning knowledge about reproduction that is required by healthcare professionals to ensure that knowledgeable and informed support and care are provided.

Patient 1.1 | Amy | 1 | 20 | 194 | 235 | **447** | 473

- 18-year-old woman
- BMI 16.3
- Downy hair on face and arms
- Referred to eating disorder clinic
- Eating under supervision to increase intake and also getting psychological support
- Also anaemic

Amy is an 18-year-old girl who has been diagnosed with anorexia nervosa. Her body mass index (BMI) was 16.3 kg/m² and she was admitted to hospital where a protocol to manage her eating disorder was put into place. This included supervised meal times and psychological support from a clinical psychologist and mental health nurses. Her menstrual periods were irregular, and she had missed periods due to a hormonal imbalance related to her low body weight and severe calorie restriction.

| Patient 2.3 | Sheila | 30 | 54 | 59 | 93 | 267 | 304 | **448** | 473 |

- 47-year-old woman
- Recent diagnosis of breast cancer
- Biological therapy with trastuzumab (Herceptin) to block HER2 action an option
- Is still offered surgery, chemotherapy and radiotherapy
- Adds trastuzumab to chemotherapy plan
- Advised about surgery: lymphoedema a possibility

Sheila has recently been diagnosed with breast cancer. Her type of breast cancer is an invasive ductal carcinoma, which means that the cancer has spread beyond the breast ducts. She will require surgery to remove the cancer, and this will be followed by a course of chemotherapy. Following consultation with her doctor and her breast care nurse, Sheila has accepted the addition of trastuzumab (Herceptin) to her chemotherapy plan as her cancer cells are *HER2* positive (see *Chapters 2* and *3*).

| Patient 4.2 | Jade and Jordon | 100 | 132 | 138 | 162 | **448** | 473 |

- 6-year-old boy and 32-year-old mother
- Jade drank alcohol excessively while pregnant
- Jordon has dysmorphic facial features and behavioural issues
- Jordon has fetal alcohol syndrome
- Jordon was small for age and given GH at age 4
- Aged 6 he is up to the 60th percentile on charts

Jade drank alcohol excessively during her pregnancy, and as a result, her son, Jordon, was born with fetal alcohol syndrome (FAS). Alcohol readily crosses the placenta from the mother to the fetus and acts as a teratogen, a substance that can cause harm to a developing fetus. The extent of the harm is determined by the amount of alcohol consumed and the stage of development of the fetus. For example, if the mother consumes excessive amounts of alcohol during weeks 6–9 of her pregnancy, her baby is likely to have the facial deformities typical of FAS because these weeks represent the critical period when facial features develop. Jordon has these features, which can include a thin upper lip, a smooth area (philtrum) between the nose and lips, a small head circumference and abnormally small, widely spaced eyes.

| Patient 5.1 | David | 138 | 161 | 195 | 237 | **448** | 474 |

- 44-year-old man
- Increased urine output; thirsty and hungry
- Blood test: low thyroxine and raised blood glucose
- Has hypothyroidism and the start of a goitre
- Given levothyroxine; dose adjusted until thyroxine levels stabilise
- Has diabetes associated with obesity – diet modified and given metformin

David has type 2 diabetes and has made a great effort to lose weight in order to improve the sensitivity of the cells to insulin and therefore to help control his blood glucose level. However, this was not successful, and over a number of years David's blood glucose levels have fluctuated considerably, requiring him to commence an antidiabetic drug. Over a period of time, David noticed that he found it increasingly difficult to achieve and maintain an erection. His concern about this was sufficient for him to seek advice from his family doctor.

| Patient 9.1 | Robert | 268 | 305 | **448** | 474 |

- 56-year-old man with family history of CVD
- First MI at 38, stent at 45, and CABG at 49
- ECG shows changes consistent with another MI; confirmed by biochemical marker tests
- Has hypotension and oedema
- Prescribed aspirin, atorvastatin, bisoprolol and perindopril
- Diet altered to reduce salt and fat and exercise levels increased

Although Robert's heart failure was controlled well through various drugs, Robert was always conscious about needing to void urine frequently and always having the sensation that he never fully emptied his bladder. At first, Robert thought this was due to his medication, but as his problems were worse during the night, disturbing his sleep, he discussed this with his family doctor. The doctor decided to perform a digital rectal examination and identified an enlarged prostate gland. The doctor therefore organized a blood test for prostate-specific antigen (PSA).

Patient 14.1 | Jess | 449 | 475

- 33-year-old woman
- Intermenstrual and post-coital bleeding
- Family doctor requests smear test
- Some dyskaryosis found

Jess is 33 years old and has been with her current partner for 1 year. She has taken the oral contraceptive pill since she was 19 and started smoking when she was 18. She has noticed that she has some bleeding between her monthly periods and also sometimes following sex. She attended her first cervical screening appointment when she was 25, but she has missed her subsequent appointments at 28 and 31 years. Her family doctor requested a smear test, which involves removing some of the cells from Jess's cervix and examining them under a microscope. Abnormal cells were discovered following the smear, and Jess was told that she had moderate changes to some of her cells, termed **dyskaryosis**.

The patients discussed in this chapter experience health problems that involve the reproductive system. They each require support to restore, where possible, normal reproductive function. For example, Amy (Patient 1.1) has an altered menstrual cycle, which is connected to her undernutrition, identifying the importance of a healthy balanced diet for reproductive health. Sheila (Patient 2.3) has breast cancer due to a mutation in her *HER2* gene, and her case highlights how surgical removal of the cancer cells, combined with chemotherapy, biological therapy and radiotherapy, can reduce the risk of her cancer returning. David (Patient 5.1) is suffering from impotence, a common problem related to alteration in blood flow arising from his diabetes. Robert (Patient 9.1) has difficulty with the voiding of urine due to an obstruction to the flow of urine from his bladder. This could be due to prostate cancer, which would have very serious consequences for his health. Jade and Jordon (Patient 4.2) highlight the importance of good antenatal guidance and support, while Jess (Patient 14.1) highlights how important regular smear tests are in order to identify changes in the shape and activity of cells and the development of cervical cancer.

14.2 What you need to know – essential anatomy and physiology

14.2.1 Structure and function of the male reproductive system

Figure 14.1 illustrates the major components of the male reproductive system. **Sperm**-producing cells are found in the testes, which are contained in the **scrotum**. A system of ducts exists to deliver sperm outside of the body. Sperm are produced in the testes (singular: testicle) and travel from the testes via the **epididymis**, the **ductus deferens (vas deferens)**, the ejaculatory duct and finally the urethra to the external opening of the penis. The paired testes are located in two separate compartments within the scrotum. Importantly, the testes are held outside of the abdominopelvic cavity in order to provide the optimal temperature for the production of sperm. Viable sperm cannot be produced in the required number if the testes are at core body temperature. The scrotum is maintained at a temperature approximately 3 °C below the core body temperature; via contraction or relaxation of the cremaster muscles, the testes can be raised or lowered to maintain the optimal temperature. Each testicle contains three to four tightly

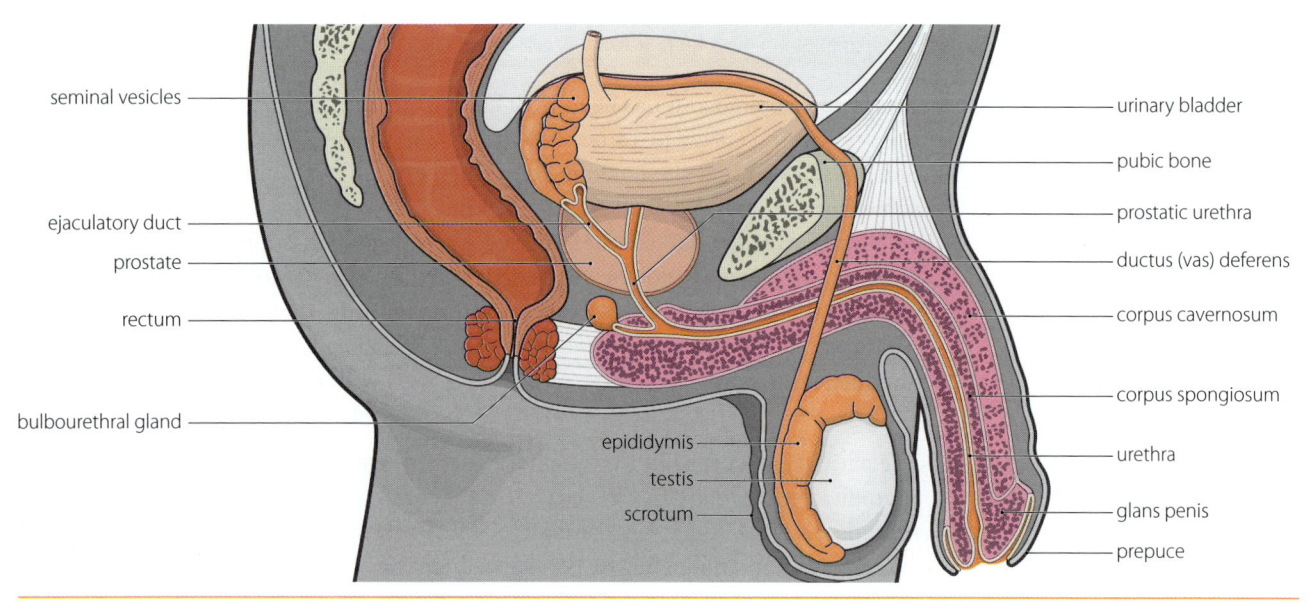

Figure 14.1 – The male reproductive organs (sagittal view).

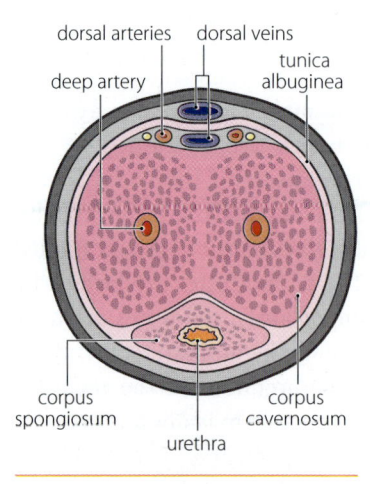

Figure 14.2 – Transverse section of the penis.

coiled **seminiferous tubules** in which sperm are produced (see *Chapter 5, Figure 5.12*). Lying in the connective tissue surrounding the seminiferous tubules are the **interstitial cells** (also called Leydig cells), which produce androgens and in particular **testosterone**.

The **penis** and the scrotum make up the external genitalia. The penis has a root and a shaft, which ends in an enlarged tip called the glans penis (see *Figure 14.1*). The loose skin (**prepuce**) covering the penis and glans penis can be pulled back to reveal the glans penis. The penis comprises the spongy urethra and three long cylindrical bodies (two called the corpora cavernosa and one called the corpus spongiosum) of erectile tissue, incorporating connective tissue, smooth muscle and vascular spaces (see *Figure 14.2*). During sexual arousal, erection of the penis is caused by filling of the vascular spaces in the erectile tissue with blood. This is due to activation of the parasympathetic nervous system (see *Chapter 4*), which promotes the release of the vasodilator nitric oxide (see *Chapter 9*). As a result, smooth muscle cells in the wall of penile arterioles relax, causing the vessels to dilate, thus increasing the blood flow to the erectile tissue. Enlargement of the penis compresses veins in the tunica albuginea, preventing venous drainage, which maintains engorgement of the corpora cavernosa. The corpus spongiosum expands to a lesser extent, which allows the urethra to remain open for ejaculation. Longitudinal and circular collagen fibres surrounding the penis ensure that the penis remains straight during intercourse. Erection is a complex process, initiated by a number of physical and emotional cues, including tactile stimulation, visual stimulation and erotic thoughts. Some men may experience erectile dysfunction where there is an inability to experience and maintain a penile erection for satisfactory sexual intercourse. This condition has many physical and psychological causes, including narrowing of the blood vessels affecting the flow of blood to the penis linked to diabetes mellitus (see David, Patient 5.1) or hypertension, following prostatic surgery, due to hormonal imbalance such as hypothyroidism (see David, Patient 5.1) and as a result of psychological concerns such as anxiety, depression and relationship problems. Other factors that may lead to erectile dysfunction include excessive alcohol consumption, some prescription drugs, recreational drugs, and pressure on nerve pathways and blood vessels from bicycle seats during long-distance cycling.

The epididymis is located on the superior surface of the testes (see *Figure 14.1*). Most of the testes comprises a highly coiled duct system. Immature, almost non-motile sperm that leave the testes are moved along the fluid of the epididymis duct; this takes about 20 days, and during this time, sperm gain the ability to swim. Sperm can be stored in the epididymis for several months. Sperm are ejaculated from the epididymis by smooth muscle contraction of the wall of the epididymis, which pushes sperm into the next duct, the ductus (vas) deferens. The ductus deferens extends upwards, over the ureter and descends behind the bladder to join the ejaculatory duct, which passes through the prostate gland and then empties into the urethra. It is the ductus deferens that is surgically cut and tied off when a man has a vasectomy. As a result, sperm cannot be ejaculated. The wall of the ductus deferens has a thick smooth muscle layer, which contracts on ejaculation, producing powerful peristaltic waves that quickly push the sperm, contained within the semen, forward along the duct into the urethra.

While erection is under the control of the parasympathetic nervous system, ejaculation occurs by the action of the sympathetic nervous system. When sensory stimuli that provoke an erection reach a peak, a spinal reflex is initiated and motor (efferent) impulses are conducted to the genital organs via sympathetic neurones. This results in:

- contraction of the bladder internal sphincter to prevent voiding of urine and the passage of semen into the bladder
- contraction of the reproductive ducts and accessory glands to propel semen into the urethra
- powerful rhythmic contraction of the bulbospongiosus muscle of the penis, triggered by semen in the urethra, to expel semen from the urethra.

These events are referred to as an orgasm. Following this, there is a period of resolution when the penis becomes flaccid and there is a latent (also called a refractory) period during which another orgasm cannot be achieved. This period varies in length from minutes to hours and the period lengthens with age.

Sperm are transported in a fluid mixture called semen, which is milky white and sticky. Semen volume on ejaculation is approximately 2–5 ml and semen contains 20–150 million sperm per millilitre. Semen provides the transport medium for sperm and contains chemicals that activate sperm and facilitate their movement. Chemicals such as prostaglandins in the semen decrease the viscosity of the mucus in the female reproductive tract; the hormone relaxin in semen enhances sperm motility, and clotting factors coagulate the semen on ejaculation to prevent loss of sperm from the vagina while the sperm are initially immobile. The semen clot is liquefied in minutes, as semen contains fibrinolysin, which breaks up the clot, releasing sperm to swim along the female reproductive tract. Semen is alkaline (pH 7.2–7.6) and this helps to neutralize the remnants of acidic urine in the urethra and the acid secretion within the vagina, providing an ideal environment for the survival of sperm.

Semen is formed by secretions from the accessory glands: the **seminal vesicles**, the **prostate** and the **bulbourethral glands** (see *Figure 14.1*). Paired seminal vesicles are located on the posterior surface of the bladder. The secretion from the seminal vesicles accounts for 60–70% of the volume of semen and contains fructose, which is used to meet the energy requirements of sperm, prostaglandins and an enzyme to activate coagulation of semen. In the ejaculatory duct, sperm mix with the fluid secretion from the seminal vesicles before flowing into the prostatic urethra. The prostate surrounds the urethra, below the bladder. The milky and slightly acidic secretion from the prostate gland accounts for approximately 33% of semen volume and contains citrate (a nutrient), enzymes including fibrinolysin, and prostate-specific antigen (PSA). The importance of PSA as a biomarker for prostate cancer is outlined in *Box 14.1*. The paired bulbourethral glands lie inferior to the prostate gland and produce a thick clear secretion that neutralizes acid urine residue in the urethra, thus ensuring a safe passage for sperm.

Spermatogenesis

Spermatogenesis occurs in the seminiferous tubules of the testes and involves a series of events resulting in the production of sperm (spermatozoa). As outlined in *Chapter 3*, male and female gametes contain the haploid number of chromosomes (23), one chromosome from each pair of chromosomes. Gamete formation involves meiosis (see *Chapter 3*). The events that occur in the seminiferous tubules to produce sperm are illustrated in *Figure 14.3*. Sperm cells develop from stem cells called spermatogonia, which are in direct contact with the epithelial layer of the wall of the seminiferous tubules. Spermatogonia divide by *mitosis* and each *mitotic* division produces two daughter cells – cell types A and B. Type A

BOX 14.1

Enlargement of the prostate, prostate cancer and prostate-specific antigen

Enlargement of the prostate includes benign prostatic hyperplasia (BPH) and prostate cancer. BPH is common in older men and does not usually present a risk to a man's life, unlike prostatic cancer. The incidence of prostate cancer varies according to race, country of origin and other factors. Prostate cancer is the most common cancer in men in the UK, accounting for 25% of all new cancers in men, and in the USA, prostate cancer is the second most common cancer after skin cancer. There is no single diagnostic test for prostate cancer, but common investigations include a digital rectal examination (DRE) to determine enlargement of the prostate and the nature of that enlargement, measurement of the levels of prostate-specific antigen (PSA) in the blood, and biopsy of the prostate. PSA levels may be raised in prostate cancer; however, there are other non-cancerous causes of a raised PSA, such as BPH and prostatitis. Factors that affect the risk of high-grade cancer are PSA level, DRE findings, age and African ethnicity, and these are incorporated into assessment tools to determine an individual's risk for high-grade cancer. Men with a high risk of cancer would undergo an investigation to biopsy the prostatic tissue. Symptoms of an enlarged prostate (whether or not due to cancer) include an alteration in urine flow (weak flow), the sensation of needing to pass urine frequently, especially during the night, difficulty in starting the flow of urine and the sensation that the bladder is never fully emptied.

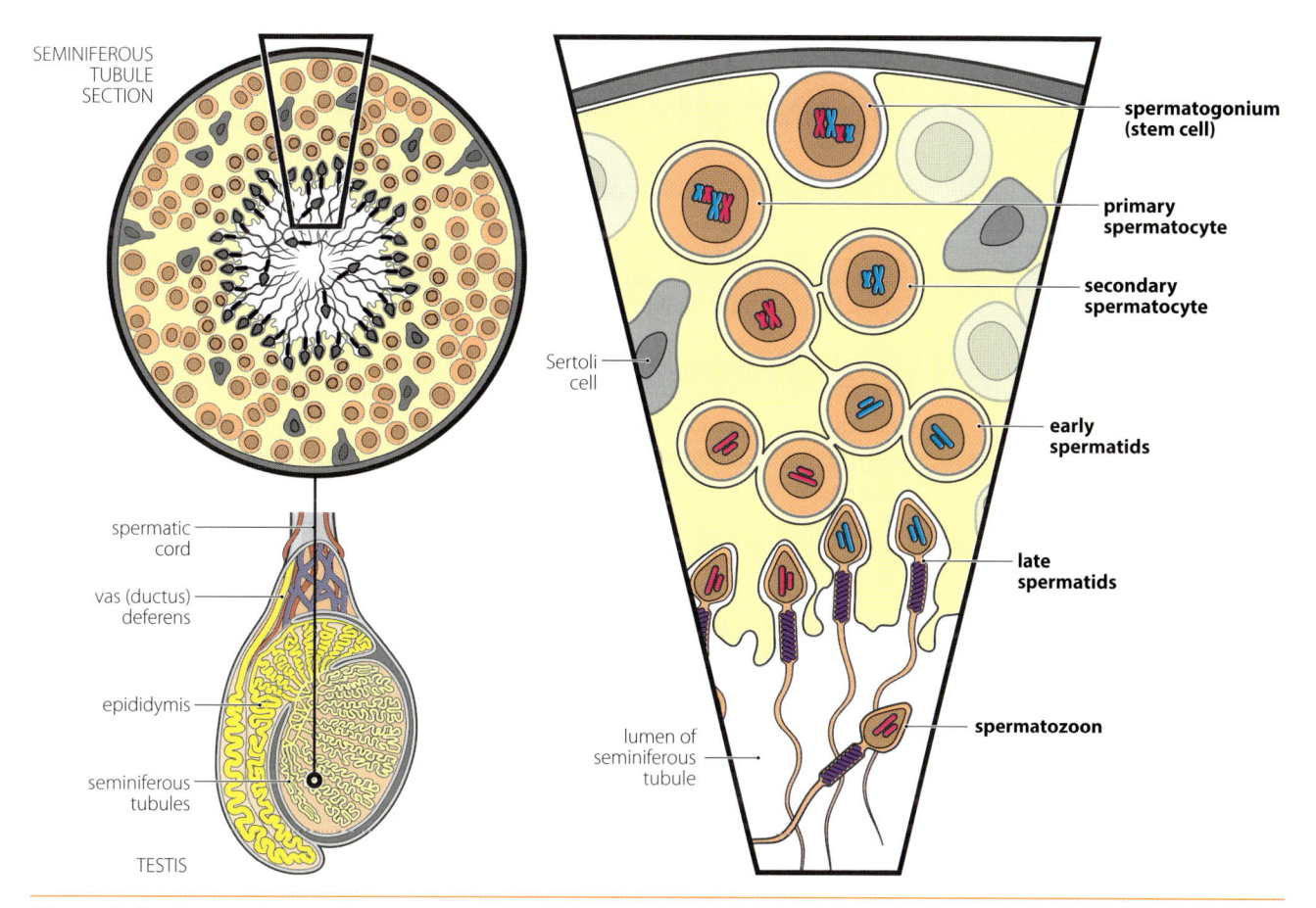

SECTION **14.2** | WHAT YOU NEED TO KNOW – ESSENTIAL ANATOMY AND PHYSIOLOGY 453

Figure 14.3 – **Spermatogenesis.**

daughter cells maintain the stem cell line, while a type B daughter cell becomes a primary spermatocyte, which ultimately will produce four sperm. Each primary spermatocyte undergoes *meiosis*, eventually resulting in the formation of spermatids, which contain the haploid number ready for fertilization. Further development of the spermatid, known as spermiogenesis, leads to elongation of the spermatid and formation of a head and tail (see *Figure 14.4*). Sperm comprise a head, containing compacted DNA, the **acrosome**, which contains enzymes that enable sperm to penetrate an ovum, a midpiece containing mitochondria for metabolic energy and a tail. Using fructose for energy, motile sperm are propelled by the whip-like motion of the tail. Spermatogenesis from the formation of a primary spermatocyte to the release of an immature sperm into the lumen of the seminiferous tubules takes approximately 64–72 days. Closely associated with spermatogonia are supporting cells called **sustentacular cells** (Sertoli cells).

Hormonal regulation of spermatogenesis and the secretion of testosterone involve interactions between the hypothalamus, the anterior pituitary gland and the testes; this interaction is illustrated in *Figure 14.5*. Spermatogenesis commences at puberty, triggered by the secretion of gonadotrophin-releasing hormone (GnRH) by the hypothalamus, which stimulates the release of follicle-stimulating hormone (FSH) and luteinizing hormone (LH) from the anterior pituitary gland.

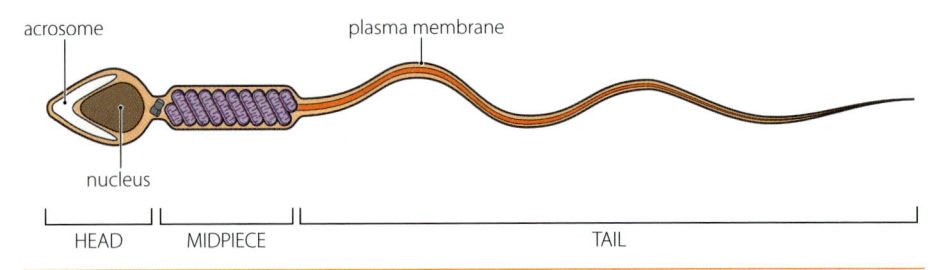

Figure 14.4 – **A spermatozoon (sperm).**

FSH stimulates sustentacular cells to release androgen-binding protein, which enables sperm-producing cells to bind testosterone to stimulate spermatogenesis. LH stimulates interstitial cells in the testes to secrete testosterone and a small amount of oestrogen. Testosterone stimulates spermatogenesis; the rising concentration of testosterone, by negative feedback, inhibits the release of GnRH, FSH and LH. In addition, when the sperm count is high, the hormone inhibin is released from the sustentacular cells, inhibiting the secretion of GnRH and FSH. As discussed in *Chapter 5*, testosterone is a steroid hormone synthesized from cholesterol. During puberty, testosterone not only stimulates spermatogenesis but also exerts more widespread effects, resulting in typical male secondary sex characteristics, including the appearance of facial, axillary and pubic hair, deepening of the voice and an increase in skeletal muscle mass.

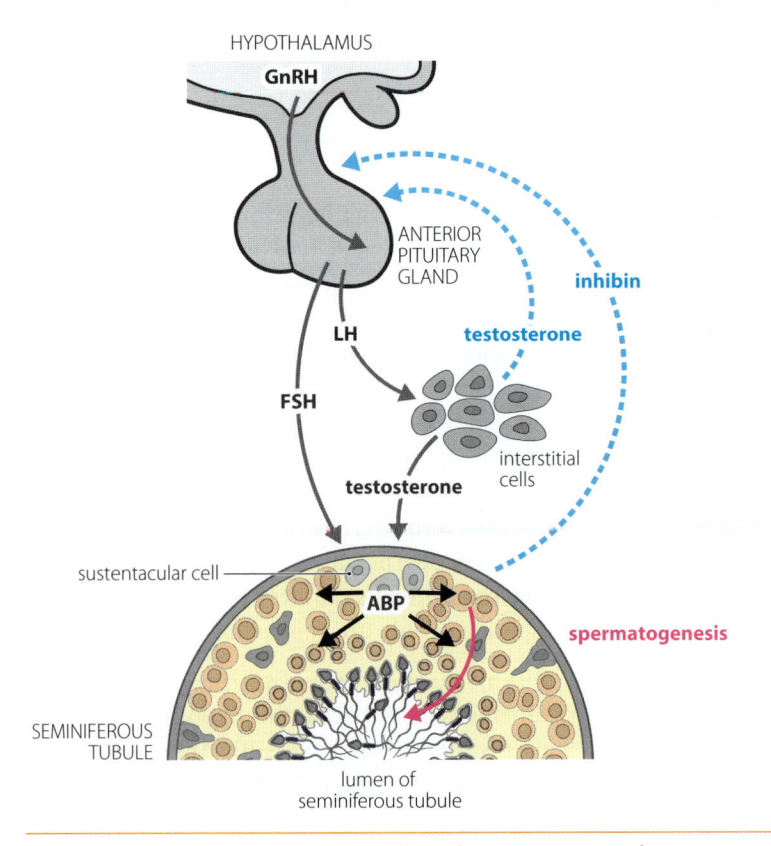

Figure 14.5 – **The hormonal regulation of spermatogenesis.**

14.2.2 Structure and function of the female reproductive system

The structures of the female reproductive system can be divided into the external genitalia and the internal genitalia. The external genitalia lie outside the pelvis and the internal genitalia lie within the pelvis.

External genitalia

The external genitalia, also known as the **vulva**, consist of a number of organs and structures (see *Figure 14.6*). The vulva is surrounded by two flaps of skin and adipose tissue called the labia majora. The labia majora form a protective cover for the rest of the genitalia and come together anteriorly to form a mass of fatty tissue called the mons pubis, which acts as a cushion over the pubic symphysis of the pelvis during sexual intercourse. The labia majora and mons pubis are covered in pubic hair following puberty.

Under the covering of the labia majora are two folds of tissue called the labia minora, which are more delicate than the labia majora and are hair free. The labia minora form the lateral borders of the vestibule, a structure that houses the external urethral and vaginal orifices. The vestibule contains mucus-producing vestibular glands, which keep the area moist and facilitate sexual intercourse.

Anterior to the vestibule lies the clitoris (see *Figure 14.6*). This is similar to the male penis in that it contains a large number of sensory nerve endings, and during intercourse it becomes engorged with blood, contributing to female sexual arousal. The clitoris is covered by a layer of skin, which is formed by the junction between the two labia minora.

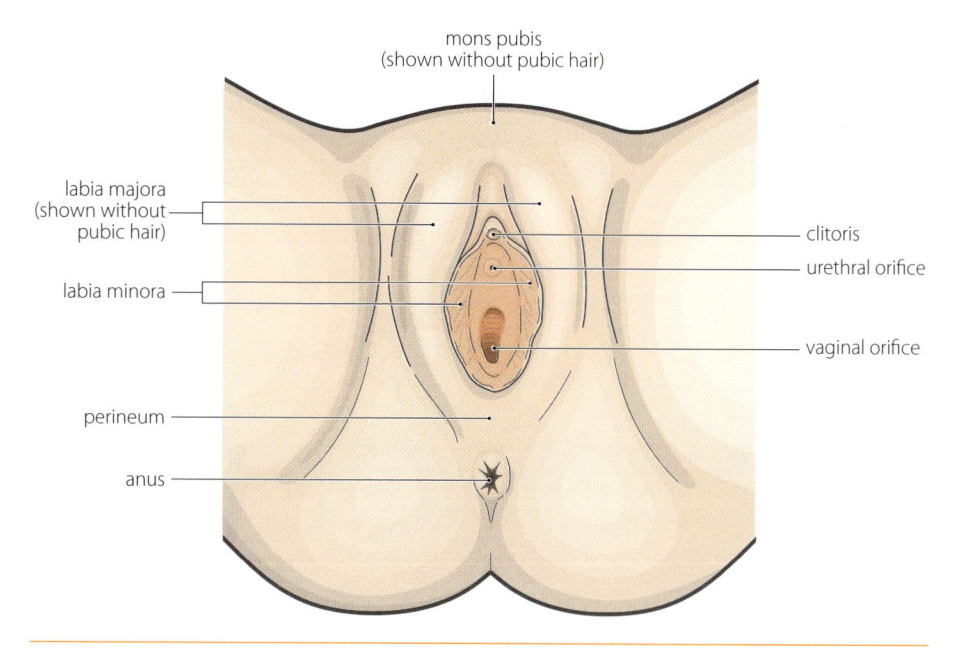

Figure 14.6 – The female external genitalia (inferior view).

The **perineum** is the muscular area between the external genitalia and the anus. This can tear during childbirth or can be purposely cut to facilitate birth. This is called an episiotomy or perineotomy.

Internal genitalia

The internal genitalia lie within the pelvic cavity and include the vagina, cervix, uterus, uterine tubes and ovaries (see *Figure 14.7*).

The vagina

The **vagina** is a tube-like structure approximately 10 cm long in an adult female. It consists of three anatomical layers: the inner mucosa, a muscularis layer in the middle and an outer adventitia of connective tissue. The mucosa consists of stratified squamous epithelium that, along with vaginal commensal organisms such as lactobacillus, is responsible for creating an acidic environment. The vagina has a pH of 4, which limits the growth of potential pathogens introduced through sexual activity. Semen neutralizes the acid for a number of hours, which facilitates fertilization. Indeed, the main role of the vagina is to receive the penis during sexual intercourse. Its tube-like structure also facilitates the passage of the baby from the uterus to the outside world during childbirth and as such is also called the 'birth canal'.

The uterus

The **uterus** is superior and posterior to the urinary bladder and consists of three parts: the fundus, the body and the cervix (see *Figure 14.7*). In adult women, it

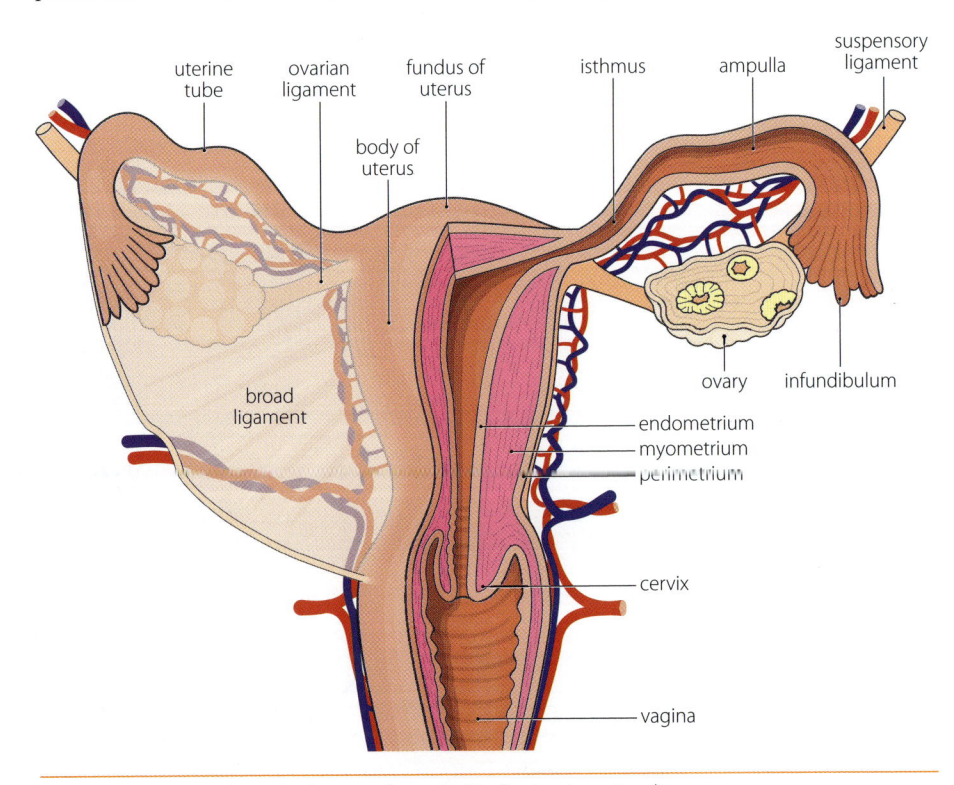

Figure 14.7 – **The female internal genitalia (anterior view).**

is approximately the size of a pear and confined to the pelvic cavity; however, it increases substantially in size and extends upwards into the abdominal cavity during pregnancy.

The position of the **fundus** during pregnancy is a useful indicator of fetal growth. As the fundus advances into the abdominal cavity to accommodate the growth of the fetus, its position or 'height' can be palpated and the distance between the fundus and the pubic bone measured with a tape measure. This measurement is used to estimate fetal growth and development.

The function of the uterus is to provide a protective cavity within which the embryo and later the fetus can grow. The embryo implants into the uterus and vascular connections develop that go on to form the placenta, the organ that connects the fetus to the inner wall of the uterus. The uterus is important during childbirth as its contractions, under the influence of oxytocin (see *Chapter 5*), help push the baby into the outside world during labour. Uterine contractions also facilitate the expulsion of menstrual blood. These contractions can be painful and are typically described as 'period pain'.

Structurally, the uterus is made up of three layers: the perimetrium, the myometrium and the endometrium. The outer **perimetrium** is connective tissue consisting of visceral peritoneum (the inner of the two peritoneal membranes), the **myometrium** consists of smooth muscle, and the inner lining of the uterus, the **endometrium**, consists of epithelial tissue.

The endometrium consists of two discrete layers: a basal layer, which is responsible for the regeneration of the endometrium every month, and a functional layer, which is shed every month during menstruation, unless the woman becomes pregnant. The cyclical nature of menstruation occurs due to the influence of specific hormones on the endometrium during the **uterine cycle** (discussed later in the chapter: see *Figure 14.10*).

The cervix

The **cervix** forms the inferior portion of the uterus, part of which protrudes into the vagina (see *Figure 14.8*) and is 3–4 cm long and 2.5 cm wide. The superior aspect of the cervix, where it joins the body of the uterus, is called the internal os, the inferior aspect of the cervix is called the external os and the cervical canal lies between the two (see *Figure 14.8*. Sperm need to travel up the cervical canal to fertilize an egg, which typically occurs in the uterine tubes. Conversely, during childbirth, the baby needs to travel down the cervical canal and through the vagina in order to be born. The cervix contains a layer of smooth muscle and dilates in order to facilitate birth. When the internal os has fully dilated and no cervix can be felt, it is less likely to tear and the woman can push her baby out. Midwives will regularly assess the degree of dilation of the cervix during labour.

A part of the cervix, the **ectocervix**, protrudes into the vagina and is distinct from the rest of the cervix, which is called the **endocervix**. The epithelial cells that make up the ectocervix are stratified squamous epithelial cells, whereas those of the endocervix are columnar epithelial cells. Where these two cell types meet is called the squamocolumnar junction (see *Box 14.2*).

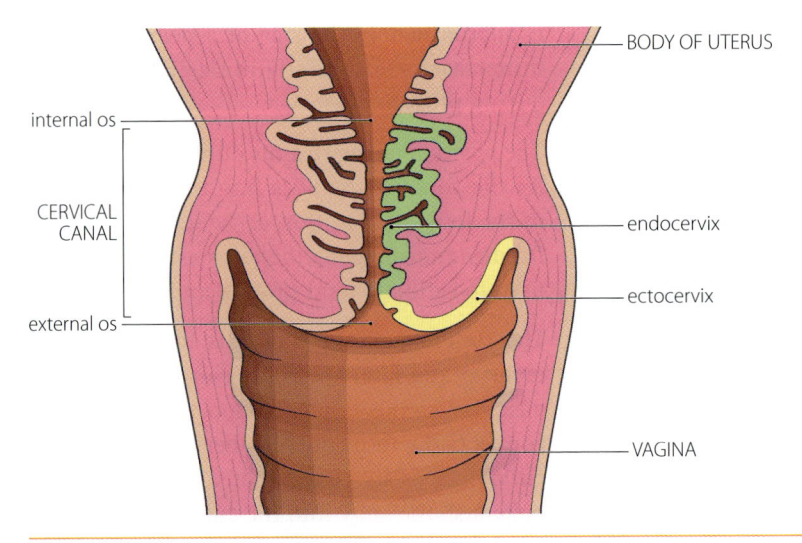

Figure 14.8 – **The cervix (anterior view).**

Cervical screening and the squamocolumnar junction

The change from one type of epithelium to another is termed metaplasia. In the cervix, this occurs usually as a response to an irritant or to changes in hormones such as in puberty, pregnancy, hormonal contraceptive use and the menopause. Hormonal changes during puberty cause the cervix to enlarge; the endocervix moves down towards the vagina, exposing the endocervix to the acidity of the vagina. This stimulates metaplastic changes to the squamocolumnar junction, whereby the columnar cells of the endocervix are replaced by non-keratinized squamous epithelium. Following the menopause, due to the reduction in levels of female reproductive hormones, the squamocolumnar junction tends to move back up to the endocervical region (away from the vagina).

The region where squamous metaplasia develops is termed the transformation zone. After the menopause and through old age, the cervix shrinks as the levels of oestrogen fall and the transformation zone begins to move partially and later fully into the cervical canal. Identification of the transformation zone is important in examination of the cervix because it is here that abnormalities in cells indicating carcinogenesis can be detected. Cervical metaplasia is a reversible adaptive process, but when promoted by chemicals or infection, in particular human papillomavirus (HPV), then metaplastic cells can progress to become dysplastic (dysplasia is a term used by pathologists to describe cells that appear abnormal), which can be an early indication of the risk of developing cancer. Thus, sampling the transformation zone of the cervix and careful examination of the cells (cytology) can be useful in estimating a woman's risk of developing cervical cancer caused by HPV infection.

Cervical screening is offered to all women in the UK aged 25–64 in order to detect and prevent the development of cervical cancer at the earliest stage. Appointments are sent to women automatically via GP patient records. After the first screen, women are invited for screening every 3 years until the age of 49, and then every 5 years up to the age of 64. Screening for the presence of HPV has now been introduced to the programme in the UK.

BOX 14.2

Following screening, the cervical cells from Jess (*Patient 14.1*) were reported by the pathologist as 'dyskaryosis present'. This term is synonymous with dysplasia but is a specific description of the abnormal appearance of the nuclei in the cells.

The uterine tubes

In an adult female, the **uterine tubes** (oviducts or Fallopian tubes) are 10–12 cm long and extend laterally from both sides of the uterus towards the ovaries (see *Figure 14.7*). They function as the duct or channel through which the oocyte or, if fertilized, the zygote passes, on its way towards the uterus.

The tubes themselves are made up of three layers: the inner mucosa, the muscularis and the outer serosa. The mucosa of the uterine tube has a folded structure, which reduces the size of its lumen. It is lined with ciliated columnar epithelial cells, the cilia of which beat in a wave-like fashion to assist the movement of the oocyte or zygote along the tube towards the uterus. The muscularis layer is composed of smooth muscle, and peristaltic contraction of this also helps propel the oocyte or zygote through the tube towards the uterus. Finally, the uterine tubes are covered by the serosa, a visceral peritoneal membrane. Each tube is divided into four sections: the infundibulum, the ampulla, the isthmus and the uterine part.

The **infundibulum** is a funnel-shaped structure, which, although not attached to the ovary, encircles it at the time of ovulation (see *Figure 14.7*). Its purpose is to capture the oocyte once it has been released from the ovary during ovulation and guide it into the uterine tube. Along its edge are finger-like folds called fimbriae, covered in cilia. Fimbriae move in a wave-like manner and the cilia beat rhythmically, drawing the oocyte towards the infundibulum following ovulation. As the infundibulum is not directly attached to the ovary there is the

---

Human papillomavirus

BOX 14.3

There are many different types of human papillomavirus (HPV) that can cause infections in humans. These range from types that cause mild infections, such as warts and verrucae, to types that are associated with cervical cancer. It is estimated that 99% of all cervical cancers are associated with infection with a high-risk type of HPV, and that of these, HPV types 16 and 18 are associated with the highest proportion of cervical cancer, at 70%.

HPV is transmitted by sexual contact, and practising safe sex can reduce the transmission of HPV; however, condoms do not cover the whole genital area where the virus may be present. A more effective way of reducing the spread of the virus and thus reducing the incidence of cervical cancer is to offer a vaccination against HPV types 16 and 18. In the UK, a national vaccination programme has operated since autumn 2008. The vaccine is offered to girls aged 12–13 years in two separate injections, typically 12 months apart. However, in the USA and Australia, the vaccine is also given to boys of this age. HPV is not only associated with cervical cancer but also with cancers of the mouth, throat, anus and penis. The vaccine is an effective prevention against HPV types 16 and 18 at all body sites, and the UK Government is investigating whether to extend the programme to boys.

Cervical screening will still be offered to women who have been vaccinated as girls because the vaccination is specific to HPV types 16 and 18 and these types are not responsible for all cervical cancers.

possibility that the oocyte may not enter the oviducts and may instead remain in the pelvic cavity. Typically, if this happens, the oocyte is resorbed. The fact that the oviducts open out into the pelvic cavity at one end and are connected to the external environment via the uterus and vagina at the other end is significant. Vaginal infections can potentially move into the pelvic cavity where they can become much more serious, causing, for example, pelvic inflammatory disease.

The **ampulla** is where fertilization most commonly occurs (see *Figure 14.7*). The resultant zygote thus begins its early stages of development as it moves down the tube towards the uterus. Once inside the cavity of the uterus the zygote implants into the endometrium. A zygote that implants in a location outside the uterus results in an ectopic pregnancy. Most commonly, this occurs within the uterine tubes, where it can cause the tube to rupture. This is treated as a medical emergency.

The **isthmus** forms the majority of the length of the uterine tube and the **uterine part** provides the entrance to the uterus and is continuous with the endometrium (see *Figure 14.7*).

The ovaries

The **ovaries** consist of a pair of oval organs, approximately 2–3 cm in length, which are found lateral to the uterus (see *Figure 14.7*). They are held firmly in place by a number of ligaments. The ovarian ligament attaches the medial edge of each ovary to the uterus, the suspensory (round) ligament attaches the lateral edge of each ovary to the pelvic wall, and the broad ligament, which consists of a broad sheet of peritoneum, covers the uterus and attaches to each ovary via the mesovarium.

A frontal section of the ovary, when viewed under the microscope, reveals an outer layer of germinal epithelial cells, with a deeper layer of connective tissue,

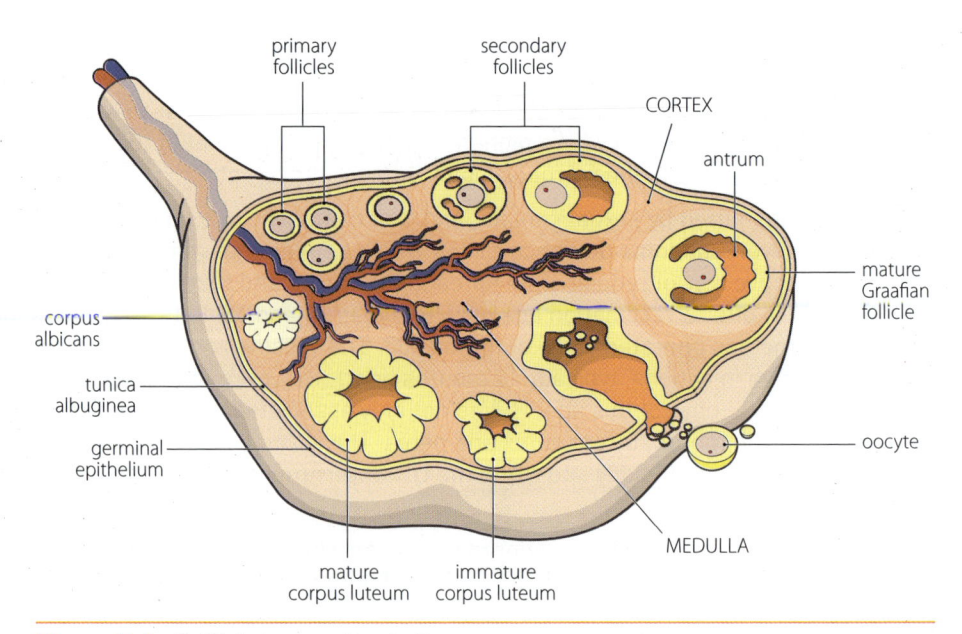

Figure 14.9 – Follicle maturation in the ovary.

the tunica albuginea, below (see *Figure 14.9*). Deep under these layers are the cortex and medulla of the ovary. The cortex contains ovarian follicles and the medulla contains blood vessels, lymphatic vessels and nerves.

The function of the ovaries is to produce female gametes, known as **oocytes**, and to produce the hormones oestrogen and progesterone. Oocytes are produced via a process called oogenesis. The germ cells that begin oogenesis are called **oogonia**, and these are present in the ovary of a woman before birth. Oogonia divide by mitosis to produce millions of primary oocytes. These primary oocytes, present at birth, contain 46 chromosomes (23 pairs), and need to undergo meiosis in order to become true haploid gametes containing 23 single chromosomes (see *Chapter 3*). Primary oocytes start to divide by meiosis, but the process is halted after the first meiotic cell division and the cells are left at this stage until puberty. This may give the impression that the ovary in a girl prior to puberty is in a completely static state; however, this is not the case. Although meiotic cell division is halted, follicles surrounding some oocytes grow and mature before degenerating and being resorbed back into the ovary. Although this follicle growth occurs, the size of the follicles is less than that found after puberty, and ovulation from the follicle does not occur.

The ovarian follicles

Follicles consist of an oocyte surrounded by follicle cells. The natural history of a follicle, following puberty, is to undergo many changes as the oocyte matures inside it and is then released, leaving an 'empty' follicle in the ovary (see *Figure 14.9*). All oocytes are produced via meiosis; however, the stages of meiosis have been arrested in immature oocytes and meiosis is only completed during the maturation process inside a follicle following puberty.

Immature follicles contain immature 'primary' oocytes, and the most immature oocyte is found in a *primordial follicle*. At birth, baby girls have approximately 1.5–2 million primordial follicles, which consist of a primary oocyte surrounded by a single layer of follicle cells. The process of meiosis has begun within the primary oocyte; however, as stated previously, it has been arrested at the first meiotic division.

Primordial follicles develop into the next stage, the primary follicle, in response to stimulation by follicle-stimulating hormone (FSH) (see *Chapter 5*) at puberty. A primary follicle typically has more than one layer of follicle cells, and also has a layer of granulosa cells, responsible for secreting the hormone oestrogen (see *Chapter 5*). Oestrogen is important as it produces the endometrial changes in the uterus required for the implantation of a fertilized egg.

Further development of the primary follicle creates the secondary follicle. Secondary follicles contain many layers of granulosa cells and are thus able to secrete a higher quantity of oestrogen. The follicle also contains a space filled with fluid called an antrum. The amount of fluid within the antrum increases as ovulation approaches.

Further development of a secondary follicle produces a mature **Graafian** or **vesicular follicle** (see *Figure 14.9*). The oocyte within it has now undergone meiosis I and is thus called a secondary oocyte. However, the cell cycle has been halted again at the second meiotic phase (meiosis II is completed following fertilization of the oocyte with a sperm). This large follicle then ruptures and releases the secondary oocyte from the ovary into the infundibulum.

Once the oocyte has left the ovary, what remains of the follicle is called a **corpus luteum** (see *Figure 14.9*). The corpus luteum starts to secrete progesterone (see *Chapter 5*) as well as oestrogen, although the amount of oestrogen is reduced. Progesterone (a 'pro-gestation' hormone) stimulates the growth of the endometrium and prepares it for the implantation of a fertilized oocyte.

If the oocyte is fertilized, the corpus luteum persists and continues to produce oestrogen and progesterone, although this role is largely taken over by the placenta after 3 months.

If the oocyte is not fertilized, the corpus luteum begins to degenerate at approximately 10 days after ovulation. Following degeneration, all that remains is a white scar made of connective tissue. This scar tissue is called the corpus albicans, and most of these are gradually resorbed over time within the ovary (see *Figure 14.9*).

In the absence of fertilization, the events above are repeated approximately every 28 days in a cycle, known as the ovarian cycle, with ovulation occurring around day 14. Usually, only one primordial follicle develops into a mature vesicular follicle, as other follicles that have started to develop at the same time begin to degenerate and undergo apoptosis. However, more than one oocyte can be ovulated at the same time, resulting in a multiple birth. This occurs in approximately 1–2% of all ovulations.

The ovarian cycle

The natural cycle of oocyte maturation and ovulation, and follicle development and degeneration is regulated by a number of hormones (see *Figure 14.10*). These are gonadotrophin-releasing hormone (GnRH), luteinizing hormone (LH), follicle-stimulating hormone (FSH), oestrogen and progesterone. The trigger for the commencement of the ovarian cycle at puberty is the hormone leptin (see *Chapter 5*). Leptin stimulates the release of GnRH from the hypothalamus, which starts the cycle. Leptin is released from adipose tissue, and girls with reduced levels of adipose tissue, who are very lean due to high physical activity levels or anorexia, often begin puberty later than their peers as a result. Similarly, if the quantity of adipose tissue in females is reduced after puberty has started, the ovarian cycle can be disrupted and stop altogether because ovulation is not stimulated (see **Amy (Patient 1.1)** who has been experiencing irregular menstrual periods and who missed her menstrual period last month).

The ovarian cycle begins on day 1 when GnRH is released from the hypothalamus stimulating the production of LH and FSH by the anterior pituitary gland (see *Figure 14.10*). FSH, as its name suggests, is responsible for stimulating the development of ovarian follicles. Once the primordial follicle has developed into a primary follicle, it is able to secrete oestrogen. The amount of oestrogen produced by the follicle increases as it matures through its stages of development from a primary to a Graafian follicle. The oestrogen acts in a positive-feedback loop to increase the secretion of GnRH, which thus increases the secretion of FSH and LH, further enhancing follicle development. The rising level of LH reaches a peak,

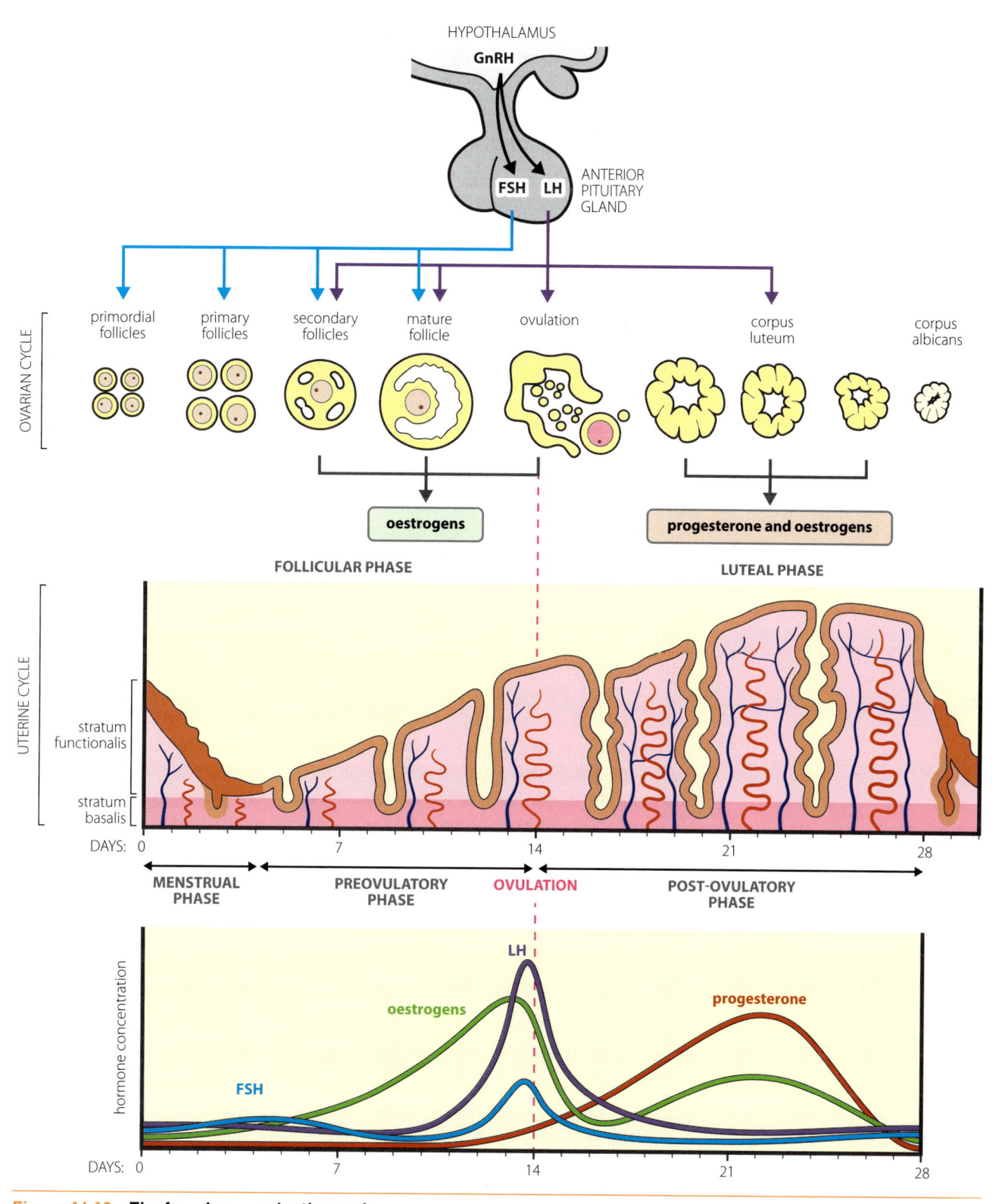

SECTION **14.2** | WHAT YOU NEED TO KNOW – ESSENTIAL ANATOMY AND PHYSIOLOGY 463

Figure 14.10 – **The female reproductive cycle.**

which triggers ovulation on or around day 14. This period of the ovarian cycle is known as the **follicular phase**.

Following ovulation, the hormones are secreted in accordance with a negative-feedback loop. The corpus luteum in the ovary begins to secrete progesterone and less oestrogen than previously due to the damage caused to the Graafian follicle by ovulation. Oestrogen, when under the influence of progesterone, reduces the secretion of GnRH and thus of FSH and LH, via negative feedback. The progesterone also reduces the secretion of these hormones via negative feedback and this usually prevents the maturation of another oocyte and follicle. A further hormone, inhibin, produced by the corpus luteum, also inhibits the secretion of GnRH, FSH and LH. If the oocyte is *not* fertilized, the corpus luteum begins to degenerate and stops producing oestrogen and progesterone. The inhibitory effect of progesterone on the production of GnRH, FSH and LH is thus removed, and the levels of these hormones once again begin to rise as another ovarian cycle begins on day 1.

The period of the ovarian cycle from day 14 (ovulation) to day 28 is known as the **luteal phase**. Although a typical ovarian cycle is repeated every 28 days, this is only true for approximately 10–15% of women. Cycles can range between 21 and 40 days. However, in this case it is the follicular phase that is either longer or shorter than 14 days; the luteal phase consistently lasts for 14 days whatever the length of the ovarian cycle.

The menstrual (uterine) cycle

At the same time as the ovarian cycle is occurring in the ovary, a cycle of events is also taking place in the uterus, which is preparing for the potential implantation of a fertilized oocyte and the resultant pregnancy. The menstrual cycle is the same length as the ovarian cycle and also begins on day 1, which signifies the start of the menstrual period when the functional layer of the endometrium is shed. Menstruation is triggered by the fall in progesterone arising from the degeneration of the corpus luteum (see *Figure 14.10*). Endometrial tissue and blood pass through the vagina for 3–5 days during menstruation, and this period is called the **menstrual phase**.

Following this phase is the proliferative (pre-ovulatory) phase, which occurs between day 6 and ovulation. As the name suggests, this phase is associated with the growth and proliferation of a new functional layer of the endometrium. This growth is stimulated by the oestrogen that is now being produced by the developing ovarian follicles (see *Figure 14.10*). The endometrium becomes highly vascularized, velvety and thick, and cells of the endometrium synthesize progesterone receptors to enable them to respond to the progesterone released after ovulation from the corpus luteum.

Following ovulation, under the influence of progesterone, the menstrual cycle enters the secretory (post-ovulatory) phase where the endometrium continues to prepare for the implantation of an embryo (see *Figure 14.10*). This phase consistently occurs from day 15 to day 28, running parallel to the luteal phase of the ovarian cycle. During this phase, the functional layer of the endometrium becomes a secretory mucosa containing glands that coil around newly developed spiral arteries. In addition, cervical mucus, which was thinned under the influence of oestrogen at the time of ovulation to facilitate the passage of sperm, now thickens to form a cervical plug. This helps block the passage of further sperm and potential pathogens into the uterus.

If fertilization *does not* occur, the corpus luteum degenerates and stops producing oestrogen and progesterone. As a result, the spiral arteries kink, the blood supply to the cells of the endometrium is reduced and the cells begin to die, sloughing off as menstrual flow.

Early hormonal changes associated with pregnancy

If fertilization *does* occur, the embryo implants into the prepared endometrium and starts to secrete the hormone human chorionic gonadotrophin (hCG). This hormone guarantees the survival of the corpus luteum for approximately 6 weeks. As a result, the corpus luteum continues to produce progesterone and oestrogen, which maintains the endometrial lining during this period. After this time, the corpus luteum degenerates and the placenta takes over, becoming the main organ producing oestrogen and progesterone in pregnancy. The specific part of the embryo that produces hCG is the chorion, one of two extra-embryonic membranes that develop from the embryo at around 12 days after implantation (the second membrane is the amnion).

The placenta

The **chorion** is the outer membrane adjacent to the endometrium (see *Figure 14.11*). It secretes enzymes that enable it to digest parts of the endometrium, creating small endometrial cavities. These cavities are then filled by chorionic projections called villi, which sit within blood-filled spaces of the endometrium, allowing intimate and maximum contact with maternal blood. Blood vessels invade the chorionic villi and become continuous with the umbilical vessels that supply the embryo and later the fetus with blood. Cells from the chorion can be sampled for genetic testing (see *Box 14.4*).

BOX 14.4

Chorionic villus sampling and amniocentesis

Cells from the chorion can be sampled for genetic testing from week 11 of pregnancy, and chorionic villus sampling is usually undertaken between 11 and 14 weeks. A tissue sample of the chorion is obtained by inserting a needle through the abdomen. The cells, which divide rapidly and are cultured in the laboratory, can then be examined. Major chromosomal abnormalities such as Down syndrome can be identified quickly, and test results are usually available to parents within a day or two. Rarer conditions are likely to take longer.

Alternatively, amniocentesis may be performed. This involves inserting a needle into the abdomen under ultrasound control and taking a sample of the amniotic fluid surrounding the fetus. Amniotic fluid contains maternal and fetal proteins along with fetal cells. Chromosomal analysis can be undertaken on such cells, which can reveal chromosomal abnormalities in the fetus. Rapid test results for major chromosomal abnormalities such as Down syndrome are available within 2–3 days; however, rarer conditions are likely to take longer. Amniocentesis is undertaken between 15 and 20 weeks of pregnancy. Both procedures are associated with a small risk of miscarriage (1–2%) and infection.

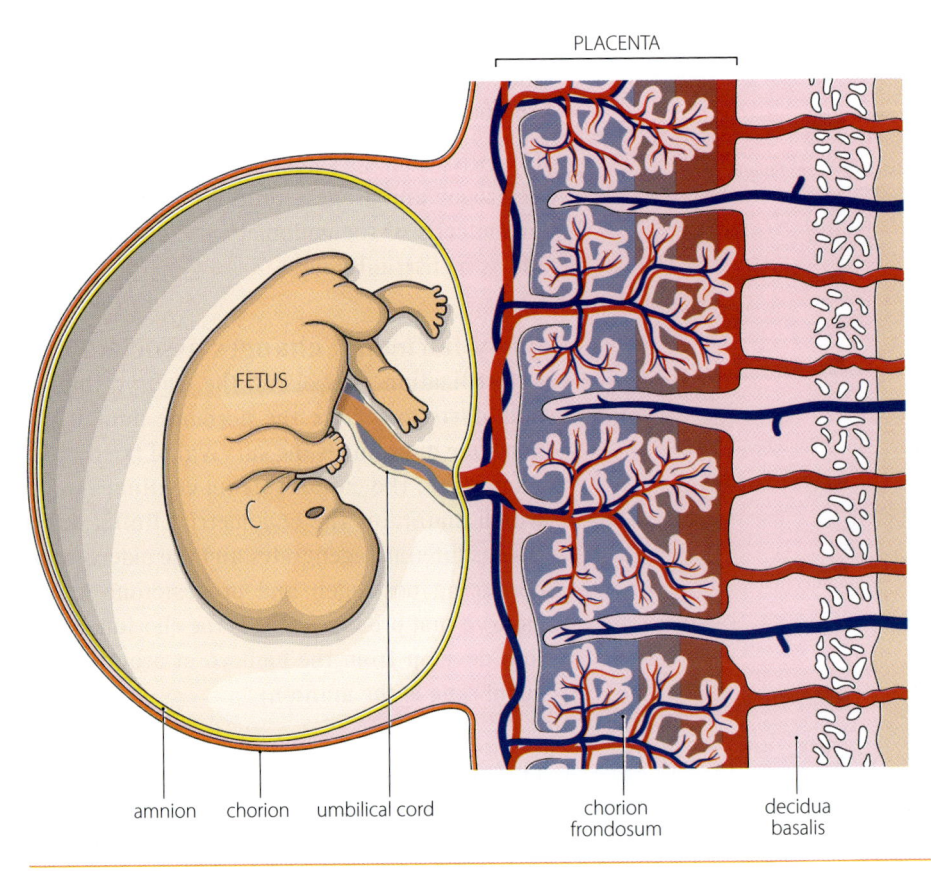

Figure 14.11 – **The chorion, amnion and placenta.**

All the **chorionic villi** that are embedded in the endometrium form a leaf-like structure called the **chorion frondosum**. The endometrium also changes following implantation of the embryo. It grows in size and its cells begin to store glycogen; it is then known as the **decidua basalis**. The chorion frondosum derived from the fetus and the decidua basalis derived from the mother together form the early **placenta** (see *Figure 14.11*). Deoxygenated blood from the fetus passes through the umbilical artery, entering the chorionic villi of the chorion frondosum. This blood circulates within the villi and is in close proximity to the maternal vessels of the decidua basalis. The close proximity facilitates the diffusion of gases, nutrients and waste between the maternal and fetal circulation. Oxygenated fetal blood, following this exchange process, then returns to the fetus via the umbilical vein. The placenta is thus the site for the exchange of gases and other molecules between the fetus and the mother.

The **amnion** is the inner of the two extra-embryonic membranes and is adjacent to the embryo (see *Figure 14.11*). Initially, it covers the embryo, but by 4–5 weeks of gestation, cells of the amnion start to produce amniotic fluid and the membrane moves away from the embryo as the quantity of amniotic fluid increases. As a result, the fetus is surrounded by a fluid-filled cavity, the amniotic cavity, for the remainder of its development. Amniotic fluid has a number of roles, which include protecting and cushioning the fetus, maintaining a constant body temperature in the fetus and allowing the fetus to practise swallowing and breathing. It also has bacteriostatic properties, protecting the fetus from infection. Amniocentesis, which involves taking a sample of the amniotic fluid for testing, is usually carried out between 15 and 20 weeks of pregnancy (see *Box 14.4*).

The decidua basalis is the part of the endometrium that lies next to the embryo. The part of the endometrium that lies next to the uterine cavity is called the decidua capsularis. The decidua capsularis expands as the fetus grows and starts to fill the uterine cavity, although the villi within it begin to degenerate and by 13 weeks have been lost altogether. Villi within the decidua basalis, however, continue to develop and branch extensively, so that by 13 weeks the placenta is fully developed and the blood vessels within it are firmly established. Although the placenta is fully developed by 13 weeks, it continues to grow throughout the pregnancy.

The placenta not only provides a site for the exchange of oxygen and carbon dioxide between the mother and the fetus but also facilitates the exchange of water, nutrients and waste products. In addition, maternal antibodies (IgG) also cross the placenta from as early as 13 weeks (see *Chapter 11*). Antibodies are large protein molecules, which are transported to the fetus by exo- and endocytosis (see *Chapter 2*), and although they begin to cross at 13 weeks, the largest amount crosses during the final 3 months of pregnancy, the third trimester, particularly after 33 weeks. This has implications for preterm babies who have lower levels of IgG and thus are more susceptible to infection.

Smaller molecules such as oxygen and glucose are transferred by established membrane transport mechanisms, such as diffusion and active transport (see

---

Fetal alcohol syndrome

BOX 14.5

A syndrome is a collection of symptoms, and fetal alcohol syndrome (FAS) describes the set of symptoms commonly found in babies born to mothers who drink alcohol during their pregnancy. There is much debate surrounding the level of alcohol consumption during pregnancy that does *not* result in FAS, and as a result the advice given to pregnant women in the UK is to avoid alcohol during pregnancy. Heavy drinking and binge drinking are known to cause the syndrome in some babies (see Jordon, Patient 4.2), although other factors such as whether the mother smokes, her nutritional status and whether she is stressed are also important to the overall health of the fetus.

Cells of the central nervous system (see *Chapter 4*) have a lower toxicity threshold for alcohol than other cells in the embryo and fetus. As a result, FAS is associated with widespread damage to the central nervous system, as alcohol impairs the development of nervous tissue in particular. Thus, along with physical abnormalities, FAS is also associated with cognitive difficulties and behavioural problems. These include learning difficulties, poor short-term memory, a reduced ability to problem solve and plan, difficulty with social interactions and hyperactivity.

Alcohol-related ill health is not linked only to FAS; alcohol misuse is also associated with an increased risk of many health problems, for example coronary heart disease, stroke, liver disease and cancers of the gastrointestinal system. Alcohol misuse is the third largest cause of avoidable ill health in England, contributing a significant burden to the NHS.

Chapter 2). Alcohol is a small molecule and is transported by diffusion from the mother to the fetus if she consumes it during her pregnancy. This occurred during Jade's pregnancy with Jordon (Patient 4.2) and resulted in him developing the symptoms of fetal alcohol syndrome (see *Box 14.5*).

As previously stated, another important role of the placenta in pregnancy is the secretion of oestrogen and progesterone. Progesterone and oestrogen help to maintain the endometrium, but they also suppress the secretion of GnRH, FSH and LH, thus stopping the ovarian and menstrual cycles described previously. In addition, they prepare the mammary glands for lactation.

It is beyond the scope of this book to discuss the physiology of pregnancy; however, the hormones associated with labour and lactation will be discussed.

Labour

Labour is initiated following a complex interplay between hormones of the mother and the fetus. It is associated with contractions of the myometrium, which push the baby into the outside world. Progesterone inhibits uterine contractions during pregnancy; however, this inhibition is overcome as labour approaches by a sharp rise in oestrogen production from the placenta. The fetus itself, through its production of cortisol, triggers the rise in oestrogen in the mother. In addition to inhibiting the effects of progesterone, the oestrogen causes an increase in the number of oxytocin receptors on the cells of the myometrium. This is important as the hormone oxytocin stimulates the uterus to contract. Rising oestrogen levels also trigger the placenta to produce prostaglandins, which also stimulate contraction of the myometrium.

The process of labour involves a positive-feedback loop (see *Figure 14.12*). Contractions of the myometrium force the head of the fetus down onto the cervix, where it stimulates stretch receptors. Stretch receptors trigger afferent sensory nerve impulses to be transmitted to the hypothalamus, stimulating the release of oxytocin by the posterior pituitary gland where it is stored. When the oxytocin reaches the myometrium, it causes more powerful contractions, which push the fetus down onto the cervix with greater force, once again stimulating stretch receptors and further oxytocin release in a positive-feedback loop.

Oxytocin stimulates the production of prostaglandins, which also stimulate contraction of the myometrium in a positive-feedback loop. Prostaglandins stimulate contraction, which stimulates more prostaglandin release, which stimulates stronger, more vigorous contractions.

Birth of the baby stops the positive-feedback loop because the stretch receptors in the cervix are no longer stimulated. However, the oxytocin in the blood continues to stimulate contractions in the myometrium, which are necessary in order to deliver the placenta and fetal membranes. An intramuscular injection of a combination of synthetic oxytocin and ergometrine (Syntometrine) may be given to speed this process along. The loss of the placenta means that there is a corresponding reduction in the levels of progesterone and oestrogen in the mother. The decline in oestrogen, in particular, stimulates the production of milk in the breast, via the hormone prolactin.

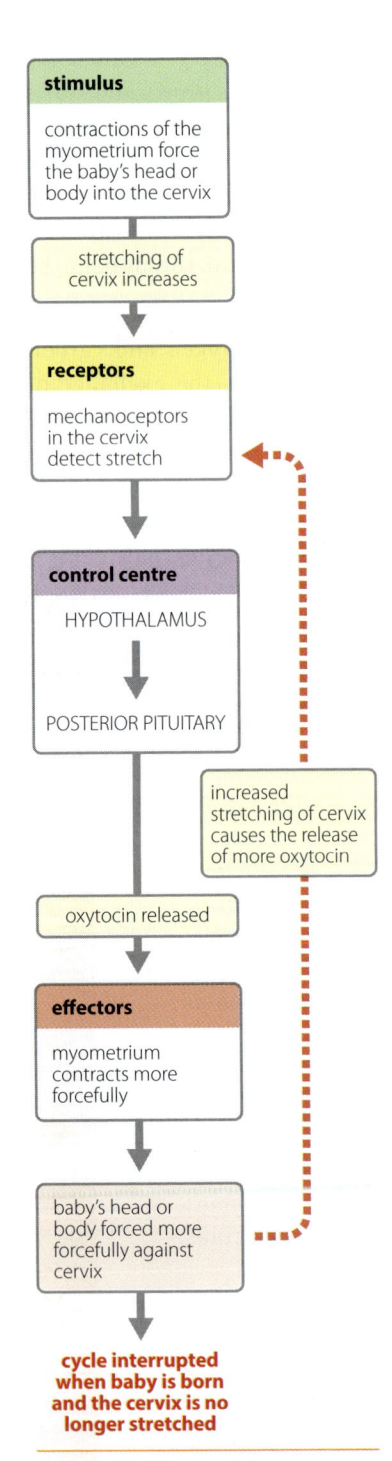

Figure 14.12 – Positive-feedback regulation of labour.

stimulus
contractions of the myometrium force the baby's head or body into the cervix

↓

stretching of cervix increases

↓

receptors
mechanoceptors in the cervix detect stretch

↓

control centre
HYPOTHALAMUS
↓
POSTERIOR PITUITARY

increased stretching of cervix causes the release of more oxytocin

↓

oxytocin released

↓

effectors
myometrium contracts more forcefully

↓

baby's head or body forced more forcefully against cervix

↓

cycle interrupted when baby is born and the cervix is no longer stretched

The menopause

The ovarian and uterine cycles continue until a pregnancy or the menopause occurs. The **menopause** is marked by the end of menstruation, although ovulation also stops as the woman has depleted the supply of oocytes she was born with. As ovulation stops, so does the production of progesterone and oestrogen, and it is primarily the fall in oestrogen that triggers the menopause. Entering the menopause is part of the natural ageing process, and it typically begins between the ages of 45 and 55.

The breast and its development

Mammary tissue in boys and girls is largely the same until puberty when a surge of oestrogen and progesterone stimulates breast development in girls. Typically, the breasts increase in size and the lobes, lobules and ductal system become apparent. However, until a pregnancy occurs and the breasts prepare for their main function, lactation, these structures are rudimental and undeveloped.

The breasts are actually modified sweat glands that form part of the skin. Their main role is to produce milk in order to nourish a newborn baby. As exocrine glands, they contain ducts through which milk can pass via the nipple to the baby during breast-feeding. The most common type of breast cancer arises in the ducts and is called ductal carcinoma (see *Box 14.6* and Sheila, Patient 2.3). Each breast

---

BOX 14.6

Ductal carcinoma of the breast

The most common type of breast cancer is found in the ducts and hence is called ductal carcinoma. There are two types of ductal carcinoma: ductal carcinoma *in situ* (DCIS) and invasive ductal carcinoma. DCIS is a very early form of breast cancer. The cancer cells are confined to the endothelial lining of the breast duct and have not spread beyond it to the local blood and lymphatic vessels. However, if the cancer is left untreated, it could become invasive and spread to other parts of the body; as a result, DCIS is usually surgically removed. Invasive ductal carcinoma is where the cancer has spread beyond the ducts to the surrounding breast tissue and as a result could spread to the rest of the body, where it is said to metastasize, via the lymphatic system (see *Chapter 11*).

Once breast cancer has been diagnosed, it is important to establish whether it has spread to the local lymphatic vessels. As a result, fine-needle aspiration of the axillary lymph nodes is commonly undertaken to see whether cancer cells are present in the aspirated lymph. Approximately 75% of the lymphatic vessels that supply the breast drain into the axillary lymph nodes, which is why these nodes are sampled in people with breast cancer. The remaining 25% drain into nodes on either side of the sternum.

If cancer cells are *not* found, this does not necessarily mean that there has been no spread. Cancer cells could be in nodes that were not aspirated, or could be absent from the aspirated fluid but still be present in the lymph nodes. It is now known that if cancer does spread to the axillary lymph nodes, it tends to spread to the closest lymph node (also termed the sentinel lymph node) first and then to more distant nodes. This node can be identified during the patient's surgery, biopsied and the results obtained during the operation. If the sentinel node is negative and found not to contain cancer cells, then it is likely the cancer has remained localized. This information is useful in guiding therapeutic options. If the node is negative, preservation of the remaining lymph nodes is possible, thus limiting the number of lymph nodes removed. This is important because if the nodes are not removed, then the likelihood of the patient developing lymphoedema in their arm is greatly reduced (see *Chapter 9*).

lies anteriorly to the pectoralis muscles of the thorax. The breasts lie between the second and sixth ribs, and extend laterally between the sternum and the axillae. Each breast contains a mammary gland surrounded by the superficial fascia, a layer of adipose tissue.

The **mammary glands** are composed of glandular tissue and adipose tissue, with the amount of adipose tissue determining the size of the breast in non-lactating women. The breasts of non-lactating women and lactating women are different in terms of their state of development. High levels of progesterone and oestrogen, produced during pregnancy, stimulate the development of breast tissue in preparation for lactation.

Structurally, the breasts are composed of lobes, which are then divided by sheaths of connective tissue into smaller lobules (see *Figure 14.13*). This connective tissue forms the suspensory ligaments, which support the weight of the breast and firmly attach it to the skin. The lobules contain secretory structures called alveoli, which produce milk when women are lactating. The alveoli are formed into clusters, and the milk they produce passes into small tubules called secondary tubules. These tubules feed into larger mammary ducts, which in turn converge into lactiferous ducts that drain into the nipple. Just behind the nipple is a small reservoir where milk collects during feeding, called the ampulla (see *Figure 14.13*). The nipple itself is surrounded by a ring of pigmented skin called the areola. The areola contains a large number of sebaceous glands (see *Chapter 12*) that secrete sebum to lubricate both the areola and nipple during breast-feeding. It is important during feeding

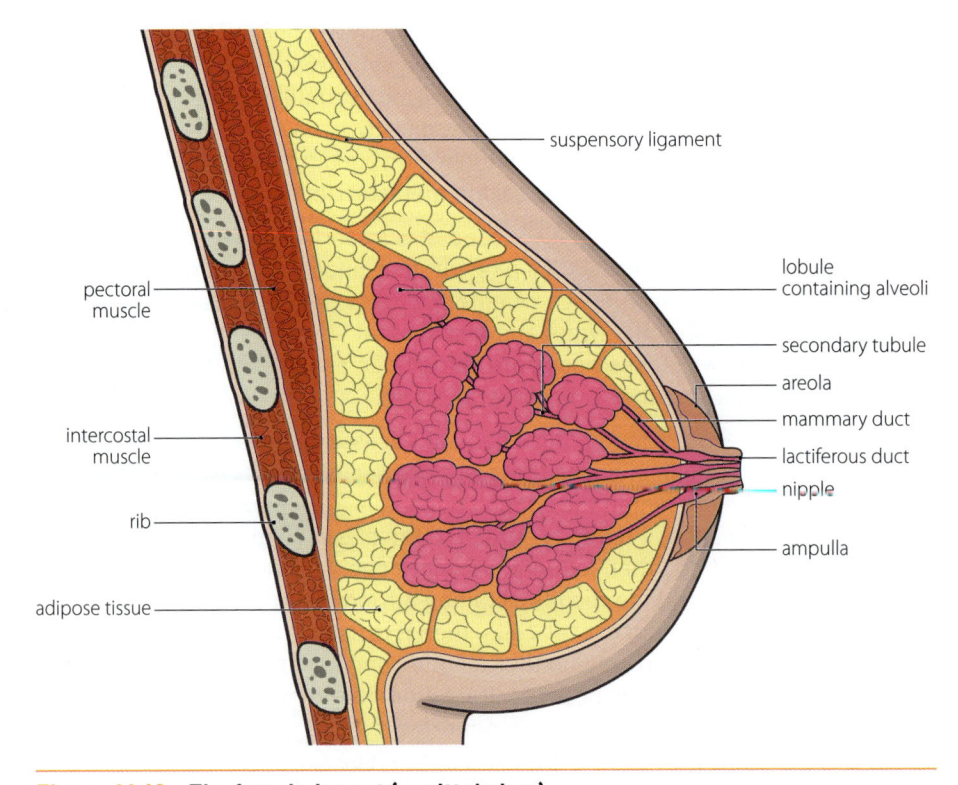

Figure 14.13 – **The female breast (sagittal view).**

that the baby 'latches on' to the areola and not just the nipple, as this ensures compression of the ampulla, releasing the milk reservoir behind the nipple.

Milk production is stimulated by the hormone prolactin, secreted via the anterior pituitary gland (see *Chapter 5*). During pregnancy, levels of prolactin are kept low as its secretion is regulated by prolactin-inhibiting hormone (PIH), which is secreted by the hypothalamus. PIH is actually another name for the neurotransmitter dopamine. Oestrogen stimulates the secretion of PIH, and so during pregnancy when oestrogen levels are high, PIH levels are also high and prolactin secretion is inhibited. Following the delivery of the placenta after the birth, oestrogen levels fall and the level of prolactin consequently rises.

Prolactin levels are also kept high by the act of breast-feeding, via a neuroendocrine reflex. Sensory nerve endings in the breast are stimulated by suckling. As a result, nerve impulses are sent to the hypothalamus, which inhibits the secretion of PIH.

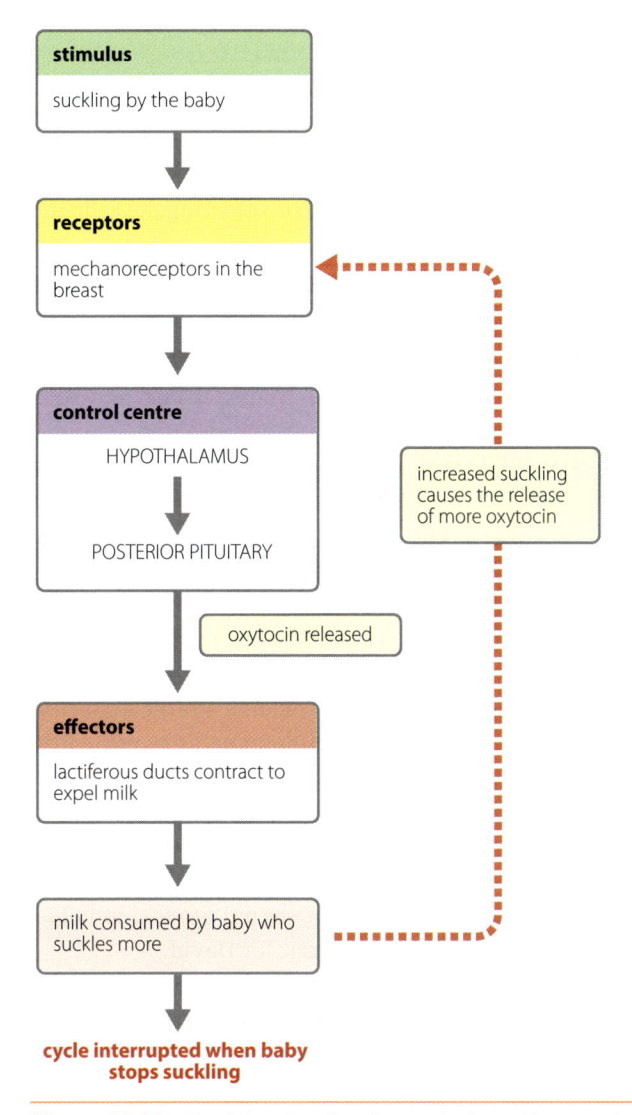

stimulus
suckling by the baby

receptors
mechanoreceptors in the breast

control centre
HYPOTHALAMUS
↓
POSTERIOR PITUITARY

oxytocin released

effectors
lactiferous ducts contract to expel milk

milk consumed by baby who suckles more

increased suckling causes the release of more oxytocin

cycle interrupted when baby stops suckling

Figure 14.14 – **Positive-feedback regulation of breast-feeding.**

Prolactin stimulates milk production and the passage of milk from the alveoli into the ducts. However, in order to eject the milk from the breast, oxytocin is needed. Oxytocin stimulates the contraction of the lactiferous ducts via a reflex, commonly known as the milk 'let-down' reflex (see *Chapter 5*). The act of suckling also triggers the production of oxytocin in a similar way to prolactin. In this case, the stimulated hypothalamus causes the posterior pituitary gland to produce oxytocin (see *Figure 14.14*).

The first milk a mother produces following the birth of her baby is called **colostrum**. This is rich in the antibody secretory IgA and other immune-related compounds (see *Chapter 11*). Breast milk is the most complete form of nutrition for babies and infants and meets all the nutritional needs of the baby for the first 6 months. Breast-feeding is also associated with a reduced incidence of breast and ovarian cancer and of osteoporosis in the later life of the mother. In addition, the act of breast-feeding helps her to bond with her baby.

14.3 Clinical application

Many factors influence reproductive physiology. The patients described in this chapter illustrate key factors that contribute to a range of problems related to the reproductive system affecting health, intimate relationships, psychological wellbeing and the ability to reproduce.

- **Amy (Patient 1.1)** has been having irregular menstrual periods and missed her last period altogether; this is termed amenorrhoea. Her amenorrhoea is a symptom of her low BMI (16.3 kg/m^2), which has occurred due to her anorexia nervosa. Amy is worried because her periods have stopped, but she understands that this relates to her eating disorder and that her periods are unlikely to resume until her weight increases and she has a BMI approaching 20, within the healthy range for her height.
- **Sheila (Patient 2.3)** has invasive ductal carcinoma of the breast, which requires surgical treatment, followed by chemotherapy, biological therapy and radiotherapy. Sheila's prognosis will be improved by her following this management plan.
- **Jade (Patient 4.2)** consumed large quantities of alcohol during her pregnancy with Jordon and as a result Jordon has fetal alcohol syndrome. The alcohol crossed Jade's placenta and acted as a teratogen, disrupting the normal growth and development of her baby while in the womb.
- **David (Patient 5.1)** has erectile dysfunction as a consequence of his long-term condition of diabetes mellitus. Restoring optimal blood flow to his penis during sexual arousal to help him achieve and maintain an erection is important for David.
- **Robert (Patient 9.1)** has problems voiding urine due to the presence of an enlarged prostate gland. Improving the flow of urine through the prostatic urethra will enable Robert to have better control over voiding urine and more effective emptying of the bladder, and he will be able to enjoy a better quality of sleep.

- **Jess (Patient 14.1)** was found to have cervical dyskaryosis following a routine smear test. Removing the abnormal cells will prevent them becoming cancerous, and following this, regular screening will identify any future cervical cell alterations. In addition, Jess will be given health promotion advice to reduce the chance of the abnormality returning.

Patient 1.1 — Amy | 1 | 20 | 194 | 235 | 447 | **473**

- 18-year-old woman
- BMI 16.3
- Downy hair on face and arms
- Referred to eating disorder clinic
- Eating under supervision to increase intake and also getting psychological support
- Also anaemic

Amy has responded to the plan to improve her heath reasonably well and she is slowly gaining weight. Her BMI has increased from 16.3 to $18.0 \, kg/m^2$ and the mental health nursing team are pleased with her progress. Amy is receiving psychological support to help her understand why she has anorexia nervosa, and cognitive behavioural therapy (CBT), which challenges the way she thinks about food, encouraging her to think differently and thus behave differently around food. This therapy also provides her with the skills to cope in environments that she had previously found difficult because of her anorexia nervosa. Her menstrual periods have restarted, although they are still irregular. Amy seems to understand better the relationship between her nutrition, her body weight and her menstrual cycle.

Patient 2.3 — Sheila | 30 | 54 | 59 | 93 | 267 | 304 | 448 | **473**

- 47-year-old woman
- Recent diagnosis of breast cancer – biopsy shows cancer cells over-express HER2 protein
- Biological therapy with trastuzumab (Herceptin) to block HER2 action an option
- Is still offered surgery, chemotherapy and radiotherapy
- Agrees to add trastuzumab to chemotherapy plan
- Advised about surgery: lymphoedema a possibility

Following Sheila's diagnosis, a fine-needle aspiration of the right axillary lymph nodes was undertaken to see whether the cancer had spread to them. Cancer cells were discovered in her lymphatic fluid, and as a result she was advised to have surgery to remove both the cancer in her breast and all the lymph nodes in her right axilla. This axillary surgery is called an 'axillary lymph node dissection'. Following her surgery, Sheila received a course of chemotherapy coupled with intravenous trastuzumab (Herceptin) to destroy any cancer cells that may already have spread via the lymphatic system. When the course of chemotherapy finished, she also received radiotherapy to the surgical site. Unfortunately, Sheila developed lymphoedema (see *Chapter 9*) in her right arm following her surgery. In spite of this, she received excellent support from her breast care nurse and also from a charity organization devoted to providing emotional and practical support for people with breast cancer following diagnosis. The charity offered complementary therapies, such as acupuncture, yoga and aromatherapy, alongside counselling and image workshops. Sheila also met other women with a similar diagnosis and gained much emotional support from them.

Patient 4.2 — Jade and Jordon | 100 | 132 | 138 | 162 | 448 | **473**

- 6-year-old boy and 32-year-old mother
- Jade drank alcohol excessively while pregnant
- Jordon has dysmorphic facial features and behavioural issues
- Jordon has fetal alcohol syndrome
- Jordon was small for age and given GH at age 4

Because Jade drank excessively while pregnant with Jordon, alcohol was able to cross the placental barrier and exert its teratogenic effects on his physical, cognitive and behavioural development. In addition, the immaturity of Jordon's liver while in his mother's uterus meant that he was unable to metabolize the alcohol and break it down himself. Jade's midwife and health visitor explained

- Aged 6 he is up to the 60th percentile on growth charts

to Jade that the alcohol she consumed while she was pregnant affected his development and that this has influenced his behaviour, intellectual ability and social relationships. They also explained that this would happen again if she continued to drink during subsequent pregnancies. Jade was quite upset at this information. She was offered support to gradually reduce her alcohol intake and was referred to her local community alcohol service where she joined a local support group and received one-to-one counselling. Jade was also offered family support from social services to help her provide a stable home environment, and Jordon was offered educational support at school.

Patient 5.1 — David — 138 | 161 | 195 | 237 | 448 | **474**

- 44-year-old man
- Increased urine output; thirsty and hungry
- Blood test: low thyroxine and raised blood glucose
- Has hypothyroidism and the start of a goitre
- Given levothyroxine; dose adjusted until thyroxine levels stabilise
- Has diabetes associated with obesity – diet modified and given metformin
- The levothyroxine helps him to metabolize food better

Following a consultation with his family doctor, it became apparent that David's erectile dysfunction was more likely to be physical, related to altered blood flow and autonomic nervous system activity associated with the effects of his diabetes mellitus, rather than due to lifestyle or psychological factors. In addition, it was recognized that while David's thyroid function was well controlled with thyroid hormone replacement therapy, hypothyroidism is a contributory factor for erectile dysfunction. His erectile dysfunction was affecting his relationship with his partner and the anxiety related to sexual activity was affecting him. This exemplifies the complex processes involved with sexual arousal and penile erection. Various approaches to helping David were discussed, and he was referred to see a specialist in erectile dysfunction, which led to him being offered a drug called sildenafil. Sildenafil belongs to a group of drugs commonly used for erectile dysfunction called phosphodiesterase type 5 inhibitors. During sexual arousal, nitric oxide is released by the action of the parasympathetic nervous system and stimulates the production of the second messenger cyclic AMP (cAMP) in the smooth muscle cells of the penile vessels, causing vasodilation and increased blood flow. cAMP is destroyed by specific enzymes and therefore the vasodilatory effect is lost. Drugs such as sildenafil block the action of these enzymes, thus prolonging vasodilation and increasing blood flow. It took some time for David to determine the optimal drug dosage (100 mg in 24 hours as a single dose), but the use of sildenafil has overcome his erectile dysfunction and transformed his self-confidence and his relationship with his partner.

Patient 9.1 — Robert — 268 | 305 | 448 | **474**

- 56-year-old man with family history of CVD
- First MI at 38, stent at 45, and coronary artery bypass graft at 49
- ECG shows changes consistent with another MI; confirmed by biochemical marker tests
- Has hypotension and oedema
- Prescribed aspirin, atorvastatin, bisoprolol and perindopril
- Diet altered to reduce salt and fat and exercise levels increased

Robert had relatively few urinary symptoms but these included hesitancy, at times urgency and also a sensation that voiding of urine was incomplete. Robert did not experience **nocturia**. A digital rectal examination (DRE) revealed a moderately large, smooth, non-nodular prostate gland with a defined furrow (called the medial sulcus) between each lateral lobe. The prostate-specific antigen (PSA) test confirmed that his PSA level was below the cut-off point for Robert's age. A diagnosis of benign prostatic hyperplasia (BPH) was made. BPH is an increase in the size of the prostate gland without a malignancy present and is common in men of advancing age. It is unusual before the age of 45 and is more common in men of African–American origin, which may be linked to higher testosterone levels, androgen receptor expression and growth factor activity. As Robert had relatively few symptoms, a watch-and-wait approach was adopted. If Robert has more severe symptoms, drugs can be given to reduce the internal sphincter muscles of the bladder neck (see *Chapter 8*). Surgery (prostatectomy) is usually reserved for those with a large prostate enlargement and severe symptoms, including severe obstruction of the urethra leading to acute retention of urine.

| Patient 14.1 | Jess | 449 | **475** |

- 33-year-old woman
- Intermenstrual and post-coital bleeding
- Family doctor requests smear test
- Some dyskaryosis found
- Abnormal cells removed via LLETZ on colposcopy

Jess underwent a colposcopy and large loop excision of the transformation zone (LLETZ), which removed the abnormal cells identified following her smear test. This treatment is usually very successful, and so it is unlikely that any abnormal cells will be detected in the future. She was reminded of the importance of attending regular smear tests following her treatment. Jess was also advised to give up smoking as the risk of cervical cancer in current smokers is estimated to be about double that of non-smokers. She was referred to her local NHS Stop Smoking service as studies have shown that people are four times more likely to quit with NHS treatment and support than without it.

Developments in the scientific understanding of reproductive physiology and associated technological advances provide both opportunities and challenges for individuals and society. For example, opportunities to overcome problems with reproduction, sexuality and forming intimate relationships can raise moral and ethical questions.

14.4 Summary

- Sperm are produced in the seminiferous tubules of the testes (see *Figure 14.2*) and exit the body, via a series of ducts, within semen, which is produced by a number of accessory glands (see *Figure 14.1*).
- Spermatogenesis is controlled via a feedback mechanism involving a number of hormones including follicle-stimulating hormone, luteinizing hormone and testosterone (see *Figure 14.5*).
- The ovarian and uterine cycles, which describe the development of an oocyte and the uterus, respectively, are regulated by specific hormones: gonadotrophin-releasing hormone, follicle-stimulating hormone, luteinizing hormone, oestrogen and progesterone (see *Figure 14.10*).
- The ovarian and uterine cycles continue until a pregnancy or the menopause occurs.
- The placenta is an important organ that allows the exchange of molecules between the mother and fetus (see *Figure 14.11*).
- Labour is initiated following a complex interplay between hormones of the mother and the fetus, which results in a sharp rise in oestrogen production from the placenta.
- High levels of oestrogen and progesterone secreted during pregnancy stimulate the development of the breast in preparation for lactation. Milk

production and ejection are stimulated by the hormones prolactin and oxytocin, respectively.

14.5 Further reading

The Cancer Research UK website provides very useful information about all types of cancer and how they can be treated and managed by healthcare professionals and patients themselves:
www.cancerresearch.org

A review of alcohol-induced nervous system defects, their physiological mechanisms and possible therapeutic targets can be found in the following article: **Muralidharan, P., Sarmah, S., Zhou, F. C. and Marrs, J. A.** (2013) Fetal alcohol spectrum disorder (FASD) associated neural defects: complex mechanisms and potential therapeutic targets. *Brain Sciences* **3**: 964–991.
Available at: www.mdpi.com/2076-3425/3/2/964/htm.

The Prostate Cancer Foundation website gives information on prostate cancer: www.pcf.org/site/c.leJRIROrEpH/b.5699537/k.BEF4/Home.htm

14.6 Self-assessment questions

Answers can be found at www.scionpublishing.com/AandP

(14.1) Select the one correct answer. With reference to spermatogenesis, the hormone testosterone:
(a) stimulates the production of sperm in the prostate gland
(b) reduces the production of sperm
(c) stimulates sustentacular cells to secrete testosterone
(d) is secreted from the interstitial cells in the testes
(e) reduces the motility of mature sperm

(14.2) Select the one correct answer. A surge in which one of the following hormones is principally responsible for stimulating the secretion of follicle-stimulating hormone?
(a) Inhibin
(b) Prolactin
(c) Luteinizing hormone (LH)
(d) Gonadotrophin-releasing hormone (GnRH)
(e) Progesterone

(14.3) Select the one correct answer. What is the name of the ruptured follicle, formed following the ejection of the oocyte?
(a) Graafian follicle
(b) Germinal follicle
(c) Pink body
(d) Corpus luteum
(e) Corpus albicans

(14.4) Rearrange the following organs and sections of the uterine tubes to describe the path taken by the oocyte following ovulation:
1 = ampulla, 2 = ovary, 3 = uterus, 4 = infundibulum, 5 = uterine part, 6 = isthmus

(a) 2, 4, 1, 6, 3, 5
(b) 2, 1, 4, 6, 5, 3
(c) 4, 2, 1, 3, 6, 5
(d) 4, 1, 2, 5, 6, 3
(e) 2, 4, 1, 6, 5, 3

(14.5) Describe the positive-feedback loop involving the hormone oxytocin that is associated with the contractions of the myometrium and parturition.

(14.6) Discuss the advantages of giving the human papillomavirus (HPV) vaccine to boys aged 12–13 as well as girls.

(14.7) Outline the key factors that influence the production of sperm.

Glossary

1,25-Dihydroxycholecalciferol – The active form of vitamin D.
Accommodation – The process of increasing the refractive power of the lens of the eye; focusing of light.
Acetabulum – A cup-like cavity on the lateral surface of the hip bone that receives the femur.
Acetylcholine – A neurotransmitter found in preganglionic sympathetic and parasympathetic neurones.
Acromioclavicular joint – A synovial joint at the top of the shoulder that forms the junction between the acromion and the clavicle.
Acromion – A bony process or outgrowth on the upper edge of the scapula or shoulder blade.
Acrosome – A membranous sac, at the tip of the head of the spermatozoa, containing the enzyme hyaluronidase.
Actin – A thin filament in muscle fibres.
Actinic purpura – Also known as senile purpura, a benign condition characterized by red-purple blotches, caused by sun-induced skin damage to connective tissue, allowing blood cells to leak into the surrounding dermis.
Action potential – A nerve impulse.
Active immunity – Immunity or resistance to infection produced by responses from immune cells.
Active transport – Transport of a substance across the plasma membrane that requires the use of metabolic energy.
Acute inflammation – A rapid immune response immediately and over days in response to tissue injury; it is characterized by a cascade of immune responses including an infiltration of neutrophils into tissues and is relatively short lived in contrast to chronic inflammation.
Acute-phase proteins – A group of proteins produced from the liver in response to pro-inflammatory cytokines to mediate a variety of local and systemic responses including fever.
Acute stress response – A psychological state that results from a traumatic event and causes activation of the sympathetic nervous system.
Adaptive immunity – A division of the immune system also known as specific or acquired immunity, characterized by highly antigen-specific responses, which include antibody production and immunological memory.
Adenine – A purine nucleotide that forms part of RNA and DNA; it is complementary to thymine and uracil and has a role in ATP production.
Adenosine diphosphate (ADP) – An intermediate during the formation of ATP from cyclic adenosine monophosphate.
Adenosine triphosphate (ATP) – An intracellular energy store that stores energy released from the metabolism of food. ATP provides energy for all synthetic cellular processes that require energy.

Adipocyte – Cells that store fat and form adipose tissue.
Adipose tissue – Tissue formed from fat cells.
Adrenaline – A neurotransmitter secreted at the end of sympathetic nerves and a neurotransmitter secreted by the adrenal medulla of the adrenal glands; also known as epinephrine.
Afferent – A directional term, conveying 'towards'.
Agglutinin – Antibody in plasma that binds to antigenic proteins (agglutinogens) on the plasma membrane of erythrocytes.
Agglutinogen – Antigen (protein) on the plasma membrane of erythrocytes that stimulates antibodies (agglutinins) in the plasma, resulting in clumping together of erythrocytes.
Agnosia – Inability to recognize objects.
Agonist – A molecule that binds to a receptor to cause a biological response.
All-or-nothing principle – A stimulus needs to be strong enough to reach a threshold in order to generate a nerve action potential that can be propagated along the entire neurone.
Allele – An alternative form or variant of a specific gene.
Allergy – A hypersensitivity disorder as a result of overactivity of the immune system.
Alpha-cell (α-cell) – Endocrine cell in the pancreas that secretes the hormone glucagon.
Alveolus – Microscopic air sac in the lung (plural = alveoli).
Amblyopia – Decreased vision without any demonstrable abnormality of the eye; often called a 'lazy eye'.
Amino acid – The building block of proteins in plants and animals and a source of nitrogen in the body.
Aminopeptidase – An enzyme that is secreted by the pancreas in exocrine pancreatic juice and is responsible for removing amino acids from the amino-terminal end of a peptide or protein.
Amnion – The inner extraembryonic membrane that initially covers the embryo.
Amphiarthroses – A slightly movable joint in which the surfaces are connected by discs of fibrocartilage.
Amphiphilic – A compound with polar (hydrophilic = *water loving*) and lipophilic (= *fat loving*) regions. These regions are responsible for the structure of plasma membranes and formation of micelles. This chemical structure is common in soaps and detergents.
Ampulla of uterine tube – The wide part of the uterine tube between the infundibulum and the isthmus.
Amylase – A carbohydrate-digesting enzyme.
Anaemia – A deficiency in the number of red blood cells or the haemoglobin content.

480 GLOSSARY

Anaerobe – A microorganism that is able to live and grow without the presence of free oxygen.

Anaerobic processes – Metabolic processes to obtain energy without the use of oxygen; metabolic processes that do not need oxygen as the final electron acceptor.

Anaphase – The fourth phase of mitosis where duplicated chromosomes are separated to opposite poles of the cell.

Anaphylaxis – A severe life-threatening allergic reaction.

Anatomical dead space – Volume of gas present in the conducting airways from the nose and mouth to the terminal bronchioles that does not participate in gas exchange.

Androgen – Steroid hormone such as testosterone that controls the development and maintenance of masculine characteristics.

Aneuploidy – An abnormal number of chromosomes in a cell.

Angiogenesis – The formation of new blood vessels from those already present; important for wound healing and also implicated in carcinogenesis.

Angiotensin-converting enzyme (ACE) – The enzyme that converts angiotensin I to angiotensin II. ACE inhibitor drugs prevent this conversion.

Angiotensin I – The precursor to angiotensin II, formed by the action of renin on angiotensinogen.

Angiotensin II – Stimulates the secretion of aldosterone from the adrenal cortex and also acts as a potent vasoconstrictor of smooth muscle.

Anhydrous – Without water.

Anions – Atoms or groups of atoms that have gained electrons and thus carry a negative charge, for example chloride ions (Cl^-) and bicarbonate ions (HCO_3^-).

Annulus fibrosus – A fibrous ring of an intervertebral disc.

Antagonist – A molecule that binds onto a receptor to prevent or reduce the effect of an agonist.

Anterior cavity – The cavity of the eye between the cornea and lens containing aqueous humour.

Anterior chamber – The chamber lying between the cornea and the iris of the eye.

Anterior fontanelle – A soft spot on the anterior top of an infant's head that bulges in a curving manner.

Antibiotic – Antimicrobial drug that targets bacteria.

Antibody – A specific glycoprotein produced and secreted by B-lymphocytes (plasma cells) in response to specific antigens; a key feature of adaptive immunity.

Anticodon – A triplet of codons present on a tRNA molecule that is able to base pair to a complementary codon.

Antigen – Any substance capable of binding antibody or a T-cell receptor.

Antigen-presenting cell (APC) – A cell that processes and presents antigens on its surface for recognition by leukocytes.

Antisense strand – See 'template strand'.

Antithrombin III – Inhibits the effects of thrombin, thus prevents blood clotting.

Aortic valve – Semilunar valve positioned between the aorta and the left ventricle.

Aphasia – Impairment of language in which both the production and comprehension of speech are affected.

Apneustic centre – A group of neurones in the pons that have a stimulatory effect on the inspiratory neurones in the medulla; promotes inspiration.

Apocrine – A type of sweat gland, typically found concentrated around the axilla, groin and areolar region of the nipples.

Apoptosis – A regulated form of cell suicide or programmed cell death.

Appendicular skeleton – The part of the skeleton consisting of the bones and cartilage that support the appendages.

Aquaporin – An integral membrane protein that forms a channel specifically for the passage of water.

Aqueous humour – Watery, clear solution that fills the anterior and posterior chambers of the eye.

Arachidonic acid – An omega-6-fatty acid found in plasma membranes. It is an important precursor molecule for the synthesis of eicosanoids.

Arachnoid mater – The middle layer of the meningeal membranes.

Arachnoid villi – Specialized protrusions of the arachnoid mater.

Astrocytes – Cells that form a selective barrier in the brain between neurones and capillaries.

Atrial natriuretic peptide – A 28-amino acid peptide that is synthesized, stored and released by atrial myocytes in response to distension of the atria and sympathetic stimulation.

Atrioventricular bundle – See 'Bundle of His'.

Atrioventricular node – Specialized cardiocytes located in the atrial septum.

Atrioventricular valves – Valves that prevent the backflow of blood from the ventricles into the atrium when the ventricles contract (mitral and tricuspid valves).

Auditory ossicles – The three tiny bones that transmit vibrations and are located in the middle ear.

Autocrine – Autocrine signalling is when a substance produced from a cell exerts an effect on the same cell that produced the substance.

Autosome – An autosome is any chromosome that does not determine sex; that is, autosomes are not sex chromosomes (allosome).

Axial skeleton – The part of the skeleton consisting of the bones of the skull and the vertebrae.

Axon – A nerve fibre that conducts electrical impulses from the cell body to axon terminals or dendrites.

Axon hillock – The area of the neurone that connects the cell body to the axon.

Ball-and-socket joint – A multi-axis joint that allows movement in all directions.

Basilar membrane – The supporting membrane that runs the length of the cochlea and supports the organ of Corti.

Basophil – A granulocyte, normally representing less than 0.5% of circulating leukocytes. Basophils release histamine and other chemical mediators and have a role in inflammation and allergies.

Beta-cell (β-cell) – Endocrine cell in the pancreas that secretes the hormone insulin.

Between brain – Another name for the diencephalon, a part of the brain consisting of the thalamus and hypothalamus, which connects the midbrain to the cerebral hemispheres.

Blood-brain barrier – A highly selective permeability barrier that separates blood from extracellular fluid in the brain and protects brain cells from undesirable substances.

Blood–CSF barrier – A barrier that isolates the central nervous system from the general circulation.
B-lymphocyte – A type of small lymphocyte that with appropriate stimulation is able to secrete antibodies, providing a humoral response of adaptive immunity.
Bohr effect – The increased oxygen release by haemoglobin in the presence of elevated carbon dioxide levels.
Bony pelvis – A bowl-shaped structure that forms the skeleton of the pelvis made up of the hip bones in front and at the sides, and by the sacrum and coccyx behind.
Bowman's capsule – The cup-shaped end of a tubule of the nephron, which encloses the glomerulus and facilitates glomerular filtration.
Brainstem – A part of the brain made up of the midbrain, pons and medulla oblongata, it is involved in arousal, attention and consciousness.
Broca's area – A language centre in the brain that enables the production of speech.
Bronchus – A branch of the bronchial tree (conduction airways) between the trachea and bronchioles (plural = bronchi).
Brownian motion – Discovered by Robert Brown (1773–1858) when studying the movement of pollen particles suspended in a fluid. It describes the continuous random movement of particles bombarded by other particles and is used to explain the process of diffusion.
B-type atrial natriuretic peptide – A 32-amino acid peptide that is secreted by the ventricles of the heart in response to excessive stretching of cardiac muscle cells (cardiomyocytes).
Bulbourethral glands – Paired accessory glands located inferiorly to the prostate gland.
Bundle of His – Specialized conducting cells in the intraventricular septum that carry the electrical stimulus from the atrioventricular (AV) node to the bundle branches; also called atrioventricular bundle.

Calcaneus – The heel bone of the foot.
Calcitriol – The hormonally active component of 1,25-dihydroxyvitamin D, which increases the amount of calcium in the blood.
Canal of Schlemm – A collection of veins at the base of the cornea that drain aqueous humour from the eye.
Canaliculus – Very small tubular channel in a tissue or organ (plural = canaliculi).
Capitulum – The lateral portion of the distal articular surface of the humerus consisting of a rounded eminence or protuberance, which articulates with another bone.
Carbaminohaemoglobin – Haemoglobin bound to carbon dioxide molecules.
Carboxypeptidase – An enzyme secreted by the pancreas in pancreatic juice that removes amino acids from the carboxyl-terminal end of peptides and proteins.
Cardiac cycle – Electrical and mechanical events associated with one heartbeat; a complete round of systole and diastole.
Cardiac muscle – Muscle unique to the heart, called the myocardium.
Cardiac output – The volume of blood ejected from each ventricle each minute (typically 5.0 L/minute at rest).
Carpals – The eight bones of the wrist.

Carrier-mediated diffusion – An arrangement of integral membrane proteins that provide a mechanism of selective transport across a plasma membrane. A substance binding to a carrier protein induces a conformational change (change in shape) in the protein, which transports the substance across the membrane. This can be either a passive (facilitated) or active transport mechanism.
Carrier protein – Integral protein within the plasma membrane that facilitates the selective transport of a particular solute across the membrane.
Cartilage – A strong and resilient supporting tissue formed by chondrocytes that is able to withstand compression.
Cartilage lacuna – Cavity in matrix that contains cartilage cells or chondrocytes (plural = lacunae).
Cascade screening – Systematic investigation of relatives for identification of family members at risk of genetic conditions.
Cataracts – Clouding of the lens in the eye.
Cathepsin – A group of degradative proteases.
Cations – Atoms or groups of atoms that have lost electrons and thus carry a positive charge, for example Na^+ and Ca^{2+}.
Cell body – The control centre of a neurone.
Cellulose – A long-chain organic linear polysaccharide of linked glucose molecules that is a major component of rigid plant cell walls.
Central (Haversian) canal – The canal in the centre of each osteon that contains nerves and blood vessels.
Central cyanosis – Bluish discoloration of the mucous membrane of the tongue and lips due to reduced oxygen concentration.
Central nervous system – The brain and spinal cord.
Centriole – A non-membranous organelle composed mainly of tubulin proteins, essential for cell division.
Centromere – A constricted region of a chromosome where a pair of chromatids is held together.
Centrosome – A region of proteinaceous material usually found close to the nucleus. It contains two centrioles important in the process of cell division.
Cerebellum – A structure found at the back of the brain involved in movement, posture and balance.
Cerebrospinal fluid (CSF) – The fluid that circulates around the brain and nourishes the brain and spinal cord.
Cerebrum – The largest and most developed part of the human brain, made up of two hemispheres.
Cerumen – Ear wax.
Cervix – The lowest part of the uterus, inferior to the body and fundus, part of which protrudes into the vagina.
Channel-mediated diffusion – A form of facilitated diffusion that involves the selective passage of molecules through the plasma membrane via channels formed by integral proteins embedded within the plasma membrane.
Channel proteins – A type of integral membrane protein that interacts with a particular solute to form a pore that, when open, allows a particular solute to be transported across the plasma membrane.
Checkpoint – A regulatory mechanism that allows interruption of cell division until favourable conditions permit it to continue.
Chemokine – A group of chemotactic cytokines.
Chemoreceptors – Receptors sensitive to various chemicals in solution, for example plasma oxygen and carbon dioxide levels.

Chemotaxis – Directional movement of a cell towards the source and along a chemical gradient.

Chief cell – Cell found in the gastric glands that produces the protein-digesting enzyme pepsin in an inactive form as pepsinogen.

Chloride shift – The movement of plasma chloride ions (Cl⁻) into the erythrocyte in exchange for bicarbonate ions (HCO₃⁻).

Chondroblast – Cell which produces the extracellular matrix of cartilage.

Chordae tendineae – Tendon-like fibrous cords that connect the atrioventricular valves to papillary muscles to ensure effective closure of the valves.

Chorion – The outer extraembryonic membrane that forms the fetal part of the placenta.

Chorion frondosum – The leaf-like structure formed from the chorionic villi that forms the fetal part of the placenta.

Chorionic villus – Projection of the external surface of the chorion that facilitates the exchange of materials between the fetal and maternal circulation (plural = villi).

Choroid – Portion of the vascular tunic (middle coat) of the eye.

Chromaffin – Neuroendocrine cells found in the medulla of the adrenal glands.

Chromatin – A complex of DNA and protein, mainly histones, within the nucleus that forms chromosomes.

Chromosome – A highly organized structure composed of chromatin.

Chyle – A milky bodily fluid consisting of emulsified fats or fatty acids, chylomicrons and lymph that results from digestion of fats in the small intestine.

Chylomicron – A lipoprotein that is assembled in the small intestine mucosa and contains apolipoprotein, triacylglycerol, cholesterol and phospholipids. Chylomicrons are secreted into the lymphatic system and blood.

Chyme – A semi-fluid substance of partially digested food mixed with gastric juices that arrives in the duodenum from the stomach.

Chymotrypsin – An enzyme secreted by the pancreas in an inactive form in pancreatic juice as chymotrypsinogen and with a role in protein digestion.

Ciliary body – A thickened region of the choroid that encircles the lens of the eye.

Ciliary process – The region of the ciliary body that is attached to the lens via the suspensory ligaments.

Ciliated columnar epithelium – Epithelial cells that are column shaped and have cilia on their free surface.

Cilium – A slender organelle that extends above the free surface of an epithelial cell and undergoes rhythmical movement; hair-like structures that move in a wave-like manner (plural = cilia).

Circadian rhythm – A 24-hour cycle of endogenously generated physiological processes in both animals and plants that can be modulated by environmental cues such as light and temperature.

***Cis* fatty acid** – A fatty acid whereby the stereochemical arrangement of the hydrogen atoms at a carbon–carbon double bond are such that both hydrogen atoms are on the same side of the double bond.

Citric acid cycle (Krebs cycle) – A degradative pathway in which ATP is synthesized and some intermediates are generated for the biosynthesis of other compounds.

Clavicles – Long horizontal bones, also known as collar bones, that lie between the sternum and the scapula (shoulder blade).

Coding strand – The strand of DNA that has the same sequence as the transcribed RNA, not to be confused with the template strand, which is complementary to the coding strand.

Codon – A sequence of three DNA or RNA nucleotides that correspond to a specific amino acid or start/stop signal.

Coenzyme – A non-protein substance such as a vitamin or mineral that activates an enzyme.

Cofactor – A metal ion or organic molecule that is needed for enzyme activity.

Collagen – A fibrous protein forming connective tissue and the most abundant protein in the body.

Collagenase – An enzyme that breaks down peptide bonds in collagen.

Collecting duct – A renal tubular structure into which a number of collecting tubules from a number of nephrons drain ultrafiltrate.

Colonize – Establish a community of microorganisms in or on the body without causing disease.

Colostrum – The first milk secreted by a mother following childbirth, rich in maternal antibodies.

Compact bone – Dense rigid bone in which the bony matrix is filled with inorganic salts and organic ground substance.

Complement – A group of proteins found in plasma; part of the innate immunity, which enhances inflammation and immune responses.

Condyle – A rounded projection of a bone that allows articulation with another bone.

Condyloid joint – A joint formed by oval surfaces allowing different angular movements.

Cone – A photoreceptor in the retina of the eye responsible for colour vision.

Conformation – The folded shape of a protein.

Conjunctiva – Mucous membrane covering the inner surface of the eyelids and the anterior surface of the eyeball to the margins of the cornea.

Connective tissue – The most abundant type of tissue; it fills the body spaces, providing structural and metabolic support.

Contractility – The ability of muscle cells to move by shortening.

Control centre – A component associated with homeostasis/ homeodynamics; it receives information from the receptors and coordinates the response of the effectors.

Cornea – The transparent portion of the fibrous tunic of the outer anterior surface of the eye.

Corneocyte – A cell type that comprises the epithelium. These cells are terminally differentiated keratinocytes which, by the time they form the stratum corneum, are flattened, full of keratin and dead.

Coronal suture – The fixed joint where the parietal bones meet the frontal bone (anterior suture).

Coronary sinus – The short trunk that receives blood from most of the veins of the heart and empties into the right atrium.

Coronoid fossa – A hollow area on the anterior surface of the distal end of the humerus where the coronoid process of the ulna rests when the elbow is flexed.

Corpus callosum – A band of thick nerve fibres that connect the left and right hemispheres of the brain.

Corpus luteum – The remains of a vesicular follicle after ovulation, which secretes progesterone and some oestrogen.

Countercurrent mechanism – The system that operates in the loop of Henle, facilitated by the flow of ultrafiltrate in opposite directions through the loop, the differences in permeability through the loop and the presence of the vasa recta, which facilitates the formation of concentrated urine.

Coxal bones – Large flat bones, also known as pelvic bones, with a constricted centre that are composed of three bones, namely the ilium, the ischium and the pubis.

Creatine phosphate – A molecule found in muscle cells which, when metabolized to create adenosine triphosphate (ATP), produces creatinine.

Creatinine – A nitrogenous waste molecule produced during the metabolism of creatine phosphate.

Cribriform plate – A portion of the ethmoid bone that contains the holes through which the axons of olfactory receptors pass to the olfactory bulbs.

Crista ampullaris – Sensory receptor complex within the ampulla of the semicircular canal.

Cristae – Folds within the inner membrane of a mitochondrion providing increased surface area to maximize efficiency of cellular respiration.

Crystallins – Proteins that fill the epithelial cells of the lens in the eye.

Cuneiform – Any of the three small wedge-shaped bones in the human foot.

Cupula – A gelatinous mass that is located in the ampulla of the semicircular canal.

Cyclic adenosine monophosphate (cyclic AMP) – A second messenger involved in many biological systems; it is formed when adenosine triphosphate is utilized as an energy source in the body.

Cyclic guanosine monophosphate (cyclic GMP) – A second messenger that is derived from guanosine.

Cyclooxygenase – Enzyme responsible for the formation of a variety of inflammatory mediators including prostaglandins, thromboxanes and prostacyclin.

Cystitis – Inflammation of the urinary bladder.

Cytochrome P450 epoxygenase (CYP) – The enzyme that converts arachidonic acid to epoxyeicosatrienoic acids.

Cytokines – A large group of small proteins important for cell signalling.

Cytokinesis – The physical process of cell division when the plasma membrane forms to separate the cytoplasm of newly divided cells.

Cytoplasm – The internal constituents of a cell; includes the cytosol and all internal structures.

Cytosine – A pyrimidine nucleotide that forms part of DNA and RNA.

Cytoskeleton – A network of intracellular protein filaments that provide structural organization to the cell.

Cytosol – The liquid portion that forms the intercellular fluid within a cell.

Cytotoxic T-lymphocyte (CTL) – A small lymphocyte that responds to intracellular antigens, important for killing body cells infected with virus.

Cytotrophoblast – The inner layer of a trophoblast.

Dalton's law – The total pressure exerted by a mixture of gases is the sum of the pressures exerted independently by each gas in the mixture; in a mixture of gases, the pressure each gas contributes to the overall gas pressure is in proportion to its relative abundance.

Damage-associated molecular pattern (DAMP) molecules – A group of molecules released from damaged body tissue, capable of causing immune responses but not inflammation (unlike PAMPs).

Decibel – A unit of measurement expressing the intensity of a sound or the power of an electrical signal.

Decidua basalis – The area of endometrium that develops following implantation of the embryo that becomes the maternal part of the placenta.

Decussation – Crossing over of nerve fibres from right side of the brain to the left side of the brain and vice versa in the medulla oblongata.

Deep sockets – Joint cavities such as the acetabulum of the hip bone where the head of the femur fits tightly, enabling the formation of a stronger and more stable ball-and-socket joint.

Deep vein thrombosis – A blood clot (thrombus) in one of the deep veins, for example in the veins of the calf muscle.

Delta-cell (δ-cell) – A cell in the pancreas that produces the hormone somatostatin.

Deltoid tuberosity – A rough or bumpy triangular side of the frontal side surface of the humerus to which the deltoid muscle is attached.

Denature – To destroy the characteristic properties of a macromolecule, disrupting its molecular conformation.

Dendrite – A branched projection or process of a neurone that propagates impulses received from the axon and axon terminals to the cell body.

Dendritic cell – An antigen-presenting cell able to process antigen and migrate to and from lymphatic tissue; important in regulating adaptive immune responses.

Dense connective tissue – Large amounts of collagen fibres with proportionally less elastic fibres forming strong structures such as tendons and ligaments.

Deoxyribonucleic acid (DNA) – A nucleic acid that is the hereditary material and provides the information for making messenger RNA.

Depolarization – A change in the electrical membrane potential of a cell due to sodium ions (Na^+) entering the cell and potassium ions (K^+) moving out of the cell.

Dermis – The layer of tissue immediately below the epidermis and on top of subcutaneous tissue.

Desmosome – A cell junction composed of thickened plasma membranes joined by filaments.

Detrusor muscle of the bladder – The smooth muscle of the bladder, which contracts to expel urine during micturition.

Diacylglycerol – A molecule of two fatty acid chains covalently bonded to glycerol.

Diapedesis – Movement of cells across blood vessels and into tissue spaces.

Diaphysis – The part of the long bone between the two extremities; also known as the shaft.

Diarthrosis – A freely movable joint such as a ball-and-socket, condyloid, gliding, hinge or saddle joint.

Diastole – The period in the cardiac cycle when the cardiac muscle is relaxed and the chambers fill with blood.
Diencephalon – A part of the forebrain containing the thalamus and hypothalamus connecting the midbrain to the cerebral hemispheres; also known as the between brain.
Dipeptidase – An enzyme secreted by the pancreas in pancreatic juice that breaks down dipeptides to amino acids.
Diploë – The spongy bone structure found in the internal structure of short, flat and irregular bones.
Diploid – A nucleus containing two copies of each chromosome.
Direct pathway – A long nerve pathway that extends from the motor cortex of the brain to the spinal cord without forming synapses.
Disaccharide – A sugar composed of simple sugars, or monosaccharides, for example lactose, maltose and sucrose.
Distal – Part of the body situated away from the centre of the body.
Distal convoluted tubule – The portion of the nephron that lies between the loop of Henle and the collecting ducts.
Dorsal horn – The posterior grey column of the spinal cord that receives and processes sensory information such as touch and vibrations from various parts of the body.
Dorsal ramus – Branch of spinal nerves containing motor and sensory axons that supplies the muscles, skin and bones of the posterior part of the head, neck and trunk (plural = dorsal rami).
Dorsal respiratory group – A cluster of neurones located in the dorsal region (towards the back) of the medulla.
Dorsal root – Contains sensory neurones that bring impulses from the peripheral regions of the body to the spinal cord; also known as the posterior root.
Ductus deferens – The tubular structure that conducts spermatozoa from the epididymis of the testicle to the ejaculatory duct – also called vas deferens.
Dura mater – The outermost layer of the meningeal membranes that surround the brain and spinal cord.
Dyskaryosis – An abnormality in the nucleus of cells, which can indicate a pre-malignant or malignant state.
Dysplasia – An abnormal change in the size, shape and appearance of cells.

Eccrine gland – The major sweat glands of the body.
Ectocervix – The part of the cervix that protrudes into the vagina.
Effectors – One of the components of a homeostatic/homeodynamic system. Effectors are typically smooth muscle, cardiac muscle or glands that produce an effect that negates the original stimulus.
Efferent – A directional term, conveying away from.
Effort – A force applied due to muscle contraction to move a load.
Eicosanoid – A signalling molecule derived from omega-3 (ω-3) or omega-6 (ω-6) fatty acids.
Elastase – A proteolytic enzyme; its main substrate is elastin.
Elasticity – The ability of tissue to return to its original shape after contraction or extension.
Elastin – An elastic protein forming part of connective tissue.
Electrolytes – Substances that ionize in ionizing solvents such as water and therefore conduct electricity, for example sodium ions (Na^+) and bicarbonate ions (HCO_3^-).

Electron transport chain – A series of mechanisms in biological systems in which electrons are transferred from an electron donor to an electron acceptor in a respiratory chain during aerobic respiration.
Embolism – Obstruction of a blood vessel by a fat globule, air bubble or blood clot (embolus) circulating through the blood.
Endocardium – Inner lining (epithelial cells) of the heart wall.
Endocervix – The part of the cervix that does not protrude into the vagina but opens into the uterine cavity.
Endochondral ossification – The embryonic formation of bone by the replacement of calcified cartilage that results in the formation of most of the skeletal bones.
Endocrine gland – A gland that secretes its hormones directly into blood instead of into a duct.
Endocytosis – A form of vesicular transport where secretory vesicles transport a substance across the plasma membrane from the surrounding space into the cell.
Endometrium – The inner lining of the uterus consisting of epithelial tissue.
Endorphin – A brain peptide or endogenous regulator of pain perception that acts like an opiate.
Endosteum – The membrane that lines the marrow (medullary) cavity of bones and consists of osteogenic cells and scattered osteoclasts.
Endotracheal tube – A specific type of tube that is inserted via the mouth or nose into the trachea to facilitate the movement of gases into and out of the lungs.
Enteropeptidase – An enzyme produced by cells in the duodenum wall that activates protein-digesting enzymes in pancreatic juice, for example activating trypsinogen to trypsin.
Enzyme – A protein that catalyses biochemical reactions.
Eosinophil – A granulocyte, responsible for extracellular killing of parasites and infection. With a role in inflammation, they are implicated in some types of allergy.
Ependymal cell – A cell that lines the cavities or ventricles of the brain and central canal of the spinal cord.
Epicardium – Serous membrane covering the surface of the heart; also called the visceral pericardium.
Epicondylar – Relating to the rounded prominence or projection at the end of long bones where ligaments and tendons are attached.
Epicondyle – A rounded protuberance or projection at the end of long bones to which ligaments, muscles and tendons are attached.
Epidermis – The outermost layer of skin cells lying on top of the dermis.
Epididymis – Coiled duct that sits above the testes, connecting the seminiferous tubules to the ductus deferens; site for maturation of spermatozoa.
Epigenetic – The control of DNA by mechanisms other than alteration of the sequence of DNA nucleotides.
Epiglottis – Plate of elastic cartilage that covers the larynx during swallowing.
Epiphyseal line – A remnant of the epiphyseal plate in the metaphysis of a long bone.
Epiphyseal plate – The site of lengthwise growth of long bones made of hyaline cartilage.
Epiphysis – The rounded end of a long bone, which usually is larger in diameter than the diaphysis or shaft.

Epithelium – A cell type that forms continuous sheets of cells forming both external and internal surfaces of the body and glands (plural=epithelia). Classified depending on morphology into four types – simple, stratified, cuboidal and columnar.

Epitope – The specific part or site on an antigen recognized by an antibody or T-cell receptor.

Epoxyeicosatrienoic acid – Signalling molecule formed by cytochrome P450 epoxygenase.

Erythrasmus – A rash due to bacterial infection often coexisting with a fungal infection associated with skin folds.

Erythrocyte – A red blood cell.

Erythropoietin – Hormone secreted by the kidney that stimulates the production of red blood cells (erythropoiesis).

Eukarya – A kingdom of life distinct from the prokaryotes, notable by being formed of larger cells containing organelles. All multicellular organisms are eukaryotic.

Eustachian tube – Passageway extending from the middle ear to the nasopharynx.

Excitability – The ability to respond to a stimulus.

Excoriation – Any loss of the surface of the skin.

Exocytosis – A form of vesicular transport where secretory vesicles transport a substance across the plasma membrane into the surrounding space.

Exon – A region within a gene, DNA or RNA transcript that remains in the final mature mRNA coding for an amino acid sequence.

Expiratory reserve volume – The maximum volume of air that can be voluntarily expelled from the lungs after a normal quiet expiration.

Expressive aphasia – The inability to produce language, either spoken or written.

Extensibility – The ability of muscle tissue to stretch when it is pulled.

Falciform ligament – A ligament that attaches the liver to the diaphragm and to the anterior abdominal wall.

False ribs – One of the last five pairs of ribs (the eighth to twelfth pairs of ribs, which are not attached to the sternum.

FAST rule – The use of the face, arms and speech as a test to diagnose whether a person has had a stroke.

Femur – A long bone of the thigh with articulations at the hip and knee.

Fibrin – Insoluble protein fibres that form the basic framework of a blood clot.

Fibrinogen – A soluble blood protein that is converted into insoluble fibrin during haemostasis (blood clotting).

Fibrinolysis – The process that removes blood clots.

Fibroblast – A type of cell responsible for producing the extracellular matrix and proteins such as collagen and elastin that form connective tissue.

Fibula – The outer of the two bones between the knee and the ankle, parallel to the tibia.

Floating ribs – Any of the lower last two pairs of ribs in humans that are attached to the spine but have no attachment to the sternum.

Fluid mosaic model – A phrase coined by Singer and Nicholson (1972) suggesting that the lipid part of the plasma membrane is fluid while the proteins embedded within it form a mosaic, both elements being movable dynamic structures.

Follicle-stimulating hormone – A hormone produced by the anterior pituitary gland whose function is to regulate the functions of the ovaries and testis.

Follicular phase of the ovarian cycle – The period of time during which the ovarian follicle develops and matures. It commences on day 1 of the menstrual period and ends at ovulation, typically day 14.

Foot – The lower extremity of the leg below the ankle that enables a person to stand and walk.

Forearm – The part of a person's upper limb extending from the elbow to the wrist and fingertips.

Fovea centralis – The portion of the retina that contains the highest concentration of cones and hence produces the sharpest vision.

Fragment antibody (Fab) – The precise region of an antibody that binds to an antigen.

Fragment crystallizable (Fc) – The part of an antibody that binds to the cell surface of an immune cell or complement, providing a mechanism for activating the immune responses.

Free radical – Any substance with an unpaired electron.

Fulcrum – A fixed point on which a lever moves when a force is applied.

Fundus of the uterus – The upper part of the uterus, superior to the body of the uterus.

GABA transaminase – An enzyme that catalyses chemical reactions in which nitrogenous groups are transferred.

Gamma-aminobutyric acid (GABA) – A neurotransmitter with inhibitory properties within the central nervous system.

Ganglion – A collection of nerve cell bodies (plural=ganglia).

Gastrocolic reflex – A process within the digestive system whereby the arrival of food in the stomach stimulates the release of the hormone gastrin, which causes the ileocaecal valve to open and allows movement of digested material from the ileum into the caecum and ascending colon.

Gene – A sequence of DNA nucleotides that provides the information for synthesis of a functional RNA molecule or the code for the amino acid sequence of a polypeptide.

Genetic code – The sequence of DNA or RNA codons that determines which nucleotide codes for an amino acid for protein synthesis.

Genome – The complete complement of DNA contained in all somatic cells with a nucleus.

Genotype – A description of the genetic composition of an organism that represents the combination of alleles present.

Glaucoma – A condition of the eye where the intraocular pressure increases to the extent that the retina and optic nerve are compressed, which can lead to blindness.

Glenoid joint – The ball-and-socket joint formed by the head of the humerus fitting into the shallow cavity of the scapula (shoulder blade).

Gliding joint – A joint formed by articular surfaces of the vertebrae.

Glomerular filtration – The first process of urine formation. It occurs between the glomerular capillaries and the Bowman's capsule of the nephron.

Glomerular filtration rate – The rate of glomerular filtration (ultrafiltrate formation) per unit of time.

Glottis – The opening between the vocal cords in the larynx.

Glucagon – The hormone produced by alpha-cells in the islet of Langerhans whose function is to lower blood glucose.

Gluconeogenesis – Synthesis of glucose from non-carbohydrate sources such as amino acids and fatty acids.

Glutathione peroxidase – An enzyme that protects cells from oxidative damage by reducing lipid hydroperoxides and hydrogen peroxides to alcohol and water, respectively.

Glycogenolysis – The breakdown of glycogen by glucagon to increase blood glucose.

Glycoprotein – A protein in which a carbohydrate such as an oligosaccharide is attached to a polypeptide chain.

Glycosuria – The presence of glucose in the urine.

Glycosylation – The addition of a carbohydrate molecule to an organic molecule. If it involves a protein, then it is an example of a type of post-translational modification.

Goblet cells – Specialized mucus-producing cells located in the respiratory epithelium.

Golgi apparatus – A series of flattened disc-like structures found close to the endoplasmic reticulum. It receives fat and proteins from the rough endoplasmic reticulum, modifies these and packages them into vesicles for transport.

Gomphosis – A joint formed by a tooth articulating in a bony socket in the skull.

G-protein – A guanine nucleotide-binding protein that acts as a molecular switch in cells and helps with signal transmission from outside to inside the cell.

Graafian follicle – A fluid-filled structure within the ovary where the oocyte develops prior to ovulation.

Granulocyte – A category of leukocyte observed by microscopy after staining to contain granules.

Granzyme – An enzyme released by cytotoxic T-cells and natural killer cells to induce apoptosis of infected body cells.

Greater trochanter – A large and irregular knob-like projection at the end of the femur.

Grey matter – A component of the central nervous system composed of neurones without myelin sheaths.

Ground substance – A gel-like material surrounding the cells that form a tissue; part of the extracellular matrix, excluding collagen and elastin fibres.

Guanine – A purine nucleotide that forms part of RNA and DNA. It is complementary to cytosine.

Gyrus – A ridge or convolution on the cerebral cortex (plural = gyri).

Haematoma – A collection of blood in a potential space within the body.

Haematopoeisis – Process for the formation of blood cellular components.

Haemocytoblast – A stem cell located in the bone marrow, division of which can lead to the various populations of blood cells.

Haemoglobin – A protein comprising four globin chains each bound to a haem unit. It is found within red blood cells.

Haemolysis – The destruction of red blood cells leading to the release of haemoglobin.

Haemophilia – A hereditary clotting disorder due to the absence of factor VIII.

Haemostasis – The cessation of bleeding through the clotting of blood.

Hamate – A wedge-shaped bone in the human wrist.

Hand – A multi-fingered organ at the end of the forearm.

Haploid – A nucleus containing a single copy of each chromosome.

Haustrum – A small pouch in the colon (plural = haustra).

Haversian canal – A microscopic canal in bone through which blood vessels and nerves run.

Haversian system – The basic unit of the structure of compact bone.

Healthy diet – A varied diet in which food components are available in the right proportions and in adequate amounts.

Helicobacter pylori – A bacterium found colonizing the mucosa of the stomach wall and associated with the development of ulcers.

Helicotrema – The opening at the apex of the cochlea through which the scala vestibuli and scala typani of the cochlea connect.

Helper T-lymphocytes (T$_H$) – A subset of T-lymphocytes with the crucial function of coordinating immune responses through cytokine production.

Hemicellulose – A polysaccharide or complex carbohydrate in plant cell walls.

Hemiplegia – Total or partial paralysis of one side of the body such as the face or limbs.

Heparin – An anticoagulant released by activated basophils and mast cells.

Hepatic – Relating to the liver.

Hepatocyte – A liver cell.

Herd immunity – Immunity that provides a measure of protection against a specific infection for the unvaccinated members of a community by virtue of vaccination of a significant portion of the community by reducing opportunities for a pathogen to spread throughout a population.

Hertz (Hz) – The standard unit of measurement for frequency; 1 Hz equals one cycle/second.

Heterozygous – A genotype containing two different alleles for a particular gene.

Hibernation – An adaptive process in which the body conserves energy by slowing metabolism and lowering body temperature.

Hinge joint – A joint allowing movement in one plane such as bending or straightening.

Hip bones – Large bones that form the main part of the pelvis on each side of the body and consist of the ilium, ischium and pubis.

Histamine – An important pleiotropic chemical mediator involved in inflammatory processes, increasing vascular permeability and vasodilation.

Histology – The microscopic study of cells and tissues.

Histopathology – The microscopic study of cells and tissues and their role in disease.

Homeodynamics – A relatively recent refinement of the concept of homeostasis, which acknowledges the homeostatic changes that occur during the lifetime of an individual and the effects of disease processes on homeostasis.

Homeostasis – The biological process that maintains the stability of the internal environment. It involves stimuli, receptors, a control centre, effectors, a communication system and negative feedback.

Homologous chromosomes – Two or more identical chromosomes present within a nucleus.
Homonymous hemianopia – The loss of vision in one side of the visual field, in both eyes.
Homozygous – A genotype containing identical alleles for a particular gene.
Hormone – A chemical substance secreted in the body that controls and regulates the activity and processes of certain specific cells and organs.
Human chorionic gonadotrophin – A placental hormone that is initially secreted by the syncytiotrophoblast.
Human chorionic somatomammotropin – A polypeptide placental hormone, also known as human placental lactogen, whose role is to modify metabolism in the mother during pregnancy to ensure an adequate energy supply to the fetus.
Human Genome Project – An international collaboration with the aim of determining the entire sequence of DNA nucleotides present within the human genome.
Human immunodeficiency virus – A virus that affects the immune system, causing patients to become immunodeficient and leaving patients at risk of opportunistic infections.
Human microbiome – All of the organisms that reside on or within the body.
Humerus – A long bone in the arm that runs from the shoulder to the elbow.
Humoral immunity – Immunity involving soluble, non-cellular components of immunity in the extracellular fluids.
Hydrogen bond – An intermolecular attraction between positively charged hydrogen ions and nearby negatively charged atoms.
Hyoid bone – A horse-shoe or U-shaped bone in the neck that supports the tongue.
Hyperaemia – An increase in blood flow to a tissue or organ.
Hypernatraemia – Elevated levels of sodium in the blood.
Hyperphosphorylation – A change in membrane potential that makes it more negative.
Hyperplasia – An increase in cell number in a normal tissue or organ.
Hyperthermia – A core body temperature that is above normal.
Hyperthyroidism – Caused by an overactive thyroid gland resulting in excess secretion of thyroxine.
Hypertonic – A solution with a higher osmotic pressure than a solution that it is compared with.
Hypertrophy – An increase in the size or volume of a tissue.
Hypodermis – The innermost and thickest layer of the skin.
Hypothalamus – A pea-like structure below the thalamus that connects the nervous system with the endocrine system via the stalk and pituitary gland.
Hypothermia – A core body temperature that is below normal.
Hypothyroidism – Caused by an underactive thyroid gland resulting in reduced secretion of thyroxine.
Hypotonic – A solution with a lower osmotic pressure than a solution that it is compared with.
Hypoxia – A deficiency of oxygen in the tissues.

Immunoglobulin – See 'Antibody'.
Incus – A small bone in the middle ear that transmits vibrations between the malleus and the stapes.
Independent assortment – The segregation of maternally and paternally derived alleles that are present on replicated chromosomes during meiosis; it is assumed to occur randomly.
Indirect pathways – Complex pathways that form many synapses within the brain.
Infarction – A process arising from obstructed blood flow that results in the death of cells.
Infundibulum – The stalk of the pituitary gland or a funnel-shaped cavity.
Infundibulum of the uterine tube – The distal funnel-shaped part of the uterine tube.
Innate immunity – A division of the immune system of cells producing chemicals and physical defences that provides an immediate and generalized defence against injury and infection.
Innate rhythmicity – The inherent ability of cardiac muscles to contract without stimulation by nerve impulses.
Inner cell mass – A mass of cells in the primordial embryo that will eventually give rise to the fetus.
Inositol triphosphate – A membrane glycoprotein that acts as an intracellular second messenger that releases calcium from calcium stores.
Insoluble fibre – A form of complex carbohydrate that does not absorb water and is not absorbed by the digestive system; it is found in seeds, skins of fruit, wholewheat bread and brown rice.
Inspiratory reserve volume (IRV) – The maximum volume of air that can be inspired after a normal, quiet inspiration.
Insula – A portion of the brain cortex folded deep within the lateral sulcus, separating the frontal and parietal lobes from the temporal lobe.
Insulin – A hormone produced by beta-cells in the islet of Langerhans whose function is to lower blood glucose.
Integral membrane protein – A protein permanently embedded as part of the plasma membrane. Some of these span the entire lipid bilayer (transmembrane protein), while others do not (peripheral membrane protein).
Intercondylar eminence – A structure of the tibia that lies between the articular surfaces of the tibia.
Interesterification – A process that modifies oils and fats by rearrangement of the fatty acids attached to the glycerol molecule.
Interferon – A type of cytokine produced in response to infection, particularly but not exclusively in response to viruses. Interferons are important modulators of immune responses.
Interleukin – A group of cytokines first identified to be produced by leukocytes.
Interlobar bile duct – A duct that receives bile from bile canaliculi, which collect bile from the liver cells.
Intermediate – Occurring in the middle of two things, a process or a series.
Internal capsule – A subcortical structure of white matter containing a large number of sensory and motor fibres that carry information to and from the brain.
Internal environment – The fluid surrounding cells in a multicellular organism; also known as extracellular fluid.
Interphase – The period between cell division.
Interstitial cells – Cells in the testes that produce testosterone and other androgens; also called Leydig cells.

Interstitial fluid – Fluid located in the interstitial space within tissues; fluid in the tissues that fills the space between cells.

Intertrigo – A rash in body skin folds, common in those who are overweight.

Intramembranous ossification – Embryonic development of flat bones such as those of the skull from embryonic connective tissue called mesenchyme.

Intrapleural pressure – Pressure in the pleural cavity.

Intrapulmonary pressure – Pressure of air in the alveoli; also called intra-alveolar pressure.

Intron – Sequences of DNA or RNA transcripts that do not code for an amino acid sequence. Introns are removed from RNA before the process of translation.

Iris – The coloured contractile portion of the eye that can be seen through the cornea.

Ischaemia – An inadequate supply of blood to an organ or part of an organ resulting in an inadequate supply of oxygen for cellular function.

Ischial tuberosity – A large swelling on the frontal part of the ischium.

Islets of Langerhans – Clusters of cells within the pancreas responsible for hormone secretion.

Isotonic – A solution with the same osmotic pressure as a solution that it is compared with.

Isotype – Antibodies are highly diverse but are grouped into one of five major classes known as isotypes. This is dictated by variation in the Fc portion of the antibody.

Isthmus of the uterine tube – The majority of the length of the uterine tube between the ampulla and uterine part.

Juxtaglomerular apparatus – An area of tissue close to the glomerulus that secretes renin in response to low plasma sodium levels, which is the first step in the secretion of aldosterone (renin–angiotensin–aldosterone system (RAAS)).

Karyotype – The chromosomal complement of a diploid cell, typically represented by the arrangement of paired chromosomes to demonstrate the number and structure of the chromosomes.

Keratin – A protein that protects epithelial cells from damage and is the key structural material found in the outer layer of the human skin.

Keratinocyte – The predominant cell type of the epidermis.

Kinocilium – A specialized cilium present within the sensory cells located in the semicircular canals of the inner ear.

Kupffer cell – A star-shaped hepatic macrophage found in the walls of sinusoids whose function is to remove debris and worn-out blood cells from blood as it flows past.

Labyrinthitis – Unilateral inflammation of the labyrinth of the inner ear.

Lactoferrin – An antibacterial protein able to sequester free iron, denying iron availability, which in some organisms is a requirement for bacterial growth.

Lactoperoxidase – A potent antibacterial enzyme that produces free radicals via hydrogen peroxide.

Lacuna – A cavity or gap in bone (plural = lacunae).

Lambdoid suture – A dense fibrous connective tissue joint found on the posterior aspect of the skull, connecting the parietal bones with the occipital bone.

Lamella – A thin plate-like structure from which bone is made from the calcified layers (plural = lamellae).

Langerhans cell – A type of antigen-presenting dendritic cell, found primarily in skin and within mucosal surfaces.

Lanugo – The soft downy hair typically found on the skin of a fetus or neonate.

Large granular lymphocyte – A granulocyte, part of innate immunity, but able to perform non-antigen-specific killing of virus-infected cells.

Larynx – The organ of voice production located between the pharynx and the trachea; a complex cartilaginous structure that surrounds the glottis and vocal cords.

Lateral – Of, at or from the side.

Lateral condyle – The lateral portion of the upper extremity of the tibia, which serves as an insertion point for some leg muscles.

Lateral epicondyle – The enlargement of bone on the lateral part of the femur but superior to the lateral condyle.

Lateral malleolus – The lower or distal extremity of the fibula.

Leg – The part of the leg from the knee to the foot whose two bones are the tibia, the larger weight-bearing bone of the leg, and the fibula.

Lens – The transparent biconvex refractive structure located in the eye between the iris and the vitreous humour.

Lesion – An abnormality in a tissue of an organism as a result of trauma or a disease process.

Lesser trochanter – The smaller posterior projecting protuberance found at the medial base of the femoral neck whose role is a site for muscle attachment.

Leukocyte – A white blood cell, a term that includes a group of cells that provide immunity.

Leukotrienes – A group of potent inflammatory mediators initially discovered in leukocytes with multiple roles in inflammation.

Levator ani – A broad, thin muscle found on either side of the pelvis whose role is to stabilize abdominal and pelvic muscles though its tonic activity.

Leydig cell – A cell type found adjacent to the seminiferous tubules of the testicles whose role is to produce testosterone when stimulated by luteinizing hormone.

Ligament – A fibrous connective tissue that connects one bone to another.

Ligands – A substance that binds to a biological molecule to form a complex; in binding, it usefully triggers an effect.

Lignin – The woody part of plants.

Limbic system – A collection of nuclei and other brain structures located under the cerebrum on either side of the thalamus that deals with emotions.

Lipase – An enzyme that digests fats.

Lipid bilayer – Two layers of lipid molecules. The plasma membrane is an example of a lipid bilayer.

Lipopolysaccharide (LPS) – The main component of Gram-negative bacteria composed of a lipid and carbohydrate molecule; also known as endotoxin.

Lipoxin – A product of the lipoxygenase pathway. Lipoxins represent a group of immunomodulatory eicosanoids with a mainly anti-inflammatory function.

Lipoxygenase – The enzyme that catalyses arachidonic acid to produce leukotrienes.
Load – The quantity that can be carried or transported at any one time.
Loop of Henle – The U-shaped part of the nephron consisting of a descending and ascending portion. It lies between the proximal convoluted tubule and the distal convoluted tubule.
Lower motor neurone – Motor neurones that arise in the ventral horn of the spinal cord and take impulses to skeletal muscles.
Lower respiratory tract – The larynx, trachea, bronchi, bronchioles and alveoli.
Lunate – A carpal bone in the human hand.
Luteal phase of the ovarian cycle – The period of time between ovulation (day 14) and the end of the ovarian cycle (day 28), when the corpus luteum secretes progesterone and some oestrogen.
Luteinizing hormone – A gonadotrophic hormone secreted by the gonadotroph cells of the anterior pituitary gland whose function is to trigger ovulation in females and testosterone production in males.
Lymphadenopathy – Enlarged lymph nodes.
Lymphocyte – A lymphocyte originating from bone marrow that differentiates within lymphoid tissue. There are three main types of lymphocyte – B- and T-lymphocytes and large granular lymphocytes.
Lymphoid tissues – Cells and organs that comprise the lymphatic system.
Lymphoma – Cancer of the lymphoid tissues.
Lysis – The rupture of a cell.
Lysosome – A vesicular organelle containing a variety of hydrolytic enzymes. Its role is to break down biological molecules.
Lysozyme – A bacteriolytic enzyme found in extracellular secretions.

Macrophage – An innate immune leukocyte able to perform phagocytosis.
Major histocompatibility complex (MHC) – A group of cell-surface proteins found on almost all cells of the body, which function to present self and non-self antigens. They are critical to the regulation of T-lymphocyte responses.
Malleolus – A bony projection or protuberance shaped like a hammer on either side of the ankle.
Mammary gland – A gland found within the breast responsible for the production and transportation of milk.
Manubrium – The uppermost portion of the sternum with which the first ribs and the clavicles articulate.
Mass movement – The movement of indigestible matter or faeces en masse in the colon by peristalsis.
Mast cell – A granulocyte important within tissues for acute inflammatory responses such as the release of inflammatory mediators, for example histamine.
Mean arterial blood pressure (MAP) – MAP is calculated using the equation: MAP = diastolic BP + ((systolic BP – diastolic BP)/3).
Medial condyle – The medial portion of the upper extremity of the tibia that serves as an attachment for the semimembranosus muscle.
Medial epicondyle – A bony protrusion located on the medial side of a bone at the distal end, which serves as a point of attachment for tendons.
Medial malleolus – A prominence formed by the lower end of the tibia on the inner side of the ankle.
Mediastinum – The middle of the thoracic cavity containing the heart, trachea, bronchi and great vessels.
Medulla oblongata – The lowest or inferior-most part of the brainstem.
Medullary cavity – The central cavity of bone shafts in which red bone marrow and/or yellow bone marrow are stored.
Meiosis – Cell division involving the production of haploid gametes.
Meissner's corpuscle – An oval receptor found in the dermis of the skin responsible for fine, discriminative touch.
Melanin – The primary pigment that determines skin and hair colour.
Melanocyte – A skin cell responsible for producing melanin.
Melanocyte-stimulating hormone – A hormone secreted by the anterior pituitary gland whose role is to regulate the synthesis of melanin.
Melatonin – A hormone found in animals (and plants) that is involved in the entrainment of circadian rhythms of different physiological mechanisms in animals.
Membrane attack complex – A part of complement-mediated immunity where a group of proteins form a pore in the membrane of a cell to cause lysis and thereby kill a pathogen.
Memory cell – A B- or T-lymphocyte primed by contact with antigen that is able to respond to future encounters with the antigen to provide protective immune responses.
Ménière's disease – A disorder of the inner ear resulting in vertigo, nausea and tinnitus.
Meninges – The three membranes that surround and protect the brain and spinal cord.
Menopause – The time in a woman's life when the menstrual (uterine) cycle and the ovarian cycle cease.
Menstrual phase of the uterine cycle – The period of time during the uterine cycle when menstruation occurs, typically days 1–5.
Merkel cell – A sensory cell present in the skin, responsive to light touch.
Merkel's disc – A cup-like receptor found in the epidermis of the skin responsible for light touch and superficial pressure.
Metacarpal – Any of the five bones of the hand located between the carpals of the wrist and the phalanges of the fingers.
Metaphase – The third phase of mitosis, where condensed replicated chromosomes can be visualized aligned along the centre of the cell.
Metaphysis – The wide portion of a long bone located between the epiphysis and the diaphysis.
Metaplasia – The change from one type of cell or tissue to another.
Metatarsal bone – Any of the five bones of the foot located between the tarsus and the phalanges of the foot.
Micelle – A spherical arrangement of amphiphilic molecules. These form spontaneously when amphiphilic molecules are within an aqueous environment.
Microglia – Glial cells found in the brain that act as macrophages to remove dead brain cells and bacteria.

Microvilli – Densely packed projections within the small intestine that increase the surface area to enable both digestion and absorption (singular = microvillus).

Mitochondrion – An organelle that extracts energy from the products of glucose and, by the process of oxidative phosphorylation, generates ATP, which is coupled to processes allowing 'cell work' (plural = mitochondria).

Mitogen – A substance that stimulates mitosis.

Mitosis – Cell division involving the production of two identical diploid daughter cells.

Mitral (bicuspid) valve – The left atrioventricular valve, which closes the orifice between the left atrium and left ventricle. It prevents the backflow of blood from the ventricle into the atrium during ventricular systole.

Monoamine oxidase – An enzyme found throughout the brain that catalyses the oxidation of some neurotransmitters such as noradrenaline and serotonin.

Monocyte – A circulating leukocyte capable of phagocytosis, which migrates into tissues and is a precursor to macrophages.

Monosaccharide – A simple sugar such as glucose, fructose or galactose that forms the building blocks for carbohydrates.

Mosaicism – A state where cells and tissues of the body possess different genotypes. It usually occurs because of chromosomal abnormalities during embryonic development.

Motor nerve – An efferent nerve that originates in the central nervous system. Motor nerves transmit impulses to muscles producing movement.

Mucosa – A mucous membrane that lines the various cavities or inside surface of some body organs such as those of the gastrointestinal tract.

Mucosa-associated lymphoid tissue (MALT) – A concentration of lymphatic tissue close to mucous membranes.

Muscarinic receptors – Acetylcholine receptors involved in many central nervous system mechanisms such as memory, arousal, attention and smooth muscle contraction, and coupled to G-proteins. There are five subtypes of muscarinic receptors.

Muscle – A tissue rich in contractile proteins that provides the facility for movement. There are three types of muscle – skeletal, cardiac and smooth.

Mutation – Any change to a sequence of DNA nucleotides.

Myeloid – The precursor stem cell line from which the granulocytes develop.

Myeloperoxidase – An enzyme responsible for the production of free radicals, especially within neutrophils.

Myenteric nerve plexus – Motor fibres that provide sympathetic and parasympathetic innervation to longitudinal and circular muscles in the gastrointestinal tract.

Myocardial infarction – An area of dead cardiac muscle cells due to prolonged ischaemia.

Myocardium – The muscle of the heart; also known as cardiac muscle.

Myofibrils – Elongated, slender and contractile threads found in striated muscle cells composed mainly of actin and myosin.

Myometrium – The inner layer of the uterus consisting of smooth muscle.

Myosin – A fibrous protein that forms thick contractile filaments of muscle cells.

Natural killer (NK) cell – See 'Large granular lymphocyte'.

Necrosis – The death of cells or tissue due to injury or disease.

Necrotic tissue – Dead tissue due to the process of necrosis.

Negative feedback – A process associated with homeostasis/homeodynamics, which maintains stability whereby the response to a stimulus negates that stimulus.

Neocortex – The largest and evolutionarily newest portion of the mammalian brain consisting of different subunits that perform different functions. It is not found in birds or reptiles.

Nephron – The microscopic functional unit of the kidney.

Neuroglia – Non-neuronal cells that provide support and protection for neurones in the central and peripheral nervous systems.

Neurohormone – A hormone produced and secreted by specialized neuroendocrine cells such as those in the hypothalamus.

Neurolemmocyte – A cell that surrounds the axons of the peripheral nervous system and forms myelin sheath; also known as a Schwann cell.

Neuromuscular junction – A synapse where an efferent (motor) neurone connects to muscle fibres and acetylcholine is released to stimulate the muscle fibres.

Neurone – A conducting cell that transmits nerve impulses.

Neutrophil – A granulocytic phagocyte, found mostly in the blood; when stimulated, it is able to migrate into tissues.

Nicotinamide adenine dinucleotide phosphate (NADPH) oxidase – A free-radical-producing enzyme especially important in the production of superoxide from activated phagocytes.

Nicotinic acetylcholine receptor – A transmembrane cation-permeable ion channel that is activated by the neurotransmitter acetylcholine and is found throughout the central and peripheral nervous systems.

Nicotinic receptor – An acetylcholine receptor that signals for muscle contraction when stimulated.

Nissl body – A cluster of rough endoplasmic reticulum found in the cell body whose function is to synthesize protein.

Nitrosative stress – An imbalance in nitrogen-based free radicals and antioxidant defences.

Nociceptor – A sensory receptor stimulated by noxious substances and injurious events leading to the perception of pain.

Nocturia – The need to wake up and pass urine at night.

Node of Ranvier – A gap in the myelin sheath that speeds up the transmission of nerve impulses.

Non-specific immunity – See 'Innate immunity'.

Noradrenaline – A neurotransmitter released at the end of sympathetic nerves; also known as norepinephrine.

Normal flora – The microorganisms that reside on or within the body without causing disease.

Nuclear pore – A complex of proteins within the membrane of the nucleus that provides selective transport of substances across the nuclear membrane.

Nucleoid – The region within a prokaryotic cell that contains genetic material. Unlike eukaryotic cells, this is not bounded by a membrane.

Nucleus
- Most commonly, the largest membrane-bound organelle within eukaryotic cells containing most of the genetic material.
- Can also describe a compact cluster of nerve cell bodies (plural = nuclei).

GLOSSARY 491

Nucleus pulposus – The inner core of a vertebral disc composed of a jelly-like material consisting of water and a loose network of collagen fibres.

Nutrient foramen – An opening on all bones for the entrance of blood vessels that carry nutrients to the bone.

Obturator foramen – A large opening created by the ischium and pubic bones of the pelvis through which blood vessels and nerves pass.

Olecranon process – A hook-like prominent bony projection of the ulna at the elbow, which serves as a point of attachment for several muscles.

Olfactory receptors – Receptors involved in the sense of smell, which are sensitive to various chemicals.

Oligodendrocyte – A type of neuroglial cell whose function is to produce the myelin sheaths that insulate axons in the central nervous system.

Oligosaccharide – A carbohydrate polymer containing a small number of simple sugars. Oligosaccharides can be found in animal cell membranes as glycoproteins and glycolipids where they enable cell-to-cell recognition.

Omega end – The methyl end of a fatty acid.

Oncotic pressure – The osmotic pressure achieved by plasma proteins alone.

Oocyte – A female gamete, which develops from an oogonium and is ovulated when mature.

Oogonium – The precursor cell from which oocytes develop (plural = oogonia).

Opsin – A member of a family of photoreceptor proteins that form the visual pigments of rods and cones.

Opsonin – A molecule that serves to enhance the process of phagocytosis or complement activation.

Optic chiasma – The point of crossing of the fibres of the optic nerves.

Organ – A group of tissues organized to undertake a physiological function.

Organ of Corti – The sensory receptor for hearing, which is supported on the basilar membrane; located in the cochlea.

Organelle – A structure within a cell with a defined function. Organelles, with just a few notable exceptions, are surrounded by a lipid membrane.

Orthostatic hypotension – A fall in blood pressure as a result of a change in posture such as standing up quickly; also called postural hypotension.

Osmolality – The number of osmoles in 1 kg of a solution.

Osmolarity – The number of osmoles in 1 L of a solution.

Osmole – A unit of measurement that defines the number of moles of a solute that contribute to the osmotic pressure of a solution.

Osseous – Consisting of bone.

Ossicles – The small bones in the middle ear involved with the conduction of sound.

Osteoblast – A bone-forming cell.

Osteoclast – A bone cell that breaks down bone tissue.

Osteocyte – A mature bone cell formed when osteoblasts have become embedded in the calcified bone matrix.

Osteoid – The unmineralized organic portion of bone matrix secreted by osteoblasts, which forms prior to bone formation. It is a gelatinous substance made up of a fibrous protein called collagen and mucopolysaccharide, an organic 'glue'.

Osteon – The structural unit of compact bone, also known as the Haversian system. These appear as elongated cylinders running parallel to the long axis of the bone and function as tiny weight-bearing pillars.

Osteoporosis – A disease of aging characterized by reduced bone density due to inadequate calcium, resulting in fractures.

Osteoprogenitor cell – A cell that differentiates from stem cells and is responsible for the synthesis of the organic components of bone matrix.

Ovarian follicle – A structures in the ovary consisting of a maturing oocyte surrounded by follicle cells.

Ovary – One of two female sex organs, responsible for the secretion of sex hormones and the development of oocytes.

Ovum – The female gamete (plural = ova).

Oxidative burst – The rapid production of free radicals from cells, typically phagocytes that have an antimicrobial action.

Oxidative stress – An imbalance of free-radical activity over antioxidant defences.

Oxyhaemoglobin – Haemoglobin bound to oxygen.

Oxyphil cell – A cell found in the parathyroid gland scattered among the chief cells whose function is unknown.

Oxytocin – A hormone released by the posterior pituitary gland during labour and after childbirth; it influences milk ejection.

Pacinian corpuscle – An oval receptor found in the deep dermis responsible for deep cutaneous pressure and vibration; also called a lamellar corpuscle.

Palm – The central region of the anterior part of the hand whose skin contains dermal papillae, which increase friction.

Paracrine – A form of cell signalling where secretion of a product from a cell has an effect on nearby cells.

Parathyroid hormone – A hormone secreted by the chief cells of the parathyroid gland whose function is to increase the concentration of calcium in the blood.

Parietal cell – A cell in the gastric glands that secretes hydrochloric acid and intrinsic factor.

Partial pressure – The pressure exerted by an individual gas in a mixture of gases.

Passive immunity – Immunity gained from humoral factors that is gained naturally via breast milk or artificially via injection of antibodies. This is a relatively short-lived gain in immunity when compared with active immunity.

Passive transport – Movement of a substance across the plasma membrane that does not require the use of metabolic energy. This is typically a form of diffusion.

Patella – The kneecap, which is a thick, circular, triangular bone that articulates with the femur and whose function is to protect the knee joint.

Pathogen – A disease-causing organism.

Pathogen-associated molecular pattern (PAMP) molecules – A group of molecules that are a part of pathogens recognized by innate immune cells.

Pathogen-recognition-receptor – A receptor on innate immune cells that is able to recognize PAMPs.

Pelvic girdle – A structure formed by a pair of hip bones that unite anteriorly and with the sacrum posteriorly; attaches the lower limbs to the axial skeleton; also known as the hip girdle.

Penis – Male organ used for urination and sexual function.

Pepsin – An enzyme found in the stomach that begins the digestion of protein and is secreted in an inactive form as pepsinogen.

Pepsinogen – An inactive form of the enzyme pepsin secreted by the chief cells of the gastric pits.

Peptide – Two or more amino acids connected by a peptide bond.

Perception – The interpretation of the world through the processing of sensory (afferent) action potentials from stimulated sensory receptors.

Perforin – A cytotoxic protein inserted into the plasma membrane causing lysis. Produced by cytotoxic T-cells and large granular lymphocytes.

Perfusion – Refers to the flow of blood through the vascular bed.

Pericardium – Double-layered membrane surrounding the heart; the two membranes are the outer parietal (fibrous) layer and the visceral (serous) layer.

Perimetrium – The outer layer of the uterus consisting of a visceral serous membrane (peritoneum).

Perineum – The area between the scrotum and the anus in males and between the vagina and the anus in females.

Periosteum – A dense fibrous membrane covering bones with the exception of joint surfaces.

Peripheral membrane protein – A protein that attaches to the plasma membrane but does not associate with the hydrophobic core or the bilayer; the attachment is sometimes temporary. Those on the outer surface generally have a role in cell signalling, whereas those on the cytosolic surface often have functions involving cytoskeletal interactions.

Peripheral nervous system – The part of the nervous system that consists of nerves and ganglia outside the brain and spinal cord.

Peripheral resistance – A measure of the amount of resistance to blood flow in all blood vessels.

Peristalsis – Wave-like contractions of smooth muscle that move foodstuff in one direction down the gastrointestinal tract.

Peyer's patch – An aggregated lymphoid nodule, found in large numbers in the ileum, the last portion of the small intestine, where they destroy bacteria.

Phagocytosis – The engulfing and destruction of extracellular material such as microorganisms or cell debris.

Phagolysosome – When a particle is phagocytosed, it is internalized into the cytoplasm held within a phagosome. This then fuses with a lysosome to form a polyphagolysosome.

Phagosome – A vesicle enclosing a particle transported into a cell by the process of phagocytosis.

Phalanges – The bones of the fingers and toes.

Pharynx – Upper expanded region of the gastrointestinal tract with the oesophagus below and the oral and nasal cavities above; also known as the throat.

Phenotype – The observable characteristics of an organism.

Phenylalanine hydroxylase – An enzyme responsible for the conversion of the amino acid phenylalanine to tyrosine.

Phosphatidyl inositol bisphosphate – A glycerol phospholipid molecule involved in lipid and cell signalling.

Phosphodiester bond – DNA or RNA nucleotides are linked together by a covalent bond between a 3′ sugar molecule on one nucleotide and a phosphate molecule on the 5′ carbon of another nucleotide. This bonding provides the basis for growing a polynucleotide chain of DNA or RNA.

Phospholipase C – An enzyme that removes or cleaves phospholipids just before the phosphate group and participates in signal transduction pathways.

Photopsin – A photoreceptor protein found in cones in the retina of the eye.

Photoreceptor – A sensory receptor sensitive to light.

Physical defences – The physical structures and responses to prevent infection, part of innate immunity and composed of barriers, chemical, mechanical and normal flora.

Pia mater – The innermost layer of the meningeal membranes that surround the brain and spinal cord.

Piloerection – Erection of hairs on the skin, commonly called goose-bumps.

Pinealocyte – A cell within the pineal gland that secretes the hormone melatonin.

Pisiform – A pea-shaped bone found in the wrist.

Pivot joint – A joint formed between the skull and the first bone of the vertebrae, known as the atlas.

Placenta – The highly vascular organ that develops from the chorion frondosum of the fetus and the decidua basalis of the mother. It enables the fetal circulation to exchange materials with the maternal circulation.

Plasma cell – An antibody-secreting B-lymphocyte.

Plasma membrane – In all living cells, the plasma membrane forms the interface between the intracellular and extracellular environments. It consists mostly of a phospholipid bilayer and proteins, and functions as a selectively permeable barrier.

Plasmid – A small piece of DNA that is not part of a chromosome, typically found within bacteria.

Plasmin – A fibrin-digesting enzyme produced when the proenzyme plasminogen is activated.

Plasminogen – A proenzyme that, once activated, produces the enzyme plasmin.

Platelet – An irregular cell fragment involved with blood clotting; also known as a thrombocyte.

Pleural membrane – The double-layered serous membrane covering each lung.

Plexus – A branching network of nerve fibres (or blood vessels).

Plicae circulares – Deep circular folds of the mucosa and submucosa that cause chyme in the small intestinal lumen to spiral, thus slowing down its movement and allowing more time for nutrient absorption.

Pneumotaxic centre – A group of neurones in the pons that have an inhibitory effect on the inspiratory neurones in the medulla.

Pneumothorax – A collection of air within the pleural cavity resulting in collapse of the lung on the affected side.

Polar molecule – A molecule where the charge due to the arrangement of electrons is unequal, resulting in the formation of an electric dipole, that is, one part of the molecule is more negative or positive than another.

Polydipsia – Excessive thirst often accompanied by excessive fluid intake.

Polymer – A natural or synthetic material that is created by the joining together of many small molecules. DNA and proteins are natural biopolymers, while plastic is a synthetic polymer.

Polysaccharide – A carbohydrate molecule made up of many sugar molecules.

Polysome – A cluster of ribosomes translating an mRNA molecule simultaneously.
Polyuria – The formation and excretion of large volumes of urine, typically 2L or more per day.
Pontine micturition centre – A group of neurones in the pons that maintain continence and coordinate micturition.
Pontine respiratory group – A group of neurones in the pons that have an inhibitory effect on the inspiratory neurones in the medulla; formerly called the pneumotaxic centre.
Portal arteriole – A branch of the hepatic artery that supplies oxygen-rich blood to the liver.
Portal triad – A structure found at each corner of a liver lobule containing a portal arteriole, a portal venule and a bile duct.
Portal venule – A small vein carrying venous blood rich with nutrients from the digestive system.
Postcentral gyrus – A convolution or ridge of the cerebral cortex in the parietal lobe of each hemisphere posterior of the central sulcus that forms the somatosensory area of the brain.
Posterior cavity – The large cavity that lies behind the lens of the eye; also called the vitreous chamber as it contains vitreous humour.
Posterior chamber – A division of the anterior cavity of the eye, which lies between the iris and the lens.
Postganglionic neurone – A neurone from the ganglion to the effector.
Post-prandial – After eating a meal.
Precentral gyrus – A convolution of the cerebral cortex in each hemisphere immediately in front of the central sulcus.
Pre-eclampsia – A condition experienced by pregnant women characterized by high blood pressure, fluid retention and protein in the urine.
Preganglionic neurone – A neurone from the central nervous system to the ganglion.
Prepuce – The fold of skin covering the head of the penis in the male and in the female the clitoris.
Presbycusis – Age-related hearing loss.
Presbyopia – Age-related long-sightedness.
Primary ossification centre – The first area of a bone to start ossifying, which in long bones is found in the diaphysis.
Primary response – The response of the adaptive immune system on the first encounter with an antigen.
Prohormone – A precursor to a hormone with minimal hormonal effects by itself.
Projection fibres – Afferent and efferent fibres that connect the cortex of the brain with lower parts of the brain and with the spinal cord.
Projection neurone – A neurone that extends its axons from the neuronal cell body in one hemisphere to one or more distant areas in the central nervous system.
Prolactin – A hormone that enables milk production by female mammals and has many other functions.
Prolapsed disc – A slipped disc that occurs when a disc between two bones of the vertebra (spine) is damaged and presses on nerves.
Proliferative phase of the uterine cycle – The period of time in the uterine cycle between the end of the menstrual phase and ovulation, typically days 5–14.
Prophase – The first phase of mitosis where replicated chromosomes can be observed to be condensed.

Proprioceptor – A sensor that provides information about muscle length and tension, which is integrated to give information about the position of a limb in space during movement.
Prostacyclin – An eicosanoid of the prostaglandin family.
Prostaglandin – A type of eicosanoid involved in inflammatory responses and pain.
Prostate – The gland at the base of the bladder in males that encircles the urethra.
Protein hormone – A hormone that has varying amino acid chain lengths and has its receptors in the cell membrane.
Proteome – The entire complement of expressed proteins present within an organism.
Prothrombin – A glycoprotein in the blood, which, in the presence of prothrombin activator, is converted to thrombin.
Proximal – Situated nearer to the centre of the body or the point of attachment.
Proximal convoluted tubule – The portion of the nephron that extends from the Bowman's capsule to the proximal straight tubule. It is a site of tubular reabsorption.
Pruritus – The sensation of itching.
Pubis – The bone that forms the anterior portion of the hip bone; also known as the pubic bone.
Pulmonary embolism – A blood clot obstructing one or more branches of the pulmonary artery.
Pulmonary valve – A semilunar valve positioned between the pulmonary artery and the right ventricle.
Pulse pressure – The difference between systolic blood pressure and diastolic blood pressure.
Purkinje fibres – Specialized cardiac muscle fibres that conduct electrical impulses throughout the ventricles.
Pyramidal cell – An excitatory neurone found in the cerebral cortex and other parts of the brain such as the hippocampus and amygdala.
Pyrexia – Fever; a rise in core temperature mediated by pyrogenic cytokines.
Pyridoxal phosphate – One form of vitamin B_6, which is an active coenzyme with a role in protein and urea metabolism.

Radial tuberosity – An eminence beneath the neck of the radius on the medial side with a rough anterior portion for the attachment of tendons of the biceps muscle (biceps brachii).
Radius – One of the two large bones of the forearm that extends from the lateral side of the elbow to the thumb side of the wrist. The other bone is the ulna.
Receptive aphasia – The inability to understand the meaning of a message received; also known as Wernicke's aphasia.
Receptor – A protein, usually on the plasma membrane, that receives a stimulus, often chemical; interaction with the chemical causes a chemical or cellular response. As such, receptors are important in cell signalling.
Recombination – The exchange of DNA molecules, most notably between homologous chromosomes during meiosis, which generates new sequences of DNA; also known as cross-over.
Regulatory-T lymphocyte – An immunosuppressive T-lymphocyte that regulates lymphocyte activity and is important in preventing autoimmune diseases.
Renal cortex – The outer layer of the kidney, which contains the glomeruli, proximal and distal convoluted tubules of the nephron.

Renal medulla – The inner portion of the kidney, which contains the collecting ducts of the nephron and is composed of renal pyramids.

Renal threshold – The concentration of a substance in the plasma above which it appears in the urine.

Renin – An enzyme produced by the juxtaglomerular apparatus of the nephron which catalyses the production of angiotensin I from angiotensinogen.

Renin–angiotensin–aldosterone system – A system of hormones that facilitates the selective reabsorption of sodium in the collecting tubules and ducts of the nephron.

Repolarization – A state in which there is a change in membrane potential, which returns it to a resting potential just after depolarization.

Residual volume – Volume of air remaining in the lung after a maximum expiratory effort.

Respiratory burst – See 'Oxidative burst'.

Resting membrane potential – The state of a neurone when it is not sending any messages and there are more sodium ions (Na$^+$) outside the cell membrane and more potassium ions (K$^-$) inside the cell membrane.

Reticular activating system – A set of interconnected nuclei in the brain whose function is to regulate wakefulness and the sleep–wake cycles.

Reticular formation – Interconnected nuclei in the brainstem together with related fibres whose role is to modulate arousal and consciousness.

Reticular tissue – A loose network of connective tissue composed of a network of fibres, which provides a space for cells within organs such as lymph nodes and bone marrow.

Retina – The neural tunic of the eye; the innermost lining of the vitreous chamber containing photoreceptors.

Retinal – A visual pigment derived from vitamin A.

Rhodopsin – The visual pigment found in the rods of the retina; it is composed of opsin loosely bound to retinal.

Ribcage – The arrangement of bones of the thorax that encloses the heart and lungs formed by the vertebral column, ribs and the sternum.

Ribonucleic acid (RNA) – A nucleic acid, formed from the information held in DNA. It forms single strands and is involved in regulating cell function and in protein synthesis.

Ribosome – A complex of protein and ribosomal RNA found either free in the cytoplasm or within the rough endoplasmic reticulum. Ribosomes are the principal site of protein synthesis.

RNA polymerase – The enzyme that synthesizes RNA from DNA during the process of transcription.

RNA splicing – Modification of a sequence of RNA nucleotides (pre-RNA) where introns are removed and exons joined to form mature messenger RNA.

Rods – Photoreceptor in the retina of the eye responsible for non-colour vision in low-intensity light.

Rough endoplasmic reticulum – An organelle with a mesh-like network of membranes studded with ribosomes involved in protein synthesis.

Rugae – Leaf-like folds found in the walls of the stomach where they help with the mechanical digestion of food.

Saddle joint – A joint formed between one bone with a concave curve and another with a convex curve.

Sagittal – An anatomical plane that divides the body into right and left halves.

Sagittal suture – A dense fibrous connective tissue joint on the superior surface of the skull joining the parietal bones.

Saltatory conduction – The propagation of an action potential from one node of Ranvier to another, which occurs in myelinated neurones.

Sarcolemma – The plasma membrane of the muscle fibre.

Sarcomere – The contractile unit of a myofibril; the skeletal muscle fibre.

Sarcoplasm – The cytoplasm of striated muscle cells (myocytes).

Satellite cells – Neuroglial cells of the peripheral nervous system that anchor neurones and surround cell bodies of sensory, sympathetic and parasympathetic ganglia.

Scaphoid bone – One of the eight small carpal bones of the wrist.

Scapulae – A pair of bones also known as shoulder blades that connect the humerus with the clavicle (collar bone).

Schwann cells – Also known as neurolemmocytes, these are neuroglial cells of the peripheral nervous system that produce myelin sheath and whose extensions wrap around individual neurones.

Sclera – The white, plaque portion of the fibrous tunic of the eye; forms the white area of the anterior surface of the eye.

Scrotum – Loose-skinned pouch in which the testes are located.

Scurvy – A disease caused by vitamin C deficiency.

Secondary ossification centre – A centre of bone formation occurring after the primary ossification centre and beginning in the epiphysis at each end with the invasion of blood vessels.

Secondary response – The second encounter with an antigen following the primary response; it is rapid, involving activation of memory cells primed during the primary response.

Secretory phase of the uterine cycle – The period of time in the uterine cycle between ovulation and the start of menstruation, typically days 14–28.

Segmentation – Backwards and forwards movement of food in a confined area of the gastrointestinal tract.

Selective reabsorption – The process that occurs in the nephron where substances that have been filtered into the Bowman's capsule are returned to the blood stream in amounts that maintain the homeostatic stability of body fluids.

Self antigen – A molecule of the body capable of stimulating an immune response; also known as an autoantigen.

Seminal vesicles – Paired glands lying on the posterior surface of the bladder which contribute approximately 70% to the volume of semen; also called seminal glands.

Seminiferous tubules – Coiled tubular structures in the testes where spermatozoa are produced.

Sensation – The immediate, unprocessed effect of stimulation of sensory receptors.

Sensory processing disorder – A neurological disorder in which there is disruption in the processing and organization of information within the central nervous system.

Sensory receptor – A sensory nerve ending that detects and responds to a stimulus in the internal or external environment of an organism.

Serotonin – A monoamine neurotransmitter also known as hydroxytryptamine (5-HT), which is derived from the amino acid tryptophan and has a role in increasing the sense of well-being.

Serum – The fluid remaining after blood has clotted. It contains no blood cells and unlike plasma does not contain clotting factors.

Sesamoid bone – A bone embedded within a tendon or muscle.

Set point – The optimum value of a variable around which fluctuations occur.

Sex chromosomes – The X and Y chromosomes, the combination of which determines sex; also known as allosomes.

Sharpey's fibres – A matrix of connective tissue, also known as perforating fibres, consisting of bundles of strong fibres of collagen that connect the periosteum to bone.

Single-nucleotide polymorphism – A change in a single DNA nucleotide base pair that occurs in more than 1% of the population.

Sinoatrial node – Mass of specialized cardiac muscle fibres located in the right atrium that generate electrical impulses that determine heart rate.

Sinusoid – A leaky capillary found between the plates of hepatocytes through which blood from the hepatic artery and portal vein passes before emptying into the central vein.

Sister chromatids – Two replicated chromosomes held together with its identical sister chromosome by a centromere.

Skeletal muscle – Striated muscle that enables voluntary movement.

Sliding filament theory of contraction – A mechanism of muscle contraction that explains how the actin (thin) filaments slide past the myosin (thick) filaments during muscle contraction.

Small lymphocyte – A lymphocyte originating from bone marrow that differentiates within lymphoid tissue. There are three main types of lymphocyte: B- and T-lymphocytes and large granular lymphocytes.

Smooth endoplasmic reticulum – An organelle with a mesh-like network of membranes involved in the synthesis of lipid- and steroid-based molecules. It is also involved with metabolic processes such as detoxification and in some cells conversion of glycogen to glucose.

Smooth muscle – Involuntary non-striated muscle.

Sodium–potassium pump – A form of active transport where two substances (sodium and potassium are exchanged across the plasma membrane. This pump is important for the regulation of many cellular functions including cell volume and the generation of nerve impulses.

Somatic hypermutation – A controlled process of mutation that occurs in antibody genes, generating diversity.

Somatostatin – A growth hormone-inhibiting peptide hormone that regulates neurotransmission and cell proliferation.

Somatotropin – A growth hormone that stimulates growth and cell reproduction.

Special senses – Refers to the four traditional senses: taste, smell, hearing and sight.

Specific immunity – See 'Adaptive immunity'.

Sperm – A male gamete; also called spermatozoa.

Spermatogenesis – The process of sperm (male gamete) formation.

Sphincter of Oddi – A muscular valve that surrounds the exit of the bile and pancreatic ducts into the duodenum.

Spine – The bones of the vertebral column stacked one on top of the other and connected by ligaments and muscles.

Spirometry – A method for performing pulmonary function assessment using a spirometer.

Squamous suture – A dense fibrous connective tissue joint found on the lateral aspect of the skull, joining the parietal bone with the temporal bone.

Stapes – A bone of the middle ear; also known as the stirrup.

Starling's law of the heart – The force of contraction of cardiac muscle is a function of the length of the muscle fibres at the end of diastole prior to ventricular systole.

Start codon – The first codon of an mRNA molecule always codes for the amino acid methionine. This marks the site of the initiation of protein synthesis.

Steatorrhoea – Fat-covered diarrhoea-like stools that arc loose, foamy and foul smelling due to malabsorption of fat.

Stellate cells – Neurones with several dendrites radiating from a cell body.

Stereocilium – An elongated microvillus present in the epithelium of the organ of Corti, portions of the ductus deferens and epididymis (plural = stereocilia).

Steroid hormone – A hormone derived from cholesterol with its receptors in the cytoplasm or nucleus of the cell.

Stimulus – A detectable change in the internal or external environment.

Stop codon – A triplet of RNA nucleotides on messenger RNA that signals synthesis of a polypeptide chain to cease.

Strabismus – Misalignment of the eyes inwards or outwards.

Stratified epithelium – Epithelium that contains multiple layers of cells.

Stratum basale – The lowest layer of keratinocyte cells of the epidermis composed of stem cells.

Stratum corneum – The outermost laycr of epidermal cells.

Stratum spinosum – The layer of keratinocytes lying immediately on top of the stratum basale. These cells begin to synthesize keratin.

Stroke – A condition arising from damage to brain cells due to either an obstruction of blood flow to the brain (thromboembolic) or haemorrhage.

Stroke volume – Volume of blood ejected from either ventricle in a single heartbeat; it is approximately 70 ml.

Stylohyoid ligament – A ligament that originates in the styloid process of the temporal bone and inserts into the lesser horn of the hyoid bone.

Styloid process – A pointed protrusion of the temporal bone of the skull. A styloid process can also be found on the radius and ulnar bones.

Subarachnoid space – A potential space between the arachnoid mater and the pia mater.

Subdural space – A potential space between the dura mater and the arachnoid mater.

Submucosa – A thin layer of dense or loose connective tissue that lies above and supports the mucosa.

Sulcus – A depression or furrow on the cerebral cortex (plural = sulci).

Surface tension – The behaviour of water molecules at the surface of a water droplet and how they cling to each other and resist being separated.

Surfactant – Lipoprotein secreted from type II pneumocytes (surfactant-secreting cells) in alveoli. In the gastrointestinal tract, bile salts act as a surfactant stabilizing the interface between fat and water molecules.

Suspensory ligaments – Small ligaments attached to the margin of the lens in the eye and ciliary body that hold the lens in place.
Sustentacular cells – Supporting cells in the seminiferous tubules of the testes; also called Sertoli cells.
Suture – An immovable fibrous joint connecting the bones of the skull.
Symphysis – A fibrocartilaginous fusion between two bones that is permanent but slightly movable.
Synapsis – The pairing of two homologous chromosomes during meiosis.
Synarthrosis – A type of joint that permits very little or no movement between the bones, such as the sutures of the skull.
Synchondrosis – A cartilaginous joint between the bones of the skull.
Syncytiotrophoblast – A cell that forms the outer layer of the trophoblast and invades the uterine wall. These cells secrete several hormones including human chorionic gonadotrophin and progesterone.
Syndesmosis – A slightly movable joint where an interosseous ligament joins the bones.
Systemic circulation – The blood vessels between the aortic valve and the entrance to the right atrium.
Systole – Contraction of the myocardium leading to expulsion of blood from the heart chambers.

Tachycardic – This refers to a person having a faster-than-normal heart rate at rest; in an adult, this refers to a heart rate of over 100 beats/minute at rest.
Tachypnoeic – This refers to a person having a faster-than-normal respiratory rate at rest.
T-cell receptor – A receptor on the surface of T-cells responsible for binding to antigen presented with major histocompatibility complex proteins.
Tectorial membrane – The membrane that covers the hair cells (stereocilia) of the organ of Corti.
Telophase – The fifth phase of cell division where a new nuclear membrane begins to form around replicated DNA that has separated to opposite poles of the cell.
Template strand – The strand of DNA that provides the sequence of nucleotides that determines the sequence of RNA nucleotides to be synthesized during transcription; it is sometimes called the antisense strand.
Teratogenic – The ability of drugs or other agents to disturb the growth and development of an embryo or fetus, resulting in congenital malformations.
Testosterone – The main androgen (male sex hormone) produced by cells in the testes.
Tetraiodothyronine – The hormone thyroxine (T4), secreted by the thyroid gland, whose function is to regulate metabolism.
Thalamus – A symmetrical structure in the brain located between the cerebral cortex and the midbrain consisting of nerve fibres that project to the cerebral cortex in all directions. It acts as a sensory and motor 'switchboard' to the cortex.
Thigh – The part of the human leg between the hip and the knee.
Thoracic cage – A bony and cartilaginous structure that surrounds the thoracic cavity; also known as the ribcage.
Thrombin – The enzyme that converts fibrinogen to fibrin.

Thrombocyte – See 'Platelet'.
Thromboxane – A type of eicosanoid that functions to cause vasoconstriction and platelet aggregation.
Thrombus – A solid or semi-solid mass formed from the constituents of blood in the vascular system; also called a blood clot (plural = thrombi).
Thymine – A pyrimidine nucleotide that forms part of DNA but not RNA.
Thymosin – A hormone produced in the thymus gland whose function is to stimulate the development of T-cells.
Thyroid-stimulating hormone – A hormone whose function is to stimulate the thyroid gland to produce its hormones; also known as thyrotropin.
Thyrotropin – See 'Thyroid-stimulating hormone'.
Tibia – One of the two bones of the leg or lower limb between the knee and the foot, and parallel to the fibula.
Tidal volume – The volume of air that is inspired or expired in a single, quiet, restful breath.
Tinnitus – A ringing in the ear; the perception of sound when there is no corresponding external sound.
Tissue – A collection of similar cells organized to provide a specific function. Multiple tissues are organized to form organs.
Tissue factor – A lipoprotein released from damaged tissue and activated platelets; also called factor III.
T-lymphocyte – A type of small lymphocyte originating from the myeloid stem cell line. See also 'Helper T-lymphocyte' and 'Cytotoxic T-lymphocyte'.
Toll-like receptor – A small group of cell-surface receptors, part of innate immunity, that detect a broad range of pathogens.
Trabecula – A plate or column of connective tissue that provides structural support to spongy bone found at the end of long bones (plural = trabeculae).
Trachea – The conducting airway extending from the larynx to the point where it divides into two bronchi.
Transcellular fluid – A component of extracellular fluid that is found within epithelial lined spaces, for example synovial fluid.
Transcription – The process by which the DNA sequence in a strand of DNA is copied into a new molecule of messenger RNA.
Transduction – The process by which cells are able to change a signal or stimulus from one form to another.
Trans **fatty acid** – A fatty acid whereby the stereochemical arrangement of the hydrogen atoms at a carbon–carbon double bond is such that the hydrogen atoms are on the opposite side of the double bond.
Translation – The process by which a protein is synthesized from the code contained in a molecule of messenger RNA.
Trapezium – An irregularly shaped carpal bone of the wrist.
Trapezoid – A small carpal bone between the trapezium and the capitate in the wrist.
Tricuspid valve – The right atrioventricular valve, which closes the orifice between the right atrium and right ventricle. It prevents the backflow of blood from the ventricle into the atrium during ventricular systole.
Triiodothyronine – A thyroid hormone whose function is to influence metabolism, growth, development and many other physiological processes; also known as T3.

Triquetral – A triangular bone that articulates with hamate, lunate and another small bone called the pisiform; also known as triquetrum.
Trisomy – An extra chromosome instead of the normal complement of two chromosomes in a diploid cell. This is a type of aneuploidy.
Trochlear – A notch that enables the elbow joint to be formed with the humerus.
Trophic hormone – A hormone that has a growth effect on tissue and causes hypertrophy or hyperplasia.
Trophoblast – The first cell type to develop from the zygote that form the outer layer of a developing embryo and provide nutrients to the embryo. Later on, these cells develop into the placenta.
Tropic hormone – A hormone that targets other endocrine glands.
Tropomyosin – A muscle protein that inhibits contraction of muscle by blocking myosin-binding sites on actin filaments, thus stopping the interaction between actin and myosin filaments.
Troponin – A globular protein in actin (thin filaments) with three subunits involved in muscle contraction.
Troponin–tropomyosin complex – A complex in which tropomyosin physically blocks the myosin-binding site on actin in the absence of calcium ions, thereby regulating skeletal muscle contraction.
Trypsin – An enzyme produced by pancreatic acinar cells that is involved in the digestion of protein in the duodenum.
Tubular reabsorption – A process whereby solutes and water that have been filtered out of the glomerular capillaries into the tubules of the nephron are transported back into the blood.
Tubular secretion – A process whereby solutes and water are transported from the peritubular capillaries of the nephron into the tubule of the nephron.
Tumour – A swelling, lump or growth of tissue.
Type 1 pneumocyte – An epithelial cell that forms the wall of the alveoli.
Type 2 pneumocyte – A type of epithelial cell found in alveoli; also called surfactant-secreting cells.

Ulna – One of the two bones of the forearm (the other being the radius), on the side opposite the thumb.
Ultrafiltrate – A solution that has passed through a semipermeable membrane, which only allows low-molecular-weight solutes through.
Upper motor neurone – A neurone with a direct pathway from the cerebral cortex to the ventral horn of the spinal cord.
Upper respiratory tract – The nasal cavity, pharynx and associated structures.
Uracil – A pyrimidine nucleotide found in RNA but not in DNA.
Urea – A nitrogenous waste molecule produced primarily in the liver from ammonia and amino acid metabolism.
Ureter – One of two fibromuscular tubes that drain urine from each kidney to the bladder.
Urinary bladder – The muscular distensible reservoir that stores urine.
Uterine cycle – The cycle of events within the uterus that occurs approximately every 28 days. It is characterized by changes to the endometrial lining of the uterus in response to changing hormone levels.
Uterine part of the uterine tube – The part of the uterine tube that provides the entrance to the uterus, between the isthmus and the uterus.
Uterine tube – The slender long tube that extends laterally from both sides of the uterus towards the ovaries.
Uterus – The hollow muscular organ that contains and nourishes the embryo and developing fetus.

Vaccination – The administration of antigens for the purpose of inducing an immune response to develop active immunity against a future exposure to the antigen.
Vagina – The tube-like structure that runs from the vaginal orifice to the cervix of the uterus.
Valsalva manoeuvre – An attempt to cause exhalation forcefully against a closed airway.
Vasa recta – Peritubular capillaries that surround the loop of Henle, which facilitate the production of concentrated urine via a countercurrent mechanism.
Ventral horn – The anterior column of the front part of the grey matter of the spinal cord where motor neurones exit the spinal cord into the periphery to innervate muscles and organs.
Ventral rami – Anterior branches of spinal nerves containing sensory and motor fibres to muscles and skin of the anterior surface of the head, neck, trunk and limbs.
Ventral respiratory group – A group of neurones found in the anterior region of the medulla activated during forced breathing.
Ventral root – The motor root of a spinal nerve that conveys information from the spinal cord to the peripheral areas; also known as the anterior division.
Vertigo – The sensation that you or the environment around you are moving or spinning.
Vesicular (Graafian) follicle – A mature follicle from which the oocyte is ovulated.
Vesicular transport – Transport across the plasma membrane involving the enclosure of a substance within a vesicle (membrane bound). It is called endocytosis or exocytosis, depending on the direction of transport.
Villus – A finger-like projection in the small intestine that facilitates the absorption of the end products of digestion (plural = villi).
Vital capacity – The greatest volume of air that can be exhaled from the lungs after a maximum inspiration.
Vitreous humour – The transparent jelly-like material found in the posterior cavity between the lens and the retina.
Vulva – The external genitalia of a female.

Wernicke's area – An area located in the temporal lobe on the left side of the brain whose function is to help with comprehension of speech.
White matter – A component of the central nervous system composed of neurones with myelin sheaths.

X-linked – Alleles present on the X chromosome, which can therefore be observed to follow a pattern of inheritance described as a sex-linked phenotype.

Zona fasciculata – The middle zone of the adrenal cortex whose function is to produce glucocorticoids, especially cortisol.

Zona glomerulosa – The outermost layer of the adrenal cortex whose function is to produce the mineralocorticoid hormone aldosterone in response to renin or decreased blood flow to the kidneys.

Zona reticularis – The innermost layer of the adrenal cortex whose function is to produce androgens.

Zygote – The cell that results from the fusion of gametes.

Index

b after a page number means the entry appear in a box, f in a figure, g in the glossary, t in a table

1,25-dihydroxycholecalciferol, 155, 211, 479g
1,25-dihydroxyvitamin D3, 155, 211, 393
20/20 vision, 174
5-hydroxytryptamine, 111
7-dehydrocholesterol, 211, 393

α-Tocopherol, 212
β-carotene, 211

Abdomen, 291
Abdominal
  aorta, 247f
  cavity, 24, 228
Abdominopelvic, 24f, 25f, 228, 449
ABO blood group system, 297, 307
Accommodation, 172, 174, 174f, 479g
Acetabulum, 424, 483, 479g
Acetylcholine, 108, 109t, 125–8, 290, 438f, 439, 479g
Acetylcholinesterase, 108, 439
Acid–base balance, 251, 255, 269, 312
Acinar cells, 224, 225
Acromioclavicular joint, 421, 479g
Acromion, 421, 479g
Acrosome, 453, 454, 479g
Actin, 433–5, 435f, 438f, 439
Actinic purpura, 380, 400, 479g
Action potential, 105, 106–9, 106f, 109f, 479g
  muscle contraction, 438f
  sensory receptors, 169, 176, 183, 185
Acute stress response, 153, 479g
Acute-phase proteins, 352, 358, 371, 479g
A-delta (δ) fibres, 187
Adenine, 63, 67f, 70b, 479g
Adenohypophysis, 148
Adenosine triphosphate (ATP), 41, 141, 196, 231, 479g
Adenylate cyclase, 141
Adipocytes, 50, 479g
Adipose tissue, 18, 50, 145t, 156, 160, 233, 470f, 479g
Adrenal
  cortex, 140, 144t, 148, 154, 259, 288
  medulla, 144, 153

Adrenaline (epinephrine), 14f, 37f, 108, 109t, 128, 142f, 153, 479g
Adrenergic receptors, 128
Afferent, 23t, 479g
  arteriole, 249f, 250f, 259
  (sensory) neurones, 10f, 16, 103, 104, 104f, 169
Agglutinins, 297, 479g
Agglutinogens, 297, 479g
Agonist, 36, 37b, 479g
Agranulocytes, 295, 296
Albumin, 293
Alcohol, 132, 448, 468
Aldosterone, 144t, 153–5, 153f, 254, 259, 260, 288f
Alkaline phosphatase, 407
All-or-nothing principle, 105, 106, 479g
Alleles, 75, 80, 82, 83, 85, 86, 366, 479g
Allergy, 351, 479g
Alopecia, 389, 391
Alveolar ventilation, 328
Alveoli, 479g
  breast, 470f
  lungs, 313, 314, 317, 317f, 318f, 321, 324
Amblyopia, 178, 479g
Amenorrhoea, 472
Amino acids, 68–70, 69b, 71f, 156, 199–202, 200f, 231f, 243t, 479g
Aminoacyl-tRNA, 68, 70
Aminopeptidase, 226, 479g
Ammonia, 224, 255, 379, 497
Amniocentesis, 456b
Amnion, 465, 466f, 479g
Amphiarthroses, 427, 429, 479g
Amphiphilic, 35, 221, 479g
Ampulla, 184, 456f, 459, 460, 470f, 471, 479g
Amygdala, 114, 114f
Amylase, 219, 224, 227t, 479g
Anabolism, 231
Anaemia, 213, 236, 263, 294, 299, 338f, 371, 479g
Anaerobic process(es), 232f, 233, 272, 480g
Anaphase, 77f, 78, 78f, 79f, 480g
Anaphylaxis, 358, 480g
Anatomic position, 22f, 26

Anatomical dead space, 321, 480g
Androgen-binding protein, 454
Androgens, 140, 154, 159, 450, 480g
Aneuploidy, 83, 480g
Angiotensin I, 154, 259, 286, 288f, 480g
Angiotensin II, 144t, 154, 259, 263, 286, 288f, 480g
Angiotensin-converting enzyme, 259, 263, 286, 288f, 306, 480g
Angiotensinogen, 154, 259, 286, 288f
Anions, 242, 480g
Annulus fibrosus, 415, 480g
Anorexia nervosa, 157, 160, 238, 387, 447, 472, 473
Antagonist, 36, 37b, 480g
Anterior, 22f, 23t
  cavity, 170, 170f, 171f, 480g
  chamber, 171f, 480g
Antibiotic, 5, 65b, 339, 345, 373, 480g
Antibody, 48b, 355f, 359, 360, 361f, 362–4, 364t, 472, 480g
  monoclonal, 3, 21, 91, 93, 338, 371
Anticodon, 68, 70, 480g
Anti-D antibodies, 299, 300, 306
Antigen, 297–9, 359–70, 383, 480g
Antigen-presenting cell (APC), 360, 365f, 383, 480g
Antioxidant, 208, 212b, 213, 356, 369, 388, 390
Antisense strand, 67, 480g
Antithrombin III, 302, 480g
Anus, 216, 228, 229, 248, 455f, 456
Aorta, 247f, 270, 275, 275f, 277, 278, 286
Aortic valve, 278, 480g
Apex – heart, 275, 282
Apocrine, 381, 384, 386, 480g
Apoptosis, 77, 88, 354, 359, 365, 392, 462, 480g
Appendicular
  region, 24
  skeleton, 404, 421, 428, 480g
Appendix, 23, 25, 228
Aqueous humour, 170, 171, 174, 480, 481, 480g
Arachidonic acid, 140, 351, 480g

Arachnoid
  mater, 119, 120, 120f, 480g
  space, 120f
  villus, 120, 120f, 480g
Archaea, 31
Areola, 149, 470f, 471
Areolar, 50, 480
Arrector pili, 14f, 18, 26, 385
Arterial baroreceptors, 286, 287f
Arterial blood gases, 313b
Artery, 270f
Arterioles, 14f, 15f, 18, 127f, 249f, 270, 271, 286–9
  efferent, 249f, 250f, 251, 254f, 259
Ascending colon, 215f, 228, 228f, 235
Assay design, 161
Asthma, 29, 53, 311, 330, 331
Astrocytes, 102, 103, 480g
Atherosclerosis, 207, 273, 273b, 302
Atmospheric pressure, 4, 319, 320, 323, 324
ATPase, 32, 36, 41, 42, 435
Atria, 274, 275f, 279, 282
Atrial natriuretic peptide, 145, 155, 260, 480g
Atrioventricular
  bundle, 281, 281f, 282, 480g
  node, 281, 281f, 480g
  valves, 275, 278, 279, 480g
Audiogram, 189f
Auditory cortex, 112f
Autocrine, 138, 351, 353, 357, 480g
Autoimmune, 339, 354, 366, 370, 441
Autonomic nervous system, 10, 26, 102f, 105, 125–7, 126f, 127f, 289
Autosomal recessive, 60, 82, 84, 85, 93, 333, 442
Autosomes, 74, 76, 480g
Avogadro constant, 244
Axial
  region, 24, 25
  skeleton, 404, 421, 480g
Axon hillock, 106, 480g
Axons, 102–4, 104f, 105–7, 111, 440b, 480g

Bachmann's bundle, 281
Bacilli, 32
Bacteria, 4, 5, 31, 338, 352
  Gram-negative, 346
  Gram-positive, 31f, 352
Balance, 115, 119, 180, 184, 185, 186b
Ball-and-socket joint, 429, 480g
Baroreceptors, 169, 286, 287f, 307
Basal ganglia, 109t, 110f, 442
Base pairing, 63
Basilar membrane, 182, 183, 480g
Basophils, 295f, 302, 349, 350, 364, 480g
Bernard, Claude, 6
Beta-adrenergic agonists, 160
Bicarbonate, 160, 243t, 251, 252f, 255, 312, 327f
Bicuspid valve, 275

Bile, 141, 145, 160, 219, 220–4
  acids, 206, 214, 220, 223, 229, 345
Bilirubin, 220, 256, 257b
Biliverdin, 220
Binary fission, 33
Biochemistry, 30, 96
Biofilm, 32
Biological fitness, 3
Biopsy, 30, 52, 54, 59, 267, 473
Biotin, 213
Bladder
  gall, 127f, 215f, 220–4, 221f
  urinary, 127f, 128, 129, 246, 247f, 424, 425, 456, 497g
Blastocyst, 158
Blood, 293–6, 293f, 294f, 295f
  clotting, 300–2, 301f, 302b, 352, 357
  groups, 297–8, 298f
  pressure, 117, 272, 284, 284t, 288, 289f, 292
  typing, 298b
  venous blood, 7, 120, 290, 291, 305
  vessels, 269, 270f, 275, 285, 289, 301, 358, 396
  volume, 153–5, 270, 280, 286, 288f, 293
Blood-CSF barrier, 119, 481g
B-lymphocytes, 360, 365, 481g
BMI, 1, 2, 3, 194, 195, 234, 447, 472, 473
Body
  cavities, 24
  mass index, see BMI
  planes, 22f, 23t
  regions, 24, 25f
  temperature, 12–19, 13b, 14f, 15f, 16b, 114, 358
Bolus, 217, 314
Bone, 51, 243, 393, 404–12, 408f, 410f, 411f
  cancellous, 407, 408f, 409, 411
  compact (dense), 406, 408f, 410, 411, 411f, 482g
  coxal, 406, 424, 483g
  ethmoid, 412, 413
  flat, 406, 407, 408, 409, 421
  hip, 24, 407, 424, 486g
  long, 51, 163, 406, 407, 421, 429
  marrow, 144, 294, 295f, 296, 342, 349, 360, 406, 410f
  metatarsal, 427, 428f, 489g
  occipital, 412
  scaphoid, 423, 424f, 494g
  sesamoid, 406f, 407t, 426, 495g
  sphenoid, 412
  spongey, see cancellous
  tarsal, 427
  see also individual bones
Bowman's capsule, 248, 249f, 250f, 251, 255, 481g
Boyle's law, 318, 319, 320
Bradykinin, 187
Brain, 51, 101, 102f, 104, 110f, 111–22
Brainstem, 111f, 114, 115–18, 128, 178, 185, 286, 318, 481g

BRCA1, 90, 91
BRCA2, 90
Breast, 90, 91, 144t, 149, 469, 470f
  cancer, 90, 91, 93, 211, 448, 469b
  milk, 369, 471f, 472
Bricks and mortar model – epidermis, 383
Broad ligament, 456f
Broca's area, 112f, 113, 130, 481g
Bronchi, 313, 314f, 316, 317, 321
Bronchial tree, 316, 317, 320, 481
Bronchioles, 29b, 313, 314f, 317, 317f, 330
Bronchoconstriction, 317, 351, 352
Bronchodilation, 317
Bronchus, 315, 481g
Brown fat, 18
Brush border enzyme, 225
B-type natriuretic peptide, 155, 260, 481g
Buffer, 160, 243, 255, 327
Bulbospongiosus muscle, 451
Bundle branches, 281f, 282
Bundle of His, 281, 281f, 481g

C3 convertase, 352, 253f
Caecum, 228, 228f
Calcaneus, 427, 481g
Calcitonin, 144t, 151, 406
Calcitriol, 151, 155, 211, 481g
Calcium, 7t, 108, 141, 151, 155, 207–8, 243t
  blood clotting, 300
  bone, 51, 211, 393, 406, 410
  muscle contraction, 434–5
  synapse, 438–9
Calmodulin, 141
Calyces, 246
Canal of Schlemm, 171, 171f, 481g
Canaliculi, 222, 223, 410, 412, 481g
Cancer, 45f, 47, 48b, 74, 87–93, 214, 351, 392, 452b, 458b, 459b
  hallmarks of, 87, 88, 93
Capillaries, 101, 225, 248, 269, 270f, 271, 272
Capillary fluid dynamics, 291–2, 292f, 306
Capitate, 423, 424f
Capitulum, 422, 481g
Carbaminohaemoglobin, 326, 327, 481g
Carbohydrates, 197, 199, 219, 220, 226, 227t
Carbon dioxide, 5f, 7t, 39, 44, 120, 233, 312, 317, 324–9, 467
Carbonic acid, 312, 326, 327
Carbonic anhydrase, 209, 312, 327
Carboxylic acid, 201, 203
Carboxypeptidase, 225, 226, 481g
Carcinogenesis, 87, 458b
Cardiac
  conducting system, 280, 281f
  cycle, 280, 282, 283f, 307, 481g
  muscle, 51, 128, 275, 276, 277f, 432, 433f, 481g
  output, 280, 285, 286, 287f, 291, 481g
Carotid bodies, 328

Cartilage, 50-1, 313, 314-17, 404, 407, 409f, 428, 429, 481g
  lacunae, 51, 481g
Catabolism, 44, 231
Cataracts, 168, 172, 173b, 173f, 188, 481g
Catecholamines, 108, 153, 154, 209
Cathelicidins, 344
Cathepsin, 355, 356, 481g
Cations, 242, 481g
CD4+ cells, 340f, 374
CD8, 366
Cell, 5f, 29-36, 44-7, 72, 76-80, 78f, *see also individual cell types*
  division, 76-9
  wall, 32, 33, 214, 324, 344, 347, 352, 354
Cellulose, 214, 481g
Central canal, 410, 481g
Central cyanosis, 331, 481g
Centriole, 34f, 45, 481g
Centromere, 78, 79, 481g
Cerebellum, 111f, 115, 116f, 185, 481g
Cerebral cortex, 111, 112-14, 113f, 116f, 169
Cerebrospinal fluid, 8, 102, 119, 120, 120f, 182, 481g
Cerebrum, 111, 114, 115, 118, 119, 179, 183, 319, 481g
Ceruloplasmin, 208, 209
Cerumen, 180, 343f, 385, 481g
Cervical
  canal, 457, 458f
  cancer, 66, 449, 458b, 459b, 476
  plug, 465
  screening, 458b
Cervix, 145, 150, 158, 449, 456f, 457, 458fb, 468f, 481g
Chain of infection, 346b
Checkpoints, 77, 481g
Chemical mediators, 272, 296, 350, 351, 357, 358
Chemokines, 354, 370, 481g
Chemoreceptors, 178, 229, 328, 328f, 329f, 481g
  central, 328, 328f
  peripheral, 16, 328, 328f
Chemosensitive area, 328
Chief cells, 151, 152, 219, 220, 482g
Chloride, 7t, 243t
  shift, 243, 327, 482g
Chloroplasts, 34
Cholecalciferol, 155, 211, 211t
Cholecystokinin, 145t, 157, 159, 160, 223, 225
Cholesterol, 35, 35f, 206-7, 224t, 306
Cholinergic system, 128, 133
Chondroblasts, 50, 482g
Chondrocytes, 407
Chordae tendineae, 279f, 482g
Chorion, 465b, 466f, 482g
  frondosum, 466f, 482g
Chorionic villi, 465, 466, 482g
Chorionic villus sampling, 465b

Choroid, 120, 170f, 171, 482g
Chromaffin, 153, 482g
Chromatin, 63, 67, 73, 78, 482g
Chromosomes, 44, 45, 61, 62f, 62t, 63, 74-9, 76f, 83, 482g
  homologous, 75, 79, 487g
Chronic kidney disease, 262b
Churning, 196, 217, 218
Chyle, 220, 482g
Chylomicrons, 227, 482, 482g
Chyme, 160, 218, 219, 220, 221, 221f, 223, 482g
Cilia, 45, 46f, 49, 102, 179, 315, 459, 482g
Ciliary
  body, 170f, 171f, 482g
  muscle, 171f, 174
  processes, 171f, 482g
  trabeculae, 171
Ciliated columnar epithelial cells, 49, 315, 459, 482g
Circadian rhythms, 146, 146b, 482g
Circulatory system, 269, 271f, 289f
Cis fatty acids, 205, 205f, 482g
Citric acid, 233, 482g
Clavicles, 420, 421, 482g
Clostridium difficile, 338, 372
Coagulation, 300-2, 301f
Cobalamin, 213, 294
Cocci, 32
Coccyx, 414, 415, 424
Cochlea, 123, 169, 181f, 182, 182f
Cochlear duct, 182, 183
Coding strand, 67, 482g
Codominance, 85
Codon, 68, 69, 70, 81, 85, 482g
Coenzyme, 213, 233, 482g
Cofactor, 202, 208, 209, 210, 213, 482g
Collagen, 50, 270, 300, 383, 396f, 406, 482g
Collagenase, 210, 482g
Collecting duct, 149, 154, 246, 249f, 254, 257, 482g
Colon, 215f, 216, 228-30, 228f
  cancer, 88-9
Colostrum, 364, 369, 472, 482g
Colposcopy, 475
Colour blindness, 176b
Columnar epithelia, 49
Comedones, 389
Commensal organisms, 456
Complement, 340f, 352, 353-4, 353f, 355f, 358, 361, 364t, 482g
Computed tomography, 24
Conduction, 14f, 17t, 107
Condyles, 422, 426, 482g
Condyloid joints, 429, 482g
Cones, 172, 175, 176, 190, 482g
Conjunctiva, 170, 482g
Connective tissue, 50, 383, 396f, 396-7, 410, 429t, 482g
Contractility, 129, 432, 482g
Control centre, 10f, 11, 12, 14f, 15f, 16, 17, 100, 103, 258f, 468f, 471f, 482g

Convection, 14f, 15f, 17t
Convoluted tubule
  distal, 149, 155, 249f, 254f, 258f, 484g
  proximal, 249f, 250f, 251, 252f, 493g
Copper, 208, 209
Core temperature, 7t, 13, 15, 16b, 17, 20, 358
Co-receptor, 366
Cornea, 170f, 171f, 174, 482g
Corneocytes, 343, 383, 482g
Coronal plane, 22f, 23t, 412, 413
Coronary
  heart disease, 273b
  sinus, 277, 482g
  veins, 277
Coronoid fossa, 422, 423, 482g
Corpora cavernosa, 450
Corpus albicans, 460b, 462, 463f
Corpus callosum, 110f, 111, 114f, 115, 118, 120f, 482g
Corpus luteum, 145, 158, 460f, 462, 463f, 464, 465, 483g
Corpus spongiosum, 450
Corticobulbar tract, 119
Corticospinal tracts, 118
Corticosterone, 154
Cortisol, 129, 144t, 154, 160, 163, 206, 468
Countercurrent mechanisms, 253, 254f, 483g
Cranial, 23, 122
  cavity, 24f
Craniosacral, 128
Cranium, 406, 412
C-reactive protein, 352, 371
Creatinine, 241, 242, 255, 256, 262, 263, 483g
Cremaster muscles, 449
Crenated, 245
Cribriform plate, 179, 483g
Cristae, 45, 233, 483g
Crista ampullaris, 185f, 483g
Crohn's disease, 3, 20, 21, 235, 236, 338, 370, 371, 372
Crystallins, 172, 483g
Cytotoxic T-lymphocytes (CTLs), 364, 365, 366, 483g
Cuboidal epithelia, 49
Cuneiform, 427, 483g
Cupula, 185, 483g
Cyclic adenosine monophosphate (cAMP), 141, 231, 483g
Cyclic guanosine monophosphate (cGMP), 141, 483g
Cyclooxygenase, 351, 352, 483g
Cystic duct, 222, 223
Cystic fibrosis, 84, 94
Cystitis, 247, 483g
Cytochrome oxidase, 208
Cytochrome P450 epoxygenase, 351, 485, 483g
Cytokine, 295f, 340f, 347, 350, 353-354, 357f, 359, 365, 368, 371, 385, 483g

Cytokinesis, 78, 483g
Cytoplasm, 33, 35f, 45, 71f, 483g
Cytosine, 63, 67, 74, 483g
Cytoskeleton, 32, 34f, 35, 36, 45, 483g
Cytosol, 32, 34f, 34, 483g
Cytotrophoblast, 158, 483g

Dalton's law, 323, 324, 483g
Damage-associated molecular patterns, 357, 483g
Decibels, 179, 189, 483g
Decidua basalis, 466f, 467, 483g
Decidua capsularis, 467
Decussation, 118, 130, 441, 483g
Deep sockets, 424, 428, 483g
Defecation, 229, 230, 230f, 231
Defences
   chemical, 338, 343
   mechanical, 343
   physical, 337, 342, 343, 346, 352, 357, 492g
Defensins, 344, 355
Degranulate, 350, 351
Delta cells, 157, 483g
Deltoid tuberosity, 422, 483g
Denature, 13, 483g
Dendrites, 34f, 34, 103, 111, 178, 349, 483g
Dendritic cells, 342, 349, 350, 359, 363, 371, 483g
Deoxyribonucleic acid, *see* DNA
Depolarization, 106-7, 106f, 281-2, 439, 483g
Dermis, 186, 381, 382f, 383-7, 388, 483g
Descending colon, 228
Desmosomes, 432, 483g
Detrusor muscle, 129, 247f, 260, 261f, 483g
Dextrinase, 226
Diabetes insipidus, 259b
Diabetes mellitus, 8, 156, 162, 163, 252, 253, 262b, 450
Diacylglycerol, 141, 483g
Diapedesis, 358, 483g
Diaphoresis, 385
Diaphragm, 24f, 123, 124, 290, 319, 320f
Diaphysis, 406, 407, 408, 409, 429, 483g
Diarrhoea, 39, 54b, 234, 236, 236b
Diarthroses, 427, 429, 483g
Diastole, 279, 280, 282, 484g
Diencephalon, 111, 114, 116, 118, 122, 484g
Diet
   Eatwell Guide, 198f
   healthy, 73, 197, 198f, 486g
Differentiation, 71, 72, 158, 210, 347, 357, 366
Diffusion, 37-9, 41, 42f, 156, 251, 252f, 317, 323, 467
   facilitated, 156, 226, 227, 481
Digestion, 215, 217-21, 227t
Dipeptidase, 226, 484g
Diploë, 406, 484g
Diplopia, 116, 188

Direct pathways, 118, 484g
Disaccharide, 197, 199, 484g
Distal, 23t, 484g
DNA, 32, 61, 62f, 62t, 63f, 63-4, 66, 71f, 483g
Docosahexaenoic acid, 206
Dominant, 82, 83, 85, 86, 93, 95
Dopamine, 108, 132, 147, 209, 404, 442, 471
Dorsal
   respiratory group, 318, 319f, 484g
   root, 124, 484g
   and ventral rami, 124, 484g, 497g
Down syndrome, 76, 83, 84, 93, 94, 465b
Ductus deferens, 449, 451, 484g
Duodenum, 215f, 218, 220, 221f, 225
Dura mater, 119, 120f, 484g
Dysarthria, 118
Dyskaryosis, 449, 459, 473, 484g
Dyspepsia, 195, 218
Dysphagia, 118

Ear, 180-5, 181f
   inner, 181f
   middle, 180, 181f
Ectocervix, 457, 458f, 484g
Effectors, 10f, 14f, 15f, 18, 100, 105, 471f, 484g
Efferent, 10, 10f, 12, 23t, 258f, 484g
Eicosanoids, 140, 206, 351, 484g
Eicosapentaenoic acid, 206
Ejaculation, 159, 450, 451
Ejaculatory duct, 449, 451, 452
Elastase, 355, 356, 484g
Elastin, 50, 270, 383, 388, 396, 484g
Electrocardiogram, 61, 95, 283b
Electrochemical gradient, 251, 252
Electrolytes, 42, 236, 242-5, 243t, 484g
Electromagnetic spectrum, 173f
Electron transport chain, 208, 233, 484g
Elongation, 66, 211, 453
Embolism, 302b, 484g
Emulsification, 219
Endocardium, 275, 276, 279, 302, 484g
Endocervix, 457, 458bf, 484g
Endocrine system, 10, 47t, 138, 139f, 143, 484g
Endocytosis, 43, 43f, 484g
Endolymph, 182, 183, 184, 185
Endometrium, 158, 456f, 457, 460, 462, 464, 465, 466, 467, 468, 484g
Endoplasmic reticulum, 34, 34f, 44, 57, 68, 78, 103, 224, 225
Endosteum, 412, 484g
Endothelins, 272
Endotracheal tube, 321, 484g
Energy, 41, 44, 196, 233, 238
Enterocytes, 225, 227
Enteroendocrine cells, 229
Enterohepatic circulation, 206, 214, 223, 345
Enteropeptidase, 225, 484g

Environment, external, 5f, 9, 10, 18, 25, 100
Enzymes, 13, 32, 44, 155, 208, 212b, 219, 484g
Eosinophils, 295, 349, 351, 364, 484g
Ependymal cells, 102, 484g
Epicardium, 277, 484g
Epicondyles, 422, 426, 484g
Epidermis, 343, 381t, 382f, 382-3, 391t, 484g
Epididymis, 159f, 449, 450f, 451, 484g
Epigastric, 25, 222
Epigenetic, 74, 484g
Epiglottis, 51, 178, 313, 484g
Epinephrine, *see* Adrenaline
Epiphyseal
   line, 407, 408f, 484g
   plate, 407, 429, 484g
Epiphysis, 406, 407, 409, 429, 484g
Episiotomy, 456
Epithelial tissue, 48, 485g
Epitopes, 363, 485g
Epoxyeicosatrienoic acids, 351, 352, 485g
Erectile dysfunction, 450, 451, 472, 474
Erythrasma, 390, 485g
Erythrocyte, 34f, 154, 293f, 294, 297, 307, 326, 327, 485g
Erythropoiesis, 296, 297f
Erythropoietin, 144t, 154, 245, 296, 485g
Escherichia coli, 228
Essential fatty acids, 206
Eukarya, 31f, 32, 32t, 485g
Eukaryotes, 31, 32, 32f, 33-5, 34f, 55
Eustachian tube, 51, 181f, 485g
Evaporation, 15f, 17t, 381
Evolution, 3, 4, 5, 81
Excitability, 432, 485g
Excoriation, 394, 485g
Exocytosis, 43, 43f, 44, 108, 109, 227, 438, 439, 485g
Exons, 66, 485g
Expiration, 318-22, 320f, 325
Expiratory reserve volume, 322, 485g
Extensibility, 432, 485g
External auditory meatus, 180, 181f, 182
External intercostal muscles, 319, 328, 470f
External os, 457, 458f
Extracellular fluid, 8f
Extrapyramidal pathways, 119
Extremophiles, 31
Extrinsic pathway, 301
Eye, 169-72, 170f, 175-8

Factor VIII, 87, 300, 302, 486
Factor X, 300
Falciform ligament, 222, 485g
Fallopian tubes, 49, 459
False ribs, 420, 485g
Familial adenomatous polyposis, 89
Fat, 50, 129, 157, 160, 203-6
Fatty acids, 39, 129, 203-6, 203f, 204f, 222f, 227t

INDEX

Feedback
    negative, 9, 10f, 12, 14f, 15f, 150, 286, 454, 464, 490g
    positive, 468f, 471f
Femur, 406, 407, 426, 485g
Ferritin, 202, 209
Fertilization, 75, 80, 158, 453, 456, 460, 462, 465
Fetal alcohol syndrome, 467b
Fetal D antigen, 299
Fetus, 83f, 158, 299, 364, 457, 465b, 466f, 466–8
Fever, 13b, 19, 338, 352, 358
Fibre (non-starch polysaccharide), 214
Fibrin, 243, 300, 301, 485g
Fibrinogen, 293, 300, 301, 301f, 302, 352, 485g
Fibrinolysin, 451, 452
Fibrinolysis, 301, 302, 485g
Fibroblast, 50, 359, 383, 388, 485g
Fibrous pericardium, 277
Fibula, 407, 426, 427, 429, 485g
Fight-or-flight reaction, 153
Filtrate, 251, 252, 253, 254, 255
Fimbriae, 459
Fitzpatrick score, 391, 392t
Flagella, 32, 45
Floating ribs, 420, 485g
Fluid mosaic model, see Plasma membrane
Folic acid, 213, 294
Follicular phase, 463f, 464, 485g
Forearm, 422, 423, 431, 437, 485g
Fovea centralis, 175, 176, 485g
Fragment antibody, 363, 485g
Fragment crystallizable (Fc), 363, 485g
Free radicals, 80, 146, 208, 209, 212b, 344, 355, 356, 485g
Frontal lobe, 112, 112f, 113, 118, 179, 261
Fructans, 199
Fructose, 197, 224, 225, 227, 452, 453
Fulcrum, 436, 437, 437f, 485g
Full blood count, 195, 348
Fundus
    stomach, 218f
    uterus, 456f, 457, 485g

G_0, 76, 77
G_1, 76, 77
G_2, 76, 77
Galactose, 197, 224, 225, 227
Gall bladder, see Bladder
Gamete, 452
Gamma-aminobutyric acid, 111, 485g, 485g
Ganglion, 102, 109t, 125–8, 126f, 175f, 176, 485g
Gaseous exchange, 325f, 327, 327f
Gastric
    acid, 145, 220, 344, 357, 369
    lipase, 220
    pits, 219, 220

Gastrin, 145t, 160, 219, 229
Gastrocolic reflex, 229, 485g
Gastrointestinal tract, 123, 159, 215–20
Gastro-oesophageal reflux disease, 218
Gene testing, 91
Genes, 61, 62f, 62t, 64, 66b, 71–4, 82, 485g
Genetic, 34, 46, 59–64, 62f, 485g
Genetically identical, 74, 76, 78, 79
Genitalia, 385, 387, 450, 455, 456
    external, 455f
    internal, 456f
Genome, 44, 61–6, 62f, 62t, 74, 81, 485g
Genotype, 64, 73, 74, 80, 84, 92, 297, 485g
Germ cells, 74, 76, 80, 81, 83, 87, 461
Ghrelin, 145t, 147, 159
Glands, 139
    bulbourethral, 450f, 452, 481g
    eccrine, 385, 386, 484g
    exocrine, 139, 224, 469
    mammary, 145, 470f, 489g
    pineal, 139f, 145t, 146
    pituitary, 139f, 140, 144t, 146, 147f, 148–50
    prostate, 159, 450f, 452, 452b, 493g
    salivary, 123, 139
    sebaceous, 381t, 385, 389, 400, 470
    sweat, 15f, 385, 387, 400
    thyroid, 139f, 140, 144t, 150–1, 150t, 152f, 161
    vestibular, 455
Glans penis, 450
Glaucoma, 168, 171, 188, 485g
Glenoid joint, 421, 422, 485g
Globular proteins, 202
Globus pallidus, 110f
Glomerular filtration, 155, 248, 250f, 262, 485g
    rate, 155, 250, 262b, 485g
Glomerulus, 248, 249f, 250f, 251, 259, 262b
Glottis, 230, 313, 485g
Glucagon, 9, 10, 11f, 12, 144t, 155, 156f, 157, 486g
Glucoamylase, 226
Glucocorticoids, 141, 153, 154, 160
Glucokinase, 156
Gluconeogenesis, 153, 154, 156, 157, 162, 233, 235, 486g
Glucose, 7t, 9–12, 11f, 44, 155–7, 199, 252f, 257b
Glucose 6-phosphate, 156, 232f
GLUT-4 transport protein, 155
Glutamate, 109
Glutathione peroxidase, 208, 486g
Gluteal tuberosity, 426
Glycerol, 203, 227, 231
Glycogen, 9, 11f, 12, 129, 199, 231
Glycogenesis, 157
Glycogenolysis, 153, 156, 157, 486g
Glycolysis, 151, 232

Glycoproteins, 35, 44, 50, 140, 197, 359, 486g
Glycosuria, 252, 486g
Goblet cells, 315, 486g
Goitre, 161, 195, 209, 237, 448
Golgi apparatus, 34f, 45f, 34, 43, 44, 78, 486g
Graafian (vesicular) follicle, 158, 460f, 461, 462, 463f, 464, 486g
Granulocytes, 295, 295f, 340f, 349, 356, 486g
Granulosa cells, 461
Granzymes, 351, 356, 365, 486g
Grey matter, 111, 115, 116, 128, 486g
Ground substance, 50, 383, 486g
Growth factors, 294, 295, 296, 347, 348, 354, 359
Guanine, 63, 67, 141, 372, 486g
Guanosine triphosphate (GTP), 141
Gums, 122, 213, 214
Gustatory cells, 178, 178f
Gyri, 111, 113, 115, 486g

Haematology, 8
Haematopoiesis, 295, 348, 406, 486g
Haematuria, 250
Haemocytoblast, 296, 486g
Haemoglobin, 4, 85, 85f, 202, 202f, 209, 210f, 294, 486g
Haemolysis, 212, 299, 486g
Haemophilia, 86, 87, 302, 486g
Haemopoiesis, 296
Haemorrhage, 213, 258, 269, 280, 285, 441
Haemostasis, 51, 87, 269, 300, 307, 486g
Hair, 18, 382f, 385, 391t
Hallux, 427
Hamate, 423, 486g
Haploid, 64, 75, 78, 79, 80, 452, 453, 461, 486g
Haustrum, 228, 229, 486g
Haversian (canal) system, 410, 411f, 486g
Hearing, 20, 179, 182, 190
Heart, 123t, 127f, 155, 274–80, 275f
    blood flow, 278f
    rate, 117, 127f, 281–2, 284t, 286, 287f
    sounds, 275, 276b
Heat loss, 12, 14, 15f, 16, 17t, 18, 19, 26
Helicobacter pylori, 217, 220, 486g
Helicotrema, 182, 183, 486g
Hemicellulose, 214, 486g
Heparin, 224, 302, 486g
Hepatic duct, 222, 223
Hepatic flexure, 228, 228f
Hepatocytes, 72, 222, 495, 486g
Hepatopancreatic sphincter, 160, 220, 224
HER2, 30, 90
Herd, 368
Heredity, 75
Hertz, 179, 486g
Heterozygous, 82, 84, 85, 486g
Hexokinase, 156

Hiatus hernia, 218
Hibernation, 235, 486g
Hinge (knee) joint, 429, 430f, 486g
Hippocampus, 115, 493
Histamine, 186, 187, 350, 351, 357, 358, 486g
Histology, 52, 277, 486g
Histone, 63, 67, 73, 74
Histopathology, 52, 486g
Homeodynamics, 6-7, 9-19, 9f, 11f, 13f, 14f, 21, 25, 39, 52, 486g
Homeostasis, 6-7, 25, 486g
Homonymous hemianopia, 177, 177b, 487g
Homozygous, 82, 84, 487g
Hormone, 16, 47, 138-61 , 142f, 144t, 145t, 271, 487g
   adrenocorticotropic, 147
   anti-diuretic (ADH), 149, 254f, 256, 257, 258f, 259b
   corticotropin-releasing, 147
   follicle-stimulating, 140, 453, 462, 463f, 475, 485g
   gonadotrophin-releasing, 147, 160, 453, 454, 454f, 462, 463f, 464, 468
   growth, 138
   growth hormone-releasing, 146
   luteinizing, 140, 149, 157, 453, 462, 463f, 475, 489g
   melanocyte-stimulating, 144t, 149, 489g
   prolactin-inhibiting, 471
   steroid, 139, 140, 141, 157, 163, 495g
   thyroid-stimulating, 139t, 140, 147, 148f, 496g
   thyrotropin-releasing, 146, 147
   tropic, 147, 497g
Human chorionic
   gonadotrophin, 158, 465, 487g
   somatomammotropin, 158, 487g
Human epidermal growth factor receptor 2, 30, 90
Human Genome Project, 64, 73, 74, 84, 91, 92, 346, 487g
Human Microbiome Project, 346
Human papillomavirus (HPV), 367, 458b, 459b
Humectant moisturizers, 394-5
Humerus, 406, 407, 421, 422, 423, 487g
Humoral, 340, 351, 352, 353, 359, 360, 487g
Hyaline, 51, 429
   cartilage, 407
Hydrochloric acid, 160, 209, 219, 243, 315, 344
Hydrogen bonds, 38b, 63, 64, 68, 201, 487g
Hydrogen ions, 7t, 243t, 262b
Hydrogen peroxide, 355, 356
Hydrogenation, 204
Hydrophilic, 34, 35, 221
Hydrophobic, 34, 35, 203, 221
Hydrostatic pressure, 248, 250f, 284, 291, 292, 305
Hydroxyapatite, 410

Hydroxyl radical, 355, 356
Hydroxylation, 211
Hyperaemia, 269, 487g
Hypercapnia, 313
Hypermethylation, 74
Hyperosmolar, 251
Hyperplasia, 148, 474, 487g
Hypertension, 285b
Hyperthyroidism, 151, 487g
Hypertonic, 245, 487g
Hypertrophic cardiomyopathy, 61, 85, 86, 93, 268, 305
Hypertrophy, 148, 433, 497, 487g
Hypochlorous acid, 356
Hypochondriac, 25
Hypodermis, 381, 382, 383, 487g
Hypoglycaemia, 117, 157
Hypophyseal portal system, 149
Hypotension, 185, 250, 291, 305, 448, 474
Hypothalamus, 13, 14f, 16, 114, 146, 258f, 463f, 468f, 487g
Hypothermia, 18, 487, 487g
Hypothyroidism, 151, 161, 195, 487g
Hypotonic, 245, 385, 487g
Hypovolaemic shock, 398
Hypoxaemia, 313
Hypoxia, 4, 154, 296, 487g

IgA, 363, 364f, 369, 472
IgD, 363, 364f
IgE, 350, 363, 364f
IgG, 363, 364f, 369, 467
IgM, 363, 364f
Ileocaecal valve, 160, 228, 228f, 229
Ileum, 145t, 157, 217, 220, 223, 228, 229, 235, 236
Iliac, 25, 28
Immunity, 338-40, 340f, 342-56, 359-69, 361f, 370t
   adaptive, 340, 340f, 359, 362f, 363, 365f, 370t, 479g
   herd, 368, 486g
   innate, 340f, 347-56, 487g
   non-specific, 339, 490g
   passive, 369, 491g
   specific, 340, 495g
Immunoglobulin, 268, 306, 350, 360, 361f, 364t, 487g
Immunosenescence, 369
Incus, 181f, 414, 415, 487g
Independent assortment, 79, 80, 96, 487g
Indirect Coombs test, 299, 300b
Infarction, 268, 272, 304, 305, 487g
Infection, 13b, 16b, 65b, 236b, 342-56
Inferior (term), 22f, 23t
Inflammation, 356-9, 357f
Infundibulum, 114, 146, 456f, 459, 462, 487g
Inhibin, 454, 464
Initiation, 66, 70, 106, 130, 353, 441
Inorganic, 30, 41, 51, 410, 435
Inositol, 199, 487

Inositol triphosphate, 141, 487g
Insensible losses, 244, 256
Insoluble fibre, 214, 487g
Inspiration, 291, 318, 319, 320, 321, 324
Inspiratory reserve volume, 322, 487g
Insula, 112, 178, 487g
Insulin, 11f, 12, 127f, 144t, 155-7, 156f, 487g
Intercalated discs, 276, 277f, 432
Intercondylar eminence, 426, 487g
Interesterification, 203, 487g
Interferons, 354, 487g
Interleukins, 354, 487g
Internal capsule, 110f, 118, 487g
Internal environment, 6-7, 8-12, 8f, 10f, 25, 73, 100, 487g
Internal os, 457, 458f
International normalized ratio, 303b
Interphase, 76, 77, 487g
Interstitial
   cells, 450, 454, 487g
   fluid, 8f, 50, 253, 291, 292f, 488g
Intertrigo, 390, 390f, 488g
Intracellular fluid, 8f
Intralobular bile ducts, 222
Intrapleural pressure, 320, 321, 488g
Intrapulmonary pressure, 320, 320f, 488g
Intrinsic automaticity, 281
Intrinsic pathway, 301, 302
Introns, 66, 494, 488g
Inulin, 199
Iodine, 208, 209
Ion channels, 32, 36
Ions, 7t, 41-2, 243t, 242-5
Iris, 170, 171, 480, 488, 493, 488g
Iron, 202f, 208t, 209, 224t, 294, 344
Ischaemia, 272, 304, 306, 488g
Ischial tuberosity, 424, 488g
Ischium, 424, 425f
Islets of Langerhans, 11, 12, 138, 155, 156, 157, 488g
Isoforms, 160
Isomalt, 197, 199
Isotonic, 244, 245, 399, 488g
Isotypes, 363, 364, 488g
Isthmus, 150, 456f, 459, 460, 488g

Jaundice, 299
Jejunum, 220, 223, 236
Joints, 404, 427, 428, 436
Jugular notch, 420f
Juxtaglomerular apparatus, 259, 286, 288, 488g

Karyotype, 75, 76, 83, 488g
Keratinocyte, 72, 382, 388, 400, 488g
Ketones, 157, 235, 256t, 257b
Kidney, 245-6, 246f, 247f, 248, 249f, 286
Kinocilium, 185, 488g
Knee joint, 430f
Krebs cycle, 232, 233
Kupffer cells, 222, 223, 488g

Labia
  majora, 455f
  minora, 455f
Labour, 468f, 475
Labyrinth, 184
Labyrinthitis, 186b, 488g
Lactase, 226
Lacteals, 225, 227
Lactic acid, 344
Lactiferous ducts, 470f, 471f, 472
Lactitol, 199
Lactoferrin, 344, 356, 369, 488g
Lacunae, 410, 488g
Lamellae, 410, 488g
Langerhans cells, 295f, 348f, 350, 383, 400, 488g
Lanugo, 194, 235, 387, 488g
Large intestine, 88, 128, 160, 199, 223, 228, 342
Laryngopharynx, 313
Laryngospasm, 313
Larynx, 51, 150, 313, 314f, 488g
Lateral (term), 22f, 23t, 488g
Lecithin, 205, 227
Lens, 170f, 171, 171f, 172, 174, 488g
Leptin, 145, 160, 462
Lesions, 116, 488g
Leukocytes, 257b, 293f, 294–6, 294f, 295f, 347–52, 358, 488g
Leukotrienes, 351, 358, 488g
Levator ani, 230, 247, 488g
Lever, 406, 436, 437, 438, 440, 443
Leydig cells, 159, 450, 488g
Ligaments, 406, 415, 422, 424, 428, 488g
Lignin, 214, 488g
Limbic system, 109, 114, 114f, 115, 179, 488g
Linea aspera, 426
Lingual lipase, 219
Linoleic acid, 204, 206
Lipases, 219, 227, 488g
Lipids, 13, 35, 39, 44, 203, 209, 383, 388, 394
Lipid bilayer, 35, 36, 41, 44, 488g
Lipogenesis, 156, 157
Lipopolysaccharide, 347, 358, 488g
Lipoproteins, 207, 224
  low-density, 207
  very-low-density, 207
Lipoxins, 351, 488g
Lipoxygenase, 351, 489g
Liver, 10, 11f, 47, 72, 215f, 221f, 222–3
Long-chain fatty acids, 227
Loop of Henle, 249f, 253, 254f, 489g
Lumbar puncture, 120, 167
Lund and Browder chart, 384b
Lungs, 38, 84, 127f, 313, 314f, 316–18, 318f
Lung volumes, 323f
Luteal phase, 463f, 464, 489g
Lymph, 292, 341, 342
  nodes, 341f, 342, 360, 363, 469

Lymphadenopathy, 342, 489g
Lymphatic
  duct, right 292, 341
  system, 292, 292f, 341, 342, 350, 351
  tissues, 340
Lymphocytes, 295–6, 295f, 342, 348f, 349t, 354, 489g
Lymphoedema, 469b
Lymphoid, 217, 341, 342, 347, 351, 359, 360
  tissues, 342, 489g
Lymphoma, 342, 489g
Lysis, 40, 344, 351, 352, 353
Lysosome, 34f, 34, 355, 489g
Lysozyme, 315, 344, 352, 356, 385, 489g

Macroelements, 207
Macromolecules, 30, 43, 44, 68, 197, 231, 359
Macronutrients, 197, 238
Macrophages, 222, 295f, 296, 349, 352, 354, 359, 365, 489g
Maculae, 184, 184f, 185, 185f
Magnesium, 207, 208, 236, 406, 410, 443
Magnetic resonance imaging, 24
Major histocompatibility complex, see MHC
Malabsorption, 212, 225, 233, 235, 236, 338
Malleolus, 427, 489g
Malleus, 181f, 414, 415
Maltase, 226
Mammary ducts, 470f
Mannose-binding protein, 352
Manubrium, 420, 489g
Mass movement, 160, 229, 489g
Mast cells, 295, 302, 350, 351, 357, 358, 364, 372, 489g
Mean arterial blood pressure, 285, 489g
Mechanoreceptors, 185, 190, 468f, 471f
Medial (term), 22f, 23t
Mediastinum, 151, 274, 316, 489g
Medulla oblongata, 109t, 111f, 115, 117–18, 123t, 286, 318, 489g
Medullary cavity, 406, 407, 408, 489g
Meiosis, 74, 78–9, 79f, 489g
Meissner's corpuscles, 186, 489g
Melanin, 391, 489g
Melanocytes, 383, 388, 391, 400, 489g
Melanoma, 392
Melatonin, 146, 492, 489g
Membrane attack complex, 353, 489g
Membrane potential, 105, 106, 107
Memory cells, 360, 494, 489g
Mendel, Gregor, 81
Ménière's disease, 186b, 489g
Meninges, 119, 120, 120f, 489g
Menopause, 90, 386, 389, 406, 410, 458b, 469, 475, 489g
Menstrual phase, 463f, 464, 489g
Menstrual (uterine) cycle, 457, 463f, 464
Menstruation, 160, 457, 464, 469

Merkel's discs, 186, 489g
Messenger RNA (mRNA), 44, 61, 62f, 62t, 68, 71f, 143f
Metabolic pathways, 4, 193, 351
Metabolism, 13, 17, 44, 64, 196, 196t, 231
Metacarpals, 422f, 423, 424f, 429, 489g
Metal-binding proteins, 352
Metalloprotein, 294
Metaphase, 75, 77f, 78f, 79, 79f, 489g
Metaphysis, 409, 489g
Meticillin, 5, 338
  meticillin-resistant *Staphylococcus aureus*, see MRSA
MHC, 80, 366, 367b, 489g,
  type I, 366
  type II, 366
Micelles, 35, 221, 227, 236, 489g
Microelements, 208
Microfilaments, 34f
Microglia, 102, 489, 489g
Micronutrients, 197, 210
Microvilli, 49, 225, 226, 251, 490g
Micturition, 51, 241, 260, 261f, 262, 265
Midbrain, 109, 111, 111f, 115, 116, 117, 122
Midsagittal plane, 22f, 23t, 24f, 25
Mineralocorticoids, 141, 153, 154
Minerals, 197, 207
Miscarriage, 456b
Mitochondria, 34f, 44–5, 63, 208, 232f, 233, 490g
Mitosis, 75, 76, 78, 490g
Mitral, 275, 278, 279, 282, 490g
Moisturizing agents, 394–5
Moles
  Avogadro constant, 244
  skin, 393b
Monoamine oxidase, 111, 490g
Monocytes, 295f, 296, 349, 354, 358, 490g
Monoglycerides, 227
Monosaccharides, 197, 199, 214, 484, 490g
Mons pubis, 455f
Mosaicism, 83, 490g
Motilin, 145t, 157, 159, 160
Motor cortex, 113, 118, 484
Motor end plate, 439
Motor pathway, 110f, 118–19
Movement, involuntary, 118, 432
MRSA, 3, 5, 20, 21, 27, 338, 339, 371
Mucins, 315, 369
Mucociliary escalator, 315
Mucosa-associated lymphoid tissue, 342, 490g
Mucous membranes, 187, 331, 345, 364, 375
Mucus, 84, 180, 219f, 220, 315, 344, 464
Multicellular organisms, 5, 25, 30, 32, 33
Multifactorial traits, 91
Multiple sclerosis, 440b, 443
Muscarinic, 128, 133, 290, 442
  acetylcholine receptors, 128, 490g

INDEX

Muscle contraction, 434–6, 436f
Muscularis, 216, 217, 246, 247, 456, 459
   externa, 216, 217
Mutation, 64, 80–1, 83, 84, 87–8, 490g
Myelin, 104, 104f, 107, 107f, 440b
Myeloid, 347, 496, 490g
Myeloperoxidase, 355, 356, 490g
Myenteric nerve plexus, 217, 490g
Myocardial infarction, 272, 273b, 296, 435, 435b, 490g
Myocardium, 275, 276, 276f, 280, 282, 490g
Myocytes, 155, 260, 281, 432
Myofibril hypertrophy, 433
Myofibrils, 433, 434, 490g
Myoglobin, 202, 209
Myometrium, 456f, 457, 468f, 490g
Myosin, 51, 433, 434, 435, 436, 436f, 490g

Na$^+$/K$^+$ pump, 32, 36, 106, 196, 243, 251
Nasal cavity, 24, 179, 190, 313, 497
Nasopharynx, 178, 181, 313, 315f
Natriuresis, 155, 260
Natural killer cells, 351, 490g
Natural selection, 3, 4, 25, 26, 366
Necrosis, 268, 272, 306, 354, 371, 441, 490g
Necrotic tissue, 272, 490g
Neocortex, 111, 115, 490g
Neonate, 18, 220, 368–9, 387, 412
Nephron, 144t, 245, 249f, 250, 253, 258f, 259, 489f, 490g
Nerve(s)
   cochlear, 183
   cranial, 116, 117, 119, 122, 133
   efferent, 10f, 16, 17
   external intercostal, 319
   facial, 178
   glossopharyngeal, 178
   optic, 168, 169, 171, 172, 176
   pudendal, 260, 261f
   thoracic, 124f, 127f
   trigeminal, 116
   trochlear, 121f, 122t
   vagus, 122, 123, 178, 290
   vestibulocochlear, 121f, 123t, 183, 184, 185
Nervous system
   central 101, 102f, 110f, 111–18, 187, 481g
   peripheral, 101, 102f, 103, 122, 133, 260, 492g
   sympathetic, 102f, 105, 116, 125–9, 126f, 126t, 127f, 289
Net filtration pressure, 250, 292
Neural layer, 175, 176
Neuroglia, 51, 101, 490g
Neurohormones, 149, 490g
Neurolemmocytes, 102, 490g
Neuromatrix theory of pain, 187
Neuromuscular junction, 105, 128, 438, 438f, 439, 490g

Neurones, 51, 101–4, 103f, 104–7, 490g
   motor, 33, 99, 104, 119
   postganglionic, 125, 493g
   preganglionic, 125, 493g
   projection, 107, 493g
   sensory (afferent), 10f, 16, 103, 104, 104f, 169
Neuropeptide Y, 145t, 160
Neurotransmitter, 107, 108, 108f, 109b, 109f, 126, 126t
Neutrophils, 294f, 295f, 296, 348f, 349, 349f, 350f, 354f, 490g
Niacin, 43, 294f, 296, 340, 347, 349t, 349
Nicotinamide adenine dinucleotide phosphate (NADPH) oxidase, 355, 490g
Nicotinic, 128
   acetylcholine receptors, 128, 490g
Nipple, 469, 470f, 471
Nissl bodies, 103, 490g
Nitric oxide, 146, 272, 273, 355, 356, 450, 474
Nitrite, 256t, 257b
Nitrosative stress, 356, 490g
Nociception, 112, 169, 186
Nociceptors, 186, 187, 190, 358, 490g
Nocturia, 474, 490g
Nodes of Ranvier, 104, 107, 490g
Non-coding RNA, 62
Non-polar molecule, 38b
Non-self, 366, 489
Non-starch polysaccharides, 197, 214, 229, 345
Non-steroidal anti-inflammatory drugs, see NSAIDs
Noradrenaline (norepinephrine), 108, 109t, 127, 140, 153, 289, 490g
Normal flora, 228, 343, 344, 345–6, 372, 373, 490g
NSAIDs, 352
Nuclei, 16, 111, 114, 116, 117, 123t
Nucleic acids, 30, 31, 61, 197, 359
Nucleoid, 32, 490g
Nucleolus, 34f
Nucleotides, 63, 67, 68, 69t, 74, 80f
Nucleus, 32, 33, 34f, 34, 44, 44f, 490g
Nucleus pulposus, 415, 418, 491g
Nutrient foramen, 406, 491g
Nystagmus, 118

Obturator foramen, 424, 491g
Occipital lobe, 112f, 114, 115, 169, 176, 177
Occlusive moisturizers, 395
Oedema, peripheral, 306f
Oesophagus, 23, 151, 216, 217, 218, 314
Oestrogen, 73, 90, 140, 144t, 157, 389, 461, 462
Olecranon
   fossa, 422, 423
   process, 422, 491g
Olfactory bulbs, 179, 180f, 483
Olfactory receptors, 179, 180f, 491g

Oligodendrocytes, 102, 491g
Oligosaccharides, 199, 226, 491g
Omega-6 (ω-6) fatty acid, 204
Oncotic pressure, 249, 250, 291, 491g
One-way valves, 290
Oocytes, 460f, 461, 469, 491g
Oogenesis, 461
Oogonia, 461, 491, 491g
Opsins, 175, 491g
Opsonins, 354, 491g
Opsonization, 353, 358
Optic
   chiasma, 122, 177, 491g
   disc, 172
   nerve, 168, 169, 171, 172, 176
Oral cavity, 24, 216
Orexins, 160
Organ of Corti, 182, 182f, 183, 183f, 185, 190, 491g
Organelles, 32, 33, 34f, 44–5, 78, 202, 231, 491g
Organism, 5, 7, 25
Oropharynx, 178, 313
Orthostatic, 291
Osmolality, 7t, 149, 244, 245, 253, 254f, 258f, 491g
Osmolarity, 244, 491g
Osmole, 244, 258, 491g
Osmoreceptors, 114, 149, 257, 258f
Osmosis, 39, 40f, 242, 244, 251, 252f
Osmotic potential, 243
Osmotic pressure, 32, 250f, 251, 291, 292, 305
Osseous, 410, 491g
Ossicles, 181, 182, 414, 415, 491g
Ossification
   endochondral, 408, 409, 484g
   primary centre, 407, 493g
Osteoblasts, 50, 393, 407, 409, 410, 412, 491g
Osteoclasts, 151, 408, 410, 412, 491g
Osteocytes, 51, 409, 410, 412, 491g
Osteoid, 407, 409, 410, 491g
Osteons, 410, 491g
Osteoporosis, 208, 393, 406, 410, 418, 472, 491g
Osteoprogenitor cells, 407, 491g
Otolith, 184, 185, 185f
Oval window, 181, 182, 183, 414, 415
Ovarian cycle, 462, 463f, 464
Ovarian follicles, 144, 158, 460f, 461, 462, 463f, 464, 491g
Ovarian ligament, 456f, 460
Ovaries, 73, 144t, 147, 157–8, 456f, 460, 460f, 491g
Ovulation, 463f
Ovum, 33, 34f, 44, 74, 75f, 78, 79, 158, 453, 491g
Oxidative stress, 356, 491g
Oxygen, 4, 7t, 38b, 197, 212, 294, 323–7, 325f
   saturation, 326

INDEX 507

Oxyhaemoglobin, 326, 491g
Oxyphil cells, 151, 491g
Oxytocin, 140, 142f, 144t, 147f, 148f, 149, 468, 491g

Pacinian (lamellar) corpuscles, 186, 491g
Pain, 109t, 186, 358, 457
Palm of hand, 422f, 423, 424f, 431t
Pancreas, 11f, 12, 127f, 144t, 155, 156f, 157, 221f
Pancreatic
　amylase, 220, 227
　lipase, 220, 227
　polypeptide, 155, 157
Pantothenic acid, 213
Papillae of the tongue, 178
Papillary dermis, 385
Papillary muscles, 275f, 279
Papillomavirus, human, 367, 458b, 459b
Paracrine, 138, 139, 140f, 353, 357, 491g
Parafollicular cells, 150, 151
Parasympathetic nervous system, 102f, 125, 126f, 126t, 127f, 128, 289–90
Parathormone, 151
Parietal
　cells, 219, 220, 491g
　lobes, 112, 112f, 113, 169, 187
　membrane, 24
　pleural membrane, 314f, 316
Parkinson's disease, 442
Parotid, 123, 217
Partial pressure, 313, 323, 324, 325f, 326, 328, 491g
Parturition, 149, 158
Patella, 407, 426, 491g
Pathogen-associated molecule patterns, 347, 491g
Pathogens, 5, 339, 340, 343, 344, 345, 491g
Peak expiratory flow rate, 311, 330, 323f
Pectins, 214
Pectoral girdle, 421
Pedigree, 81, 82, 83, 86, 87, 96
Pelvic cavity, 24, 424, 425, 456, 457, 460
Pelvic diaphragm, 247
Penis, 159, 449, 450, 450f, 451, 455, 456, 472, 491g
Pepsin, 160, 220, 482, 492g
Peptide, 492g
　bond, 70, 201, 202f
　hormones, 140, 141
Peptidoglycan, 344, 352
Peptones, 220
Perception, 169, 176, 177, 178, 179, 186, 492g
Percutaneous coronary intervention, 273b, 274f
Perforin(s), 351, 356, 365, 492g
Perfusion, 269, 272, 303, 307, 311, 324, 385, 492g
Pericardial
　cavity, 24
　fluid, 277

Pericardium, 275, 276f, 277, 492g
Perilymph, 182, 183
Perimetrium, 456f, 457, 492g
Perineotomy, 456
Perineum, 455f, 456, 492g
Periosteum, 406, 407, 408f, 410, 411f, 428, 492g
Peripheral resistance, 285, 286, 289, 492g
Peristalsis, 160, 217, 229, 246, 492g
Peritoneum, 217, 222, 224, 457, 460
Peritubular capillaries, 249f, 251
Peroxisomes, 34
Peyer's patch, 217, 342, 360, 492g
Phagocytosis, 43, 349, 351, 353f, 354, 355f, 358, 361, 396, 492g
Phagolysosome, 355f, 492g
Phagosome, 43, 354, 355f, 356, 492g
Phalanges, 405f, 422f, 423, 424f, 427, 492g
Pharmacogenetics, 73
Pharynx, 123, 178, 313, 315, 315f, 492g
Phenotype, 64, 74, 75, 82, 83, 84, 91, 297
Phenylalanine hydroxylase, 201, 492g
Phenylketonuria, 94, 201
Phosphate, 34, 63, 151, 243t
Phosphatidyl inositol bisphosphate, 141, 492g
Phosphodiester, 63, 492g
Phospholipase C, 141, 492g
Phospholipids, 34, 35f, 56, 205
Phosphorus, 207, 208, 406, 443
Phosphorylation, 141
Photo-damage, 391
Photolesions, 392
Photons, 169
Photopsins, 175, 176, 492g
Photoreceptors, 169, 173f, 174, 175, 176, 492g
Phylloquinone, 211, 212
Pia mater, 120f, 492g
Pigmented layer, 175
Piloerection, 18, 26, 492g
Pinealocytes, 146, 492g
Pinna, 51, 180
Pisiform, 423, 492g
Pivot joints, 429, 492g
Placenta, 158, 299, 369, 465–7, 466f, 492g
Placental lactogen, human, 158, 487
Plasma, 8, 8f, 9, 293f, 298
　cells, 360, 492g
Plasma membrane, 33, 34f, 34, 35f, 36, 38, 39, 492g
　fluid mosaic model in, 34, 55, 485g
Plasmids, 32, 492g
Plasmin, 301, 302, 492g
Plasminogen, 301, 302, 492g
Platelets, 273, 293, 294, 296, 300, 301, 347, 352, 492g
Pleural cavity, 316, 321, 488, 492
Pleural membranes, 314f, 316, 319, 320, 321, 492g
Plexus, 124, 217, 490, 492g
Plicae circulares, 225, 492g

Pneumocytes, 317, 321
Pneumotaxic centre, 319, 492g
Pneumothorax, 321, 492g
Polar molecule, 38b, 39, 41, 242, 263, 492g
Polarization, 243
Polydipsia, 253, 492g
Polygenic, 91
Polypeptides, 71f, 201, 227t
Polyps, 88, 89
Polysaccharides, 199, 214, 492g
Polysome, 70, 493g
Polyuria, 253, 493g
Pons, 111f, 115, 116, 116f, 122, 123t, 260
Pontine micturition centre, 261, 261f, 493g
Pontine respiratory group, 319, 493g
Portal triad, 222, 223, 493g
Portal venules, 222, 493g
Postcentral gyrus, 112, 493g
Posterior (term), 22f, 23t
　cavity, 170, 171f, 493g
　chamber, 170, 171, 493g
Post-prandial sugar spike, 214
Postsynaptic membrane, 108, 438f, 439
Post-translational modification, 70, 202, 486
Potassium, 7t, 42, 105, 106f, 208t, 243t, 255
Precentral gyrus, 112, 112f, 118, 493g
Pre-eclampsia, 211, 493g
Pregnancy, 243t, 458b, 465, 465b, 467b, 471
Prepuce, 450, 493g
Presbycusis, 183b, 493g
Presbyopia, 174, 493g
Presynaptic membrane, 439
Primary
　immune response, 361f, 363, 367, 493g
　spermatocyte, 453
　structure, 201
Primordial follicle, 461, 462
Procarboxypeptidase, 225
Pro-erythroblast, 296
Progesterone, 140, 144t, 157, 461, 462, 463f, 464, 468
Prohormone, 140, 493g
Prokaryotes, 32
Prokaryotic, 31, 32, 33, 490
Prolactin, 90, 109, 140, 144t, 149, 468, 471, 472, 493g
Proliferative (pre-ovulatory) phase, 463f, 464, 493g
Promoter region, 67
Prone (term), 22
Prophase, 77f, 78, 78f, 79f, 493g
Prostacyclin, 351, 352, 493g
Prostaglandins, 187, 351, 352, 358, 451, 452, 468, 493g
Prostate-specific antigen, 452
Protease inhibitors, 352
Proteases, 209, 219, 225, 355, 356

Protein
  clotting, 87, 301
  hormones, 139, 141, 151, 493g
  plasma membrane, 35f, 36, 42f
  synthesis, 44, 62, 68
Proteinuria, 250, 262b
Proteome, 64, 493g
Prothrombin, 212, 293, 300, 301, 301f, 305, 493g
  activator, 301, 301f
Proton pump(s), 220
  inhibitors, 220
Proximal, 23t, 493g
Pruritus, 186, 188, 364, 385, 493g
Puberty, 145t, 154, 159, 458b, 461, 469
Pubis, 424, 425f, 455, 493g
Pulmonary
  arteries, 275f, 277, 278, 282, 289f, 325f
  circulation, 271f
  embolism, 276, 302, 305, 493g
  valve, 277, 493g
  veins, 278, 291
  ventilation, 311, 318
Pulse
  oximetry, 326, 326b
  pressure, 284, 493g
Pupil, 116, 171f, 172, 174
Purkinje fibres, 281, 281f, 282, 493g
Putamen, 110f
Pyloric antrum, 160
Pyramidal cells, 107, 118, 119, 493g
Pyrexia, 19, 493g
Pyridoxine, 213
Pyruvic acid, 232, 233

Quadrants, 25
Quaternary structure, 202

Radial muscle fibres, 172
Radial tuberosity, 422, 493g
Radiation, 14f, 15f, 17t
Radius, 407, 422, 423, 429, 431, 437, 493g
Raffinose, 199
Reactive oxygen or reactive nitrogen species (ROS/RNS), 356
Receptive zone, 175
Receptors, 9, 10f, 12, 14f, 15f, 36, 37b, 48, 169, 493g
Recessive trait or allele, 82, 84
Recombination, 80, 493, 493g
Rectum, 128, 228, 229, 230, 424, 425
Red blood cells, 293, 294, 294f, 296, 297f
Reflex arc, 124, 125
Refraction, 174
Relaxin, 158, 451
Renal
  cortex, 154, 245, 246f, 254f, 493g
  medulla, 155, 245, 246f, 253, 254f, 494g
  pelvis, 245, 246f, 248
  pyramids, 245, 246f, 494
  sinus, 245, 246f
  threshold, 252, 494g

Renin, 144, 154, 243, 259, 286, 288f, 494g
Renin-angiotensin-aldosterone system, 259, 288f, 494g
Repolarization, 106, 494g
Reproductive system, 449, 455, 472
Residual volume, 322, 494g
Respiration, 318–21
Respiratory
  burst, 355
  centres, 319f, 318–19
  pump, 290
  tract, lower, 313, 489g
  tract, upper, 181, 313, 314, 497g
Resting membrane potential, 105, 106, 494g
Reticular, 50, 494
  activating system, 109t, 116, 494g
  formation, 115, 116, 494g
Reticulocyte, 296
Reticulospinal tract, 119
Retina, 169, 170f, 171, 171f, 172, 174, 175f, 176, 177, 494g
Retinal ganglion, 176
Retinoic acid, 210, 211
Retinol, 210, 211
Retinol-binding protein, 210, 211
Rhamnose, 214
Rhesus system, 298, 299f
Rhodopsin, 175, 176, 494g
Rhythmicity, innate, 432, 487g
Ribcage, 314f, 319, 405f, 494g
Riboflavin, 213
Ribosomes, 34f, 44, 46, 57, 68, 70, 96, 494g
RNA (ribonucleic acid), 31, 61, 494g
  polymerase, 67, 67f, 68, 494g
  splicing, 68, 494g
Rods, 172, 175, 175f, 176, 494g
Round window, 181, 182, 415
Rubrospinal tract, 119
Rugae, 218, 246, 247f, 260, 494g

S cells, 160
S phase, 77, 79
Saccule, 184
Sacrum, 414, 415, 424
Saddle joint, 429, 483, 494g
Sagittal plane, 22, 23, 25, 246f, 412, 431, 450, 470f
Salbutamol, 37b
Saliva, 130, 178, 217, 219, 344, 364, 403, 441
Salivary amylase, 219
Saltatory conduction, 107, 107f, 494g
Sarcolemma, 433, 439, 494g
Sarcomere, 432, 433, 436f, 494g
Sarcoplasm, 433, 494g
Satellite cells, 102, 103, 494g
Saturated carrier proteins, 252
Saturated fats, 204, 205, 206
Scala
  media, 182, 182f
  tympani, 182, 182f
  vestibule, 182, 182f

Scapula, 421, 421f, 422, 494g
Schwann cells, 102, 103f, 104, 494g
Sclera, 170, 170f, 171f, 494g
  venous sinus, 171
Scrotum, 449, 450f, 494g
Scurvy, 213, 390, 494g
Sebum, 344, 381t, 385, 389, 470
Second messenger, 141, 142, 157, 474
Secondary
  active transport, 251
  oocyte, 461, 462
  immune response, 361, 363, 364, 367, 494g
  structure, 201
Secretin, 145t, 157, 160, 225
Secretory phospholipase A2, 356
Segmentation, 218, 494g
Selective reabsorption, 254, 494g
Selenium, 208
Self antigens, 366, 494g
Semen, 8, 159, 248, 451, 452, 475, 494
Semicircular canals, 181f, 184, 184f, 185, 186b
Semilunar valves, 275, 279
Seminal vesicles, 450f, 452, 494g
Seminiferous tubules, 159f, 450, 452, 453f, 494g
Senile purpura, 380
Sensation, 169, 190, 381, 494g
Sense strand, 67
Senses, 169
  special, 169, 187, 188, 495g
Sensory cortex, 112f, 113f, 169, 187
Sensory processing disorder, 113, 494g
Sensory receptors, 100, 169, 184, 494g
Septum, 274, 281, 282, 289
Serosa, 216, 217, 246, 247, 459
Serotonin, 100, 108, 133, 146, 300, 494g
Serous pericardium, 277
Sertoli (sustentacular) cells, 453, 453f
Serum, 298b, 495g
  amyloid A, 352
Set point, 7, 9, 13, 13b, 495g
Sex chromosomes, 74, 75, 495g
Sexual reproduction, 34, 96
Sharpey's fibres, 406, 495g
Shell temperature, 16
Shivering, 14f, 17
Sickle cell disease, 70, 84, 85f, 307f
Sigmoid
  colon, 128, 228
  flexure, 228f
Simple epithelia, 49
Sine wave, 180f
Single nucleotide polymorphisms, 81, 495g
Single-celled organisms, 5, 32
Sinoatrial node, 129, 280, 281f, 495g
Sinusoids, 149, 222, 223, 488, 495g
Sister chromatids, 78, 495g
Skeletal muscle, 49f, 51, 102, 105, 109, 433–4, 495g
  pump, 290

Skeleton, 404, 405f, 412, 421–7
Skin, 382–7, 382f, 387–95
Skull, 407t, 412, 412f, 413f, 414f
Sliding filament theory, 434, 436, 495g
Small intestine, 123t, 127f, 215f, 220, 225–6
Smell, 178–9, 180f
Smoking, 130, 131, 389, 475
Smooth muscle, 37, 51, 123t, 432, 433f, 434, 495g
Soaps, 394
Sodium, 7t, 40b, 42, 207t, 242t, 256–60
Soft palate, 178
Soluble fibre, 214
Solute, 39, 40f, 41, 149
Solvent, 38b, 39, 214, 242, 244, 253
Somatic
  cells, 47
  hypermutation, 362, 495g
  nervous system, 102f, 125
Somatosensory area, 112, 113, 169, 493
Somatostatin, 145, 156f, 157, 160, 495, 495g
Somatotropin, 148, 495, 495g
Sorbitol, 199
Spasticity, 439, 440, 443
Specific gravity (urine), 256t, 257b
Speech centre, 113, 130
Sperm, 44, 62, 74, 78, 79, 449, 450, 451, 452–3, 454f, 495g
Spermatids, 453
Spermatogenesis, 452, 453, 453f, 454f, 475, 495, 495g
Spermatogonia, 452, 453, 453f
Sphincter
  external urethral, 247f, 261f
  internal anal, 230
  internal urethral, 247f, 260, 261f
  lower oesophageal, 218
  oesophageal-gastric (or cardiac), 218
  of Oddi, 160, 220, 221, 495g
Spinal
  cavity, 24f
  column, 404, 405, 415, 417
  cord, 101f, 102f, 111, 111f, 118–19
  reflex, 124–5
Spinothalamic tract, 119
Spirilla, 32
Spirometry, 322, 323f, 495g
Spleen, 50, 215f, 341f, 342, 360
Splenic flexure, 228, 228f
Squamocolumnar junction, 458b
Squint, 177
Stapes, 181f, 495g
Stachyose, 199
Staphylococci, 32
Staphylococcus aureus, 3, 4, 5, 338
Starling's Law of the Heart, 279, 495g
Stellate cells, 107, 495g
Stem cells, 47, 72, 80, 294, 347
Stereocilia, 182f, 183, 185, 185f, 495g
Sternal angle, 420

Sternum, 405f, 407t, 419, 420, 420f, 421
Stomach, 123t, 127f, 145t, 160, 215f
Strabismus, 177, 178, 495g
Stratified epithelia, 49, 382, 400, 495g
Stratum basale, 382, 383, 495g
Stratum corneum, 382, 382f, 383, 495g
Stratum spinosum, 383, 495g
Streptococci, 32
Stretch reflex, 124, 125
Stroke, 120, 130, 131b, 177, 495g
  volume, 279, 280, 285, 290, 291, 305, 306, 495g
Strong ligaments, 424
Styloid process, 422, 495g
Subarachnoid space, 120, 495g
Subcutaneous fat, 13, 19, 20, 383
Subdural space, 120, 120f, 495g
Sublingual, 123, 217
Submandibular, 123, 217
Submucosa, 216, 217, 225, 246, 495g
Substantia nigra, 132, 442
Sucrase, 226
Sudoriferous, 18, 385
Sulci, 111, 112, 495g
Sulphur, 207
Sunscreen, 393, 399, 400
'SunSmart' campaign, 393
Superior (term), 22f, 23t
Superoxide, 208, 355, 356
Superoxide dismutase, 208
Supine, 22, 24
Suprarenal, 152
Surface tension, 320, 321, 322b, 495g
Surfactant, 221, 321, 322, 496g
Survival advantage, 3, 5, 84, 88, 363
Suspensory ligaments (of eye), 170f, 171f, 174, 470f, 496g
Suspensory (round) ligament (of uterus), 456f, 460
Sustentacular (Sertoli) cells, 453, 453f, 454, 496g
Sweating, 15f, 18, 385
Synapse, 107, 108f, 108–9, 109f, 128, 133, 187, 438f, 439
Synaptic cleft, 108f, 109, 438f, 439
Synaptic knob, 104, 108f
Synarthroses, 427, 429, 496g
Syncytiotrophoblast, 158, 496g
Syncytium, 276
Synovial
  fluid, 428
  joint, 428, 428f
  membrane, 428, 428f
Systemic circulation, 270, 278, 282, 288, 289, 307, 496g
Systole, 280, 281, 282, 283f, 305, 481, 496g

T-helper lymphocyte (TH), 360, 365, 365f
Tachycardia, 4, 30, 53, 290, 448
Tachycardic, 331, 496g
Tachypnoeic, 331, 496g
Tamoxifen, 90

Taste, 178, 190
  buds, 178, 178f
TATA box, 67
T-cell receptor, 32, 36, 359, 365, 496g
Tectorial membrane, 183, 183f, 496g
Telophase, 77f, 78, 78f, 79f, 496g
Template, 46, 67
Temporal lobe, 112, 112f, 113, 182, 183, 190
Teratogen, 132, 162, 448, 472, 496g
Terminal bronchioles, 317
Termination, 66, 69
Tertiary structure, 202
Testes, 144t, 148, 159, 159f, 449, 450f, 452
Testosterone, 144t, 159, 160, 206, 453–4, 454f, 496g
Tetraiodothyronine, 151, 496g
Thalamus, 109t, 110f, 111, 114, 115, 116, 178, 187, 496g
Thermogenesis, 14f, 17, 18
Thermoreceptors, 14f, 15f, 16, 17, 26, 114, 169
Thermoregulation, 14f, 15f, 269
Thiamine, 213, 233
Thigh, 124, 426, 431, 496g
Thin filaments, 434f, 435f
Thirst centre, 114, 257, 259
Thoracic
  cavity, 24f, 319, 322
  duct, 227, 292, 341
  organs, 15, 24
Thorax, 123, 274, 290, 313, 320, 341
Thrombi, 275, 276, 302, 496
Thrombin, 301, 301f, 302, 305, 496g
Thrombocytes, 51, 293f, 294, 296, 307, 496g
Thrombolytic, 274, 302
Thromboxanes, 351, 352, 496g
Thrombus, 273, 274, 296, 302, 320b, 496g
Thymine, 63, 67, 496g
Thymosin, 151, 496g
Thymus, 139f, 151, 152, 342, 360
Thyrotropin, 146, 147, 148, 496, 496g
Thyroxine, 14f, 17, 36t, 140, 144t, 151, 161, 209
Tibia, 407, 426, 427, 429, 485, 487, 488, 489, 496g
Tidal volume, 321, 322, 355, 496g
Tinea pedis, 386
Tinnitus, 183b, 188, 189, 496g
Tissue factor, 301, 496g
T-lymphocyte, 152, 360, 364–6, 365f, 367b, 370t, 496g
Tobacco, 73, 80
Toll-like receptor, 347, 496g
Touch receptors, 185
Trabeculae, 407, 408, 409, 410, 411, 412, 496g
Trace elements, 208, 209, 236
Trachea, 313–16, 314f, 316f, 496g
Traits, 3, 82, 83, 91, 96

Trans fatty acids, 205, 496g
Transamination, 201
Transcellular fluid, 8, 9, 496g
Transcription, 66, 67, 496g, 496g
    factors, 67, 73, 143
Transduction, 169, 183, 496g
Transfer RNA, 68, 71f
Transferrin, 202, 209
Transformation zone, 258b
Transforming growth factor-beta, 359
Transfusion, 268, 297, 298
Translation, 66f, 68, 71f, 73, 143, 496g
Transmembrane conductance transporter, 84
Transport
    active, 41, 42f, 196, 251, 255, 479g
    passive, 37, 42f, 491g
Transverse
    plane, 22f, 23t, 24, 25
    colon, 215f, 228, 228f
Trapezium, 423, 496, 496g
Trapezoid, 423, 496g
Treg, 365
Trehalase, 199
Tricarboxylic acid cycle, 151, 232, 233
Tricuspid valve, 275f, 276, 277, 282, 496g
Triglyceride(s), 203, 204, 227, 231, 233, 268
Trigone, 246, 247f, 260
Triiodothyronine, 151, 497g
Triquetral, 423, 497g
Triquetrum, 423
Trisomy, 76, 83, 93, 94, 497g
Trochanter
    greater, 426, 486g
    lesser, 426, 488g
Trochlea, 422f, 423f, 497g
Trophic, 148
Trophoblast cells, 158, 497g
Tropins, 147, 148
Tropomyosin, 434, 435, 435f, 435b, 497g
Troponin, 434, 435f, 435b, 497g
Troponin-tropomyosin complex, 435, 497g
True ribs, 420
Trypsin, 220, 225, 497g
Trypsinogen, 220, 225
Tubular
    reabsorption, 248, 497g
    secretion, 248, 255, 497g
Tumour necrosis factor, 354, 371
Tumour suppressor, 88, 90
Tumours, 87, 91, 92, 497g
Tunica adventitia, 269, 270
Tunica albuginea, 450, 460f, 461
Tunica intima, 269, 275
Tunica media, 269
Tympanic membrane, 16b, 180, 181f, 182

Ulna, 405f, 407t, 422, 422f, 423, 423f, 497g
Ultrafiltrate, 250, 252f, 497g
Umbilical
    artery, 466
    cord, 466f
Umbilicus, 25
Unicellular microorganisms, 31
Unmyelinated C fibres, 187
Unsaturated fatty acids, 203
Uracil, 67, 479, 497g
Urea, 7t, 224, 245, 252f, 253, 254f, 255, 256, 262b, 497g
Ureter, 241, 245, 246f, 247f, 451, 497g
Urethra, 247f, 248, 256, 260, 262, 450f, 451, 452, 455f
Urinalysis, 241, 252, 256, 257b, 265
Urinary bladder, *see* Bladder
Urine, 42, 245, 248, 250, 253, 255-6
Urobilinogen, 256t, 257b
Urogenital diaphragm, 247f
Uterine
    cycle, 457, 463f, 464, 497g
    tubes, 456f, 457, 459, 460, 497g
Uterus, 49, 144t, 158, 456f, 457, 459, 464, 468, 497g
Utricle, 184

Vaccination, 366, 367, 368, 459b, 497g
Vagina, 451, 452, 455f, 456f, 457, 458fb, 460, 464, 497g
Valsalva manoeuvre, 230, 497g
Vas deferens, 450f, 449
Vasa recta, 249f, 253, 254f, 497g
Vasectomy, 451
Vasoactive
    inhibitory polypeptide, 157
    intestinal peptide, 160
Vasoconstriction, 14f, 18, 270, 285, 286, 287f, 289, 291, 352
Vasodilation, 15f, 18, 155, 270, 287f, 289, 291, 352, 358
Vasodilator, 272, 352, 358, 450
Vasopressin, 149, 256, 265, 271
Veins, 270, 270f
Vena cava, 222, 236, 247f, 277
Venous circulation, 271, 277
Venous return, 290, 290f
Ventilation, 318, 320f, 328
Ventral
    horn, 118, 119, 497, 497g
    respiratory group, 318, 319f, 497g
    root, 124, 497g
Ventricles
    brain, 49, 110f, 120, 120f
    heart, 129, 155, 274, 275f, 276b, 282
Venules, 291
Verbascose, 199

Vertebral column, 119, 124f, 407t, 414-15, 416f, 417f, 418f, 419f
Vertigo, 186b, 497g
Vesicle, 34f, 43, 43f, 44, 108f, 109f, 140f, 438f, 439
Vesicular follicle, 460f, 461, 462, 497g
Vestibular
    apparatus, 182, 183f, 184, 190
    system, 184
Vestibulospinal tract, 119
Villi, 120, 225, 226f, 227, 465, 466, 467, 497g
Virus, 66, 351, 354, 360, 364-5, 369, 375
Viscera, 104
Visceral
    membrane, 24
    pleural membrane, 314f, 316
Viscosity, 285
Vital capacity, 322, 497g
Vitamins, 35, 197, 210-13, 211t
    A, 175, 210, 211
    B_{12}, 213
    B_6, 213
    C, 209, 213, 236, 390
    D, 151, 206, 211, 245, 381, 392, 393, 394, 400
    D_3 receptor, 393
    E, 212
    fat-soluble, 210, 211t
    K, 212, 300
    water-soluble, 211
Vitreous humour, 8, 170, 174, 497g
Vocal cords, 113, 313
Voluntary movement, 118, 432, 441, 443
Vulva, 455, 497g

Wallace's rule of nines, 384b
Warfarin, 95, 268, 302, 305
Water, 9, 19, 38b, 39, 40f, 40, 214-15, 242-5
Water-soluble vitamins, *see* Vitamins
Wernicke's area, 112f, 113, 130, 497g
White matter, 110f, 111, 111f, 115, 118, 125f, 497g
Wound healing, 395, 396f

Xiphisternal joint, 420f
Xiphoid process, 420f
X-linked, 86, 497g
X ray, 22, 300, 399

Yellow body, 158

Zinc, 208, 209, 210
Zona fasciculata, 154, 498g
Zona glomerulosa, 154, 498g
Zona reticularis, 154, 498g
Zygote, 75, 140, 459, 460, 498g